Saunders Nursing Guide to

Laboratory and Diagnostic Tests

Saunders Nursing Guide to

Laboratory and Diagnostic Tests

Louise M. Malarkey, EdD, RN
Professor, Department of Nursing,
College of Staten Island,
City Univerisy of New York,
Staten Island, New York

Mary Ellen McMorrow, EdD, RN, CCRN
Professor, Department of Nursing,
College of Staten Island,
City University of New York,
Staten Island, New York

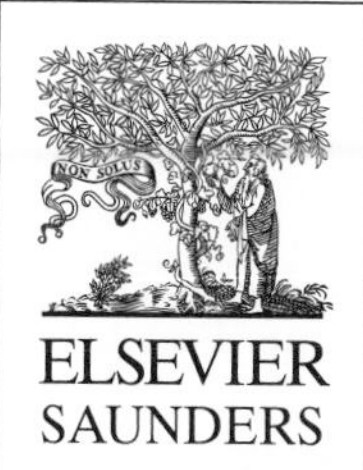

ELSEVIER
SAUNDERS

ELSEVIER
SAUNDERS

11830 Westline Industrial Drive
St. Louis, Missouri 63146

SAUNDERS NURSING GUIDE TO LABORATORY AND DIAGNOSTIC TESTS ISBN 1-4160-0205-7

NOTICE

Nursing is an ever-changing field. Standard safety precautions must be followed, but as new research and clinical experience broaden our knowledge, changes in treatment and drug therapy may become necessary or appropriate. Readers are advised to check the most current product information provided by the manufacturer of each drug to be administered to verify the recommended dose, the method and duration of administration, and contraindications. It is the responsibility of the licensed prescriber, relying on experience and knowledge of the patient, to determine dosages and the best treatment for each individual patient. Neither the publisher nor the author assumes any liability for any injury and/or damage to persons or property arising from this publication.

International Standard Book Number 1-4160-0205-7

Managing Editor: Brian Dennison
Associate Developmental Editor: Betsy Stream
Publishing Services Manager: Jeffrey Patterson
Senior Project Manager: Mary G. Stueck
Design Manager: William Drone

Printed in the United States of America

Last digit is the print number: 9 8 7 6 5 4 3 2 1

This book is dedicated to our families

To my sons, Frank and Charles
L. M. M.

To my sisters, Lydia, Peggy, and Ruth
and my daughter, Mary
M. E. M.

Preface

The *Saunders Nursing Guide to Laboratory and Diagnostic Tests* is designed to provide the student nurse and the nurse in clinical practice with easily accessible information about laboratory tests and diagnostic procedures. The content of the book includes specific tests and procedures that are frequently encountered in patient care settings. The major strength of the book is its emphasis on the nursing care related to laboratory and diagnostic tests.

PART 1

Part 1 of the text addresses the overall responsibilities of the nurse in laboratory and diagnostic testing. Additionally, there is discussion of the nursing role and the patient-nurse interactions in the pretest period, during the test, and in the posttest period. This content is written in the nursing process format so that the student or clinical nurse can use critical thinking abilities to provide accurate care. Also, a separate chapter addresses the procedures used by the nurse to accurately collect the various specimens of blood, feces, or urine.

PART 2

The largest section of the book contains material related to specific laboratory tests and diagnostic procedures. The tests and procedures are presented in alphabetical order so the reader can locate the information rapidly. The information for each test is provided in a consistent format so that the student or nurse can access it more easily.

Comprehensive Scope

The content is appropriate and useful for student nurses throughout their program of study and as a reference for nurses in the varied areas of clinical practice. The text is comprehensive in the array and number of tests and procedures presented. The tests and procedures include those used in cardiopulmonary, gastrointestinal, renal, hepatobiliary, gynecological, obstetrical, pediatric, hematological, vascular, orthopedic, neurological, oncological, and endocrine disorders, as well as infectious diseases. This book includes genetic tests since they are used to identify the DNA or RNA of infectious organisms, in prenatal screening, and in illnesses caused by inherited disorders.

New Tests

The array of specific laboratory and diagnostic tests also include the newest tests approved for clinical use as well as more familiar tests that have been approved for expanded uses. Some of these include the *Helicobacter pylori* antigen test, cardiac troponin, Alzheimer's disease testing of cerebrospinal fluid for the presence of β amyloid$_{(1\text{-}42)}$ and T-tau; videofluorographic swallowing study for swallowing disorders; virtual colonoscopy that uses a CT scan instead of an endoscope; DNA testing for *Chlamydia trachomatis*; rapid HIV antigen testing; ambulatory esophageal pH monitoring; positron emission tomography (PET) testing; prenatal screening for the gene of cystic fibrosis and quadruple marker screening for Down syndrome; fetal fibronectin; and SARS testing protocol.

Organization

This text uses a consistent format for every test or procedure. This allows the reader to become familiar with the format, comfortable with the content, and acccess the material more readily. Generally, reference content on laboratory and diagnostic testing written by physicians can be difficult for the nursing student to understand because of the numerous synonyms and abbreviations, as well as technical content and the vocabulary of the different medical specializations. This text provides summary background information from various medical disciplines but emphasizes the content relevant in the nursing care of the patient.

Synonyms, Abbreviations, and Pronunciation

The beginning of each test or procedure introduces the reader to the various names and abbreviations of the test that may be used in the patient's record or on the laboratory reports. The pronunciation guide gives a phonetic spelling of the test name, which will help the student read the content more easily.

Purpose of the Test

This section briefly describes what the test does and why it is used.

Basics the Nurse Needs to Know

This section provides a summary explanation of how the test relates to the underlying pathology. The pathophysiologic basis of abnormal, elevated, or decreased values is explained. When there are multiple tests that give information to help diagnose a problem, as in human immunodeficiency virus (HIV) tests, they are differentiated and explained. In diagnostic procedures there may be several components of the test; for example, the entry for angiography discusses imaging, contrast medium, and puncture site. All of these components are important considerations for nursing assessment in the posttest period.

Normal Values

The laboratory test results are presented in conventional units and in international units (SI units). When appropriate, the different values for gender and age are included. The reference values may differ from those used in particular institutions or laboratories because of different methodology or analyzer equipment. The normal values presented in this book are useful as a frame of reference for the reader, but the values determined by the laboratory that performed the test should be used when referring to a specific patient.

Critical values, sometimes called "possible panic values" are also presented for those tests that are relevant. The critical value is the extreme elevation or decline in value that indicates a life-threatening situation. The identification of this extreme result helps the student or clinical nurse to recognize the acuity of the problem and the need to quickly notify the physician of the test result.

How the Test is Done

This section briefly states how the specimen is collected or the diagnostic procedure is performed. It helps the reader understand what the patient will experience and how the results are obtained.

Significance of Test Results

This section lists the medical diagnoses associated with elevated, decreased, or abnormal results. It helps the student relate the abnormal test findings to the patient's illness and the severity of the condition.

Interfering Factors

In the pretest period there may be substances, food, activities, medications, or other factors that would alter the test results or cause them to be invalid. For a specific test, the nurse can use the information to teach the patient to follow pretest instructions and avoid the pertinent interfering factors.

Nursing Care

Nursing care is presented in three diagnostic phases: Pretest, During the Test, and Posttest, with an emphasis on nursing responsibilities in each of these phases. In the pretest phase the nurse provides the preparatory care to the patient, particularly for a diagnostic procedure. During the test, the nurse may be present to assist, particularly for diagnostic procedures as biopsy, endoscopy, and others. In the posttest phase, the nurse provides care that relates to recovery.

Patient Teaching. Patient teaching is a special feature that describes the role of the student or nurse in preparing the patient for the testing and for the patient's discharge. The need for patient teaching has increased because many patients have their diagnostic workup done in outpatient settings. The patient may be at home until the day of the procedure, and he or she often returns home after the procedure is completed. Patient teaching and communication are needed so that the patient can assume responsibility for self-care.

Three additional subcategories of nursing care appear in the nursing care content of specific tests and procedures, as applicable: Health Promotion, Nursing Response to Critical Values, and Nursing Response to Complications.

Health Promotion. Health promotion discussions cover those tests recommended for health screening and preventive health care. Based on national guidelines, the information includes who should have the test, what age to start testing, the frequency of testing, and the benefits of early detection and follow-up care. The student and nurse can use this information for teaching the public about effective measures to monitor health and the need to seek early medical treatment when the results are abnormal. Screening tests such as routine Papanicolaou smear, prostatic specific antigen, fecal occult blood test, colonoscopy, mammography, lead levels, electrocardiogram, cholesterol, and bone densitometry are part of current health promotion recommendations.

Nursing Response to Critical Values. The nursing response to critical values applies to laboratory tests with identified values that indicate a life-threatening situation. An extreme elevation or decline in test result values requires a rapid medical response. This text provides information about the significance of the critical value, the necessary nursing assessments of the patient, and possible nursing interventions that can be performed while awaiting medical evaluation of the patient.

Nursing Response to Complications. The nursing response to complications applies to the posttest phase of various diagnostic procedures, with the more common complications presented and described. The focus is on the nursing assessments that monitor for possible complications and the nursing interventions that can be used while awaiting medical evaluation of the patient. Complications of invasive diagnostic procedures are possible and, depending on the procedure, could result in an allergic reaction or anaphylaxis, stroke or thrombosis, infection, cardiac disturbance, respiratory impairment, bleeding, perforation, shock, or other problems. The complications often occur during the posttest period while the patient is being cared for by a nurse.

This book presents information in a clear, consistent, and precise manner so that the reader can maximize his or her learning. Included are numerous illustrations that help the student or nurse visualize how the procedure is performed. There are also diagnostic images, including x-ray, CT scan, MRI, PET scan, ultrasound, nuclear scan, and ECG tracings, to show the types of abnormalities that can occur. The combination of written explanation and illustrations enable the reader to grow in understanding of the tests the patient must undergo and the significance of the test results.

FOR THE INSTRUCTOR

Additional materials can be found on the Instructor's Resource CD, which was created to support instructors by providing additional tools for teaching laboratory and diagnostic testing procedures. The Instructor's Resource CD offers critical thinking questions and discussion as well as a test bank with rationales provided for the correct answers. It also includes approximately 100 images of laboratory and diagnostic procedures and equipment to help instructors make lectures more visual and engaging.

As nursing faculty members, we have endeavored to write this book for nursing students and for nurses in clinical practice. Their learning needs were prominent in our minds as the book was developed. As authors, we have endeavored to write to and for this audience so that their learning would be enhanced and satisfying.

Louise M. Malarkey
Mary Ellen McMorrow

Acknowledgments

This book was written with the help and support of many people who provided guidance, shared expertise and offered encouragement to us. The authors wish to thank them for their assistance.

Nursing students are a constant source of delight because they seek knowledge, ask questions, and work diligently to learn. Their high level of motivation is a constant stimulus to us in our teaching and writing activities. Nursing faculty members and colleagues at the College of Staten Island are thanked for their encouragement and ongoing support. Their high level of nursing expertise and commitment to effective teaching are sources of motivation and renewal for us. We also want to thank the nursing reviewers of the manuscript: Pamela D. Korte, Monroe Community College, Rochester, New York; Patricia K. O'Brien, Penn Valley Community College, Kansas City, Missouri; Deborah Shows-Rushing, Troy University, Troy, Alabama. Their expertise and input were appreciated.

The writing of a textbook requires extensive library work and facility with electronic databases. We appreciate the assistance of the librarians and library staff of the College of Staten Island who helped us to locate the many publications and sources of information that were obtained. Particular recognition goes to Wilma Jones, chief librarian, Raja Jayatilleke, and Angela DeMartinis for their assistance, expertise and support.

Special recognition and appreciation is extended to Brian Dennison, our editor at Elsevier. His vision, communication, support, and encouragement were very positive influences on our writing and completion of the project. We also want to acknowledge the work of Mary Stueck, Senior Project Manager and Betsy Stream, Associate Developmental Editor, for their work to convert this manuscript into a completed book.

Contents

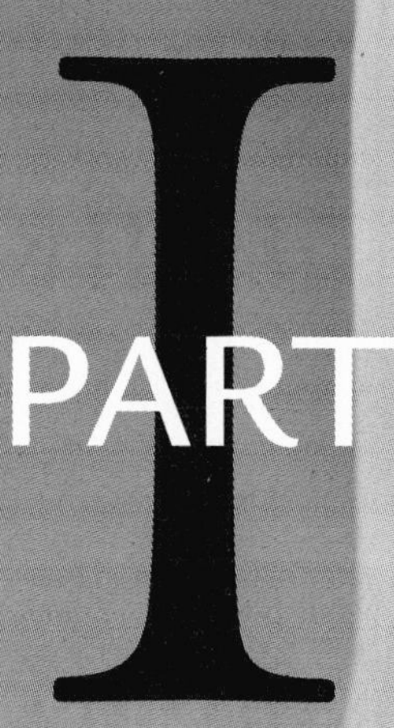

PART I

Nursing Responsibilities in Laboratory Tests and Diagnostic Procedures

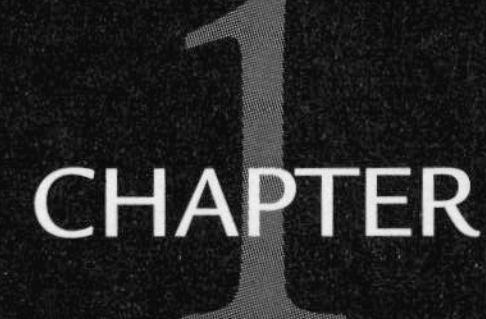

CHAPTER 1

The Nursing Role

Laboratory tests and diagnostic procedures involve two broad areas of nursing performance. The first area pertains to the procedure itself and to the nursing measures that ensure completion of the testing in an accurate and timely manner. The second area concerns the nursing interactions with the patient who must undergo the diagnostic test or procedure. The nursing process is used to organize patient care and meet the patient's needs.

The nursing role in patient care for individuals undergoing diagnostic tests and procedures may be direct or indirect. Often, it involves an interdisciplinary approach to the planning and implementation of care.

Direct care is provided by the nurse when the patient is hospitalized or enters an outpatient setting for performance of the laboratory or diagnostic test. The nurse may perform some aspects of the care or supervise paraprofessional workers in the delivery of care, particularly during the pretest and posttest periods. For some of the more complex or invasive tests, a nurse is present during the procedure to provide care to the patient and assist the physician who performs the test.

Indirect care often occurs when the patient is at home for the pretest and posttest phases of the diagnostic testing. The nurse may be responsible for guiding or instructing the patient in preparing for the test or in recovery after the test. The patient performs self care, or a family member assists the patient according to the instructions that are given.

In many instances, diagnostic work is an interdisciplinary function that involves coordination and communication among the nurse, several physicians, and technicians of the laboratory, radiology department, or diagnostic specialty units. The nurse's role is often pivotal in the transmission of information to and from the testing center. The nurse must explain the pretest laboratory or diagnostic requirements to the patient or must perform specific pretest procedures on the patient. Additionally, the specific needs or problems of the patient are explained to the testing center personnel. The goal is to accomplish the diagnostic work accurately, safely, and in a timely manner.

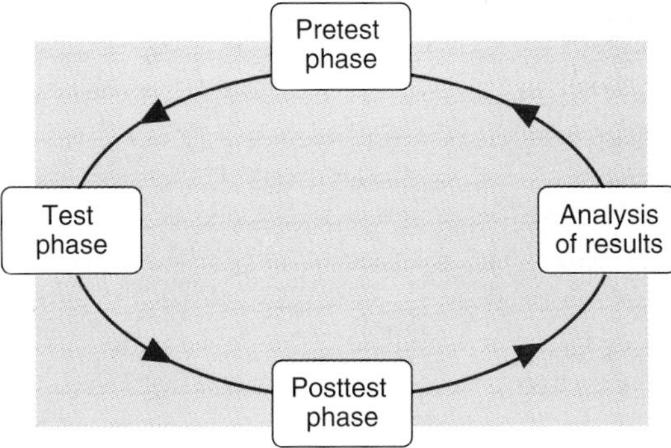

Figure 1. The cycle of laboratory or diagnostic testing. Both the nurse and the patient are involved in each phase of the cycle. After analysis of the test results, the cycle may be restarted for additional testing, as needed.

The process of laboratory or diagnostic testing can be conceptualized as a cycle that has four phases of operation: (1) the pretest phase, (2) the test phase, (3) the posttest phase, and (4) analysis of the results (Figure 1). Appropriate nursing roles and responsibilities for the test or procedure, as well as appropriate aspects of nursing care for the patient, are pertinent to each phase.

PROCEDURAL ROLE AND NURSING RESPONSIBILITIES

Pretest Phase

Scheduling of a Diagnostic Test

This involves communication among the individual who prescribes the test, the patient, and the individual who performs the test. The nurse or unit coordinator is often responsible for accurate transcription of the orders, completion of the requisition form, and scheduling of the test.

When multiple tests are prescribed, it is sometimes necessary to prioritize the test schedule, because the method of conducting one test can interfere with the results of another. For example, x-ray studies that use iodinated contrast medium are performed before x-ray studies that use barium contrast material. This timing is necessary because residual barium remains in the intestine for several days, and its opacity obscures the view of the other tissues, such as the biliary tract and abdominal vasculature. Likewise, blood tests that use a radioimmunoassay method of analysis must be performed before or 7 days after a nuclear scan, because the radioisotopes of the scan would interfere with the radioimmunoassay method of analysis of the blood and alter the test results.

When these interfering factors involve tests performed by a single department, such as the laboratory, the priorities are routinely sorted out by the laboratory personnel. When the interfering factors involve two departments, such as the laboratory and the radiology department, the nurse consults with the departments to clarify the priorities and to plan appropriately.

Some priorities in scheduling are determined by the acuity of the patient. Particular test results are needed rapidly for the assessment of the patient's status, for correct medical diagnosis and treatment, or for evaluation of the patient's response to treatment. Blood tests may be performed serially, for example, every hour for 4 hours; at frequent intervals such as daily; or immediately (stat). The request may specify the urgency and the desired times for the tests.

The nurse monitors each situation, ensuring that the tests are performed on time and that the results are reported to the physician or posted in the patient's chart, or both, as quickly as they become available. When a test with an immediate or urgent priority is ordered, the laboratory or diagnostic unit is notified by telephone, the scheduling arrangements are confirmed, and the tests are completed as requested.

Some tests can be performed at the bedside with immediate results, such as the basic metabolic panel and coagulation tests. Other tests are specialized, and the final results may not be available for several days or more.

Nonroutine or special tests must be scheduled in advance. For example, positron emission tomography (PET), a nuclear scan, is performed in large medical centers on a particular day of the week, because the radioisotopes must be made in a special laboratory. Fertility and genetic tests are other examples of tests that must be scheduled. The analysis may involve one or more laboratories with specialized equipment and personnel.

Whenever questions exist about scheduling, priorities, the availability of the test, or even the type of specimen container to be used, the nurse can consult the printed hospital reference manual or communicate with the appropriate laboratory or diagnostic unit for assistance.

Requisition Forms

These forms must be completed accurately because they are often the only form of communication used to request a test, and they are part of the identification process that ensures that the correct test is performed on the correct patient. The requisition form is used to request the specific test, including the time and date that it should be performed. The form contains patient information, including the patient's name, identification number, and hospital room number, and the name of the physician. Some agencies require additional information, such as the patient's birth date, to help ensure correct identification.

The requisition slip includes additional information that is appropriate to the test as determined by the physician or the individual who prescribes the test. Examples include the patient's age and gender, date of the last menstrual period, gestation of the pregnancy in a pregnant woman, pertinent medical history, and suspected diagnosis. The information is used in the analysis of the specimen and in the interpretation of the results.

Test Phase

The procedural responsibilities of the nurse vary considerably with different tests, and they vary somewhat among different institutions or units within an institution. When the specimen collection is performed by the physician or technician, the nurse may have only indirect responsibility for ensuring that the test is performed, that the specimen is labeled properly, and that it is sent to the laboratory.

If the hospitalized patient must go to the radiology department or to a special diagnostic unit, the nurse ensures that patient care is completed and that the patient is prepared for transport to the unit. Equipment, such as an intravenous line or a drainage system, must be functional and secured properly. The patient's chart goes with the patient.

In some cases, the nurse is directly involved in the collection of specimens. This may include the collection of blood, urine, stool, and culture specimens, as well as assistance with the collection of a sample of tissue or other body fluids. In these processes, the nurse shares in the responsibility for maintenance of quality controls, proper performance of the equipment, and accurate identification of the patient.

Identification Procedures

It is essential to perform a correct identification before collecting the specimen and starting a diagnostic procedure. To identify the patient, the person who performs the test compares the data on the patient's identification band (name, room number, bed number, and other data) with the data on the requisition slip. Also, the patient is asked to state his or her full name. If the patient cannot respond, the staff nurse or a relative is asked to verify the identity.

Once the specimen is obtained, the label is compared with the requisition slip and the patient's identification band. All three must be identical. Before leaving the patient's bedside or the examining room, the nurse applies the label to the specimen container. For specimens of tissue or body fluid, the labels and requisition slips must identify the source of the specimen, as paracentesis fluid or liver biopsy tissue.

Alternative-Site Testing

Alternative-site laboratory testing refers to choices about where laboratory testing is performed. In the past, a central laboratory and its subsections were housed in a single location, often in a hospital or a single community location. Today, a growing move toward decentralization has resulted in an increase in the sites of laboratory services inside the hospital and outside the institution. Technologic improvements have created miniature, computerized, desktop analyzers and handheld analyzers that bring laboratory testing and analysis nearer to the patient.

For some tests, it is possible to obtain the specimen and the analysis of results within a very brief time, usually 10 minutes or less. When point-of-care technology is used, it provides immediate information about the patient's condition. There is rapid turnaround time between obtaining the specimen and receiving the test results. Medical diagnosis and treatment is based on real-time values and will be more accurate than when there has been a long delay before the laboratory data are available.

Point-of-Care Testing

Point-of-care (POC) testing refers to methods of testing and analysis that bring the laboratory services nearer to the patient. This type of testing, also known as bedside testing or near-patient testing brings laboratory testing and analysis nearer to the patient or to the bedside. In many cases, satellite laboratories are established near or next to operating rooms, intensive care units, and emergency rooms. Sometimes one or more desktop analyzers are used in a clinic, an ambulatory care setting, a physician's office, or even the patient's home. The automated analyzers are used to perform certain laboratory tests rapidly and with increased efficiency. Patient benefits include rapid turnaround time (the results are known within minutes), more prompt treatment, a smaller amount of blood loss with a decreased specimen volume requirement, and possibly lower costs and a shorter hospital stay.

In critical care units, emergency rooms, operating rooms, and other hospital settings in which patients are acutely ill, the common tests that are performed and analyzed at the bedside include determination of blood gases, electrolytes, acid-base balance, osmolarity, and glucose levels; blood chemistries, coagulation studies; and determination of the red blood cell count, platelet count, hemoglobin, and hematocrit values. When the patient is critically ill, many tests are performed at frequent intervals.

In addition to other laboratory test responsibilities, the nurse must ensure that all the results are charted in the correct order and time sequence. When computerized charting is used, the laboratory results must be transferred electronically to central computer systems.

With point-of-care methodology, some reference values are different from the values of the same tests analyzed in the central laboratory. Different reagents, test equipment, and procedures can create the differences in values. The nurse refers to the reference values provided by the laboratory or the manufacturer of the point-of-care equipment for correct analysis of the data. Sometimes, the manufacturer provides a printed conversion table to translate the data to a common reference value.

Another category of point-of-care testing refers to the testing that is performed with small handheld instruments that analyze the patient's blood in a few minutes. The specimen is obtained and the blood analyzed wherever the patient is located, including the home or the workplace. The patient may be the one who performs the test as part of self-care responsibilities.

Expanded Nursing Role

Point-of-care testing involves an expanded role for nurses that overlap with that of laboratory technicians. The nurse may collect the blood sample, perform the analysis, and produce the test results. When the diabetic patient uses the glucometer, the nurse may have to teach the patient these same functions or evaluate the patient's performance and accuracy in using the equipment. In addition, nurses are involved in the selection and maintenance of the equipment located in the patient care units.

In some institutions, laboratory technicians are responsible for point-of-care testing; in other places, nurses, as the providers of direct patient care, use the automated analyzers. As part of the cross-training approach that is being used in hospitals, the nurse who uses this equipment must have formal training, certification that the training has been completed satisfactorily, and periodic reevaluation of performance. Without the training of non-laboratory personnel, a high incidence of inconsistency of performance and inaccurate test results exists. Because of the turnover or rotation of nursing staff, the nurse manager of the unit must monitor the ongoing staff needs for continuing education.

Infection Control: Standard Precautions

Standard precautions must be used when obtaining or handling a blood or body fluid specimen. Gloves must be worn during the collection procedure. If splashing or contact with a mucous membrane is anticipated, the nurse wears a mask, protective eyewear, and a gown or protective clothing in addition to the gloves.

All specimens of blood or body fluids are placed in the correct containers with tightly fitted lids to prevent leakage during transport of the specimen to the laboratory. After the completion of the procedure, the gloves and disposable clothing are removed and discarded. Hands are washed with soap and water.

Precautions are taken to prevent the puncture or cutting of one's own skin with a contaminated needle, scalpel blade, or sharp instrument. To prevent needlestick injury, the needle-and-syringe unit is disposed of in a puncture-resistant container. The needle is not recapped, broken, bent, or removed from the syringe because of the risk of accidentally puncturing the hand.

Special reusable needles, such as those for a spinal tap or aspiration of a joint, are placed in puncture-resistant containers for transport to an area where they are cleansed and sterilized. After use, reusable instruments and diagnostic equipment are also cleansed and sterilized or disinfected according to established procedures.

The use of standard precautions is based on the premise that all patients are potentially infectious and that there is a risk of transmission of infection after exposure to blood or other body fluids. The precautions are used to protect all health care workers against blood-borne pathogens, including HIV.

Posttest Phase

Transport of the Specimen

The specimen is generally transported to the laboratory as quickly as possible. Some laboratory or pathology specimens become unstable shortly after they are collected. Specific factors, such as exposure to sunlight, warming, refrigeration, and exposure to air, can cause alteration or deterioration of particular specimens. For many blood tests, the untreated specimen will begin to deteriorate within a few hours. The nurse must ensure that all specimens are delivered to the laboratory for immediate processing.

When a fresh tissue sample must be analyzed for cytologic features, the specimen cannot be placed in fixative or preservative. Because the specimen will dry out after some exposure to the air, it may be delivered directly into the hands of the pathologist or technician as soon as it is obtained. This coordination of activity provides immediate transport and tissue preparation so that the quality of the specimen is maintained.

Rejection Criteria

When an unsatisfactory specimen is delivered to the laboratory, rejection criteria are applied. The causes of rejection are presented in Box 1. The nurse or staff member who is responsible can help ensure acceptance of the specimen by collecting a sufficient quantity, by complying with the written protocol of the test, and by carefully labeling the specimen container.

BOX 1 Criteria for Rejection of an Unsatisfactory Laboratory Specimen

- Improper labeling of the specimen
- Lack of a label on the specimen
- Improper collection of the specimen
- Lack of a preservative
- Delay in delivery of the specimen to the laboratory
- Improper preservation of the specimen
- Improperly completed requisition form
- Insufficient volume or quantity of the specimen
- Inadequate pretest preparation of the patient

Analysis of the Results

Reference Values

Normal values, or reference values, are often given in a range from the lower to the upper limits of normal. The reference values are used to interpret the results of the test, assist in making an accurate diagnosis, and evaluate the patient's response to treatment.

The reference values for a test vary with the different methods of analysis and different quantitative measurements that are used. For example, the test that measures the 5′-nucleotidase enzyme may be reported with different numeric reference values. The results can have different measurements, and the values are reported as units per liter (U/L), units per milliliter (U/mL), units (U), or Bodansky units. The nurse can use the reference values in this text as a general guide, but the reference values provided by the laboratory that performed the test are the most appropriate values for interpreting the findings in the clinical setting.

For some tests, there is no normal value because the particular substance should not be present at all. When it is not present, the result is described as negative. When it is found, the result is abnormal. The finding may be described as "present" or "positive," or it may be measured with a numeric value that quantifies the amount of substance found.

Variables

The normal reference values are determined by research studies that use human subjects with varying characteristics. These include the variables of demographics, age, gender, and race. Some of the tests, however, have additional reference values for particular groups of individuals because their normal values are influenced by differences in physiology.

Age differences create distinct sets of reference values for some tests. At one end of the life cycle, some reference values are different for the fetus, newborn, and child. In children, the reference values for some tests are different at particular ages. At the other end of the spectrum, age differences result in some variation of reference values in the older adult. For example, hormonal values in the postmenopausal woman are measurably different from those in the younger adult woman.

Gender is another variable that produces some differences in reference values. When differences between men and women occur, the variations are probably the result of increased muscle mass in men and differences in hormones and hormone secretion between men and women.

Additional variations in the reference values for some tests are the result of differences in body weight, position (whether the patient is lying down or seated at the time of specimen collection), and pregnancy.

SI Units

The International System of Units (Systeme International d'Unites or SI) is a system that reports laboratory data in terms of standardized international measurements. This system of measurement is currently used in a number of countries, with the goal of worldwide use in the near future. Throughout this text, whenever possible, the reference values are presented in conventional units and their SI equivalents.

Critical Values

The phrases of *critical value* or *possible panic* value refer to a test result that is extremely abnormal and indicates that the patient's life or health is in imminent danger. The value may be markedly elevated or decreased. Identification of these extreme results helps the nurse and physician differentiate between abnormal results and the extremes that indicate a crisis. When a test result has reached the level of a critical value, the nurse must notify the physician immediately. Medical diagnosis and treatment are needed to correct the imbalance before the patient's acute condition worsens.

Verbal Reports

When a laboratory test result is in the critical value range or when the laboratory test or diagnostic procedure was ordered on a stat basis (to be done immediately), the laboratory or diagnostic unit personnel will phone the physician and the nurse to report the results. When the nurse receives a verbal report, there is risk of error because of a potential misunderstanding of what was heard. The procedure the nurse follows is to first write down the name of the test and the results and then to read back the information to the caller. This provides for confirmation of the accuracy of the message or opportunity to correct a misunderstanding. The nurse must then call the physician and report the information and the read-back procedure is again followed. The nurse should treat all verbal reports of results of diagnostic tests or laboratory tests as critical values and contact the physician without delay.

PATIENT-NURSE INTERACTIONS

Dimensions of Nursing Care

The range of interactions between the patient and the nurse varies considerably with the complexity of the test or procedure. Laboratory tests that use specimens of blood, urine, or feces require some nursing intervention to ensure adequate patient preparation or accurate patient ability to collect the specimen. Diagnostic procedures, however, require increased interaction with the patient, particularly when they are invasive.

Nursing responsibilities involve physical and psychosocial dimensions of patient care, with particular concern for the patient's safety.

Patient-nurse interactions involve direct or indirect care in the pretest, test, and posttest phases of the diagnostic procedure. The nursing process is applicable as a guide to the identification of the patient's needs and the development of the appropriate nursing interventions that lead to a positive outcome (Figure 2).

Changes in Health Care Delivery

These changes have resulted in shorter hospital stays for patients. Shorter periods of hospitalization limit the time for direct care during the acute phase of illness. For the acutely ill hospitalized patient, numerous diagnostic tests or procedures are often scheduled during a concentrated period. In addition to the routine pretest and posttest assessments of the patient, the nurse assesses for actual or potential complications related to the invasive diagnostic procedures.

Changes in health care delivery have resulted in many diagnostic tests being performed on an outpatient basis. The patient has been given greater self-care responsibility for pretest preparation and posttest recovery. The direct nursing interactions with the patient are often short-lived and may be limited to a brief pretest phase, the test phase, and the immediate posttest phase.

When a diagnostic procedure is performed in the outpatient setting, the patient receives pretest planning information and instructions regarding special requirements necessary before or after the procedure. The clearly stated instructions are given to the patient or the family member who assists with the patient's care. If the instructions are complex, they should be given in writing so that the patient can refer to them as needed. Also, the patient needs the address and location of the laboratory or diagnostic unit, as well as the time and date for which the test is scheduled.

In procedures requiring sedation or light anesthesia, the patient is instructed in advance that a responsible individual will be required to provide transportation home at the end of the test. When a delayed complication in the posttest period is possible,

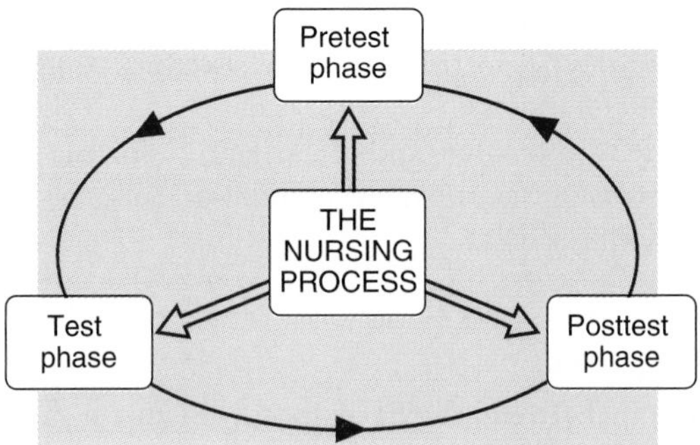

Figure 2. Application of the nursing process. In each phase of diagnostic testing, the nursing process is applied to provide safe, accurate, complete, and effective nursing care.

the patient receives instruction so that he or she will recognize abnormal symptoms and notify the physician if they occur. All these measures are designed to provide continuity of care, even when the patient is some distance from the health care provider.

Pediatric Patients

Modifications in communication and safety measures are required for pediatric patients. These measures should be compatible with the age and behavior of the child. When explanations can be understood, time should be taken to prepare the young child for the test or procedure. Honest, friendly explanations help the child cope with and endure the test. The child may fear pain, injections, the large equipment of the radiology department, or even the strangers who perform the test. Explanations are given simply and briefly. In some cases, the parents help prepare the child and provide calming reassurance.

Infants or active small children usually require restraints to protect them from harm and to maintain immobility during the test or procedure. The choice of restraint is based on the particular need and are used for tests of short duration. The choices include a sheet restraint, a mummy-style restraint, or a special commercial restraint that holds the patient in a particular position.

When the procedure requires a prolonged period of immobility, sedation is often used for infants and small children. Because of their young age, children cannot be expected to remain still for a long time. The procedures that use sedation in children include nuclear medicine scans, computed tomography, magnetic resonance imaging, electroencephalography, echocardiography, and some ultrasound procedures.

Geriatric Patients

Older adult individuals may have certain needs that are age related or caused by a specific disease process. For the confused or depressed patient, instructions may need to be given slowly or repeated several times. The patient may have a hearing deficit or difficulty understanding speech or language. Alternative communication measures may include written pretest and posttest instructions, inclusion of a family member in the communications, or providing an interpreter to help the patient.

The elderly patient may take a wide range of medications, and some of them can interfere with particular laboratory tests. The physician is consulted regarding any alteration in the medication schedule, such as withholding the medication for a specified period.

Frail, elderly patients are at risk for injury from a fall. The common underlying problems include visual impairment, stiffness, weakness, mental confusion, dizziness, and the effects of medication. Care is taken to prevent accidental injury or a fall by assisting the patient out of the wheelchair and onto or off a gurney, examining table, radiography table, or toilet.

The elderly individual is often uncomfortable when lying on an x-ray table for a long time. The table is hard and the patient's joints are often stiff with arthritis. The room is usually cool, and some older patients complain that they feel cold. It may not be possible to change the patient's position during x-ray studies or other diagnostic procedures because of the requirements of the test; however, warm blankets are usually provided so that at least the discomfort of chilling is removed.

Pretest Phase

Nursing Assessment

This assessment consists of the appraisal of the patient's physical and psychosocial status in relation to the requirements of the test. Pertinent findings in the psychosocial and physical history include any problems with the patient's vision, hearing, mobility, and comprehension of instructions. Current medications are listed. When iodinated contrast medium is used in the radiologic study, the nurse assesses for any history of allergy to shellfish or iodine or of a previous reaction during a radiology test. Allergies to other foods and medications are also documented. If a female of childbearing age needs an x-ray study, she is questioned to determine whether there is any possibility of pregnancy.

Vital signs are taken to establish baseline values, particularly for invasive procedures or for when contrast medium, sedation, or anesthesia is used. The infant's or child's weight is recorded when the dose of medication or contrast medium must be calculated according to body weight.

For the purposes of consent, the patient is assessed for knowledge about the procedure, the pretest preparation, and other information that has been explained by the physician.

The nurse assesses the patient for signs of anxiety or fear. The cause can be apprehension about the test or procedure, or it may be fear of abnormal test results that indicate serious illness. If signs of distress are noted, the nurse asks about the cause or source of the anxiety.

The nurse also reviews the laboratory and other diagnostic test results and ensures that they are placed in the patient's record. Some tests, such as prothrombin time, complete blood cell count, chest radiograph, and electrocardiogram, must verify a health clearance before some of the more invasive diagnostic tests are undertaken.

Nursing Diagnoses

Once the nursing assessment is completed, the nurse formulates nursing diagnoses that are appropriate to the patient who will undergo a procedure. The pretest-phase nursing diagnoses are presented in Table 1.

Expected Outcomes

During the pretest period, the expected outcomes include the following:

1. When conscious sedation or anesthesia is anticipated, the patient arranges for a family member or friend to provide transportation home from the ambulatory test center.
2. The patient shows no signs or symptoms of infection.
3. The patient communicates any history of allergic reaction to iodine, other allergens, and medications.
4. The patient's vital signs, test results for coagulation studies, and other blood profiles remain within normal limits.
5. The patient requests information or clarification regarding the test and any special measures required in preparation for the test.
6. The patient, a family member, or a significant other demonstrates comprehension of the test and its preparation requirements.

TABLE 1 Pretest-Phase Nursing Diagnoses

Nursing Diagnosis	Defining Characteristics	Related Factors
Risk for injury	Presence of risk factors such as developmental age, psychological factors, or physical factors such as sensory or motor deficit	
Risk for infection or allergic reaction	Presence of risk factors such as altered immune function, history of chronic illness, impaired oxygenation of tissues, external factors such as allergens or infectious agents	
Protection, ineffective	Presence of risk factors such as altered clotting factors, immunosuppression, myelosuppression, altered cardiovascular status, or disorientation	Developmental or age-related factors
Impaired verbal communication	Unable to speak dominant language, speaks with difficulty, disorientation, difficulty in comprehending	Cultural, developmental, or age-related factors; psychological barriers, physiological conditions
Anxiety	Presence of increased tension, uncertainty, fear of unspecific consequences, cardiovascular excitation, facial tension, insomnia, confusion	Threat to or change in health status

Nursing Intervention

The nurse notifies the physician of abnormal pretest results that indicate infection, clotting abnormality, fever, or irregularity in the vital signs. The diagnostic procedure may have to be postponed until the abnormality is corrected.

If the patient has allergies to food, medication, or contrast medium, the nurse posts an allergy warning sticker on the outside of the patient's record.

The nurse provides pretest instructions that can be understood by the patient. Pretest instructions often include the discontinuation of food and fluids for a specified period. They may also involve modification of activity or the temporary stoppage of one or more medications for a specified period. Some abdominal or intestinal tests require a cleansing of the bowel by enema or cathartic, or both.

When indicated, the nurse obtains the patient's signature of consent for the test or procedure. The patient should have received the physician's explanation of the procedure, the method of performing the test, and the potential risks involved. If the patient cannot give consent because of age or physical or mental impairment, obtain the signature of the person who is legally responsible for the patient's health care decisions. Once the consent form is signed and witnessed, the nurse enters it into the patient's record.

The nurse provides reassurance or information, as needed, to help reduce the patient's anxiety. This is best done by communication with and assistance to the patient in an attentive and caring manner.

Nursing Evaluation

The pretest phase is completed successfully when the following have been accomplished:

1. The patient has followed all the pretest instructions accurately.
2. The patient's blood values, vital signs, and temperature measurement are within normal limits.
3. The patient appears calm and accepting about the test.

Test Phase

Nursing Assessment

The nursing assessment during the test phase begins with the correct identification of the patient and the verification of the procedure and the area to be tested (such as right or left leg, arm, breast, or lung).

Monitoring of the physiologic status of the patient is carried out by a variety of measurements, depending on the complexity of the procedure and the use of conscious sedation or light anesthesia. Ongoing assessment of the patient may be performed through observation of the level of consciousness, repeated monitoring of vital signs, pulse oximetry, cardiac monitoring, or, in pregnant patients, fetal monitoring.

The skin is assessed for signs of infection or trauma, particularly at the site of intended venipuncture. The patient's chart is also reviewed for the most recent laboratory findings and the pretest vital signs.

The nurse observes the patient for signs of discomfort, including shivering, trembling, pain, and tension. To encourage communication of any problems or concerns, the patient is asked how he or she feels.

Nursing Diagnoses

Once the nursing assessment is completed, the nurse formulates nursing diagnoses that are appropriate to the patient who undergoes the procedure. The test-phase nursing diagnoses are presented in Table 2.

Expected Outcomes

During the test period, the outcomes include the following:

1. The patient maintains adequate skin circulation and tissue perfusion.
2. Cardiopulmonary stability is maintained. Vital signs and the results of the monitoring devices are in a normal range.
3. The puncture wound or incision remains clean and free from infection.
4. The patient expresses any pain or discomfort, including the location and characteristics of the sensation.
5. The patient verbalizes any feelings of apprehension and helps identify the cause of those feelings.

Nursing Intervention

The nurse positions the patient correctly for the procedure. Use padding, supportive devices, or restraints to promote safety and protect the patient's tissue against injury.

TABLE 2 Test-Phase Nursing Diagnoses

Nursing Diagnosis	Defining Characteristics
Risk for impaired skin integrity	Disruption of the skin surface Presence of internal or external risk factors, including skin compression, immobility, or altered circulation
Decreased cardiac output	Variations in blood pressure readings, arrhythmias, color changes of the skin, decreased peripheral pulses, dyspnea, increased heart rate
Impaired gas exchange	Cyanosis, restlessness, dyspnea, hypoxemia Risk factors: administration of sedative analgesic medications, contrast medium, and potential allergic reaction
Risk for infection	Presence of risk factors such as inadequate primary defenses and performance of invasive procedures
Pain	Verbal report or expressive behavior, such as moaning, crying Observed evidence, such as guarding behavior or grimacing
Anxiety	Verbalization of feelings about the test or its potential findings, changes in cardiovascular and respiratory rates

The patient's cardiopulmonary status is monitored continuously, including assessment of skin color and integrity, vital signs, breathing status, and level of consciousness.

The nurse keeps the emergency cart in a nearby location.

The nurse ensures that all invasive equipment is sterile or has been properly cleaned and disinfected. Before the skin is punctured or opened, ensure that the skin is appropriately cleansed. Draping the area with sterile towels may also be indicated.

Verbal or physical support is offered to the patient by the nurse, particularly when the patient appears distressed by the procedure.

The nurse administers prescribed pain medication as indicated.

Nursing Evaluation

The test phase is completed when the following has been accomplished:

1. The patient demonstrates normal cardiopulmonary function, as measured by normal vital signs and normal readings on all monitoring devices.
2. The patient maintains normal skin color and tone, with palpable peripheral pulses.
3. The patient experiences a lessening of pain, anxiety, or discomfort.
4. The patient has a clean, dry dressing with no signs of renewed bleeding, hematoma, swelling, or redness.

Posttest Phase

Nursing Assessment

The assessment after the test is completed is focused on the patient's physiologic, emotional, and mental status. Physiologic assessment is essential after an invasive procedure, conscious sedation, or anesthesia. The nurse assesses the expected alterations that occur because of the procedure or medications and the potential complications.

When cardiac monitoring, fetal monitoring, and pulse oximetry are used during procedures, they are usually continued into the posttest period until the results are stable and remain in a normal range. Vital signs are taken to ensure that the hemodynamic status remains stable.

A risk of complications from an allergic response to the contrast medium and a risk of an embolus to a more distal location exist when an invasive neurologic, cerebrovascular, or peripheral arterial study is performed. Neurovascular assessments are performed to assess the integrity of the distal arterial blood flow and the responses of the neurologic tissues that are supplied by that blood flow. Vital signs also are monitored frequently to identify any untoward changes in cardiorespiratory status.

The nurse also uses observation to perform many assessments. When the diagnostic procedure is invasive, the nurse examines the site of the incision, penetration of the needle, or insertion of the instrument. The tissue is examined for signs of swelling, discharge, bleeding, or discoloration. Some pain or soreness may be present because of the incision or the manipulation of internal tissue. The nurse asks the patient to describe and locate the pain or tenderness. Sometimes the patient does not have immediate pain because of the lingering effects of the anesthetic or narcotic-analgesic medications. The nurse also examines the dressings. They should be clean, dry, and intact.

The nurse can usually perform an emotional assessment by asking general questions about how the patient feels and observing the patient's responses. Most patients are relieved to have completed the test and are ready to return to their hospital rooms or to their residences. If there has been a period of fasting, they often express the desire to eat.

The assessment of mental status is appropriate when the patient has received conscious sedation or anesthesia or after a cerebrovascular invasive test. The nurse assesses the level of consciousness as well as clarity of thinking and speech. During the initial recovery from conscious sedation or anesthesia, the patient may be somewhat confused or drowsy, with diminished affect. As the medications are metabolized and excreted, increasing responsiveness and clarity of thinking are noted.

Before discharge, the patient who has had an invasive procedure is assessed for knowledge about continued requirements for care at home until healing is complete. The patient may be able to perform self-care, or there may be a need for family assistance for the remainder of the day. Assessment for infection or inflammation continues for several days, because the symptoms take time to develop. The patient or family member is taught to continue this assessment at home.

Nursing Diagnoses

Once the nursing assessment has been completed, the nurse formulates nursing diagnoses that are appropriate to the patient during the posttest phase of care. The posttest-phase nursing diagnoses are presented in Table 3.

Expected Outcomes

During the posttest period, the outcomes include the following:

1. The patient is conscious and alert.
2. Oxygenation and tissue perfusion are sustained, including circulation to the extremities.
3. Adequate cardiac output is maintained.
4. The skin remains warm, with normal color and no evidence of swelling or bleeding.
5. The patient does not fall or experience trauma.
6. After medication is given, the patient expresses relief from pain.
7. The site of puncture or incision remains free from infection.
8. The patient or family member verbalizes understanding of posttest instructions regarding patient care.

Nursing Intervention

After the completion of a diagnostic procedure in which conscious sedation or a light anesthesia was used, position the patient on his or her side to maintain a patent airway.

Oxygen may be administered, and the intravenous fluid replacement continues until the patient is able to drink fluids.

Administer the prescribed pain medication as needed. To help relieve discomfort, encourage the patient to change positions. Provide support with pillows.

Maintain sterile technique in the assessment of the wound or in changing the dressing.

To prevent a fall or an injury, assist the patient off the x-ray or examining table; also help the patient to the bathroom or with dressing in street clothes, as necessary.

TABLE 3 Posttest-Phase Nursing Diagnoses

Nursing Diagnosis	Defining Characteristics
Altered tissue perfusion: cerebral, cardiopulmonary, peripheral	Changes in skin temperature, blood pressure changes, arrhythmias, dyspnea, decreased peripheral pulses, altered mental status
Pain	Verbal report about pain or discomfort Alteration in muscle tone, movement, or facial expression Expressive behavior, such as moaning, grimacing, and crying
Risk for injury	Presence of risk factors such as immobility, developmental age, or sensory-motor deficit
Risk for infection	Presence of risk factors such as exposure to pathogens, immunosuppression, or broken skin
Knowledge deficit regarding care after procedure	Verbalization of the problem, inaccurate follow-through on instructions
Anxiety	Expressed concerns or uncertainty about the findings of the test or procedure, sleep disturbance, increased tension, worry

The patient may experience stiffness, pain, or drowsiness or may have diminished mental acuity as the result of the medication or procedure.

Inform the patient that the physician will discuss the diagnostic results with him or her as soon as this information is available. The patient with sutures is instructed to make an appointment with the physician for the evaluation of the incision and removal of the sutures.

Before discharge, instruct the patient about any recommended restrictions, such as instructions regarding activity, bathing, resumption of medication, the intake of fluids, or care of the incision.

Nursing Evaluation

The posttest phase is completed when the following have been accomplished.

1. The patient demonstrates normal vital signs, responsiveness to questions, and normal skin color and temperature.
2. The patient experiences a lessening of pain, anxiety, or discomfort.
3. The patient has a clean, dry dressing with no signs of renewed bleeding, hematoma, swelling, or redness.
4. The patient verbalizes his or her understanding of the discharge instructions.

Analysis of the Results and the Significance in Nursing Practice

The nurse who cares for the patient reads the laboratory results and reports of the diagnostic procedures that provide additional objective assessment information. The information helps confirm the patient's medical diagnosis and severity of the pathophysiologic changes. When repeat testing is done, the results are compared to previous results to monitor the patient's response to treatment.

In the diagnostic workup, the physician or the nurse practitioner uses the tests to confirm the medical diagnosis and estimate the severity of the condition. Often several tests are needed to identify the illness the patient has and to rule out other conditions. Also, many illnesses cause alterations of more than one organ or body system. For example, a diagnosis of pneumonia can be confirmed by a chest x-ray, but the patient also has infection, dehydration because of fever and a lack of fluid intake during the infection, and alteration of blood gases because of impaired gas exchange in the lungs. Thus, the nurse will review the x-ray report, and identify abnormalities in white blood count, the serum electrolytes, acid-base balance, arterial blood gases, specific gravity of the urine, and the results of a sputum culture or DNA identification of the microbe that caused the pneumonia.

When repeat tests are used to monitor the patient's response to treatment, the nurse monitors the changes that indicate an improving condition. For example, during or after a severe bleeding episode from a duodenal ulcer, the patient will have stool specimens that are positive for blood and there will be a sudden decline in the red blood cell count, the hemoglobin, and hematocrit values. Medical treatment of the illness and nursing interventions to implement the prescribed treatment are designed to stop the bleeding and, possibly, administer a blood transfusion to replace the lost blood. The follow-up testing confirms successful treatment and patient healing, as evidenced by a rising red blood cell count, hematocrit, and hemoglobin. Additionally, the feces become negative for blood.

The nurse also can use his or her knowledge of the significance of test findings to help patients in other ways. The patient may be apprehensive about the possibility of abnormal findings or in need of counseling, clarification, or reassurance regarding abnormal results of a test. For example, a patient who was diagnosed and treated for ovarian cancer, now has follow-up testing with the blood test for cancer antigen 125 (CA-125). The physician told the patient that the test value is now elevated and its significance. The patient is troubled and wants to talk to the nurse about her condition. The nurse knows that this level is severely elevated and the elevation indicates that the cancer is progressing. The nurse can help the patient with emotional support by listening and providing calm and caring responses. The nurse also can try to determine what the patient knows about the meaning of the test and what she wants to do about it. Finally, the nurse also provides hope by encouraging the patient to return to the physician to discuss again treatment options and to follow-up with additional treatment.

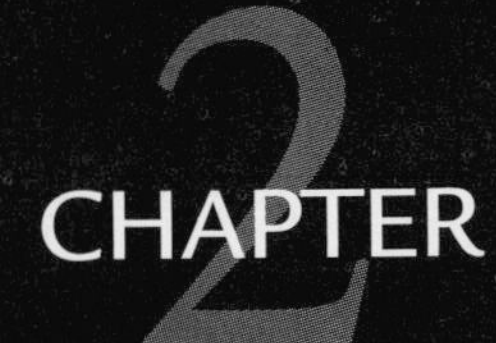

CHAPTER 2

Specimen Collection Procedures

Three major sources of specimen samples are blood, stool, and urine, with most tests performed on blood. The laboratory performs biochemical and microscopic analysis of these body substances to provide objective data about the patient's health and to identify disease processes.

In collection procedures, accurate technique is essential for obtaining a valid specimen and to prevent patient injury. In addition, quality control measures are used in maintaining accuracy in the identification of the patient and the specimen, in the method of obtaining the specimen, and in the transportation of the specimen to the laboratory.

BLOOD COLLECTION PROCEDURES

Arterial Puncture

ahr-tee-ree-uhl punk-chur

SPECIMEN OR TYPE OF TEST: Arterial blood

PURPOSE OF THE TEST

Arterial puncture is used to obtain a sample of arterial blood for analysis of blood gases and acid-base balance.

BASICS THE NURSE NEEDS TO KNOW

Arterial blood specimens are obtained for blood gas studies, including the measurement of oxygen, carbon dioxide, and pH. The assessment of arterial blood is usually performed on the patient who has an actual or potential problem with oxygenation.

The nursing diagnoses may include ineffective airway clearance, ineffective breathing pattern, impaired gas exchange, and altered tissue perfusion: cardiopulmonary.

The procedure of arterial puncture is technically more difficult than that of venipuncture, but arterial blood is far more accurate for the measurement of oxygenation throughout the body. The usual puncture site is either the radial or the brachial artery, with the radial artery being preferred. The femoral artery can be used; however, the risk of hemorrhage at that site is greater.

Before an arterial puncture of the radial artery is carried out, the *Allen test* is performed to verify the presence of collateral circulation to the hand. If arterial occlusion of the radial artery occurs after arterial puncture, the presence of collateral circulation protects the hand from ischemic damage. The Allen test procedure is presented in the content on Arterial Blood Gases (p. 99).

Some institutions and settings permit the nurse with specialized training to draw blood through an arterial puncture. Refer to the institutional or laboratory protocol to determine who may do this procedure.

HOW THE TEST IS DONE

A heparinized syringe and needle is used to collect 3 mL of arterial blood. For radial artery puncture, a 23- to 25-gauge needle is used. For brachial artery puncture, an 18- to 20-gauge needle is used. In many institutions, a prepackaged kit provides the equipment for blood gas studies.

INTERFERING FACTORS

- Poor collateral circulation to the extremities
- Inability to puncture the artery or withdraw blood
- Air mixed in with the blood specimen

NURSING CARE

Pretest

- Identify the patient by asking his or her name, checking the identification bracelet, and comparing the identification bracelet with the name on the requisition form.
- When the radial artery is to be used, palpate the pulse of each wrist to select the site with the stronger circulation. Perform the Allen test to assess the collateral circulation to the hand. Position the hand so that the wrist is in slight dorsiflexion.
- Explain to the patient that a sharp pain will be felt as the needle punctures the blood vessel. In some cases, a local anesthetic may be given beforehand.

During the Test

- The interior of the syringe and needle must be coated with heparin. The syringe in the blood gas kit may be heparinized already. If heparin must be added, 1 mL (1000 or 5000 units/mL) is drawn into a 10-mL syringe. After the syringe is rotated to coat the entire interior surface, the heparin is expelled. A small amount of heparin remains in the dead space and within the shaft of the needle.

Continued

NURSING CARE—*cont'd*

During the Test—*cont'd*

- Clean the skin over the pulse point with povidone-iodine, using sterile gauze. Remove this solution by wiping the skin with 70% alcohol. Allow the skin to dry.
- With the bevel of the needle up and the syringe placed at a 45- to 60-degree angle, slowly insert the needle into the artery (Figure 3). Blood will pulse into the syringe without your having to draw back on the plunger.
- Once the required amount of blood is in the syringe, remove the needle. The amount is usually 3 mL, but the volume can vary according to the type of syringe and the test protocol.

Posttest

- Use sterile gauze to apply immediate pressure to the puncture site for 5 minutes. Blood flow from the artery and hematoma formation are more likely to develop because of the pressure within the arterial walls. Pressure on the puncture point lessens the tendency of excess bleeding.
- Remove the needle from the syringe. If there is air in the syringe, expel it. Place the airtight cap on the tip of the syringe. These measures limit or eliminate possible alteration of blood gas values because of contamination of the blood by the oxygen and carbon dioxide gases in the air.
- Place the syringe on ice and arrange for immediate transport of the specimen to the laboratory.
- Once the bleeding from the puncture site has stopped, the nurse applies a small sterile bandage and continues to assess the wrist and hand for signs of complications. It is common for the patient to complain of some temporary discomfort, such as aching, throbbing, or tenderness at the puncture site.

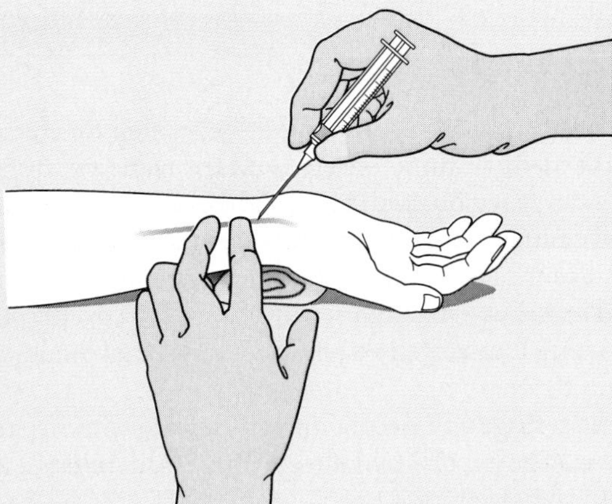

Figure 3. Technique for arterial puncture. Puncture of the radial artery can be performed only when both the radial and ulnar arteries provide adequate circulation to the hand.

NURSING CARE—*cont'd*

 **Nursing Response to Complications**

The three complications of arterial puncture are bleeding, infection, and thrombus formation, but the incidence is low.

Bleeding. The most common sign of bleeding is hematoma formation. The tissue becomes tense and somewhat swollen in the area of bleeding and spreads through the tissue by gravity. The nurse looks for bruising around the puncture site and at the tissue on the underside of the extremity.

Infection. If the patient develops an infection, the puncture site may become tender, reddened, and swollen. Systemically, the patient develops a fever and the white blood count rises above normal values.

Thrombus formation. The nurse assesses for signs of an obstruction in the circulation distal to the puncture site. This may include loss of a distal pulse when a brachial or femoral puncture site is used. In addition, the distal parts, such as fingers, feel cool or cold and appear pale or cyanotic. The patient complains of pain in the area where there is loss of circulation.

Capillary Puncture

ka-puh-le-ree punk-chur

Also called: Microcapillary Puncture; Skin Puncture

SPECIMEN OR TYPE OF TEST: Capillary blood

PURPOSE OF THE TEST

Capillary blood collection is used when a small amount of blood is sufficient or the venipuncture method is not feasible.

BASICS THE NURSE NEEDS TO KNOW

The traditional use of the capillary puncture is for patients with small or inaccessible veins. This method is useful in burn patients, in those who are extremely obese, and in patients who have a tendency toward thrombus formation. It is the method of choice for obtaining blood samples from premature infants, neonates, and young babies. It may be used to preserve the total blood volume of the infant or small child, particularly when there is a need for repeated blood testing.

Because capillary blood is similar in composition to venous blood, capillary blood collection may be performed for a complete blood cell count, hematocrit determination, blood smear, coagulation studies, and most blood chemistry tests. The specimen source is always identified on the requisition slip, because there may be differences between venous and capillary blood values for calcium, glucose, potassium, and total protein.

Site of Collection

The available sites for collection of capillary blood include the finger, heel, and earlobe. The finger is often used for adults or older children. The locations most often used are the distal tips of the third and fourth fingers, slightly to the side (Figure 4). Few calluses are located on the sides of the fingers, and the lancet can puncture the skin more easily. The frontal tips or pads of the fingers are not used because many nerve endings are located there, and the puncture would be more painful.

The heel is used for premature infants, neonates, infants, and small children and for special cases, such as patients with thermal injury. With the heelstick technique, the medial or lateral plantar surface of the foot is used (Figure 5). The heel and big toe are preferred. The central area of the plantar surface of the foot is never used. There is a risk of damage to the calcaneus bone, Achilles tendon, or other tendons, nerves, and cartilage that are located in the central area of the foot.

The earlobe may be used as the alternative puncture site of last resort in adults and older children, but it cannot be used for infants and neonates. It is a preferred site for obtaining arterialized blood for measurement of pH and partial pressure of carbon dioxide (Pco_2), because it is highly vascular tissue with few metabolic requirements. However, the blood values obtained from an earlobe site are unreliable in cases of low cardiac output and vasoconstriction. If the earlobe is used, the soft fleshy part is punctured, and the area of cartilaginous tissue is avoided.

In the selection of the skin puncture site, the tissue should not be edematous, inflamed, or recently punctured. These factors cause increased interstitial fluid to mix with the blood, and they also increase the risk of an infection.

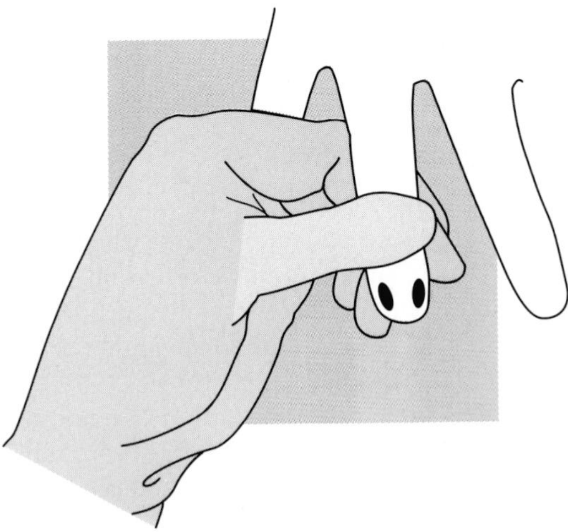

Figure 4. Capillary puncture sites in the finger. In adults, the middle or ring finger is the preferred site for a capillary blood sample. The sterile lancet punctures the skin in the distal tip slightly to the side of the finger pad.

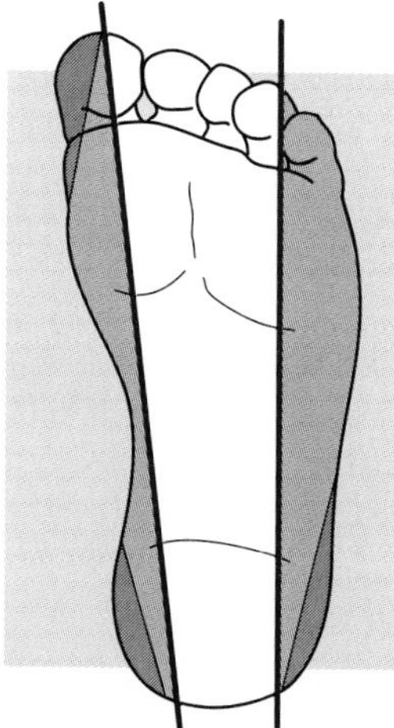

Figure 5. Heelstick sites for capillary puncture. The shaded areas are appropriate sites for neonates and infants, but the best sites are the heel and big toe, as indicated by areas of darker shading.

The heelstick method is preferred for sampling blood in the premature baby and infant. It is technically easier to perform and avoids the significant complications that can occur with arterial or venous puncture. Some special considerations must be made, however, because of the number of heelstick punctures performed and the small size of the patients.

Increasingly, infants are discharged from the nursery after a short stay. This means that additional blood tests for bilirubinemia, phenylalanine, hemoglobinopathy, and galactosemia, as well as other screening tests, are performed on an outpatient basis. Some of these tests are performed serially, meaning that multiple blood samples are taken over time. The nurse in the outpatient setting assesses the heels of the infant for signs of complications that can occur from repeated punctures.

The premature infant also needs special consideration when multiple blood samples are obtained by the heelstick technique. The premature infant may weigh as little as 500 g. The heels are small, and there is little depth to the tissue for the many punctures and tests that are needed. Additionally, blood flow is often inadequate, and two or three punctures may be needed to obtain the required amount.

To help prevent injury to the calcaneus, the depth of the lancet must be controlled, and careful selection of the tissue site must be carried out. To help prevent infection and hematoma, aseptic technique and gentle handling of the tissue are needed whenever blood is drawn. Because of repeated trauma to the heels of the premature infant, the nurse assesses this tissue for signs of localized complications. These complications can occur during the stay in the neonatal unit, or they can develop years later.

HOW THE TEST IS DONE

A sterile lancet is used to collect capillary blood from a skin puncture site. The blood is blotted onto special filter paper (Figure 6) or collected in a narrow-diameter glass tube. The tube is called a micropipette, microtube, or capillary tube.

INTERFERING FACTORS

- Reduced cardiac output
- Vasoconstriction

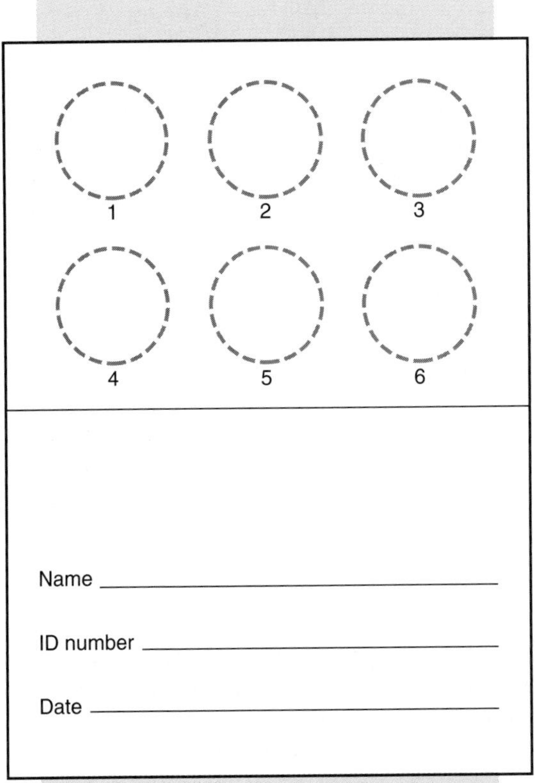

Figure 6. Capillary blood filter paper. Droplets of blood are blotted onto the filter paper at each circle. The nurse must saturate each circle before moving on to fill the next one. The nurse must not partially fill some circles and then return to complete them later. To promote blood flow, the hand is kept lower than the heart, and the finger is stroked in a distal direction.

NURSING CARE

Pretest

- Identify the patient and check the requisition form with the patient's identification bracelet. Inform the patient that blood needs to be drawn from the designated site.
- Particularly with small children, provide reassurance to help limit anxiety.
- If pretest fasting or dietary restriction is required, verify that the instructions were followed for the correct period.
- Assemble the equipment and put on a pair of gloves.
- The patient may be seated or in the supine position.

During the Test

- Assess the skin site for color and temperature and the absence of infection and edema. If the skin is cool or pale, the circulation may be diminished. Put the hand in warm water or apply a warm, moist compress to the site for a few minutes. This helps increase circulation to the skin.
- Use gauze and 70% alcohol to cleanse the skin site. Allow the skin to dry.
- Holding the tissue between the thumb and the forefinger, use a firm, quick stroke to puncture the skin with the sterile lancet.
- Wipe away the first drop of blood, because it contains tissue fluids. Collect the subsequent drops of blood in capillary tubes or on the blotting paper.
- To help obtain more blood, the finger may be massaged gently. The tissue near the puncture should not be squeezed because tissue fluids will mix with the blood, and the blood will clot quickly.
- The capillary tubes are held horizontally to prevent air bubbles. They should be filled two-thirds to three-quarters full and then sealed with clay.
- The circles on the filter paper are filled one at a time, until they are fully saturated. Allow the blood on the paper to air-dry for 10 minutes before it is placed in a collection envelope.

Posttest

- Once the specimen collection is completed, wipe the puncture site with alcohol.
- Place sterile gauze on the site and instruct the patient to apply pressure until the bleeding stops.
- If the infant or small child is crying, provide comfort.
- Label all specimens and arrange for their prompt transport to the laboratory.

◆ Nursing Response to Complications

The nurse inspects the infant's feet daily for damage to the skin in the sites of capillary punctures. The abnormal findings are documented in the patient's record and the physician is notified.

Infection. The most serious but infrequent complication of heelstick puncture in infants is infection. The infection is usually localized in the soft tissue, and the most common causative organism is *Staphylococcus aureus*. Weeks later, however, the infection can develop into osteomyelitis. The source of the infection is poor aseptic technique, a contaminated lancet, or injury to the bone during the skin puncture.

Continued

NURSING CARE—*cont'd*

Infection is characterized by localized redness and swelling. The area is tender or painful. In more advanced infection, there may be purulent drainage or abscess formation. Because of the risk that the infection could spread to the bone, x-rays of the heel and foot may be ordered.

Hematoma and bruising. Bruising, pain, scarring, and hematoma formation are more frequent complications. They occur from frequent skin punctures or excessive squeezing of the tissues during the collection of the blood samples.

When blood has leaked from the puncture site into tissue, the area becomes bruised and discolored. There may be leakage of blood onto the skin. The nurse should handle the baby's foot gently during the examination because the area is swollen and painful.

Venipuncture

vee-ni-punk-chur

Also called: Phlebotomy; Venous Blood Collection

SPECIMEN OR TYPE OF TEST: Whole blood, serum, plasma

PURPOSE OF THE TEST

Venipuncture is used to obtain a venous blood sample for laboratory analysis. The serum component of the blood is used for most of the chemistry analyses.

BASICS THE NURSE NEEDS TO KNOW

Venipuncture is performed by drawing and collecting a specimen of blood from a superficial vein. It is a quick method of obtaining a larger sample of blood, and the specimen can be used to perform many different laboratory analyses. Depending on the test to be performed, the analysis is carried out on whole blood, serum, or plasma.

Whole blood contains all the blood components. A centrifuge is used to separate the blood components and obtain either serum or plasma. If the blood has been collected in a tube containing anticoagulant, the centrifuge process produces plasma. If whole blood is collected in a tube without anticoagulant, the centrifuge process yields serum. Plasma is serum that contains fibrinogen.

Site of Collection

The most common site for venipuncture is the antecubital fossa, because several large superficial veins are available. The most commonly used veins are the median cubital, the basilic, and the cephalic veins (Figure 7). Veins of the wrists, hands, or ankles may also be used.

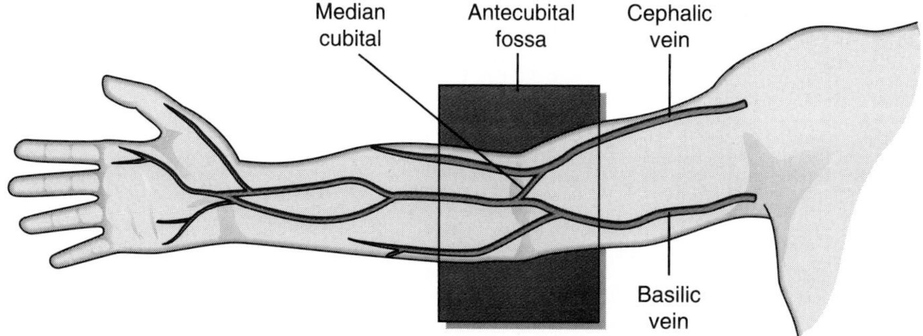

Figure 7. Preferred sites for venipuncture. The three primary veins in the antecubital fossa are preferred because they are usually visible and fixed in place by surrounding tissue. *(Reproduced with permission from Lehmann, C. A. [1998].* Saunders Manual of Clinical Laboratory Science *[p. 7]. Philadelphia: W. B. Saunders.)*

Intervening Variables

When an intravenous line, shunt, or other intravenous device has been placed in one arm, the opposite arm or another venous site must be selected. The reason for avoiding these sites is that the administration of intravenous fluids alters the composition of the blood specimen. Additionally, venous shunts are established for specific treatments, and they can be damaged by excessive punctures.

For a variety of physiologic and age-related reasons, locating a suitable vein is sometimes difficult. When the patient is severely dehydrated or hypotensive, or both, the veins have less fluid volume. They are less visible and less palpable and may be partially collapsed. Reduced cardiac output also diminishes the volume of blood in the peripheral veins.

Severe obesity can be a problem, because the overlying layers of fat interfere with the location and palpation of a suitable vein. In the elderly, the superficial veins of the hands are highly visible and prominent, but it is difficult to use these sites. The veins are fragile, and venipuncture can cause a hematoma to form. Additionally, these veins move during the venipuncture process, making it difficult to enter the lumen of the vein. The excess movement is caused by the loss of supportive muscle and connective tissue associated with aging.

In the premature and newborn infant, the veins are small. Frequent venipuncture can cause severe complications, including damage to the veins and surrounding tissue.

If any of these factors cause difficulty with venipuncture, capillary puncture may be an acceptable alternative. If the hand veins are selected for venipuncture, a butterfly needle and a syringe are used to obtain the blood.

HOW THE TEST IS DONE

Either a vacuum tube system or a needle, syringe, and test tube containers are used to collect the blood sample. The selection of the color-coded specimen tube is based on the requirements of the specific test. Each laboratory blood test discussed in this text lists the correct test tube to be used for that test.

INTERFERING FACTORS

- Dehydration
- Hypotension
- Obesity
- Fragility of veins
- Prematurity and infancy

NURSING CARE

Pretest

- Identify the patient, and check the requisition form with the patient's identification bracelet.
- Inform the patient that blood needs to be drawn from the designated site. Provide reassurance to help limit anxiety.
- If pretest fasting or dietary restriction is required, verify that the instructions were followed for the correct period.
- Assemble the equipment and put on a pair of gloves.
- The patient may be seated or in the supine position. The patient's arm is in extension, with easy access to the antecubital fossa.

During the Test

- Inspect the antecubital fossae of both arms to select the best vein for the venipuncture. Ask the patient to open and close the hand a few times to help make the veins more visible.
- Gently palpate the vein to determine its location, direction, width, and depth.
- Cleanse the skin with 70% alcohol and allow it to air-dry.
- Apply the tourniquet about 2 to 3 inches above the antecubital fossa.
- Using your fingertips, anchor the vein above and below the puncture site.
- With the bevel up, insert the needle at a 15-degree angle along the pathway of the vein (Figure 8).

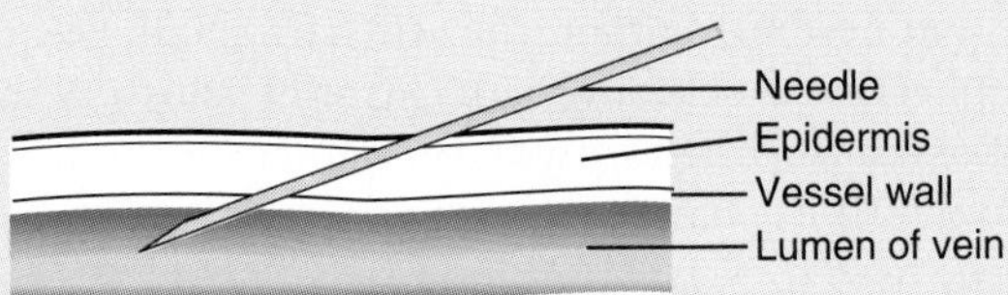

Figure 8. Needle placement during venipuncture. To obtain good blood flow, the needle is positioned correctly in the vein lumen. The needle should not rest against the upper wall of the vein or puncture through the vein wall on the opposite side.

Continued

NURSING CARE—*cont'd*

Syringe method. Once the needle is in the vein, gently aspirate blood into the syringe. Collect the volume of blood that is needed.

Vacuum tube system method. Once the needle is in the vein, hold it firmly in place. Push the blood collection tube fully into the holder so that the blood flows through the needle and into the vacuum tube (Figure 9). When multiple specimens are needed, remove each full tube and insert the next tube firmly into the holder. After all blood has been collected, release the tourniquet. Place sterile gauze over the puncture site. Remove the needle. Use the gauze and your finger to compress the puncture site.

When blood is drawn by syringe or the vacuum tube system method, the tourniquet should not remain tied for more than 1 minute. The prolonged compression of the vein and stasis of the blood flow results in clumping or hemolysis of the erythrocytes. Hemolysis and clumping interfere with the laboratory analysis and alter some test results.

Posttest

- Instruct the patient to continue compression of the puncture site for 2 to 5 minutes or until the bleeding stops.
- If a syringe and needle were used, transfer the blood to the appropriate test tube containers.

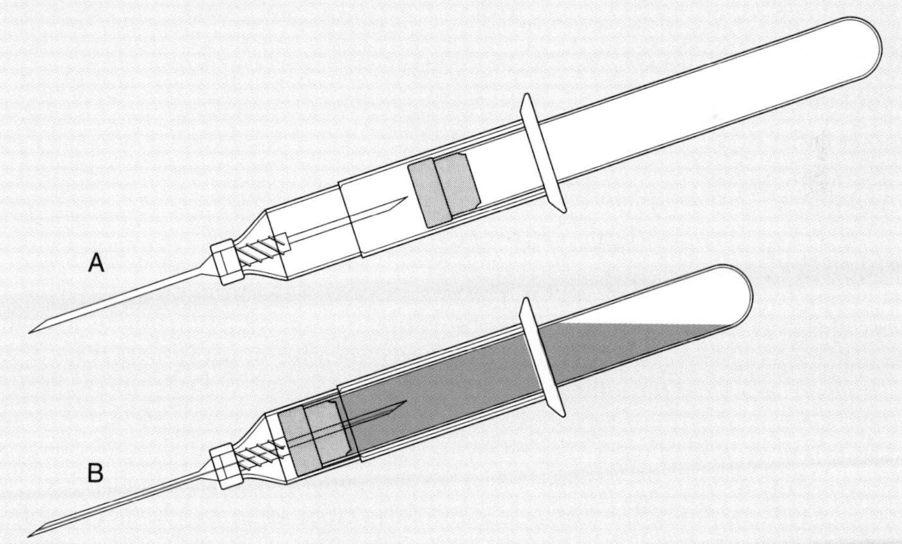

Figure 9. Function of the vacuum tube collection system. *A,* Before venipuncture, the vacuum tube is placed into the holder, resting on the tip of the sterile needle. *B,* Once the needle enters the vein, the tube is pushed to the front of the holder, and the needle penetrates the stopper of the tube. Because of the negative pressure in the tube, the blood is pulled from the vein, through the needle, and into the vacuum tube.

Continued

NURSING CARE—*cont'd*

- Label every vial of blood with the patient's name and identification number, the time, and the date.
- Perform any special measures needed to protect the specimen from deterioration. These measures are test specific and are described throughout this text.
- Assess the patient's arm to ensure that the bleeding has ceased. Apply an adhesive bandage as needed.
- Remove gloves and wash your hands.
- Arrange for prompt transport of the specimen to the laboratory.

◇ Nursing Response to Complications

Hematoma. Hematoma formation occurs when the vein continues to leak blood under the skin.

The nurse assesses for a bruised area in the site of the venipuncture. The problem can be prevented by continued compression of the puncture site until clotting occurs. The patient can also elevate the arm and rest it on top of the head. This reduces the blood volume and pressure on the walls of the vein, promoting clotting.

STOOL COLLECTION PROCEDURE

Stool Collection

stool kuh-lek-shun

Also called: Stool Specimen

SPECIMEN OR TYPE OF TEST: Feces

PURPOSE OF THE TEST

Analysis of feces is used to screen for intestinal disease in an asymptomatic individual and to help identify abnormal intestinal function or abnormal function of the gallbladder, liver, or pancreas. It is also used to detect microbes or parasites that reside in the intestinal tract and cause infection.

BASICS THE NURSE NEEDS TO KNOW

The laboratory testing of fecal matter may involve chemical analysis that identifies the abnormal composition of the feces or may involve microbiologic analysis that identifies infectious organisms. Once the abnormality has been identified, additional diagnostic tests or procedures are often needed to determine the cause and location of the problem.

One group of abnormal fecal test results is caused by diseases that damage the intestinal mucosa, alter the integrity of the intestinal tissue, or interfere with the functions of digestion, absorption, and elimination. The fecal changes may include the presence of blood or an alteration in the composition of the feces. Examples of these diseases include malignancy of the stomach or colon, peptic ulcer, regional ileitis, celiac disease, or scleroderma.

A second group of abnormal fecal test results is caused by abnormality in the organs and ducts that secrete into the intestinal tract. These organs include the liver, pancreas, and gallbladder. The fecal changes can include excess fat in the stool or a lack of fecal urobilinogen. Examples of these conditions include cystic fibrosis, pancreatic cancer, hepatitis, and bile duct obstruction.

A third category of abnormal fecal test results is caused by infectious organisms that infect the intestinal tract. The organisms are discovered by microscopic examination of the stool or stool culture. The infection may be of bacterial, viral, parasitic, or other origin, often infecting the small or large intestine. Sometimes the infection causes damage to the intestinal mucosa or underlying tissue, resulting in blood in the stool.

HOW THE TEST IS DONE

A half-pint waterproof container that is clean and dry and has a wide mouth with a tight-fitting lid is used to collect approximately 1 to 2 oz of fecal matter.

INTERFERING FACTORS

- Improper specimen collection
- Contamination of the specimen with water or urine
- Delay in transport of the specimen
- Failure to follow pretest dietary instructions
- Pretest ingestion of antibiotics, cathartics, or barium, or administration of an enema

NURSING CARE

Pretest

- Ask the patient if he or she has had a recent barium x-ray study or recent treatment with oral antibiotics. After ingestion, barium sulfate interferes with the analysis of feces for approximately 2 weeks. Stool culture is less likely to demonstrate the causative organism when antibiotics have been taken during the preceding 3 to 4 weeks. Schedule the stool collection accordingly.
- ***Patient Teaching.*** The nurse instructs the patient about any dietary restrictions that are part of specific test preparations. For some of the tests, such as those looking for fecal fat and fecal occult blood, pretest dietary modifications are required or recommended. The patient is also instructed not to ingest castor oil, mineral oil, antacids, or antidiarrheal medications or to administer an enema before the test. These substances would appear in the fecal matter and interfere with the chemical or microscopic analysis.

During the Test

- ***Patient Teaching.*** The nurse instructs the patient to evacuate directly into the container or a clean, dry bedpan. Tongue blades can be used to transfer a small amount of feces from the bedpan into the collection container. Urine, water, or toilet paper must not be mixed in with the fecal specimen.
- Once the specimen is obtained, place the lid on the container and hands are washed.

Continued

NURSING CARE—*cont'd*

Posttest

- The nurse labels the container with the patient's name and other appropriate data. Mark the time and date of the collection on the container and requisition slip.
- Arrange for transport of the specimen within 30 minutes. If there is a delay before transport, store the specimen in the refrigerator. The cool temperature preserves any microorganisms that may be present.

URINE COLLECTION PROCEDURES

BASICS THE NURSE NEEDS TO KNOW

Urine provides a major source of data about the status and function of the urinary tract. In addition, because urine is an ultrafiltrate of the plasma, it is used to assess various homeostatic and metabolic processes of the body. Urine is easily collected, but the procedure must be performed completely and accurately. If there is an error in procedure, false or invalid test results can occur.

The four basic urine collection procedures, which are based on the time or duration of the collection period, are as follows: the first morning specimen, the random specimen, the fractional specimen, and the timed specimen. Because the purposes and methods vary, each of these procedures is discussed separately in subsequent sections of this chapter.

In addition to spontaneous voiding, several other possible methods of collection are available. A description of the special collection methods is presented here. When urine cannot be collected by normal voiding, these special methods are used for any of the basic collection procedures.

Special Collection Methods

Catheterization

A catheterized specimen is used when the patient cannot void or when an indwelling catheter is already in place. For straight catheterization, a sterile catheter is inserted through the urethra and into the bladder. The urine flows from the bladder, through the catheter, and into the specimen container. Once the bladder has been emptied, the catheter is removed.

For a patient with an indwelling catheter, fresh urine is collected directly from the catheter in all types of tests except the timed specimen. For the single urine specimen collection, the catheter is clamped below the port temporarily. After a short interval, a sterile needle and syringe are used to remove the urine sample through a special port in the catheter. After the sample is taken, the clamp is removed, and the urine flow to the collection bag resumes. A timed specimen has a much longer collection period and requires a larger volume of urine. At the start of the test, a new, empty collection bag is attached to the indwelling catheter and its tubing. The urine is removed from the collection bag at intervals and is added to the specimen collection container until the time period is completed.

Pediatric Specimens

If the child is toilet trained and can follow directions, the nurse can provide instructions to the parent or assist the child in the collection of the urine. For the infant or child who cannot control the release of urine voluntarily, a pediatric collection bag is used. The perineum is cleansed and dried, and then the bag is applied and fixed with an adhesive strip. For the male infant, the bag is placed over the penis. For the female infant, the bag is applied over the labia and perineum. In each gender, the rectum must be excluded to prevent the mixing of fecal matter with urine. Once the bag is in place, it is checked every 15 minutes until the urine is collected.

Suprapubic Aspiration

This method is used when an anaerobic culture is required or when there is a problem with external contamination of the urine culture, such as in infancy. With the use of sterile technique, the suprapubic aspiration is performed by the physician. A sterile needle is inserted through the abdominal wall above the symphysis pubis and then is advanced into the full bladder. A syringe is used to aspirate the urine specimen. The specimen is placed into a culture container, and the needle is removed.

First Morning Specimen

furst mohr-ning spes-i-men

SPECIMEN OR TYPE OF TEST: Urine

PURPOSE OF THE TEST

The first morning specimen is used for routine urinalysis that includes chemical and microscopic analysis. This specimen is also used to identify orthostatic proteinuria.

BASICS THE NURSE NEEDS TO KNOW

The first morning specimen is the first urine to be voided after the patient awakens from sleep. This urine has been retained in the bladder for about 6 to 8 hours. Because of the lack of fluid intake or exercise during the period of sleep, the urine is concentrated and somewhat acidic.

This type of specimen is preferred for routine screening. It is also preferred for the detection of specific substances, including nitrites, protein, and microorganisms. Concentrated urine or an incubation period is needed to readily detect these substances in the urine.

HOW THE TEST IS DONE

A clean, dry plastic or glass container with a lid is used to collect a midstream urine specimen.

INTERFERING FACTORS

- Menstrual secretions
- Delay in the analysis of the urine
- Inadequate labeling of the specimen

NURSING CARE

Pretest

- The nurse provides the patient with a urine container with a lid.
- ***Patient Teaching.*** Instruct the patient to collect a midstream voided specimen. A midstream void means that the patient begins to urinate, and about halfway through the process the specimen is collected. With this method, the initial urine flow washes the bacteria out of the distal urethra before the specimen is collected.
- ***Patient Teaching.*** In some protocols, a midstream clean-catch method is used. If this is the case, provide the patient with the materials and instructions, as presented in Box 2.

Posttest

- The nurse seals the lid of the container completely to prevent leakage.
- The container must be labeled appropriately with the patient's name and other pertinent information, including the date and time of the collection. The information should not be placed on the lid.
- The nurse ensures that the specimen is delivered to the laboratory immediately. If a delay is anticipated, the specimen must be refrigerated or a preservative added to the urine container. If there is a delay of 2 hours or longer before analysis is performed, a warm, unpreserved specimen will undergo a number of changes. The changes vary among the individual specimens, but almost every laboratory value can be altered.

BOX 2 Midstream Clean-Catch Urine Procedure

Purpose

This method of urine collection reduces the external sources of contamination before the urine is collected. The contaminants are the bacteria and secretions of the skin that surround the urethra and reside in the distal portion of the urethra.

Procedure

Cleansing process: Male

The glans is exposed and cleansed with the use of three sterile cotton balls or gauze squares moistened with a mild antiseptic solution.

The first cotton ball cleanses the tissue from the urethral meatus to the ring of the glans in a single stroke. The cotton ball is then discarded. The process is repeated with the other two cotton balls, cleansing the remaining areas of the glans.

If the male is uncircumcised, the foreskin must be retracted and the tissue under the foreskin cleansed thoroughly before the preceding steps are taken.

BOX 2 Midstream Clean-Catch Urine Procedure—*cont'd*

Cleansing process: Female

The labia minora are separated to expose the urinary meatus. They must then remain separated throughout the cleansing process and urine collection phase.

The exterior mucous membranes and the meatus are cleansed, with the use of three sterile cotton balls or gauze squares moistened with a mild antiseptic.

The first moist cotton ball cleanses the tissue on one side of the urinary meatus with a single stroke from front to back. The cotton ball is discarded. The second cotton ball cleanses the other side of the meatus with the same motion and direction. The third cotton ball cleanses the center of the meatus, wiping in a single motion, also from front to back.

Midstream collection

The patient begins to void into the toilet or bedpan. The urine washes residual bacteria and secretions from the distal urethra.

At about the midpoint of voiding, the urine stream is interrupted. On release of the urine, 1 to 3 oz of urine is collected in the specimen container.

The container must not touch the perineal tissues or hair either during or after collection. The patient's fingers must not touch the inside of the container or lid.

Once the amount of urine in the container is sufficient, the patient finishes voiding into the toilet or bedpan, and the remaining amount is discarded.

Random Specimen

ran-duhm spes-i-men

SPECIMEN OR TYPE OF TEST: Urine

PURPOSE OF THE TEST

The random specimen is used for routine urinalysis that includes chemical and microscopic examination. This method of collection is also used for bacterial culture and cytologic studies to help identify the cause of disease in the urinary tract.

BASICS THE NURSE NEEDS TO KNOW

The random urine specimen can be collected at any time. It is easy and convenient for the patient because there is no need to plan or schedule the test. Even though the daytime activities of fluid intake and exercise alter the composition of the urine, there is no need to control these variables. The specimen is usually satisfactory for the purposes of screening or routine urinalysis.

Cytologic studies are also performed on random urine samples. For this test, the patient must drink extra fluids before each of several urine sample collections. The goal is to flush out an increased number of cells so that the detection of abnormal cells is enhanced. Random samples are also used for urine cultures, with the goal of identifying microbial growth and the presence of infection.

HOW THE TEST IS DONE

For routine urinalysis or a random urine screen, a clean plastic or glass container with a lid is used to collect a urine sample at any time. A midstream clean-catch method is used (see Box 2).

For bacterial, fungal, or viral culture, a sterile plastic or glass container with a lid is used to collect the random urine sample. The midstream clean-catch method is used. In special cases, a catheter or suprapubic aspiration is used to obtain the random specimen.

For cytologic studies, the midstream clean-catch method is used to collect each specimen in a clean plastic or glass container with a lid. Daily specimens are collected for 3 to 5 consecutive days.

INTERFERING FACTORS

- Menstrual secretions
- Delay in the analysis of the urine
- Inadequate labeling of the specimen
- Contamination of the specimen

NURSING CARE

Pretest

- ***Patient Teaching.*** The nurse provides written and verbal instructions regarding how to cleanse the urethral meatus and surrounding tissue and how to collect the specimen. The patient is given the appropriate collection container or containers.
- ***Patient Teaching.*** For cytologic studies, the nurse instructs the patient to drink 24 to 32 oz of water each hour for 2 hours before voiding. In some laboratory protocols, the patient is also instructed to exercise for 5 minutes by skipping or jumping rope before voiding. The activity and fluid volume should increase the yield of cells needed for the study. This process is repeated daily for 3 to 5 days to provide for the analysis of three to five consecutive urine specimens.

Posttest

- The lid of the container must be closed completely to prevent leakage.
- The nurse labels the container appropriately with the patient's name and other pertinent information, including the date and time of the collection. The information is not placed on the lid.
- The nurse ensures that the specimen is delivered to the laboratory immediately. If there is an anticipated delay, the specimen must be refrigerated or a preservative added to the urine container. If a delay of 2 hours or longer occurs before analysis is performed, the warm, unpreserved specimen can undergo a number of changes. The changes vary among the individual specimens, but almost every laboratory value can be altered.

Fractional Specimen

frak-shun-uhl spes-i-men

Also called: Double-Voided Specimen

SPECIMEN OR TYPE OF TEST: Urine

PURPOSE OF THE TEST

Fractional collection is used to compare blood and urine values in screening for diabetes mellitus and in the diagnosis of some liver and kidney disorders.

BASICS THE NURSE NEEDS TO KNOW

A fractional collection of urine is a method used to compare a particular component of the urine with the serum level of that component. Blood samples and urine samples are collected at specific times, and the laboratory analysis measures the amount of the component found in each specimen.

The serum sample is measured for the blood level during controlled conditions, such as in a fasting state or after administration of a dye or solute. The urine samples are measured for the baseline and renal threshold values. One example of fractional collection is the Glucose Tolerance Test (p. 356).

HOW THE TEST IS DONE

Generally, baseline blood and urine specimens are obtained first. The patient then receives a measured intravenous or oral substance such as food, dye, or glucose. Thereafter, timed blood and urine specimens are collected.

INTERFERING FACTORS

- Failure to complete the pretest preparation
- Failure to collect all urine specimens
- Failure to obtain all urine specimens at the correct times
- Failure to label all specimens accurately

NURSING CARE

Pretest

- ***Patient Teaching.*** The nurse provides the patient with written and verbal instructions. Some of these tests require nothing-by-mouth (NPO) status for 6 to 8 hours before the test. Some have instructions to void and discard the first morning specimen. The instructions are specific to the test.

During the Test

- The nurse administers the prescribed oral glucose solution, injectable dye, or other measured substance used in the test.
- Each urine specimen is collected in a separate container at the specific time interval required by the protocol.

Continued

NURSING CARE—*cont'd*

During the Test—*cont'd*

- The nurse labels each container with the patient's name and other appropriate identifying information. The time of each voided specimen is also recorded on the container (e.g., ½-hour specimen, 1-hour specimen). The information is not written on the lid.

Posttest

- The nurse sends all specimens to the laboratory together without delay. If a delay of more than 2 hours occurs, the specimens must be preserved by refrigeration. Many components of urine are altered when the specimen remains warm and a delay occurs in performing the analysis. In particular, the level of urinary glucose becomes falsely decreased because of cellular and bacterial glycolysis.

Timed Specimen

taimd spes-i-men

SPECIMEN OR TYPE OF TEST: Urine

PURPOSE OF THE TEST

The timed collection is used to perform quantitative urine assays and clearance tests and to identify abnormal cytology, or ova and parasites in the urine.

BASICS THE NURSE NEEDS TO KNOW

Timed collection is used for the quantitative analysis of a specific urinary component. Circadian rhythms, diurnal rhythms, metabolism, exercise, and hydration all affect the excretion rate of substances in the urine. At certain times during a 24-hour period, the excretion of substances such as electrolytes, hormones, proteins, and urobilinogen increases, and at other times excretion decreases. By collecting the quantity of urine over a specified period, accuracy of measurement is greater than that with a random specimen.

Sometimes, an abnormal substance is not present consistently in the urine. Thus, the urine is collected for a longer period to try to identify the small amounts of the component that are occasionally present. Urine cytologic testing requires a 2-hour collection period repeated over several days. The parasites *Schistosoma* and *Onchocerca* are detected in urine that is collected over a 24-hour period.

Time Intervals

The designated time period for a urine collection depends on the specific component to be tested. Some tests are for a *predetermined length of time*, such as a 2-hour, 12-hour, or 24-hour urine collection. Other tests are for a *specific time of day*, such as 12 PM to 4 PM. In these instances, the time frame reflects when the substance is maximally excreted in the urine each day.

HOW THE TEST IS DONE

A large (3000-mL) clear or brown glass or plastic container with a lid is used to collect all urine within the designated period.

INTERFERING FACTORS

- Failure to discard the first voided specimen before the procedure begins
- Failure to collect all the urine voided during the test period
- Failure to refrigerate or preserve the urine specimen
- Improper labeling

NURSING CARE

Pretest

- *Patient Teaching.* The nurse provides both written and verbal instructions regarding the collection of the urine. These instructions must include the specific times for the collection period. For a 24-hour urine collection, the nurse instructs the patient to moderately limit fluid intake during the collection period. Alcohol intake should be avoided for 24 hours before and during any timed collection of urine. Other restrictions are part of specific test protocols. Some tests have specific dietary restrictions, and some medications need to be withheld for a specific period. Any special restrictions or modifications are included in the patient's pretest instructions.
- *Patient Teaching.* When the patient works or is in school, the nurse advises that the easiest time to collect the specimen is on the weekend.

During the Test

- For all timed collections, the nurse or the patient maintains the specimen and container on ice or in the refrigerator during the collection period. Such measures prevent deterioration of the specimen.
- During the time period, all urine is added to the collection container. If any urine spills or if a specimen is discarded accidentally, the test is invalid. The stored specimen is discarded, and a new collection period is started the next day.
- For the 24-hour urine collection, the first void of the morning is discarded, and the urine collection period begins at 8 AM. Place all urine for 24 hours into the container. This includes the first voided specimen of the next morning.

Posttest

- The nurse labels the container with the patient's name and other appropriate identifying data. Include the time and date of the start and the completion of the urine collection period. No information is placed on the lid of the container. The nurse also arranges for prompt delivery of the specimen to the laboratory.

PART II

Laboratory Tests and Diagnostic Procedures

A

Acid Phosphatase

See Prostatic Acid Phosphatase on p. 543.

ACTH Stimulation Test

See Adrenocorticotropic Hormone Stimulation Test on p. 49.

Activated Clotting Time

ak-tiv-ay-ted klot-ing taim

Also called: (ACT); Activated Coagulation Time

SPECIMEN OR TYPE OF TEST: Whole blood

PURPOSE OF THE TEST

The activated clotting time is used to measure the anticoagulation effect during therapy with high-dose heparin.

BASICS THE NURSE NEEDS TO KNOW

When the patient receives very high doses of heparin medication, frequent monitoring of the anticoagulation effect is required. This high-dose heparin therapy is often used during cardiopulmonary bypass surgery, cardiac angioplasty, hemodialysis, and vascular therapy. If the anticoagulant effect of the heparin is insufficient, the clotting time will be lower than the therapeutic value, and the patient may form a blood clot. If the anticoagulant effect of the heparin therapy is beyond the therapeutic range, the patient may develop a hemorrhage. This blood test measures the time it takes for the blood to form a clot.

When high doses of heparin are given, the therapeutic values are elevated because it takes a longer time for the blood to coagulate. This is a desirable goal because the patient is protected from formation of a thrombus or embolus during the surgery or procedure. The therapeutic values vary with the type of procedure and coagulation risk that is involved. Generally, the therapeutic goal of anticoagulation during cardiopulmonary bypass surgery is longer than 400 to 500 seconds and during cardiac angioplasty, the therapeutic value is longer than 350 seconds. Prolonged clotting times are indicated for vascular surgery, with a therapeutic goal of 275 to 350 seconds.

The specimen for the activated clotting time is analyzed in point-of-care testing. This means that the analyzer instrument is at the patient's bedside or near the patient care unit so that test results can be obtained without delay. Several types of analyzer instruments are available. The test method and the test values vary with the analyzer instrument used. The nurse should refer to the instructions and normal values determined by the institution's laboratory and the manufacturer.

NORMAL VALUES 70–180 sgeconds

HOW THE TEST IS DONE

A small amount of blood is collected in a special tube that contains a coagulation activator substance.

SIGNIFICANCE OF TEST RESULTS

Elevated Values

Anticoagulation with heparin
Severe deficiency of coagulation factors of the intrinsic pathway (except Factors VII and VIII)

INTERFERING FACTORS

- Contamination with heparin in the intravenous line

NURSING CARE

Nursing actions are similar to those used in other venipuncture procedures (see Chapter 2), with the following additional measures.

Pretest

- The nurse uses a flow sheet that provides for documentation of the time, amount, and route of heparin administration, as well as the time and result of ACT testing.

During the Test

- If the nurse collects the specimen of blood, the intravenous line that contains heparin or heparin infusion should not be used. Select a vein in the opposite arm because the heparin in the intravenous line or catheter would falsely elevate the test result. Some specimen tubes require vigorous shaking to mix the blood with the activator in the tube. Other tubes require gentle mixing. The nurse should refer to the specific manufacturer's instructions for reference information. Once obtained, the specimen should be placed in the analyzer, without delay.

Posttest

- Using sterile gauze, the nurse applies pressure on the venipuncture site until bleeding ceases. There is a tendency to bleed for a longer time than usual because the patient is very anticoagulated.
- The nurse frequently assesses for signs of abnormal bleeding, as into the urine or from the gingivae and mucosa in the mouth. The skin is assessed for bruising, bleeding, and petechiae.
- Each ACT test result is posted in the patient's record and on the flow sheet.

▼ Nursing Response to Critical Values

When the activated clotting time result is elevated, the patient may begin to bleed or hemorrhage. The nurse performs frequent assessment for signs of bleeding and monitors the values of ACT test results.

The nurse keeps protamine sulfate on hand for use in case of hemorrhage. The action of protamine sulfate is to neutralize heparin, usually within 5 minutes after it is administered. If prescribed, this medication would be given slowly, intravenously, over a period of 1 to 3 minutes. It may be administered in an undiluted form or

Continued

NURSING CARE—*cont'd*

diluted with 5% dextrose in normal saline. When protamine sulfate is administered, the nurse monitors the vital signs because if it is administered too rapidly, this medication can result in severe hypotension, bradycardia, and dyspnea. Thereafter, ACT values are monitored because of a potential heparin rebound effect that can occur several hours later. Protamine sulfate would lower the ACT value; a heparin rebound effect would again raise the ACT value.

Adrenocorticotropic Hormone, Plasma

a-dree-noh-kohr-ti-koh-tro-pik hohr-mohn, plaz-muh

Also called: (ACTH); Corticotropin

SPECIMEN OR TYPE OF TEST: Plasma

PURPOSE OF THE TEST

A plasma ACTH determination is obtained to diagnose Cushing's disease and differentiate primary and secondary adrenal insufficiency.

BASICS THE NURSE NEEDS TO KNOW

Adrenocorticotropic hormone (ACTH) is produced and secreted by the anterior pituitary gland. Its secretion is under the control of the hypothalamus and the central nervous system by neurotransmitters and corticotropin-releasing hormone (CRH). ACTH, in turn, regulates the secretion of the glucocorticoids and androgens from the adrenal cortex.

The mechanisms of regulation of CRH, ACTH, and the adrenal hormones are multiple, and patterns of secretion of these hormones vary within the individual and among individuals. CRH and ACTH are excreted episodically and by circadian rhythm. Increases in ACTH levels cause increased levels of glucocorticoids and androgens in the blood within minutes. Generally, CRH, ACTH, and cortisol (the major glucocorticoid) levels are low in the evening and continue to decline for the first few hours of sleep. After 3 to 5 hours of sleep, the levels of the hormones increase and then peak after 6 to 8 hours of sleep. On waking, the hormone levels begin to decline. Superimposed on this circadian rhythm are episodic secretions. The hormone levels increase with exercise, eating, and stress.

A feedback mechanism also regulates the hypothalamic-pituitary-adrenal hormonal responses. As the cortisol level increases in the plasma, it inhibits both ACTH secretion by the pituitary gland and CRH secretion by the hypothalamus (Figure 10). The nurse needs to be aware of the feedback inhibition of CRH and ACTH, which occurs with exogenous administration of glucocorticoids.

An increase or decrease in the production of ACTH will cause an increase or decrease in the glucocorticoid levels. A deficiency of ACTH will cause secondary adrenal insuffi-

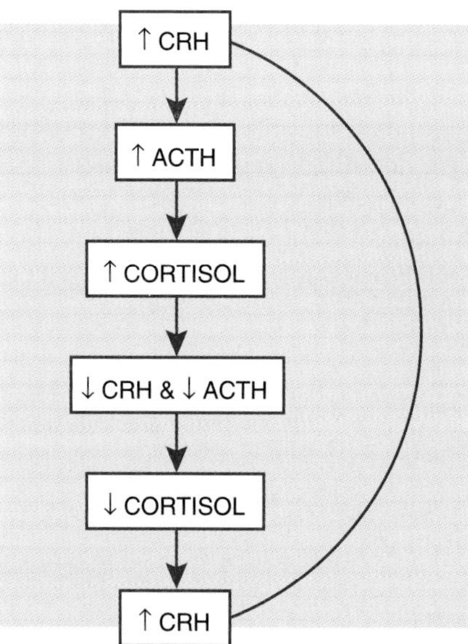

Figure 10. Hypothalamic-pituitary-adrenal axis. Hypothalamic control of adrenal hormone secretion occurs through release of corticotropin-releasing hormone (CRH), which stimulates the secretion of adrenocorticotropic hormone (ACTH) by the pituitary gland. ACTH stimulates the adrenals to increase their secretion of cortisol. By a negative feedback mechanism, the increase in serum cortisol level suppresses the release of CRH and ACTH.

ciency. An increase in ACTH will cause Cushing's disease (Cushing syndrome is a primary adrenal disorder).

NORMAL VALUES

Adult
In morning (6 AM–10 AM): 25–100 pg/mL *or* SI: 25–100 pmol/L
In evening (9 PM–12 AM): 0–50 pg/mL *or* SI: 0–50 pmol/L

HOW THE TEST IS DONE

A venipuncture is done with chilled syringe and blood placed in 2 lavender-topped tubes. Test tubes are placed on ice and sent immediately to the lab.

SIGNIFICANCE OF TEST RESULTS

Elevated Values
Primary adrenal insufficiency
Cushing's disease
Congenital adrenal hyperplasia
Ectopic ACTH syndrome

Decreased Values

Primary adrenal hypersecretion
Cushing syndrome
Tumors of the adrenal gland may suppress the ACTH level if they produce glucocorticoids; however, not all adrenal tumors do.

INTERFERING FACTORS

- Noncompliance with medication, diet, or activity restrictions
- Administration of radioactive scans within 7 days
- Pregnancy
- Traumatic venipuncture
- Ingestion of alcohol, amphetamines, calcium gluconate, corticosteroids, estrogen, lithium, or spironolactone

NURSING CARE

Nursing actions are similar to those used in other venipuncture procedures (see Chapter 2), with the following additional measures.

Pretest

- ***Patient Teaching.*** The nurse explains to the patient the need to obtain two specimens of blood, one in the early morning and one in the evening. The early morning specimen reflects the peak secretion time and the evening specimen, the low secretion time for ACTH. Instruct the patient to ingest nothing by mouth for 12 hours before the test. Some physicians recommend a low-carbohydrate diet for 2 days before the test.
- Check with physician if cortisol levels are to be obtained at the same time.
- The nurse obtains a medication history and asks the physician if any interfering drugs should be withheld. The nurse also inquires and notes on the requisition slip if the patient is pregnant, because this may affect test results.

During the Test

- Have a glass heparinized syringe, and ice available.
- After blood is obtained by venipuncture, place the specimen on ice and immediately send it to the laboratory.
- The nurse notifies laboratory personnel that the specimen is being transported, because it should be frozen until a radioimmunoassay analysis (RIA) can be performed.

Posttest

- The patient resumes a normal diet, activity, and medication regimen. The nurse notifies the dietary department to bring the patient his or her meal.

Adrenocorticotropic Hormone Stimulation Test

a-dree-noh-kohr-ti-koh-tro-pik hohr-mohn sti-myoo-lay-shun test

Also called: ACTH Stimulation Test; Rapid or Short ACTH Test; Corticotropin Stimulation Test; Cosyntropin Test; Cortrosyn Stimulating Test

SPECIMEN OR TYPE OF TEST: Plasma, serum

PURPOSE OF THE TEST

The ACTH stimulation test is performed to diagnose primary and secondary adrenal insufficiency.

BASICS THE NURSE NEEDS TO KNOW

ACTH is secreted by the pituitary gland. Its target organ is the adrenal cortex, where it stimulates the secretion of the glucocorticoids, aldosterone, and androgens. Synthetic ACTH, known as cosyntropin (Cortrosyn), normally has the same effect. It causes an increase in adrenal cortex hormones. A normal response excludes the diagnosis of primary adrenocorticoid insufficiency, because the gland was able to respond. A normal response will also rule out complete ACTH deficiency (secondary adrenocorticoid failure), because complete lack of ACTH causes adrenal atrophy, and the gland is unable to respond.

In an abnormal response, primary or secondary adrenal insufficiency may be present. To distinguish between the two forms, aldosterone levels may be measured. If no change occurs in the aldosterone levels after cosyntropin is given, primary adrenal insufficiency is present. With secondary adrenal insufficiency, aldosterone levels will increase by more than 4 mcg/dL.

NORMAL VALUES Within 30–60 minutes, plasma cortisol increases to 18–20 mcg/dL *or* SI: 500–550 npmol/L.

HOW THE TEST IS DONE

After the baseline plasma cortisol level is obtained in a red top tube, then cosyntropin is given intravenously. Cosyntropin may be given intramuscularly if the patient is not hypotensive. After 30 to 60 minutes, another plasma cortisol level is obtained. Occasionally, instead of cosyntropin, insulin may be used.

SIGNIFICANCE OF TEST RESULTS

Elevated Values

Normal response

Unchanged Values

Addison's disease
Adrenal atrophy
Hypopituitarism

INTERFERING FACTORS

- See section on Cortisol, Total p. 238.

NURSING CARE

See section on Cortisol, Total p. 238.

Pretest

- The nurse explains to the patient the need for more than one venipuncture procedure.
- If insulin is being used as the stimulant, the nurse instructs the patient to fast overnight.

During the Test

- If insulin is used as the stimulant, nurse observes the patient for clinical manifestations of hypoglycemia.

Posttest

- The nurse ensures that the patient eats, especially if insulin was used as the stimulant.

Alanine Aminotransferase

al-uh-neen am-in-oh-trans-fuhr-ays

Also called: (ALT); Glutamic-Pyruvic Transaminase

SPECIMEN OR TYPE OF TEST: Serum

PURPOSE OF THE TEST

The ALT test is used to detect hepatocellular injury (damage to liver cells). It is the most specific of the transaminase enzyme tests to detect acute hepatitis from a viral, toxic, or drug-induced cause.

BASICS THE NURSE NEEDS TO KNOW

Alanine aminotransferase (ALT) is a transaminase enzyme that is found in the cells of the liver and to lesser extents in the cells of the kidneys, heart, skeletal muscle and red blood cells. When injury or necrosis (cell death) occurs in hepatocytes (liver cells), the ALT enzymes leave the cytoplasm, pass through damaged cell membranes and enter the serum. In acute hepatitis, the serum level rises dramatically, to a level of 20 times the normal value. In cases of obstructive jaundice, cirrhosis, and liver tumor, the ALT level rises mildly or moderately, from two to four times the normal value.

The ALT value also rises slightly as a result of myocardial infarction, congestive heart failure, and shock. Skeletal muscle injury, as from trauma or surgery also causes a mild to moderate rise in the ALT level.

NORMAL VALUES

Average adult range: 4–36 international units/L at 37° C
Male >60 years: 13–40 international units/L at 37° C
Female >60 years: 10–28 international units/L at 37° C
Male infant–adult <60 years: 15–35 international units/L at 37° C
Female infant–adult <60 years: 15–35 international units/L at 37° C
Male newborn–1 year: 13–45 international units/L at 37° C
Female newborn–1 year: 15–45 international units/L at 37° C

HOW THE TEST IS DONE

A venipuncture is performed to collect 10 mL of venous blood in a red-topped tube.

SIGNIFICANCE OF TEST RESULTS

Elevated Values

Acute or chronic hepatitis
Liver cell necrosis
Acute pancreatitis
Cirrhosis
Infectious mononucleosis
Biliary obstruction
Obstructive jaundice
Liver tumor
Fatty liver
Chronic alcohol abuse
Myocardial infarction
Shock
Muscle trauma
Recent surgery
Pregnancy induced hypertension
Hemolytic anemia

INTERFERING FACTORS

- Hemolysis

NURSING CARE

Nursing actions are similar to those used in other venipuncture procedures (see Chapter 2), with the following additional measures.

Pretest

- Many medications cause an elevated test result. If they cannot be discontinued for 12 hours, list the medications on the requisition slip.

A

Albumin, Serum

See Protein, Total, Serum on p. 549.

Albumin, Urinary

al-byoo-min, yur-i-ner-ee

Also called: Protein Screen; Urine Screen for Albumin

SPECIMEN OR TYPE OF TEST: Urine

PURPOSE OF THE TEST

Urinary excretion of albumin is evaluated to assess renal function, determine effectiveness of therapy, and differentiate renal disorders. It is being increasingly used to screen for the complications associated with diabetes mellitus.

BASICS THE NURSE NEEDS TO KNOW

Evaluation of protein in the urine is done as part of a urinalysis. Normally in the healthy adult, the excretion of protein is so small that it is undetectable by routine methods of analysis. Because albumin can be tested by the use of reagent strips, urinary albumin testing is frequently used in the management of urinary disorders. Studies have shown that albumin in urine can be used as a predictor of complications associated with diabetes mellitus.

NORMAL VALUES

Microalbumin: <2 mg/dL
Reagent strip: Negative

HOW THE TEST IS DONE

Various methods are available for assessing urinary excretion of albumin, including radioimmunoassay (RIA), turbidimetric, and chemical methods and reagent strips. Reagent strips are sensitive to albumin, but not at very low levels. To evaluate microalbuminuria, laboratory analysis is necessary. If the specimen is being sent to the lab, it is kept refrigerated until it is sent. The specimen should be sent to the lab within 2 hours of its collection.

For a reagent strip analysis of albumin, a random urine specimen is collected in a clean container. A first voided urine specimen is preferred.

For microalbuminuria, the procedure varies with the method of analysis. With the turbidimetric method, a 24-hour specimen of urine is used with no preservative in the collection container.

SIGNIFICANCE OF TEST RESULTS

Elevated Values

Amyloidosis
Cystic kidney

Cystitis
Diabetes mellitus (complications of)
Glomerulonephritis
Heavy metal poisonings
Multiple myeloma
Nephritis
Nephropathies
Pyelonephritis
Renal transplant rejection
Urinary tract malignancies

INTERFERING FACTORS

- *With reagent strips*: Highly concentrated urine; highly alkaline urine; specimen contaminated with bacteria, blood, ammonia compounds, or chlorhexidine
- *With turbidimetric method*: Ingestion of cephalosporin, penicillin, sulfonamides, or tolbutamide; recent administration of radiocontrast dyes

NURSING CARE

Nursing actions are similar to those used in other urine collection procedures (see Chapter 2), with the following additional measures.

- ***Health Promotion.*** The nurse may need to instruct patients who have renal disorders or possible diabetes mellitus complications to test their urine daily for albumin using a reagent strip.

Pretest

- Care is dependent on the method of analysis. Check with the laboratory regarding the method and specimen required.

Posttest

- ***Patient Teaching.*** If the patient is going to be assessing his or her own urinary albumin at home, the nurse will assess the patient's understanding of the purpose of home testing and the need to notify the physician if albumin is spilled or if its concentration increases. Instruct the patient to use the first voided urine in the morning. Warn the patient that any vigorous exercise will increase the excretion of albumin in the urine, thus affecting results. Teach the patient how to follow the manufacturer's instructions for using the dipstick. Timing varies by manufacturer. Instruct the patient to keep the top on the reagent strip container. Warn the patient that abnormal results must be checked by laboratory analysis of urinary albumin, because changes in specific gravity may affect results.

A

Aldosterone, Serum

al-dos-tuh-rohn, seer-um

SPECIMEN OR TYPE OF TEST: Serum, plasma

PURPOSE OF THE TEST

The aldosterone level is used in the work-up for hypertension and in the diagnosis of aldosteronism.

BASICS THE NURSE NEEDS TO KNOW

Aldosterone is a mineralocorticoid produced by the adrenal cortex and controlled primarily by the renin-angiotensin system. Renin secreted by the kidneys acts on angiotensinogen to convert it to angiotensin I. Later, angiotensin I is converted to angiotensin II. Angiotensin II stimulates the adrenal cortex to produce and secrete aldosterone. The aldosterone acts on the renal tubules to (1) increase sodium retention and thus increase fluid retention, which increases plasma fluid volume and blood pressure, and (2) increase potassium excretion in the urine (Figure 11).

Another stimulant for aldosterone secretion is the serum potassium level. When serum potassium levels are elevated, increased secretion of aldosterone occurs, promoting greater urinary excretion of potassium.

The presence of high levels of aldosterone is called *aldosteronism*. Primary aldosteronism often is caused by adrenal adenoma (Conn syndrome). This condition is characterized by hypertension with hypokalemia and urinary potassium loss. Secondary aldosteronism is caused by nonadrenal disease that stimulates the adrenal cortex to produce and secrete excessive aldosterone.

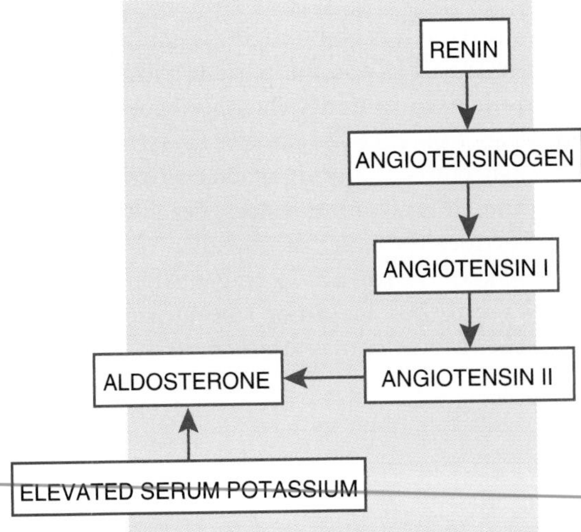

Figure 11. Primary regulation of aldosterone secretion.

In testing for serum aldosterone levels, a number of variables must be controlled to provide accurate results. A low-salt diet, an upright position, and stress all produce increased levels of aldosterone. A high-salt diet and a supine position decrease the serum levels. With the administration of fludrocortisone acetate (Florinef) or intravenous saline, the secretion of aldosterone is suppressed in normal patients and in patients with secondary aldosteronism, but serum levels rise in patients with primary aldosteronism.

NORMAL VALUES

Adult (Average Sodium Diet)

Peripheral blood, supine position: 3–10 ng/dL *or* SI: 0.08–0.27 nmol/L

Peripheral blood, upright position: 5–30 ng/dL *or* SI: 0.14–0.83 nmol/L

After fludrocortisone acetate (Florinef) suppression or intravenous saline infusion: <4 ng/dL *or* SI: <0.11 nmol/L

Adrenal vein: 200–800 ng/dL *or* SI: 5.54–22.16 nmol/L

Child

11–15 years: <5–50 ng/dL *or* SI: <0.14–1.39 nmol/L

3–11 years: <5–80 ng/dL *or* SI: <0.14–2.22 nmol/L

1–3 years: 5–60 ng/dL *or* SI: 0.14–1.7 nmol/L

1 week–1 year: 1–160 ng/dL *or* SI: 0.03–4.43 nmol/L

HOW THE TEST IS DONE

A red-topped or green-topped heparinized tube is used to collect venous blood. If a renin level is being done at the same time, a lavender-topped tube is used. The specimen is sent immediately on ice to the lab. The vascular site may be any peripheral vein. The patient may be in a supine or an upright position. A blood sample from the adrenal vein may be done to confirm the diagnosis of adrenal adenoma.

Other diagnostic methods include administering 2 L of normal saline over 4 hours before the blood test or drawing the blood on the third day after the administration of fludrocortisone acetate, a synthetic mineralocorticoid.

SIGNIFICANCE OF TEST RESULTS

Elevated Values

Primary Aldosteronism

Adrenal adenoma (Conn syndrome)
Adrenal hyperplasia

Secondary Aldosteronism

Laxative abuse
Excessive diuretic therapy
Nephrotic syndrome
Renal juxtaglomerular hyperplasia
Renin-producing renal tumor
Bartter syndrome
Toxemia of pregnancy

Decreased Values

Addison's disease
Turner syndrome
Aldosterone deficiency
Diabetes mellitus
Renin deficiency
Acute alcoholic intoxication

INTERFERING FACTORS

- Licorice intake
- Uncontrolled sodium intake
- Postural changes
- Warming of the specimen
- Recent radioisotope administration
- Loop diuretics

NURSING CARE

Nursing actions are similar to those used in other venipuncture procedures (see Chapter 2), with the following additional measures.

Pretest

- ***Patient Teaching.*** The nurse instructs the patient to follow a normal sodium intake (3 g/day) for 2 to 4 weeks, if not contraindicated by clinical status. The nurse also instructs the patient to discontinue all diuretics, antihypertensives, cyclic progesterone, estrogens, and licorice for 2 to 4 weeks if ordered by the physician.
- The nurse administers potassium replacement, as ordered.
- Any radioactive scans are scheduled for a time after the aldosterone level is obtained.

During the Test

- The nurse needs to make sure the position used and the site of the sample is standardized.
  - *Supine Position:* On the morning of the test, instruct the hospitalized patient to remain flat in bed until the specimen is drawn.
  - *Upright Position:* On the morning of the test, the nurse instructs the patient to remain seated in a chair for 2 hours until the blood is drawn.

Posttest

- Place the blood specimen on ice and arrange for its immediate transport to the laboratory.
- The nurse ensures that the requisition slip contains the following information: the time and date of the test, the venous source of the blood, the patient's position, the pretest diet, and the time and date of administration of fludrocortisone acetate or intravenous saline infusion.
- Since hepatic perfusion is the primary determinant of aldosterone metabolism, the nurse knows that interpretation of test results is influenced by any disorder that can interfere with liver blood flow, such as congestive heart failure.

Aldosterone, Urinary

al-dos-tuh-rohn, yur-i-ner-ee

SPECIMEN OR TYPE OF TEST: Urine

PURPOSE OF THE TEST

The main use of the urine aldosterone test is to help identify primary hyperaldosteronism caused by adrenal adenoma.

BASICS THE NURSE NEEDS TO KNOW

Aldosterone is a mineralocorticoid produced by the adrenal cortex. Its synthesis and release are controlled primarily by the renin-angiotensin system. Aldosterone acts on the renal tubules to resorb greater quantities of sodium, and therefore water, and increases the excretion of potassium into the urine. Elevated levels of urinary aldosterone may be caused by excess secretion of aldosterone by the adrenal glands, excessive secretion of renin, or conditions that result in decreased kidney perfusion.

NORMAL VALUES

2–26 mcg/24 hr *or* SI: 6–72 nmol/24 hr
Normal values for this test vary among laboratories

HOW THE TEST IS DONE

A 24-hour urine specimen is collected in a clean plastic container. Some laboratories add a measured quantity of preservative (boric, acetic, or hydrochloric acid) to the container before the start of the collection period.

SIGNIFICANCE OF TEST RESULTS

Elevated Values

Aldosterone-producing adrenal adenoma (Conn syndrome)
Adrenal hyperplasia
Nephrotic syndrome
Renin-producing renal hyperplasia or tumor
Renal hypertension
Bartter syndrome
Preeclampsia

Decreased Values

Addison's disease
Aldosterone deficiency
Renin deficiency
Diabetes mellitus
Acute alcoholic intoxication

INTERFERING FACTORS

- Excess salt intake
- Recent administration of radioisotopes

- Licorice intake
- Failure to collect all the urine
- Warming of the specimen
- Diuretics (loop or thiazides)
- Lithium
- Oral contraceptives

NURSING CARE

Nursing actions are similar to those used in other 24 hour urine collection procedures (see Chapter 2), with the following additional measures.

Pretest

- ***Patient Teaching.*** The nurse instructs the patient to follow a normal (3 g/day) sodium diet for 2 to 4 weeks. Excessive sodium intake suppresses aldosterone secretion and causes a false decrease in the aldosterone value. Instruct the patient to discontinue all diuretics, antihypertensives, and oral contraceptives for 2 weeks, if ordered. These medications interfere with the test results.
- The nurse checks the patient's serum potassium level and administers prescribed potassium to correct any deficiencies that may be present.
- Schedule any radioisotope scan for after the urine test is completed.

During the Test

- At the start of the test, the nurse instructs the patient to void at 8 AM and discard this urine. The collection period starts at this time, and the patient collects all the urine for 24 hours, including the 8 AM specimen of the following morning.
- On the requisition slip and specimen label, the nurse writes the patient's name and the time and date of the start and finish of the test period.
- The nurse ensures that the urine is kept refrigerated or on ice throughout the collection period.

Posttest

- On the requisition slip, write the pretest sodium diet.
- Arrange for prompt transport of the cooled specimen to the laboratory.

Alkaline Phosphatase

al-kah-lin fos-fah-tays

Also called: (ALP)

SPECIMEN OR TYPE OF TEST: Serum

PURPOSE OF THE TEST

Serum alkaline phosphatase (ALP) testing is a nonspecific indicator of liver disease, bone disease, or hyperparathyroidism. It is part of a battery of tests that evaluate liver function. It also serves as a tumor marker by indicating rapid cell growth or accelerated function caused by malignancy of the liver or bone.

BASICS THE NURSE NEEDS TO KNOW

ALP is an enzyme located in the osteoblast cells of the bone, in liver cells, and in the intestines, kidney, and placenta. The enzyme is normally excreted via the biliary tract. The function of any enzyme is to activate particular chemical reactions in cells in which the enzyme is located. A high level of any enzyme usually means that a specific organ or tissue has increased the manufacture or release of the enzyme.

The ALP level will rise with increased activity from liver disease or bone disease. When the cause arises from liver disease, other liver enzyme tests—alanine aminotransferase (ALT) and aspartate aminotransferase (AST)—also are mildly elevated. Bone disease, however, causes no elevation of the ALT or AST levels.

NORMAL VALUES

20–130 Unit/L at 37° C *or* SI: p20–130 Unit/L at 37° C

HOW THE TEST IS DONE

A venipuncture is performed to collect 10 mL of venous blood in a red-topped tube.

SIGNIFICANCE OF TEST RESULTS

Elevated Values

Cancer of the liver
Cirrhosis
Acute fatty liver
Infectious mononucleosis
Infiltrating liver disease (abscess, sarcoidosis, tuberculosis)
Paget's disease
Osteogenic sarcoma
Bone metastases
Rickets
Healing bone fracture
Acromegaly
Sclerosing cholangitis
Biliary obstruction (gallstones or pancreatic cancer)
Cholestasis
Myelofibrosis
Hyperthyroidism
Hyperparathyroidism

Decreased Values

Malnutrition (protein deficiency, magnesium deficiency or both)
Hypophosphatemia
Hypothyroidism

INTERFERING FACTORS

- Healing bone fracture
- Pregnancy
- Fatty food intake, 2 to 4 hours before the test

NURSING CARE

Nursing actions are similar to those used in other venipuncture procedures (see Chapter 2), with the following additional measures.

Pretest

- ***Patient Teaching.*** Instruct the patient to discontinue food intake for 12 hours before the test, as indicated by laboratory policy. Foods in general and fatty foods in particular, can elevate the test results in some individuals.

Alpha-Fetoprotein

al-fuh–fee-toh-proh-teen

Also called: (AFP), α-fetoprotein

SPECIMEN OR TYPE OF TEST: Serum

PURPOSE OF THE TEST

In the nonpregnant patient, AFP is a tumor marker for primary cancer of the liver (hepatoma). It is used to help with the diagnosis and to monitor the effect of chemotherapy treatment on that tumor. It is also used as a tumor marker and to help with diagnosis and staging of some types of testicular cancer.

In a pregnant woman, serum AFP serves as a screening test for neural tube defects in the fetus. Neural tube defects in the fetus include spinal bifida, myelomeningocele, and anencephaly. It is also part of the multiple marker screening test that detects fetal Down syndrome in the pregnant woman.

BASICS THE NURSE NEEDS TO KNOW

In the blood of healthy, nonpregnant adults, AFP is present in very small amounts. If the liver has been injured by trauma, exposure to chemical toxins or the hepatitis virus, the AFP level will rise moderately as healing and regeneration of liver cells occurs.

As a tumor marker for primary hepatoma, the serum level rises to values of 1000 ng/mL (SI: 1000 mcg/mL) or dramatically higher. When the test is used to monitor the response of the testicular tumor to chemotherapy treatment, a rising AFP value indicates additional growth of the tumor and a falling value indicates a favorable response to the chemotherapy treatment.

In a pregnant woman, the fetus produces the AFP and it is, therefore, present in the amniotic fluid and the maternal serum. The maternal serum level increases throughout the pregnancy and in the third trimester rises to 500 ng/mL (SI: 500 mcg/mL). The pregnant African American woman has a normal value that is 10% to15% higher than the white American woman throughout the pregnancy. The normal value for the pregnant woman who has insulin-dependent diabetes is 20% lower than the average normal value.

For prenatal screening, the best time to draw the maternal blood is in the 16th to 18th week of the pregnancy, but the specimen can be drawn during time period of the 15th to

21st week. An abnormally elevated value occurs with open neural tube defect and some other congenital defects in the fetus. The test, however, can have false positive results because the calculation of the normal result is based on the gestational age of the fetus.

The gestational age is best measured by ultrasound. Often, however, the calculation is based on the mother's estimate of when her last menstrual period occurred and this may not be precise. Because of the possibility of error, a positive screening test result is considered to be only suggestive of abnormality of the fetus. Additional evaluation by ultrasound is recommended and based on the results of the pregnancy ultrasound, amniocentesis may be needed. With follow-up pregnancy ultrasound, the examination focus is on the fetal spine and cranium. With amniocentesis, the analysis of the amniotic fluid would provide accurate information about the condition of the fetus. Normal findings of these additional tests demonstrate that no neural tube defect exists (Figure 12).

Multiple Marker Screening for Down Syndrome

Pregnant women can now be tested for fetal Down syndrome in the second trimester, using the triple or quadruple marker screening test. This blood test is offered in the 15th to 22nd week of the pregnancy. The triple marker screening test consists of alpha-fetoprotein, human chorionic gonadotrophin, and unconjugated estriol. The newest, improved method is to use the quadruple marker screening test, consisting of the above three tests and adding a fourth test, inhibitin A.

When Down syndrome affects the fetus, the quadruple marker screening test demonstrates characteristic changes in the second trimester of pregnancy. The alpha-fetoprotein result is 25% lower than normal and the unconjugated estriol result is 30% lower than normal. Both human chorionic gonadotrophin and inhibitin A rise to twice

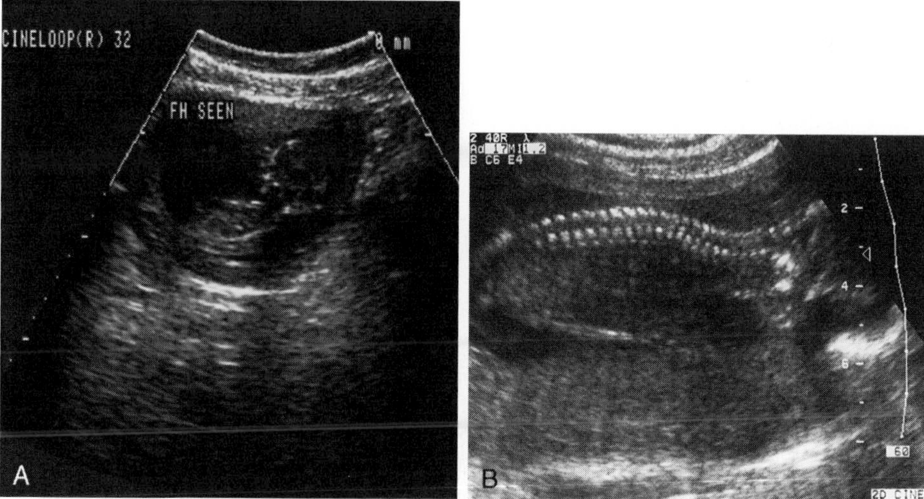

Figure 12. Pregnancy ultrasound. The varying densities and compositions of tissue allow visualization of the uterine contents. *A,* A normal 4-month-old fetus. The fetal heart (FH) is identified. *B,* The normal spinal structure of a 4-month-old fetus.

A

the normal value. Pregnancy ultrasound must be done first, to obtain an accurate gestational age. The quadruple marker screening test detects 80% of fetal Down syndrome pregnancies, with a 5% false positive rate of error. It is a very useful test for pregnant women younger than age 35, because there is a high rate of Down syndrome that occurs in pregnancies of younger females and amniocentesis is not done routinely to detect the problem.

NORMAL VALUES

Adult: <15 ng/mL *or* SI: <15 mcg/mL
Pregnancy: <15–500 ng/mL *or* SI: <15–500 mcg/mL (result rises to the high-end value in the third trimester of pregnancy)

HOW THE TEST IS DONE

A venipuncture is performed to collect 10 mL of venous blood in a red-topped tube.

SIGNIFICANCE OF TEST RESULTS

Nonpregnant State

Liver cancer
Gonadal germinal tumor
Liver trauma
Hepatitis
Cirrhosis

Pregnant State

Spinal bifida
Myelomeningocele
Anencephaly
Intrauterine fetal death
Esophageal atresia
Oligohydramnios
Congenital nephrosis
Multiple pregnancy

INTERFERING FACTORS

- Recent radioisotope scan

NURSING CARE

- ***Health Promotion.*** The nurse teaches the patient that all pregnant females are encouraged to have the AFP blood test screening during the 15th to 18th week of gestation to help ensure that the fetus is healthy and developing normally. Generally, the blood is drawn during a routine prenatal visit.

For the AFP test itself, nursing actions are similar to those used in other venipuncture procedures (see Chapter 2), with the following additional measures.

NURSING CARE—*cont'd*

Pretest

- For the pregnant woman, include the following data on the requisition slip: gestational age, maternal weight, maternal race, and diabetic status. These are variables that affect the interpretation of the test results.

Posttest

- If there is an elevated AFP value that is suggestive of fetal abnormality, prospective parents often react with fear and anxiety. The physician gives the initial explanation of the findings and stresses the importance of follow-up testing with fetal ultrasound and amniocentesis. There is the possibility that the screening test result is a false positive because of error in determining the gestational age of the fetus. The prospective parents, however, experience emotional distress and may not be listening or understanding the information. A one-time explanation by the physician may not be sufficient.
- The nurse can help the expectant parents to minimize maternal anxiety, particularly during the waiting time before follow-up testing is performed. The expectant mother often seeks more information and clarification. The nurse can help the patient understand the information that was provided by the physician and prepare a list of additional questions to ask the physician.
- Emotional support is needed when the prospective parents think about possible abnormality of the fetus. They may consider possible decisions and outcomes prematurely. The nurse should remind the parents that this AFP test is a screening test and no plans should be made until additional test results and information are known. Prompt scheduling for follow-up testing with ultrasound and possible amniocentesis will be very helpful.

Ammonia

am-mohn-yuh

Also called: NH_3

SPECIMEN OR TYPE OF TEST: Plasma

PURPOSE OF THE TEST

The ammonia level is used to evaluate or monitor severe liver failure, hepatic encephalopathy, and the effects of impaired portal vein circulation. It also may be used to monitor patients on hyperalimentation therapy. It may help identify some rare forms of inborn errors of metabolism that can affect a neonate and may be used to help diagnose Reye syndrome, a childhood disorder that results in an acute fatty liver and encephalopathy.

BASICS THE NURSE NEEDS TO KNOW

As proteins are digested and metabolized or broken down into amino acids in the intestine, ammonia is produced as a by-product. The ammonia enters and circulates in the bloodstream until the liver removes it from the portal circulation. Liver cells then

A

convert the ammonia to urea. Ultimately, the kidneys remove the urea from the circulation and excrete it in urine.

The two most common causes of an elevated ammonia level are the failure of the hepatic cells to function in the conversion of ammonia to urea and the impairment of the portal vein circulation, which prevents the ammonia from reaching the liver tissue.

NORMAL VALUES

Adult: 20–120 mcg/dL *or* SI: 12–70 µmol/L
Child: 29–70 mcg/dL *or* SI: 21–50 µmol/L
Neonate: 90–150 mcg/dL *or* SI: 64–107 µmol/L

HOW THE TEST IS DONE

An arterial puncture or a venipuncture is performed to collect 7 to 10 mL of blood in a grey-, lavender-, or green-topped tube. The tube must be filled completely and the stopper kept in place at all times.

SIGNIFICANCE OF TEST RESULTS

Elevated Values

Liver failure (hepatic necrosis or terminal cirrhosis)
Hepatic encephalopathy
Portal hypertension
Portacaval shunting of the blood
Inborn errors of metabolism that affect the urea synthesis cycle
Reye syndrome

INTERFERING FACTORS

- Tobacco smoke
- High protein intake
- Gastrointestinal hemorrhage
- Hyperalimentation (total parenteral nutrition)
- Ureterosigmoidostomy
- Hemolysis

NURSING CARE

Nursing actions are similar to those used in other arterial puncture or venipuncture procedures (see Chapter 2), with the following additional measures.

Pretest

- ***Patient Teaching.*** Instruct the patient not to smoke before the test. The smoke itself will elevate the results falsely. If venipuncture will be used to collect the specimen, instruct the patient not to clench the fist.

Posttest

- Ensure that the specimen is placed in a bed of ice and sent to the laboratory immediately.
- If the specimen is allowed to warm, it will produce falsely elevated results.

Amniocentesis and Amniotic Fluid Analysis

am-nee-oh-sen-tee-sis and am-nee-ah-tik floo-id an-al-uh-sis

SPECIMEN OR TYPE OF TEST: Amniotic fluid

PURPOSE OF THE TEST

Amniocentesis is the procedure to obtain a sample of amniotic fluid and fetal cells. The analysis of the amniotic fluid is used to detect genetic or chromosomal abnormalities in the fetus. It is also used to assess fetal maturity or fetal distress in the management of a problem pregnancy.

BASICS THE NURSE NEEDS TO KNOW

When the purpose of the amniocentesis is to screen for fetal abnormality, it is performed early in the second trimester. Usually, the procedure is performed in the 15th to 17th weeks of gestation, when the risk to the fetus is lower and sufficient time is available to provide the appropriate counseling and discuss treatment alternatives (Table 4). When the purpose of the amniocentesis is to evaluate a problem pregnancy or to identify a change in the health status of the fetus, the procedure is performed in the late part of the second trimester or during the third trimester. In high-risk pregnancy, it may be advisable to terminate the pregnancy by delivery of the preterm infant. Severe maternal illness can adversely affect the fetus. The analysis of the amniotic fluid provides information about the health and development of the fetus.

Chromosomal analysis identifies genetic abnormalities that are present in the fetal cells of the amniotic fluid. A *karyotype* is the complement of chromosomes. In humans, the normal karyotype consists of 46 chromosomes aligned in a standard sequence, with defined location, size, structure, and banding patterns.

Trisomy 21 (Down syndrome) and other trisomy conditions caused by the translocation of genes have an identifiable incidence in women older than age 35. Chromosomal analysis also can detect genetic abnormalities that cause more than 80 different types of inborn errors of metabolism. They include disorders of lipid, carbohydrate, glycoprotein, mucopolysaccharide, amino acid, and organic acid metabolism. The use of gene probe technology can also identify other autosomal recessive genetic mutations and sex-linked autosomal recessive genetic disorders.

Alpha-fetoprotein (AFP) testing of the amniotic fluid is the more accurate follow-up test when the maternal serum test is positive (see Alpha-Fetoprotein, Serum, p. 60). When the amniotic fluid value of the AFP is >2.1 multiple of median value (MoM), the result is considered abnormal. If the value is 7 MoM, it is considered positive for spinal bifida. If the value is at 20 MoM, it is considered positive for anencephaly. The calculation of the test value is based on the ultrasound measurement of the gestational age of the fetus.

Acetylcholinesterase is an enzyme present in cerebrospinal fluid. If the fetus has an open neural defect, this enzyme enters the amniotic fluid and the test result is positive.

Bilirubin causes the amniotic fluid to change to a dark yellow or amber color. When the maternal blood is Rh negative or contains atypical antibodies, there is potential for

TABLE 4 Amniocentesis: Timing, Purposes, and Potential Findings

Gestation	Indications	Potential Abnormalities
15–17 wk	Maternal age >35 yr	Trisomy 21 (Down syndrome) Neural tube defect (spina bifida, anencephaly)
	Sex determination of the fetus	Sex-linked recessive disorders (hemophilia, Duchenne's muscular dystrophy)
	Family history of chromosomal abnormality	
	Family history of metabolic disorder	Inborn errors of metabolism (Tay-Sachs disease, Gaucher's disease, Niemann-Pick disease; galactosuria, maple syrup disease, homocystinuria)
	Family history of hemoglobinopathy	Hemoglobin disease (thalassemia, sickle cell anemia)
20–42 wk	Management of a problem pregnancy	Maternal heart disease, diabetes, endocrine disorder; analysis of amniotic fluid for fetal thyroid hormone, glucose, estriol, L/S ratio*
	Assessment of fetal distress	Rh incompatibility, infection, fetal pulmonary immaturity

**L/S ratio,* Lecithin-sphingomyelin ratio.

the fetus to develop hemolytic disease of the newborn (erythroblastosis fetalis). In this disorder, the erythrocytes of the fetus undergo hemolysis and bilirubin is released. An abnormal test result is usually followed up with Percutaneous Umbilical Cord Blood Sampling (see p. 508) to obtain a direct sample of the fetal blood.

Lecithin/sphingomyelin (L/S) ratio is a major indicator of fetal pulmonary maturity. The test is used to help determine the best time for the physician to do the obstetrical delivery of a problem pregnancy that is threatening the health of the mother, the fetus, or both. When the L/S ratio reaches a value of 2 or higher, the fetal lungs are mature. An L/S ratio of 1.5 to 1.9 is the indicator of fetal lung immaturity, with the increased likelihood that the newborn infant will experience respiratory distress syndrome.

Phosphatidylglycerol is a component of pulmonary surfactant that normally appears in the amniotic fluid after the 35th week of gestation. It is a major indicator of fetal lung maturity. Once it appears, little risk exists that the fetus will experience respiratory distress syndrome (hyaline membrane disease). Generally, this test is used with the L/S ratio determination to assess fetal lung maturity.

Pulmonary surfactant is a substance produced by the mature epithelial cells of the alveoli that enables the walls of the alveoli to expand and contract in the function of respiration.

One way to measure pulmonary surfactant is with the *foam stability index* (FSI). An FSI value of 0.47 or more indicates fetal lung maturity.

NORMAL VALUES	Chromosome analysis: Normal karyotype Alpha-fetoprotein: <2.0 multiple of median value (MoM) Acetylcholinesterase: Negative Bilirubin: 0.01–0.03 mg/dL *or* SI: 0.02–0.06 µmol/L Lecithin-to-sphingomyelin ratio: >2 Phosphatidylglycerol: Present Pulmonary surfactant: Positive; foam stability index: 0.47
▼ Critical Values	L/S ratio: <1.5

HOW THE TEST IS DONE

Ultrasound is used to locate the position of the fetus, the placenta, and the pool of amniotic fluid. Using sterile technique, the physician passes a long, sterile needle through the abdominal wall and into amniotic fluid. Syringes are used to aspirate 12 to 20 mL of amniotic fluid from the uterus (Figure 13). The fluid is placed in sterile brown plastic containers for transport to the laboratory.

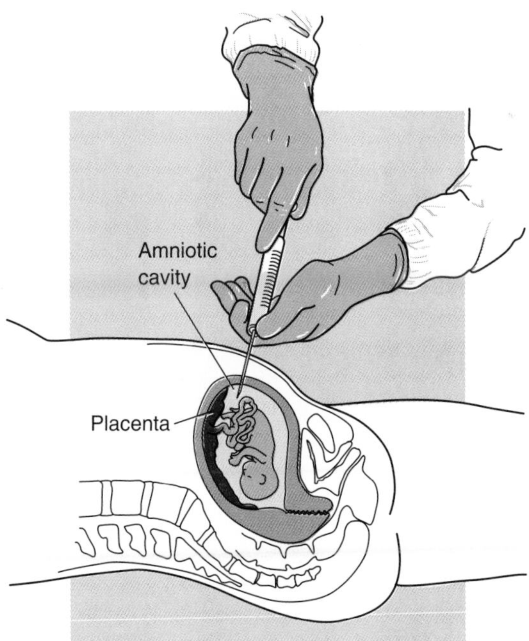

Figure 13. Amniocentesis. Once the needle is inserted through the skin and the uterine wall, a sample of amniotic fluid is aspirated with a syringe.

SIGNIFICANCE OF TEST RESULTS

Abnormal Findings

Chromosomes

Cystic fibrosis
Sickle cell anemia
Muscular dystrophy
Hemophilia A, B
Inborn errors of metabolism
Down syndrome
Retinoblastoma
Wilms' tumor
Thalassemias
Phenylketonuria
Enzyme G-6-PD deficiency

Elevated Values

Alpha-Fetoprotein

Neural tube defects: anencephaly, spinal bifida, myelocele, hydrocephaly

Acetylcholinesterase

Neural tube defect

Bilirubin

Rh incompatibility
Hemolytic disease of the newborn

L/S Ratio

Maternal diabetes

Pulmonary Surfactant

Maternal diabetes

Decreased Values

L/S Ratio

Fetal lung immaturity

Phosphatidylglycerol

Fetal lung immaturity

Pulmonary Surfactant

Fetal lung immaturity
Polyhydramnios

INTERFERING FACTORS

- Exposure of specimen to sunlight
- Contamination of specimen (blood, meconium)
- Recent radioactive isotope scan
- Position of the placenta

NURSING CARE

Pretest

- After the patient receives a complete explanation of the amniocentesis procedure from the physician, obtain the patient's written consent for the procedure and the chromosomal (genetic) analysis.
- ***Patient Teaching.*** Provide instructions regarding pretest preparation. These instructions vary, depending on the gestation of the pregnancy. For a pregnancy that is less than 20 weeks of gestation, instruct the woman to drink extra fluids 1 hour before the test and not to urinate until the test is completed. A full bladder raises the uterus up and out of the pelvis so that the uterine contents can be visualized. For a pregnancy that is greater than 20 weeks of gestation, no requirements exist for fluid intake. Instruct the woman to void before the procedure begins. With the larger size of the uterus, an empty bladder is less likely to be punctured during the procedure.
- Assist the patient in removing her clothes, putting on a hospital gown, and lying supine on the examining table.
- Obtain and record vital signs, including the blood pressure, temperature, pulse, respirations, and fetal heart rate. This establishes the baseline values that are needed for comparison in the posttest period.
- Provide emotional support for the patient. Anxiety about the procedure and the status of the fetus' health is common.

During the Test

- Position the patient with her hands behind her head to help prevent contamination of the sterile field.
- After ultrasound images have located the position of the fetus, the placenta, and the pool of amniotic fluid, the nurse washes the abdomen with povidone-iodine solution and helps drape the sterile field.
- The nurse comforts the patient as the physician administers the local anesthetic in the intended area of the abdomen. The patient will feel some stinging during the injection.
- After the fluid sample is withdrawn by the physician, the nurse assists with its placement in the sterile specimen container. Glass containers cannot be used because the cells would adhere to the surface of the glass. A brown container is used to protect the fluid and bilirubin from sunlight. If a brown container is not available, a clear container may be used. After the fluid is inserted, the container must be covered by aluminum foil immediately to prevent oxidation by sunlight. Ensure that the specimen is correctly labeled. The requisition slip should state the source of the fluid, the maternal age, and the period of gestation of the pregnancy. Additional information includes the reason for the study and relevant patient history, medication and transfusion history.
- Once the needle is withdrawn, a small adhesive bandage is placed over the site of the needle puncture.

Continued

NURSING CARE—*cont'd*

Posttest

- The nurse monitors and records the maternal blood pressure, pulse, respirations, and fetal heart rate every 15 minutes for 30 to 60 minutes. They should remain within normal limits and be comparable to the pretest data.
- If the patient feels faintness, nausea, or cramps, the nurse places her on her right side to relieve the uterine pressure.
- After amniocentesis, all nonsensitized patients with an Rh_o(D) negative blood type should receive immunization. The nurse administers the intramuscular injection of Rh_o(D) immune globulin (Win Rho SD), as prescribed. This helps prevent hemolytic disease of the newborn (erythroblastosis fetalis) in future pregnancy.
- ***Patient Teaching.*** At the time of discharge, instruct the patient to rest at home until the cramping subsides. Light activity can then resume. Posttest activity restrictions for the next several days include no bending at the waist, no lifting of anything heavier than 20 pounds, and avoidance of strenuous exercise. Provide the patient with written instructions to notify the physician immediately about any symptoms of itching, fever, leakage of fluid, severe abdominal pain, or unusual (increased or decreased) fetal activity.
- Once the test results are known, the patient (or the prospective parents) meets with the physician. In early stage amniocentesis, when a genetic abnormality is encountered, the parents need comprehensive information about the health status of the fetus. They need to make an informed decision about the pregnancy, and the choices are painful. The alternatives include termination of the pregnancy or completion of the pregnancy with preparation for the special health care needs of the newborn. Genetic counseling precedes the amniocentesis and is also provided when a genetic abnormality is encountered. The nurse uses listening skills and a supportive approach in communication and interactions with the patient. The patient may need clarification, time for additional discussion, or to express feelings and concerns. The nurse may need to refer the patient to appropriate health care personnel for in-depth information.

Nursing Response to Critical Values

A low L/S ratio indicates fetal lung immaturity. If delivery occurs at this time, the test value is a predictor that the fetus will develop respiratory distress syndrome (RDS). Usually, this value is correlated with a gestation of 34 weeks or less. The nurse informs the physician of the test result. Medical and nursing interventions will be specific to each patient, depending on the physical condition of the mother and fetus. When delivery is anticipated before the fetal lungs are mature, the mother is usually given prescribed antenatal glucocorticoid therapy that will stimulate fetal lung maturity.

Nursing Response to Complications

The overall incidence of complications from amniocentesis is less than 0.5%. The complications include spontaneous rupture of the membranes, premature labor, bleeding from a traumatic tap, and infection.

NURSING CARE—*cont'd*

Ruptured membranes, premature labor, bleeding, infection. The patient is asked to describe the symptoms that she is experiencing. Her vital signs are taken, including temperature. The nurse assesses for signs or bleeding or leakage of amniotic fluid from the puncture site or the vagina and asks about any leakage of fluid, blood, or passage of clots that occurred at home. The nurse also questions the patient about cramping or contractions, including the intensity, frequency and duration. Assessment findings are reported to the physician and entered into the patient's record.

Amylase, Serum

am-uh-lace, seer-um

SPECIMEN OR TYPE OF TEST: Serum

PURPOSE OF THE TEST

Serum amylase can help diagnose acute pancreatitis, particularly when the specimen is drawn within 6 to 48 hours of the onset of abdominal pain. It is used together with serum lipase, to investigate the cause of epigastric pain, nausea, and vomiting.

BASICS THE NURSE NEEDS TO KNOW

Amylase enzymes function to act on dietary starch and convert it to maltose. Amylase is produced by the parotid glands and the pancreas, but pancreatic amylase performs most of the digestive work on the starch. In normal physiology, the acinar cells of the pancreas produce the amylase and the enzymes flow out through the pancreatic ducts, the common bile duct, and the ampulla of Vater, to empty into the duodenum.

Many methods of laboratory analysis are used for serum amylase, with a range of normal values based on the method used. The nurse uses the specific laboratory report to obtain the reference value for a particular patient.

Elevated Values

Inflammation or obstruction in any part of the pancreas or the common bile duct causes obstruction of the flow of amylase and a backup of the enzyme in the pancreatic tissue. The amylase is absorbed into bloodstream, with resultant hyperamylasemia (elevated level of amylase in the blood). In acute pancreatitis, the serum amylase value starts to rise within 2 to12 hours of the onset of the inflammation. The level peaks in 12 to 72 hours and returns to normal in 3 to 4 days. Intestinal diseases that cause inflammation of the pancreas or blockage of the common bile duct also cause the serum amylase to rise. Acute inflammation of the parotid glands, as in parotitis (mumps) can cause an elevated serum amylase from a salivary source.

Decreased Values

Mucoviscidosis is a congenital pancreatic disease that causes dysfunction of the mucus secreting glands. Thick mucus obstructs the pancreatic ductal system, causing acinar cell atrophy. In children or adults who have advanced cystic fibrosis, the serum amylase levels are decreased.

NORMAL VALUES	Adult: 16–120 Somogyi units/dL or SI: 30–220 units/L The normal values depend on the method of analysis
Critical Values	An increase of three to five times the upper limit of the normal value.

HOW THE TEST IS DONE

A venipuncture is performed to collect 10 mL of venous blood in a red-topped tube.

SIGNIFICANCE OF TEST RESULTS

Elevated Values

Acute pancreatitis
Other pancreatic disorders (trauma, abscess, pseudocyst)
Obstruction at ampulla of Vater
Intestinal obstruction
Obstruction of the common bile duct
Perforated peptic ulcer
Parotitis

Decreased Values

Cystic fibrosis
Chronic pancreatitis
Pancreatic cancer
Cirrhosis
Hepatitis

INTERFERING FACTORS

- Drinking alcohol before the test
- Recent use of morphine

NURSING CARE

Nursing actions are similar to those used in other venipuncture procedures (see Chapter 2), with the following additional measures.

Pretest

- ***Patient Teaching.*** Instruct the patient not to drink alcohol for 24 hours before the test. Alcohol stimulates the secretion of salivary amylase. No other fasting measures are required.

NURSING CARE—*cont'd*

- Before the test, the administration of morphine, codeine or meperidine (Demerol) may be omitted. The recent administration of narcotics would close the sphincter of Oddi, with the effect of falsely raising the amylase level.

Posttest

▼ Nursing Response to Critical Values

Severe increases in serum amylase are considered significant and the physician must be notified. The sudden rise is usually caused by acute pancreatitis or an acute surgical condition of the abdomen.

When the serum amylase value rises to three to five times the upper limit of normal, according to the reference value of the laboratory that performed the test, the nurse should assess the patient for signs of acute abdominal pain, including location and any increase in intensity. Ecchymosis (bruising) may appear in the flank or around the umbilicus. Vital signs must to be taken to help evaluate for shock. Tachycardia, hypotension, and respiratory distress are indicators of severe, acute pancreatitis.

Amylase, Urine

am-uh-lace, yur-in

SPECIMEN OR TYPE OF TEST: Urine

PURPOSE OF THE TEST

Urinary amylase is used to help diagnose acute and relapsing pancreatitis, particularly when the serum value is borderline or normal.

BASICS THE NURSE NEEDS TO KNOW

Amylase is cleared from the body in the urine. When the serum amylase level is elevated, the filtration rate by the kidneys increases and a greater rate of amylase clearance occurs. The amount of amylase clearance is measured in units per urine volume in a specific collection period. After the onset of acute pancreatitis, urinary amylase levels remain elevated for up to 2 weeks, as compared with the serum level that declines after 3 to 4 days.

NORMAL VALUES

Adult, 2-hour collection period: 35–260 Somogyi units/hour *or* SI: 6.5–48.1 Units/hour

The reference range varies with the laboratory method of analysis.

HOW THE TEST IS DONE

Urine is collected for a specific time period. The most common period is 1 or 2 hours, but 6- , 8- , or 24-hour collection periods are sometimes used.

A

SIGNIFICANCE OF TEST RESULTS

Elevated Values

Acute pancreatitis
Cancer of the head of the pancreas
Pancreatic pseudocyst
Gall bladder disease
Obstruction (pancreatic ducts, intestine, salivary glands)
Parotitis (mumps)

Decreased Values

Alcoholism
Chronic pancreatitis
Hepatitis
Cirrhosis
Liver cancer or abscess

INTERFERING FACTORS

- Heavy menstrual flow
- Bacterial contamination of the urine
- Salivary amylase contamination of the specimen
- Omission of any voided specimen in the collection period
- Failure to cool the specimen

NURSING CARE

Nursing actions are similar to those used in other timed urinary collection procedures (see Chapter 2), with the following additional measures.

Pretest

- ***Patient Teaching.*** Instruct the patient not to drink alcohol for 24 hours before the test. Alcohol stimulates the secretion of salivary amylase. Just before the start of the test, instruct the patient to void and discard the specimen. This urine has been in the bladder for an unknown period.

During the Test

- Write the date and time for the start and finish of the test on the specimen label and the requisition slip.
- During the collection period, refrigerate the urine or place the container in a bed of ice. Amylase is unstable in acidic urine. The patient and personnel must be careful not to cough, sneeze, or talk near the open collection container. Their saliva will add amylase to the content of the specimen.

Posttest

Maintain refrigeration of the specimen until it is sent to the laboratory.

Angiography, Cerebral

an-jee-ah-gruh-fee, suh-ree-bruhl

SPECIMEN OR TYPE OF TEST: Radiography

PURPOSE OF THE TEST

Cerebral angiography identifies abnormalities of the vasculature and the blood flow in the neck and brain. When intracranial or extracranial vascular surgery is indicated, the procedure is used preoperatively to provide a precise image.

BASICS THE NURSE NEEDS TO KNOW

Angiography of the brain, head, and neck provides clear x-ray imaging of intracranial and extracranial vascular abnormalities and their locations. Although the less invasive procedures of computed tomography (CT) and magnetic resonance imaging (MRI) have surpassed angiography for the imaging of tumors and trauma to the brain, cerebral angiography remains a mainstay in the investigation of the cerebral vasculature.

Two new imaging modalities use a combination of methods to perform cerebral angiography. *Computed tomography angiography* (CTA) uses CT scanning with contrast medium to provide very clear and accurate images of the vasculature of the brain. *Magnetic resonance angiography* (MRA) uses MRI sometimes combined with contrast medium to obtain images of aneurysm, vascular malformation, and obstruction in blood vessels of the brain (Figure 14).

In addition to the visualization of the vasculature of the head, neck, and brain, cerebral angiography demonstrates the location and characteristic vascular patterns of different types of brain tumors. It locates and defines the source of a subarachnoid hemorrhage and identifies vascular malformation. Thrombosis, embolic occlusion, or atheromatous stenosis can be seen when it occurs in a major extracranial or intracranial artery. Subdural hematoma also is visualized, because no contrast material is circulating in the space between the skull and the displaced brain tissue.

Some infrequent but devastating complications can occur with cerebral angiography. Many of the patients are elderly and in poor general health, with extensive arteriosclerotic disease, heart disease, or both. These problems make the patients more vulnerable to complications after the procedure.

NORMAL VALUES No abnormalities of the tissue or vasculature are visualized.

HOW THE TEST IS DONE

The femoral artery is the most common approach to inject the contrast medium. The physician passes a long, thin catheter through the vasculature until the tip reaches the internal carotid, external carotid, and vertebral arteries. Radiopaque contrast material is injected arterially. Rapid serial x-ray films are taken to image the contrast medium as it moves through the circulation of the neck and intracranial blood vessels.

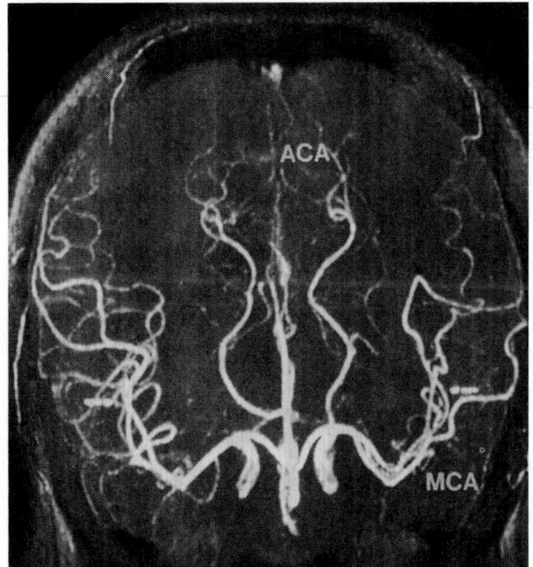

Figure 14. Magnetic resonance (MR) angiogram. An anterior view of the head showing intracerebral vessels, including the anterior cerebral artery (ACA) and the middle cerebral artery (MCA). These images were obtained without injection of any contrast agent. *(Reproduced with permission from Mettler, F. A. [1996].* Essentials of radiology [p. 9]. *Philadelphia: W. B. Saunders.)*

SIGNIFICANCE OF TEST RESULTS

Abnormal Values

Brain tumor
Arteriovenous malformation
Arteriosclerosis
Atherosclerotic plaque
Vasospasm, arteritis, stenosis
Cerebral aneurysm
Intracranial hemorrhage
Vascular occlusion, stroke

INTERFERING FACTORS

- Movement of the head during imaging
- Metal objects in the x-ray field
- Vomiting during the imaging process
- Allergy to iodine

NURSING CARE

Pretest

- Ask the patient about a history of allergy to iodine, including allergic reactions to shellfish or to iodine during a previous x-ray studies that used contrast medium. Document the results. The nurse verifies that recent reports of the complete blood count (CBC), blood urea nitrogen (BUN), creatinine, prothrombin time (PT), and partial thromboplastin time (PTT) are placed in the chart. These laboratory tests are needed because the patient must have adequate renal function to filter and remove the contrast at the end of the study. Additionally, there should be no coagulation disorder that would contribute to bleeding after an arterial puncture. The nurse reviews these preliminary laboratory values and notifies the physician of abnormal results.
- Once the physician has informed the patient about the procedure, obtain written consent from the patient and enter the signed document in the patient's record.
- ***Patient Teaching.*** The nurse instructs the patient regarding the food and fluid restrictions to be implemented before the test. Instruct the patient to discontinue food intake for 6 to 8 hours before the test. The contrast medium can cause nausea. If food is in the stomach, vomiting would result in head movement during the imaging process and blurring of the photographic results. Most protocols permit the intake of clear fluids during the fasting period because the extra intake of fluids promotes hydration and renal excretion of the contrast medium. When this test is to be performed on an outpatient or ambulatory basis, instruct the patient to have a responsible person available for transportation home after the test. The sedative effects of the medications will remain for several hours after the test is completed.
- Assist the patient in removing all clothing and putting on a hospital gown. All metal objects are removed from the head, mouth, hair, neck, and upper torso. These include hair ornaments or pins, removable metal dental appliances, jewelry, and body-piercing items.
- Take baseline vital signs and assess the peripheral pulses. Record the results. With peripheral pulses, the nurse assesses pulse points distal to the arterial site of the catheter insertion and compares the pulses of both right and left extremities. For a femoral catheter approach, the pulse points that are assessed are the femoral, popliteal, and pedal pulses. If the patient has an elevated blood pressure, this finding is reported to the physician.
- About 1 hour before the procedure, the patient receives medication for sedation and analgesia. The purpose of the medications is to decrease central nervous system activity, anxiety, tension, physical activity, and potential agitation.

During the Test

- Establish an intravenous line for fluid replacement and the electrocardiogram leads for monitoring the heart rate and rhythm. Monitor vital signs at appropriate intervals.

Continued

NURSING CARE—*cont'd*

- The site for the arterial puncture and passage of the arterial catheter is shaved and scrubbed with antibacterial soap solution.
- The patient is placed in the supine position. Instruct the patient to keep the head and neck absolutely still during the injection of contrast material and the imaging sequence. The head is immobilized in a support device and restraints to the forehead and chin are used to prevent movement of the head.
- Inform the patient that he or she may experience a temporary flushing or burning sensation, a salty taste, headache, or nausea as the contrast medium is injected.

Posttest

- After the catheter is removed from the artery, use sterile gauze to apply pressure to the puncture site for 10 minutes. This should prevent bleeding or hematoma formation. If swelling or redness occurs, apply ice to the area.
- The patient must remain supine for 4 hours, without bending the extremity used for the procedure. The nurse continues to monitor vital signs at frequent intervals until they are stable and in a normal range. The nurse also assesses the extremity used for the arterial injection. Adequate circulation and mobility and intact neurologic function should be present. There should be minimal to no bleeding to the site of the arterial puncture.
- ***Patient Teaching.*** Before discharge, the nurse instructs the patient to remain on bedrest for the remainder of the day. The extremity used for the arterial injection should be maintained in extension. By the next day, most physical activities may be resumed, but vigorous exercise should be avoided for an additional day or two.

◆ Nursing Response to Complications

After cerebral angiography, the overall incidence of complication is 0.5% to 3%. Complications include stroke, leg ischemia, excessive bleeding, a reaction to the contrast medium, and possible death. In most instances, the complication related to allergy occurs rapidly after the contrast medium is injected. The others occur within 1 to 2 hours after the test. If any of the nursing assessments demonstrate abnormality associated with complication, the nurse immediately informs the physician.

Vascular occlusion, stroke. The nurse continues to assess for signs of vascular occlusion in the extremity, as evidenced by tissue that is cold, pale or cyanotic, painful and has lost sensation or motor ability. Signs of vascular occlusion in the brain are the same as those of a stroke. The nurse assesses the patient for changes in the level of consciousness, loss of motor or sensory ability on one side of the face, and alterations of pupillary responses.

Mild allergic reaction. In a mild allergic reaction, nursing assessment findings include urticaria (hives and itching), angioedema (diffuse swelling of the skin), hoarseness that results from swelling of the larynx and trachea, wheezing and coughing, and nausea and vomiting. The patient seems apprehensive.

Severe allergic reaction. Severe allergic reaction begins as a mild allergic response, but progresses rapidly to greater severity. The nurse assesses the patient's breathing ability, because swelling and bronchospasm can result in pallor, cyanosis, dyspnea, and respiratory failure. Shock can occur, as evidenced by hypotension and tachycardia.

NURSING CARE—*cont'd*

If the severe reaction cannot be reversed, the patient can develop seizures, coma, and then die. The nurse assists the physician with the administration of steroid medication and subcutaneous injections of epinephrine (adrenaline). The emergency cart should be on hand, as it may be necessary for the physician to insert an endotracheal tube. Cardiopulmonary resuscitation may be necessary.

Angiography, Coronary

See Catheterization, Cardiac on p. 187.

Angiography, Fluorescein

an-jee-ah-gruh-fee, floo-o-res-een

Also called: (IVFA); Intravenous Fluorescent Angiography

SPECIMEN OR TYPE OF TEST: Photography with contrast

PURPOSE OF THE TEST

This test is used to visualize retinal circulation as part of the evaluation of retinopathy. The retinal pathology can be the result of a systemic, intraocular, or retinal disease.

BASICS THE NURSE NEEDS TO KNOW

When disease alters the retinal circulation, the changes can be seen in the retina and the blood vessels. Fluorescein angiography is used to image and document the changes, including the location and extent of the circulatory abnormality.

In the examination, the intravenous dye illuminates the blood vessels by its fluorescence. The dye leaks into the vitreous humor where there is a rupture or leakage from the damaged blood vessel. The leakage produces a hyperfluorescent area. Alternatively, an area of hypofluorescence or prolonged venous drainage is visualized when there is obstruction of the circulation from retinal artery stenosis or occlusion. Abnormal vascular patterns are characteristic of other retinal and circulatory problems, including atherosclerosis, arteriosclerosis and diabetes mellitus.

NORMAL VALUES

Retinal blood vessels are intact, with normal circulation and no evidence of leakage or obstruction.

HOW THE TEST IS DONE

After the pupils are fully dilated by mydriatic drops, the fluorescent dye is injected intravenously. A rapid series of 20 to 30 images are taken at 1- to 2-second intervals to document the retinal circulation. After a rest period, a second series of images may be obtained to document additional retinal findings.

A

SIGNIFICANCE OF TEST RESULTS

Abnormal Values

Microaneurysm
Arteriovenous shunt
Occlusion (arterial, venous)
Neovascularization
Tortuosity of blood vessels
Capillary hemangioma
Hypertensive retinopathy
Tumor
Edema (retinal, macular)
Ruptured blood vessel
Papilledema

INTERFERING FACTORS

- Allergy to the iodinated contrast medium
- Cataracts
- Insufficient dilation of the pupils
- Movement of the head, eyes, or eyelids

NURSING CARE

Pretest

- After the physician describes the procedure to the patient, a written consent is required and placed in the patient's record.
- The nurse asks the patient about any past history of allergy to iodine or seafood or of a previous reaction to contrast material during a radiographic examination. The nurse also assesses the patient's baseline vital signs and records the results.
- ***Patient Teaching.*** If the patient has glaucoma, instruct him or her to omit eye drop medication on the morning of the test. Glaucoma medication constricts the pupils, so the pupillary dilation needed for the test would be difficult to accomplish.

During the Test

- The nurse dilates the pupils with mydriatic eye drops, as prescribed. The nurse inserts an intravenous line into a vein of the antecubital fossa for the purpose of administration of the contrast material.
- Instruct the patient to sit in a chair with the chin and forehead resting against supports. The camera is positioned in front of the eye and is focused on the retina. The patient is told to keep the head immobile and to stare straight ahead. Normal breathing and blinking are permitted during the photography phase. The nurse informs the patient that nausea, hot flashes, or a sensation of warmth may be experienced as the fluorescein dye is injected. Vomiting may occur.
- After the photographs are taken, remove the intravenous needle and instruct the patient to rest for 20 to 60 minutes. If a second series of photographs is taken after the rest interval, no additional dye is needed. This is because the dye continues to circulate and the retinal vessels remain clearly visible.

NURSING CARE—*cont'd*

Posttest

- In preparation for discharge, the nurse teaches the patient that the skin and sclera will become bright yellow because the dye circulates throughout the body before excretion. The yellow color will disappear in 4 to 6 hours. The urine will become fluorescent yellow-orange for about 24 hours as the dye is excreted from the body. The patient is taught to drink extra fluids to help with the renal clearance of the dye.
- Because the pupils remain dilated for a few hours, the nurse instructs the patient to wear sunglasses to protect the eyes from the glare of sunlight. The nurse also advises the patient to avoid driving a car until the vision becomes clear.

◆ Nursing Response to Complications

The complication of allergic reaction to the dye can occur. The fluorescein dye contains iodine. In most instances, the complication related to allergy occurs rapidly after the contrast medium is injected. Should any of the nursing assessments demonstrate abnormality associated with allergic response, the nurse immediately informs the physician.

Mild allergic reaction. In a mild allergic reaction, nursing assessment findings include urticaria (hives and itching), angioedema (diffuse swelling of the skin), hoarseness that results from swelling of the larynx and trachea, wheezing and coughing, and nausea and vomiting. The patient seems apprehensive. A mild reaction will generally respond to the prescribed intravenous or intramuscular administration of the antihistamine diphenhydramine hydrochloride (Benadryl).

Severe allergic reaction. Severe allergic reaction begins as a mild allergic response, but progresses rapidly. The nurse will assess the patient's breathing ability, because swelling and bronchospasm can result in pallor, cyanosis, dyspnea, and respiratory failure. Shock can occur, as evidenced by hypotension and tachycardia. If the severe reaction cannot be reversed, the patient may develop seizures, coma, and then die. The nurse assists the physician with the administration of steroid medication and subcutaneous injections of epinephrine (adrenaline). The emergency cart should be on hand, as it may be necessary for the physician to insert an endotracheal tube. CPR may be necessary.

Angiography, Pulmonary

an-jee-ah-gruh-fee, pul-muh-ne-ree

Also called: Pulmonary Arteriography

SPECIMEN OR TYPE OF TEST: Radiography

PURPOSE OF THE TEST

Pulmonary angiography is used primarily to confirm the diagnosis of pulmonary embolism. It may be performed to diagnose congenital or acquired abnormalities of pulmonary vasculature.

BASICS THE NURSE NEEDS TO KNOW

Pulmonary angiography is an invasive diagnostic procedure in which radiocontrast medium is injected into the pulmonary artery or its branches to visualize the pulmonary vascular bed. It is usually performed when a pulmonary embolism is suspected and other less invasive procedures cannot exclude or confirm the diagnosis.

Risks are involved with pulmonary angiography; however, most of the problems are manageable, such as dysrhythmias, an allergic response to the contrast medium, and infection of the venous access site. There is no absolute contraindication for pulmonary angiography, but certain conditions may require adaptations of the technique used. These conditions include systemic anticoagulation, pregnancy, an uncooperative patient, severe hypoxia, pulmonary hypertension, right-sided endocarditis (risk of dislodging vegetation), left bundle branch block (risk of complete heart block), and amiodarone pulmonary toxicity.

NORMAL VALUES Pulmonary vessels fill quickly and symmetrically, with no filling defects, narrowing, or obstruction.

HOW THE TEST IS DONE

The procedure is performed in an angiography laboratory in which cardiac monitoring equipment and emergency equipment are available. With the patient supine, a catheter is inserted via the antecubital or femoral vein into the right or left pulmonary artery, or both (the decision is based on previous testing). Multiple films are taken after the dye is administered through the catheter.

Additional imaging techniques are available in some laboratories and may be part of the angiography. These techniques include *high-resolution cineangiography, balloon occlusion angiography,* and *digital subtraction angiography.* Cineangiography has the advantage of delineating flow and motion and helping to distinguish questionable filling defects and overlapping structures. Balloon occlusion angiography involves occlusion of the pulmonary artery with a balloon catheter. A smaller amount of contrast dye is needed with balloon occlusion angiography, which permits excellent opacification. Digital subtraction angiography allows dye to be inserted into the superior vena cava or right atrium; thus, the procedure is less invasive.

SIGNIFICANCE OF TEST RESULTS

Pulmonary embolism
Pulmonary artery stenosis
Pulmonary arteriovenous fistula

INTERFERING FACTORS

- Uncooperative patient
- Noncompliance with dietary restrictions

NURSING CARE

Pretest

- Perform and document baseline assessments.
- Ensure that informed consent has been obtained.
- The nurse checks blood test results for PT, PTT, and platelet determinations. Ensure that a baseline electrocardiogram and electrolyte, blood urea nitrogen, creatinine, and arterial blood gases (ABG) determinations are performed, that the results are in the patient's chart, and that abnormalities are reported.
- The nurse checks with the patient for a history of allergic reaction to contrast dyes or shellfish. The nurse also reports and documents the allergies according to hospital protocol.
- If a femoral vein is to be used as the access site, shave the area, if necessary. If the patient is taking anticoagulants, the angiography procedure is usually performed with the antecubital approach.
- The nurse ensures that the patient maintains adequate hydration. A peripheral intravenous line is usually inserted.
- ***Patient Teaching.*** Instruct the patient about the procedure. Warn the patient that a warm, flushed, or nauseated feeling may ensue when the dye is injected but that this feeling passes quickly.
- ***Patient Teaching.*** The nurse instructs the patient not to eat or drink, except for sips of water, for 4 to 6 hours before the procedure.

During the Test

- The patient is awake and will need reassurance and explanations by the nurse during the procedure.
- Place the patient on a cardiac monitor and observe cardiac rhythm during the procedure.
- Place the patient in the supine position. The site of venous entry is exposed, and the patient is draped.
- After a local anesthetic is given, right-sided heart catheterization is performed under electrocardiographic monitoring and intermittent fluoroscopy. As the catheter is inserted, the nurse records pressure readings.
- Contrast dye is warmed to body temperature. The nurse again reassures the patient that any discomfort felt when the dye is administered is temporary.
- The nurse continuously monitors the patient for complications related to the dye (allergic reaction, anaphylaxis, or bronchospasms) or to catheterization (dysrhythmias, cardiac perforation).

Posttest

- Maintain the patient on bedrest for 2 to 4 hours. Keep the patient warm.
- Apply pressure to the site for a minimum of 5 minutes. The nurse checks the venous access site for hemostasis, and assesses distal pulses.

Continued

NURSING CARE—*cont'd*

Nursing Response to Complications

The nurse monitors for indications of complications following pulmonary angiography; such as bleeding and arterial occlusion. In addition, observe for hypotension caused by osmotic diuresis and any delayed allergic reaction to the dye.

Bleeding. The nurse observes for overt and covert bleeding. Vital signs may indicate tachycardia and hypotension. The nurse should also observe for restlessness, confusion, pallor, cool skin, and decreased urinary output. The nurse immediately notifies the physician and anticipates an order for hemoglobin and hematocrit. A blood typing and cross-matching may also be ordered.

Arterial occlusion. A hematoma may form at the site of the arterial insertion site. The nurse will assess for distal pulses and the temperature and color of the skin distal to the insertion site. If the nurse identifies decreased perfusion distal to the arterial access, the physician is notified immediately.

Angiography, Vascular

an-jee-ah-gruh-fee, vas-kyuh-luhr

Also called: Arteriography

SPECIMEN OR TYPE OF TEST: Radiography

PURPOSE OF THE TEST

Angiography is used to investigate arterial vascular disease, to provide visualization of the arteries during treatment procedures, and to evaluate the effectiveness of vascular surgery in the postoperative period.

BASICS THE NURSE NEEDS TO KNOW

Angiography is an invasive test that uses an arterial injection of contrast medium to visualize the lumens of arteries. Multiple radiographic images are taken with fluoroscopy and x-ray to illustrate the arterial abnormality. Common abnormalities include atherosclerosis, embolus, aneurysm, stenosis, arteriovenous fistula, and arteriovenous malformation. Angiography can provide a view of the arterial circulation of specific sites or organs including the heart, brain, lung, kidney, liver, spleen and pancreas.

Technique of Angiography

Angiography is performed using a 2% lidocaine solution for local anesthesia. The patient may also receive sedative-analgesia to promote relaxation. The procedure is performed under sterile conditions to minimize the risk of septicemia.

Arterial access is achieved by the use of a special needle or catheter that passes through the skin and is inserted directly into an artery. When a needle is used, the access is by puncture technique. Once the needle has been properly placed in the lumen of the artery, the contrast medium is instilled by an automatic injection through the hollow core of the needle. When a catheter is used, a small incision in the skin is made. The catheter with guidewire is carefully manipulated by the physician and advanced through the arterial structure until the tip reaches the area to be examined (Figure 15). After the guidewire is removed, the contrast medium is injected by automated technique.

The arterial puncture site is usually the common femoral artery because the artery has a wide lumen and is superficial in location. In the transfemoral approach, the puncture or incision site is in the groin on the side with the best pulse (Figure 16). When this site is not suitable, the physician may use the transaxillary or translumbar approach. The nurse must know the location of the arterial entry site because in the posttest period, the site must be assessed for the presence or absence of distal pulses, potential bleeding and possible neurologic deficits.

Contrast Medium

A variety of intravascular agents can be used to provide the arterial radio-opacity needed for imaging. When the contrast medium is injected into the patient by the physician, it is common and normal for the patient to experience brief pain, heat, a warm feeling, or a burning sensation. Some of the contrast medium preparations

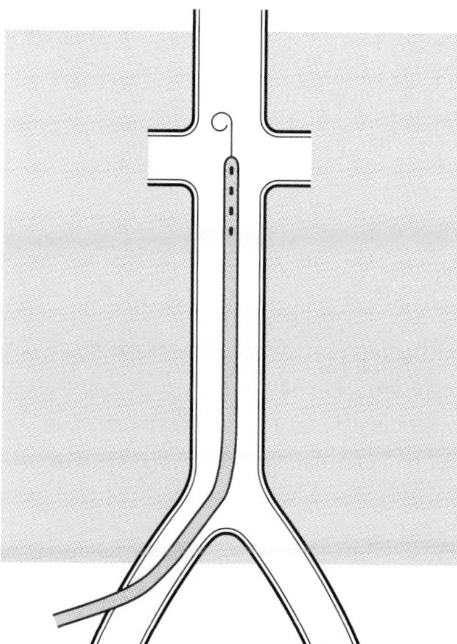

Figure 15. Transfemoral catheterization of the abdominal aorta. Once the catheter is inserted into the femoral artery, it is advanced in a retrograde direction through the aorta until it reaches the desired level.

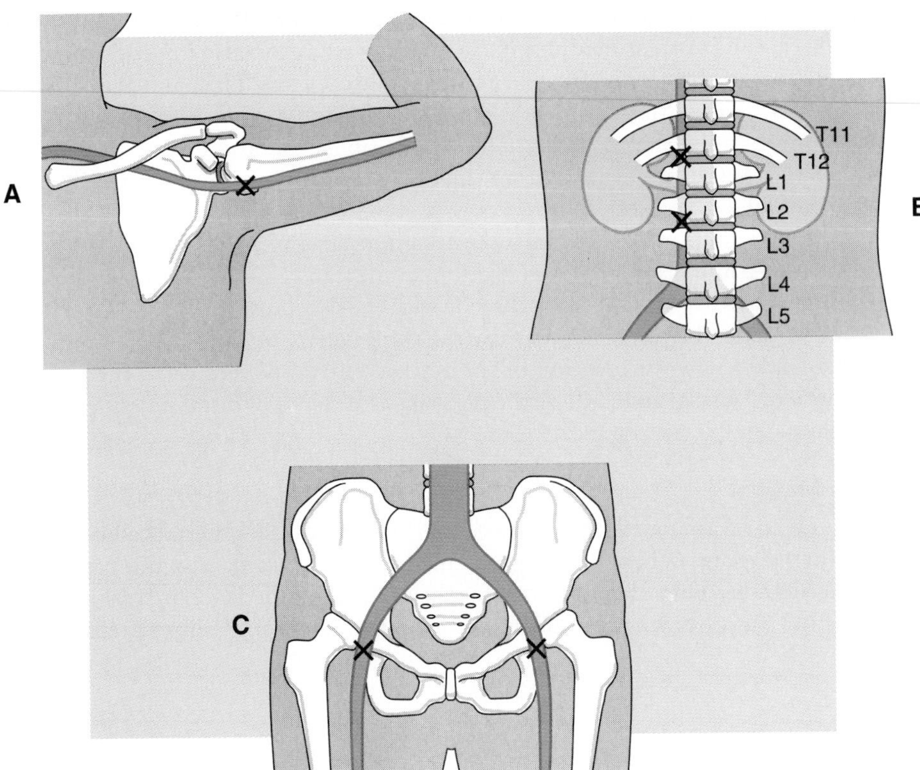

Figure 16. Arterial access sites for angiography. *A,* Transaxillary arterial puncture, frontal view. *B,* Translumbar aortography arterial puncture, dorsal view. *C,* Femoral arterial puncture, frontal view.

contain iodine. The noniodinated contrast is sometimes selected by the physician for patients who are at increased risk for an allergic reaction, including hives, urticaria, flushing, and nausea. However, both the iodinated and the noniodinated contrast preparations can cause severe cardiorespiratory complications. The more uncommon, but severe reactions include bronchoconstriction, laryngeal edema, and cardiopulmonary arrest.

The contrast medium is excreted from the body by the kidneys. In almost all cases, the contrast is eliminated without renal damage, but the iodinated contrast is somewhat nephrotoxic. Occasionally renal failure occurs after the angiographic procedure is completed. The cause is not clearly understood, but the nurse maintains the patient's hydration status before, during, and after the procedure to promote complete excretion of the contrast medium.

NORMAL VALUES No anatomic or functional abnormalities of the arteries are noted. No stenosis, occlusion, aneurysm, or bleeding is visualized.

HOW THE TEST IS DONE

Contrast medium is injected into an artery via a needle or an arterial catheter. Fluoroscopic images and serial x-ray films are taken to demonstrate the vasculature and any arterial abnormalities that are present. The procedure requires 30 to 90 minutes to complete.

SIGNIFICANCE OF TEST RESULTS

Abnormal Values

Peripheral vascular disease
Arterial occlusion
Aneurysm
Vascular fistula
Traumatic arterial injury
Thromboangiitis obliterans
Fibromuscular dysplasia
Collagen vascular disease
Arterial spasm
Tumor
Arteriovenous malformation
Inflammatory vasculitis
Giant cell arteritis
Raynaud's disease or phenomenon

INTERFERING FACTORS

- Severe allergy to contrast medium (iodine)
- Recent myocardial infarction
- Coagulation disorder
- Renal failure
- Sickle cell disease
- Homocystinuria

NURSING CARE

Pretest

- ***Patient Teaching.*** To help reduce distress and anxiety, the nurse instructs the patient regarding the procedure. Most patients do not know much about the test and will benefit from information. The discussion can help with accurate expectations and reduction of the anxiety associated with the unknown. In addition, the patient teaching provides information so that the patient follows the required preparation measures.

Continued

NURSING CARE—*cont'd*

- ***Patient Teaching.*** The patient is taught to drink extra fluids on the days before and after the test. No food can be taken after midnight or 8 hours before the test, but clear liquids and medications (except heparin) can be continued during this time.
- ***Patient Teaching.*** The nurse informs the patient that analgesic and sedative medication usually is given in the pretest period to help with relaxation. A local anesthetic will be injected to numb the tissue surrounding the arterial puncture site.
- ***Patient Teaching.*** The patient is informed that he or she will lie on the radiography table and be unable to move during the test. There is equipment in the room for imaging, computer calculations, and radiographs. The patient will hear clicking and whirring sounds during the procedure. As the contrast medium is injected, the patient may feel a burning sensation or heat, pain, or nausea. Although momentary discomfort occurs, the sensations are normal and brief.
- During the assessment interview, the nurse identifies and reports any patient history of allergy to iodine or shellfish or of previous reaction to a radiologic procedure that used a contrast medium or dye. Once the physician has explained the procedure, a written consent form must be signed by the patient.
- The nurse ensures that recent laboratory test results are posted in the patient's record. Blood urea nitrogen and creatinine determinations are needed to verify adequate renal function. Activated partial thromboplastin time, prothrombin time, and platelet determinations are needed to verify adequate clotting ability. The nurse notifies the physician of abnormal values.
- The nurse monitors the vital signs and records the results in the chart. Hypertension should be under control before this test is performed. On the morning of the test, the peripheral pulses are assessed and the findings are recorded. A small ink mark should be placed on the skin to record the distal sites of pulsation.
- ***Patient Teaching.*** The patient is instructed to void to empty the bladder before going to the radiology department. The contrast medium acts as a diuretic and can cause the discomfort of a full bladder. The patient receives assistance, as needed, to remove all clothing and put on a hospital gown. All metal objects, such as jewelry, must be removed from the area of the x-ray field.
- The nurse administers the on-call pretest sedation. This usually consists of an intramuscular injection of the narcotic analgesic meperidine (Demerol) and a sedative-relaxant such as midazolam (Versed) or diazepam (Valium).

During the Test

- Intravenous fluids are administered during the test and an intravenous line is established before the test begins. Instruct the patient to remain motionless on the narrow table during the imaging procedure.

Posttest

- The nurse places the patient on bedrest for 6 to 8 hours. The punctured extremity is to be kept straight. When the aorta has been used as the puncture site, the patient must remain in the supine position for the same amount of time.
- The nurse assesses the vital signs and peripheral pulses every 15 minutes for 1 hour and every hour for 2 hours. With a femoral puncture site, the pertinent pulses are

NURSING CARE—*cont'd*

those of the popliteal, dorsalis pedis, and posterior tibialis arteries on the affected side. With an aortic puncture site, the bilateral pulses include the femoral sites as well as those of the lower extremities. With an axillary puncture site, the brachial, radial, and ulnar pulses are significant.

- The nurse assesses and compares the extremities bilaterally for signs of occlusion of the circulation and neurologic deficit. The data include color, warmth, movement, and the absence of neurologic signs, such as pain or paresthesias.
- The pressure dressing and the tissue surrounding the puncture site are observed frequently for signs of swelling or hematoma. Gentle palpation of the tissue near the puncture site also may be performed.
- Extra fluid intake is essential to prevent nephrotoxicity from the contrast medium. The patient should drink extra fluids to achieve a 2000- to 3000-mL intake in the 24-hour posttest period. Because of the high volume of fluids and the diuretic effect of the contrast material, the patient will experience a frequent need to urinate. Remind the patient that a urinal or bedpan must be used during the period of bedrest. Intake and output measurements are recorded.

◆ Nursing Response to Complications

The overall complication rate for the angiography procedure is 1% to 3%. Complications at the puncture site are the largest group of problems and consist of hemorrhage or hematoma formation. Thrombus or embolus also may occur because thrombi tend to form at the puncture site, on the catheter or guidewire, or at the area of arterial wall abnormality. Neurologic complications are varied, depending on the underlying cause or location. If hemorrhage or hematoma compresses the nerve or nerve plexus, the compression can result in paralysis of the distal extremity. When cerebral angiography is performed, the patient can experience cerebral ischemia or a stroke, caused by a thrombus or embolus. Reaction to the contrast medium consists of an allergic response, cardiorespiratory complications, and renal failure. The nurse monitors and assesses for complications and calls the physician immediately should abnormal findings appear.

Hematoma and bleeding. When hematoma or hemorrhage occurs, there are ecchymosis and swelling near the puncture site. The patient may complain of severe pain or paresthesias (numbness and tingling) in the distal extremity. If the bleeding is severe, the patient may develop signs of shock, including hypotension and tachycardia. Until the physician can evaluate the situation, ice can be applied to the puncture site to slow the bleeding.

Vascular occlusion. In the event of formation of a thrombus or embolus, the assessment findings reveal diminished or absent pulses distally. The distal extremity becomes cool, dusky, and cyanotic. The patient may report loss of sensation or paresthesias in the distal extremity. There may be a loss of motor function and the patient may experience pain distally.

If there is an embolus or thrombus in the cerebral circulation, the nursing neurologic assessment monitors for a change in the level of consciousness and changes in the functions of the cranial nerves.

Continued

NURSING CARE—*cont'd*

Mild allergic reaction. A mild allergic reaction to contrast medium consists of skin that is red with swelling and itching from hives. The nurse prepares to counteract this reaction with the administration of diphenhydramine hydrochloride (Benadryl), as prescribed.

Severe allergic reaction. If the reaction to the contrast medium becomes severe, the nurse begins frequent and specific assessment for potential respiratory and cardiac complications. Respirations are monitored for abnormal rate, rhythm, and effort, particularly dyspnea. The lungs are assessed for the presence of wheezes, crackles, or rhonchi. The patient may develop shock with hypotension and tachycardia. If this very serious anaphylactic reaction occurs, it is usually rapid and unrelenting. Because complete obstruction of the airway can occur, the nurse brings the emergency cart to the patient's bedside. To assist the patient with breathing, the nurse prepares to administer oxygen and places the patient in full Fowler's position. The nurse also prepares to assist with additional treatments, including probable administration of steroids, and possible insertion of an endotracheal tube. It is essential that the physician assess the patient immediately and begin to treat the complication before the airway closes completely and the heart develops severe arrhythmia or cardiac standstill. CPR may be necessary.

Angiotensin-Converting Enzyme

an-jee-oh-ten-sin kuhn-vur-ting en-zaim

Also called: (ACE); Serum Angiotensin-Converting Enzyme (SACE)

SPECIMEN OR TYPE OF TEST: Serum

PURPOSE OF THE TEST

ACE levels are determined to evaluate possible cause of hypertension and to diagnose and treat sarcoidosis.

BASICS THE NURSE NEEDS TO KNOW

Angiotensin-converting enzyme (ACE) is found primarily in the pulmonary epithelial cells. ACE converts angiotensin I to angiotensin II. Angiotensin II stimulates the adrenal cortex to produce and secrete the hormone aldosterone and is also a powerful vasoconstrictor. Because angiotensin II is a vasopressor, ACE levels are determined as part of the diagnostic work-up for hypertension.

ACE levels increase with sarcoidosis, a disease that causes widespread granulomatous lesions that may affect any organ, including the lungs. When sarcoidosis is suspected, ACE levels are determined to diagnose the disorder, assess its severity, and evaluate its therapy.

NORMAL VALUES

Adult male: 12–36 international units/L *or* SI: 12–36 international units/L
Female: 10–30 international units/L *or* SI: 10–30 international units/L
Children and adolescents: 15–50 international units/L *or* SI: 15–50 international units/L

HOW THE TEST IS DONE

A venipuncture is performed to collect a sample in a red-topped tube. If a delay is expected in sending the specimen to the laboratory, place the specimen on ice.

SIGNIFICANCE OF TEST RESULTS

Elevated Values

Cirrhosis
Gaucher's disease (familial disorder of fat metabolism)
Hansen's disease
Histoplasmosis
Hodgkin's disease
Hyperthyroidism
Myeloma
Pulmonary fibrosis
Sarcoidosis
Scleroderma

Decreased Values

Adult respiratory distress syndrome
Diabetes mellitus
Hypothyroidism
Tuberculosis

INTERFERING FACTOR

- Steroids

NURSING CARE

The nursing actions are similar to those for other venipuncture procedures, as presented in Chapter 2.

A

Anion Gap

an-yuhn gap

Also called: Electrolyte Gap; Ion Gap

SPECIMEN OR TYPE OF TEST: Serum

PURPOSE OF THE TEST

The anion gap is calculated to determine the cause of metabolic acidosis.

BASICS THE NURSE NEEDS TO KNOW

The anion gap is the sum of unmeasured anions in the serum: phosphates, sulfates, ketones, proteins, and organic acids. It is used to distinguish among causes of metabolic acidosis. The anion gap is used to determine if the metabolic acidosis is a result of the accumulation of hydrogen ions or due to a loss of bicarbonate.

The major determinant of the anion gap is protein. A significant decrease in plasma protein causes a large decrease in the anion gap.

In addition to disease states that cause an increase or decrease in anions or cations, or both, in the blood, fluid volume also affects the anion gap, because it may cause hemoconcentration (higher sodium and potassium concentration) or hemodilution (dilutional hyponatremia).

NORMAL VALUES

3–11 mEq/L *or* SI: 3–11 mmol/L, *or*
10–15 mEq/L *or* SI: 10–15 mmol/L, depending on laboratory methodology

HOW THE TEST IS DONE

The anion gap is determined by subtracting the sum of measured anions (bicarbonate [HCO_3] and chloride [Cl]) from the measured cations (sodium [Na] and potassium [K]).

SIGNIFICANCE OF TEST RESULTS

Elevated Values

Hypernatremia
Hyperosmolar coma
Hypocalcemia
Hypomagnesemia
Ketoacidosis
Lactic acidosis
Starvation

Decreased Values

Hypercalcemia
Hypermagnesemia
Hypoalbuminemia

Hyponatremia
Multiple myeloma

INTERFERING FACTORS

- Dehydration
- Ingestion of licorice
- Excessive ingestion of antacids, ethylene glycol, methanol, paraldehyde, or salicylates
- Use of medications such as adrenocorticotropic hormones, antihypertensive agents, bicarbonates, chlorpropamide, diuretics, lithium, Na penicillin, phosphates, steroids, sulfates, and vasopressin

NURSING CARE

After the results of blood electrolyte determinations are obtained, calculate the anion gap during the test with the following formula:

$$(Na + K) - (HCO_3 + Cl) = \text{Anion gap}$$

Antidiuretic Hormone

See Vasopressin on p. 665.

Anti-DNA

an-tai-dee-en-ay

Also called: DNA Antibody; Antibody to Double-Stranded DNA (Anti-ds-DNA); Antibody to Native DNA (n-DNA)

SPECIMEN OR TYPE OF TEST: Serum

PURPOSE OF THE TEST

The anti-DNA test helps confirm the diagnosis of systemic lupus erythematosus (SLE). It is also used to monitor the response to treatment.

BASICS THE NURSE NEEDS TO KNOW

In autoimmune disease, antibodies attach to and destroy nuclear or cytoplasm antigens in one's own body tissue. The autoimmune response causes inflammation, fibrosis, and destruction of a single target organ, or the process becomes disseminated, meaning that it affects many different organs or tissues.

Elevated Values

Anti-DNA is one of the specific antinuclear antibody (ANA) tests. Antibody to double-stranded DNA is highly elevated in the serum of 75% to 90% of patients with active systemic lupus erythematosus at some time during an active phase of illness. It is present to a much lesser degree in patients with other collagen vascular or autoimmune diseases. By enzyme-linked immunosorbent assay, a value of 25 to 30 international units/mL is considered to be a borderline result, and a value of 31 to 200 international units/mL or more is positive. When the value is in the high or very high range, it is specific for SLE. It may take several years before a medical diagnosis of SLE can be made, based on this test, other antibody tests and clinical symptoms of the illness.

SLE is a disease of exacerbation and remission, meaning there are "flare-ups" of active illness and quiet periods when there is less disease activity. The level of anti-DNA is much higher during exacerbations. To monitor the patient during an active phase, this test may be ordered every 1 to 3 months; during remission, it may be ordered every 6 to 12 months.

NORMAL VALUES Enzyme immunoassay method: Negative; <25 international units/mL

HOW THE TEST IS DONE

A red-topped tube is used to collect 10 mL of venous blood.

SIGNIFICANCE OF TEST RESULTS

Active systemic lupus erythematosus
Discoid lupus erythematosus
Rheumatoid arthritis
Other collagen vascular or rheumatic disorders
Chronic active hepatitis (lupoid hepatitis)

INTERFERING FACTORS

- Administration of radioactive isotopes in the preceding 7 days
- Warming of the specimen

NURSING CARE

Nursing actions are similar to those used in other venipuncture procedures (see Chapter 2), with the following additional measures.

Pretest

- Schedule this test before any radioactive isotope test.

Posttest

- Arrange for prompt transport of the specimen to the laboratory, because the specimen will require chilling.
- The nurse can assist by obtaining a history of the patient's symptoms. The patient with SLE complains of fatigue, fever, muscle aches, and pains in small joints, including those of the feet and hands. There is a characteristic rash across the bridge of the nose and on both cheeks. It is called a butterfly rash because of its characteristic

NURSING CARE—*cont'd*

shape. The exacerbation of illness often occurs with exposure to sunlight, stress, infection, and treatment with antibiotic therapy. The nurse also notes the patient's recent use of medications, because some of them can cause drug-induced lupus, a temporary condition. Medications include procainamide hydrochloride (Pronestyl), hydralazine hydrochloride (Apresoline), and chlorpromazine (Thorazine).

Antiglobulin Tests

an-ti-glo-byuh-lin tests

Also called: (DAT); Antiglobulin Test, Direct; Direct Coombs' Test; (IAT); Antiglobulin Test, Indirect; Indirect Coombs' Test

SPECIMEN OR TYPE OF TEST: Blood

PURPOSE OF THE TEST

The *direct antiglobulin test* is part of the posttransfusion work-up to detect red blood cell incompatibility between donor and recipient blood. It is also used to help diagnose erythroblastosis fetalis, or hemolytic disease of the newborn, and helps confirm the diagnosis of hemolytic anemia.

The *indirect antiglobulin test* is used as an antibody screen in type and crossmatch testing in preparation for blood transfusion. It detects maternal-fetal blood incompatibility and predicts the hematologic risk to the fetus. It is used to evaluate the need for $RH_0(D)$ immune globulin administration and helps confirm the diagnosis of hemolytic anemia.

BASICS THE NURSE NEEDS TO KNOW

The antiglobulin tests consist of direct and indirect tests. They are used to detect the presence of antibodies in the serum and antigens on erythrocytes (Figure 17). When an antigen-antibody reaction has occurred in the blood, the erythrocytes become coated with antibody globin, and the erythrocytes agglutinate (clump together). In severe conditions, lysis of the coated erythrocytes occurs. The lysis of many erythrocytes results in hemolytic anemia.

Direct Antiglobulin Test

The direct antiglobulin test detects antibodies attached to red blood cells. In this antigen-antibody reaction the coated cells are "sensitized" and then clump together in the process called *agglutination*. The severity of the reaction depends on the number of antibodies produced and the number of erythrocytes affected. This test would detect the antigen-antibody reaction during the transfusion of incompatible blood of the donor to the recipient. It also detects the Rh_0 incompatibility between the expectant mother and the fetus. Because the blood types of the mother and fetus are incompatible, the

A

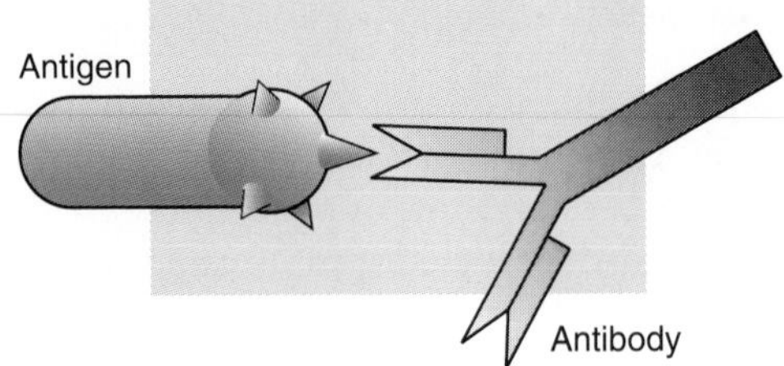

Figure 17. Antigen and antibody. A specific antibody matches the antigen based on the characteristic shape that protrudes from the antigen surface. Once the antibody locks onto the antigen, the antigen is destroyed by phagocytosis, an enzyme toxin from complement, or other biochemical response of the immune system.

maternal antibodies attack the erythrocytes of the fetus. As the erythrocytes of the fetus become coated, agglutinate, and undergo hemolysis, erythroblastosis fetalis or hemolytic anemia of the newborn develops.

Some medications also cause elevation of the direct antiglobulin test. Methyldopa (Aldomet), acetaminophen, and quinidine are the medications often involved, but others are penicillin, cephalosporin, tetracycline, sulfonamides, levodopa, and insulin. Protein in the medication is the antigenic substance, and IgG or complement causes the erythrocytes to become coated. In most of these cases, the direct antiglobulin test result is elevated, but in a few cases, hemolytic anemia results.

Indirect Antiglobulin Test

The indirect antiglobulin test detects the presence of antibodies in the patient's serum.

In the first trimester of pregnancy, this test is used to screen the expectant Rh negative mother for potential blood incompatibility with the fetus. When the test result is negative, the test is repeated in the 28th week of pregnancy and at delivery. Whenever the test becomes positive for the presence of antibodies, it is followed up with antibody identification, a titer reading, and possible amniocentesis. The development of maternal antibodies occurs in the Rh-negative mother who carries an Rh-positive fetus. The antibodies cross the placental barrier, enter the fetal circulation, and result in the coating and agglutination of fetal erythrocytes.

Methyldopa is a common drug cause of elevated indirect antiglobulin test results.

NORMAL VALUES

Negative

HOW THE TEST IS DONE

Direct Antiglobulin Test

One red-topped tube and one lavender-topped tube are used to collect 10 mL and 7 mL, respectively, of venous blood. In the newborn, venous cord blood may be collected.

Indirect Antiglobulin Test

A red-topped tube is used to collect 10 mL of venous blood.

SIGNIFICANCE OF TEST RESULTS

Positive Values

Direct Antiglobulin

Autoimmune hemolytic anemia
Hemolytic transfusion reaction
Hemolytic disease of the newborn
Sensitivity to particular medications

Indirect Antiglobulin

Maternal-fetal blood incompatibility
Autoimmune hemolytic anemia
Sensitivity to particular medications

INTERFERING FACTORS

- Hemolysis
- Inadequate identification of the specimen

NURSING CARE

Nursing actions are similar to those used in other venipuncture procedures (see Chapter 2), with the following additional measures.

Pretest

- Include the following information on the requisition form: recent history of blood transfusion or plasma expanders, obstetric history, and the pertinent medications taken by the patient.

Posttest

- Ensure that the specimen label and requisition slip include the patient's name and identification number and the source of the blood (venous, cord).

Antinuclear Antibody

an-ti-noo-klee-er an-tib-od-ee

Also called: (ANA); Fluorescent Antinuclear Antibody, (FANA)

SPECIMEN OR TYPE OF TEST: Serum

PURPOSE OF THE TEST

The ANA test is used as a screen to detect systemic lupus erythematosus and other connective tissue disorders.

BASICS THE NURSE NEEDS TO KNOW

An autoimmune disease is a disorder caused by an immunologic reaction against one's own tissue antigens. When the antibodies attack one or more antigens in the cell nuclei, the antibodies are called *antinuclear antibodies,* or ANA. Of the many different autoimmune disorders, some affect cell nuclei of a single organ and others cause systemic disease, affecting the cell nuclei of many tissues.

Positive ANA results identify the presence of the antibodies of various systemic rheumatic diseases, but ANA cannot identify a specific disease. As a screening tool, however, ANA is particularly relevant in the detection of systemic lupus erythematosus. A titer of 1:320 or higher is considered a very significant indicator of systemic lupus erythematosus.

Antinuclear Antibody Subtypes

For more specific information, a *precipitin panel* of antibody subtypes may be ordered to follow-up on a positive ANA test result. These subtypes include anti-ds-DNA, anti-Ro, anti-La, anti-nRNP, and anti-Smith autoantibody. When positive, the subtype is highly specific for a particular connective tissue disease.

The ANA test can produce false-positive results because of medications, including procainamide (Pronestyl) and hydralazine (Apresoline), and a number of other drugs. It can also produce false-positive results in normal individuals, particularly normal elderly individuals. In these cases, however, the titer elevation is low.

NORMAL VALUES

Negative; titer by immunofluorescent assay: <1:40

HOW THE TEST IS DONE

A red-topped tube is used to collect 10 mL of blood.

SIGNIFICANCE OF TEST RESULTS

Elevated Values

Systemic Autoimmune Diseases

Systemic lupus erythematosus
Rheumatoid arthritis
Polymyositis
Dermatomyositis
Progressive systemic sclerosis (scleroderma)
Mixed connective tissue disease
Sjögren syndrome

Autoimmune Diseases of the Blood and Target Organs

Hashimoto's thyroiditis
Myxedema
Thyrotoxicosis
Hepatic or biliary cirrhosis
Leukemia
Chronic renal failure
Multiple sclerosis
Pernicious anemia
Regional ileitis
Ulcerative colitis

Gluten-sensitive enteropathy
Pemphigus vulgaris

INTERFERING FACTORS

- Hemolysis of the specimen of blood

NURSING CARE

Nursing actions are similar to those used in other venipuncture procedures (see Chapter 2), with the following additional measure.

Pretest

- On the laboratory requisition slip, list any medications taken by the patient.

Antithrombin III

See Coagulation Inhibitors on p. 209.

Arginine Vasopressin

See Vasopressin on p. 665.

Arterial Blood Gases

ahr-tee-ree-uhl blud ga-sez

Also called: ABGs

SPECIMEN OR TYPE OF TEST: Arterial blood

PURPOSE OF THE TEST

ABG determinations are obtained for a variety of reasons, including the diagnosis of chronic and restrictive pulmonary disease, adult respiratory failure, acid-base disturbances, pulmonary emboli, sleep disorders, central nervous system dysfunctions, and cardiovascular disorders such as congestive heart failure, shunts, and intracardiac atrial or ventricular shunts, or both.

ABG determinations also are used in the management of patients on mechanical ventilators and during the weaning process from the ventilators.

BASICS THE NURSE NEEDS TO KNOW

ABGs provide valuable information about the acid-base balance, ventilatory ability, and oxygenation status of the individual. The data derived from blood gas determination support clinical assessments and are invaluable in evaluating medical treatment and nursing interventions. ABG determinations provide the pH, partial pressure of carbon dioxide (pCO_2), partial pressure of oxygen (pO_2), bicarbonate (HCO_3), O_2 saturation (SaO_2), and base excess/deficit levels.

The pH (the partial pressure of hydrogen [H^+] ions in the blood) reflects the acid-base balance of the blood. A narrow normal range of pH reflects the body's need to maintain a relatively constant internal environment. An inverse relationship exists on the pH scale between H^+ concentration and pH. As the H^+ ion concentration goes up, the pH goes down. As the H^+ ion concentration increases in solution, H^+ ions can be given up. This is *acidosis*. As the H^+-ion concentration decreases in solution, H^+ ions may be taken on (H^+-ion receiver). This is *alkalosis*.

The pH of human blood is normally 7.35 to 7.45, which on the pH scale of 1 to 14 is above the neutral point of 7 and therefore slightly alkaline. In the clinical setting, however, a pH of 7.35 to 7.45 is used as the neutral state. A pH below 7.35 is acidotic, and a pH above 7.45 is alkalotic. One must remember that other body fluids have a different normal pH.

To maintain a normal pH, the body has evolved several mechanisms, including buffering systems and the respiratory and renal systems. Within seconds, the body buffers respond to changes in pH. Within minutes, the respiratory system adapts to changes in H^+-ion concentration, and in days, the kidneys respond to the acid-base needs of the body. These changes reflect the body's ability to compensate for deviations in the acid-base balance and the need to maintain that balance within a narrow range.

The pCO_2 value reflects the ventilatory ability of the body to maintain a normal pH. Carbon dioxide (CO_2) in blood travels as an acid (carbonic acid) until it dissociates in the lungs to be exhaled as CO_2. If the blood becomes acidotic, the respiratory system increases its rate and depth of ventilation to blow off CO_2 and thus reduce the acid load in the blood. If the blood becomes alkalotic, the respiratory system hypoventilates to retain CO_2 and thus move the pH toward normal. Pathologic conditions of the pulmonary system may interfere with this normal compensatory action. When an individual cannot adequately ventilate, CO_2 is retained, and acidosis occurs. Because this acidosis results from a pulmonary cause, it is called *respiratory acidosis*. If the lungs blow off too much CO_2, respiratory alkalosis occurs. Table 5 presents causes of respiratory acid-base imbalances and the nursing assessments for the imbalances.

The bicarbonate ion concentration in the blood (HCO_3) reflects the renal system's response to the acid-base balance. HCO_3 is made by the kidneys, and its production is increased whenever acidosis is present. However, it takes several days for the kidneys to respond fully to changes in pH. If the kidneys are unable to make HCO_3 to buffer the acid in the blood, the patient will be in a state of metabolic acidosis. If the patient has too much HCO_3 or has lost acid from the gastrointestinal or genitourinary tract, a state of metabolic alkalosis occurs. Table 5 presents causes of metabolic acid-base imbalances and the nursing assessments for the imbalances.

The pulmonary and renal systems are constantly balancing and adapting to maintain a normal pH. An abnormality in pH initiates a compensatory mechanism to restore the pH to normal or to achieve at least a partial compensation. For example, a patient with chronic obstructive pulmonary disease retains CO_2 and thus experiences respiratory acidosis. The kidneys respond to the decrease in pH and increase their production of HCO_3. This response results in a normal pH and high pCO_2 and HCO_3 levels

TABLE 5 Causes and Assessments of Acid-Base Imbalances

Cause	Clinical Assessment
Respiratory Acidosis	
Respiratory center dysfunction	Dyspnea
Opiates, anesthetics, sedatives	Tachycardia
Oxygen-induced hypoventilation	Headache
Central nervous system lesions	Confusion
Disorders of the respiratory muscles	Pallor
or chest wall	Diaphoresis
Myasthenia gravis, amyotrophic lateral sclerosis	Apprehension
Kyphoscoliosis	Restlessness
Pickwickian syndrome	Lethargy
Splinting caused by pain	Drowsiness
Disorders of gas exchange	Coma
Chronic obstructive pulmonary disease	Hypertension
Acute pulmonary edema	Papilledema
Asphyxia	
Hypoventilation while on a mechanical ventilator	
Respiratory Alkalosis	
Hyperventilation	Restlessness
Atelectasis	Dizziness
Severe anemia	Agitation
Pulmonary emboli	Tetany
Anxiety	Numbness
Central nervous system disorders	Tingling
Brain stem dysfunction	Muscle cramps
Subarachnoid hemorrhage	Seizures
Salicylate poisoning	Increased deep tendon reflexes
Hypermetabolic states	
Fever	
Thyrotoxicosis	
Sepsis	
Hyperventilation while on mechanical ventilation	
Metabolic Acidosis	
Diabetic ketoacidosis	Lethargy
Lactic acidosis	Nausea
Cardiac arrest	Vomiting
Anaerobic metabolism	Dysrhythmias
Ingestion of acid	Coma
Salicylates	Hypotension
Ethylene	Hyperventilation

Continued

TABLE 5 Causes and Assessments of Acid-Base Imbalances—*cont'd*

Cause	Clinical Assessment
Metabolic Acidosis—*cont'd*	
Ingestion of acid—*cont'd*	
Methanol	
Paraldehyde	
Loss of bicarbonate	
Diarrhea	
Fistulas	
Renal failure	
Metabolic Alkalosis	
Loss of acid	Dullness
Vomiting	Weakness
Excessive gastric suction	Dysrhythmias
Urine loss	Tetany
Diuretics	Hypokalemia
Excessive corticosteroids	Hyperactive reflexes
Exogenous	
Endogenous	
Hypokalemia	
HCO_3 overload	
Excessive ingestion of $NaHCO_3$*	
Massive blood transfusions	
Excessive ingestion of licorice	
Nonparathyroid hypercalcemia	

*$NaHCO_3$, Sodium bicarbonate.

(Figure 18) for the process used to assess acid-base balance). A serious clinical problem occurs with mixed acid-base imbalances, in which the patient has either respiratory and metabolic acidosis or both respiratory and metabolic alkalosis, because compensation cannot take place.

The partial pressure of oxygen in the blood (pO_2) is the amount of O_2 dissolved in the plasma. SaO_2 is the percentage of hemoglobin saturated with O_2. Together, the pO_2 and the SaO_2 form the O_2 *content,* the total amount of O_2 in the blood.

When interpreting the O_2 levels in the blood, barometric pressure must be considered. At sea level, barometric pressure is 760 mm Hg; at 5000 feet above sea level, barometric pressure is 630 mm Hg; thus, the norms for pO_2, SaO_2, and O_2 content must be adjusted. Use the normal values of the laboratory doing the testing to interpret oxygen levels.

The base excess or base deficit on the ABG determinations reflects the metabolic non-respiratory contribution to the maintenance of normal pH. With a base excess, a positive balance greater than 2 correlates with metabolic alkalosis, and with a base deficit, a negative balance less than −2 correlates with metabolic acidosis.

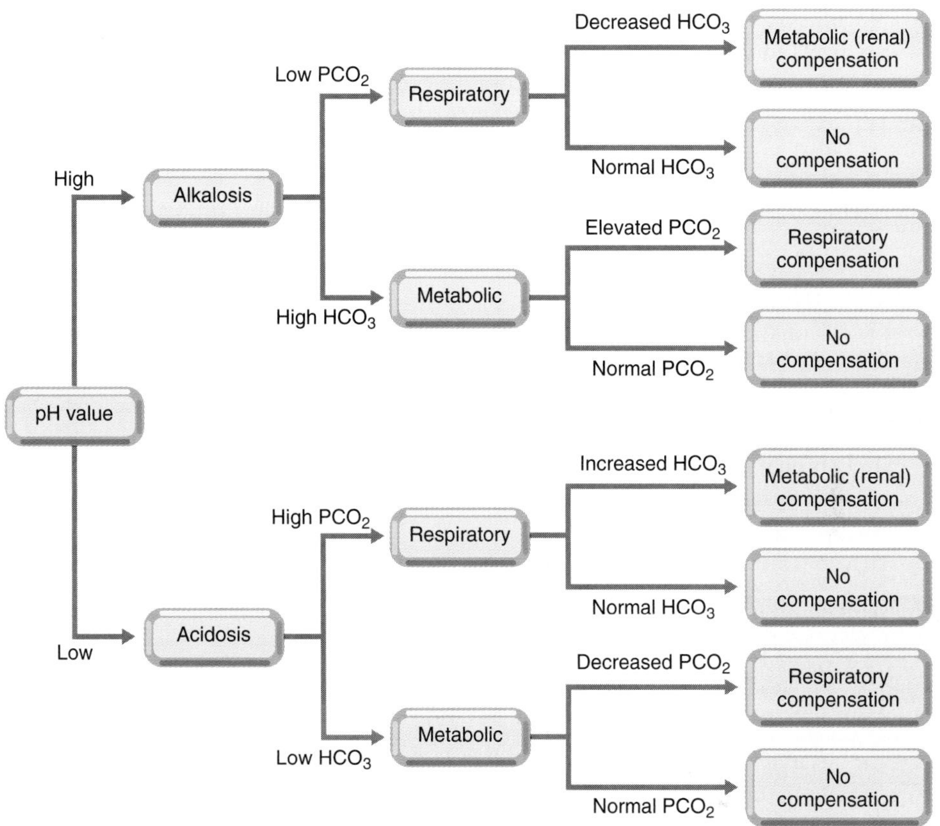

Figure 18. Evaluation of arterial blood gas results. *(Reproduced with permission from Lehmann, C. A. [Ed.]. [1998].* Saunders manual of clinical science [p. 163]. *Philadelphia: W. B. Saunders.)*

NORMAL VALUES

pH: 7.35–7.45 *or* SI: 7.35–7.45
pCO_2: 35–45 mm Hg *or* SI: 4.7–5.3 kPa
HCO_3: 21–28 mEq/L *or* SI: 21–28 mmol/L
pO_2: Adult: 80–100 mm Hg *or* SI: 10.6–13.3 kPa
  Newborn: 60–70 mm Hg *or* SI: 8.0–10.33 kPa
SaO_2: Adult: >95% *or* SI fraction saturated >0.95
  Newborn: 40%–90% *or* SI fraction saturated 0.40–0.90
Base excess/deficit: ±2 mEq/L *or* SI: ±2 mmol/L

HOW THE TEST IS DONE

An arterial blood sample of 5 mL is obtained via an arterial puncture or arterial line. The radial or femoral artery is usually used in adults, whereas the temporal artery is used in infants.

A

Continuous intra-arterial blood gas monitoring is a new technology that provides paO_2, $paCO_2$, and pH levels to be displayed. In addition, derived parameters of O_2 saturation, bicarbonate, base excess, and total CO_2 content are calculated and displayed every 20 to 30 seconds. With continuous intra-arterial blood gas monitoring, a sensor is inserted into a radial or femoral artery via an 18- or 20-gauge arterial catheter. The tip of the sensor is advanced 1 to 2 inches beyond the tip of the catheter, so it is exposed to arterial blood that is not heparinized. This method decreases the number of blood samples needed, thus conserving patient's blood.

SIGNIFICANCE OF TEST RESULTS

Acid-base imbalances (see Table 5.)
Hypoxia

INTERFERING FACTORS

- Noncompliance with proper collection procedure, including air bubbles in syringe and hemolysis of sample
- Low hemoglobin level
- With continuous intra-arterial blood gas monitoring, clot formation at sensor tip, sensor lying against arterial wall, and transition periods, when a change in FiO_2 occurs

NURSING CARE

Nursing actions are similar to those used in other arterial puncture procedures (see Chapter 2), with the following additional measures.

Pretest

- Before a radial artery puncture is executed or a radial arterial line is inserted, perform an Allen test to ensure adequate collateral circulation to the hand. With the Allen test, occlude the radial and ulnar arteries with the fingertips while instructing the patient to tighten the fist (Figure 19). Ask the patient to open the fist and remove pressure from the ulnar artery while maintaining pressure on the radial artery. If color returns to the palm and fingers within 5 seconds, adequate ulnar circulation exists.
- Prepare ice and heparinized syringe.
- Excessive amounts of heparin or an air bubble in the syringe will cause inaccurate results. Draw 1 mL of heparin up into a 5- to 10-mL glass syringe or plastic syringe with vented plunger. The plunger is pulled back to coat the barrel of the syringe. Excess heparin is ejected, leaving the syringe coated with heparin. A 22- or 25-gauge needle is used.
- The patient's temperature affects results because the ABG machines are calibrated using gases at 37° C. The nurse writes on the requisition slip the patient's temperature at the time the blood is drawn.

NURSING CARE—*cont'd*

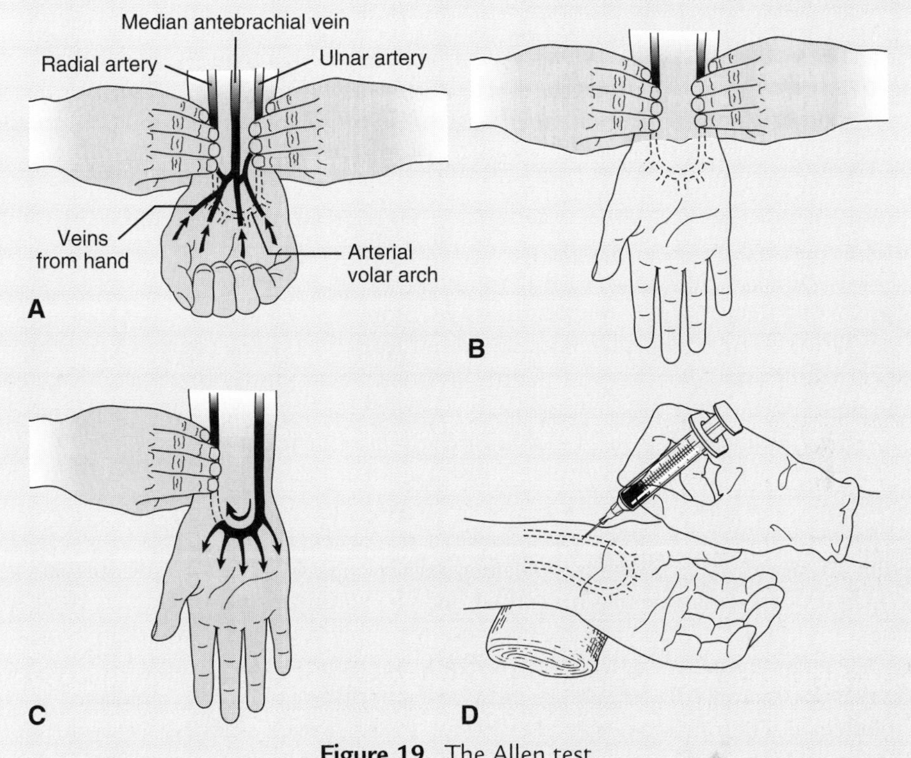

Figure 19. The Allen test.

- The nurse reassures the anxious patient, since arterial punctures are painful and hyperventilation may occur, giving false readings because CO_2 is blown off.
- Do not obtain an ABG reading for 20 to 30 minutes after a procedure or event that does not reflect the patient's current status (e.g., suctioning).

During the Test

- Nurses in specialized units may perform arterial punctures. The procedure is usually performed by a physician or a respiratory therapist. In critical care units, nurses usually obtain samples from arterial lines.
- If a radial artery is used, the wrist is hyperextended and the arm is externally rotated.
- Palpate the artery for the point of maximal impulse. Cleanse the site with an alcohol swab.
- The needle is inserted at a 45- to 90-degree angle at the point of maximal pulsation.
- Observe the syringe; the plunger will move upward under arterial pressure.
- Withdraw the needle and cork the syringe with the airtight rubber stopper.
- Roll the syringe between your palms to mix the blood with the heparin.
- Label the syringe and place it on ice.

Continued

NURSING CARE—*cont'd*

During the Test—*cont'd*

- Send the specimen to the laboratory immediately with a requisition slip marked with the patient's temperature, the FiO_2 value, and the time.
- Care of the continuous intra-arterial blood gas line is similar to care of any arterial line.

Posttest

- Immediately after the needle is withdrawn, exert pressure on the arterial site for a minimum of 5 minutes. If the patient is taking anticoagulants, pressure on the site should be maintained for at least 10 minutes.

◆ Nursing Response to Complications

Complications from ABG determination result from the trauma of arterial puncture. They include arterial occlusion from hematoma formation or thrombosis, bleeding, and infection.

Arterial occlusion. The nurse needs to check sites distal to arterial puncture for pulse, skin color, and temperature. If distal site is cold, pale, or if patient reports numbness, report findings immediately to the physician.

Bleeding. Bleeding may be overt or a hematoma may occur at the site of the arterial puncture. Keep site visible, except if femoral artery is used. Check site frequently. Palpate around site for hematoma formation. A hematoma may press on the artery, so assess for arterial occlusion. If bleeding occurs, apply pressure; notify the physician immediately if bleeding does not stop or significant blood has been lost. If a hematoma is causing a decrease in perfusion to distal parts, notify the physician immediately.

Infection. The nurse assesses the site for inflammation (redness, warmth) and patient complaint of discomfort or pain at the arterial site.

Arthrocentesis and Synovial Fluid Analysis

ahr-throh-sen-tee-sis and si-noh-vee-uhl floo-id an-al-uh-sis

Also called: Joint Fluid Analysis

SPECIMEN OR TYPE OF TEST: Synovial fluid

PURPOSE OF THE TEST

Synovial fluid analysis helps in the diagnosis of rheumatic diseases, infection, or other diseases that cause swelling of the joint, increased production of fluid, or damage to the joint space.

BASICS THE NURSE NEEDS TO KNOW

Arthrocentesis, needle aspiration of the joint, is used to obtain a sample of synovial fluid. Normally, the joint contains little fluid volume. In inflammation, infection, trauma, or irritation of the joint, cartilage, or synovial membrane, the fluid fills or distends the joint capsule. Analysis of the aspirated fluid provides data regarding the cause of the swelling and the increased fluid production.

Few to no red blood cells should be present in the fluid. If the specimen is grossly bloody, it indicates hemorrhage into the joint, such as from fracture, hemophilia, trauma, or a traumatic tap. An abnormal leukocyte (white blood cell) count can be mildly to severely elevated.

Protein increases in the synovial fluid because of inflammation. When the patient has gout, the uric acid level is elevated. The glucose level should be equivalent to the blood glucose value. A decrease in the synovial fluid glucose level is indicative of inflammatory arthritis. For the glucose analysis, the patient is usually in a fasting state before the test is performed. This provides a stable baseline value for both the blood and the synovial fluid.

A mucin clot and a favorable string test are indications of normal viscosity. Inflammation and excessive synovial fluid lessen the viscosity, so that when the fluid is poured, only a short string can form.

Culture of the fluid may identify the pathogen that caused the infection. Microscopic examination of the fluid is also performed to identify cells, sediment, or crystals in the fluid.

NORMAL VALUES

Synovial Fluid Analysis
Appearance: Crystal clear, pale yellow
Viscosity: High
Volume: <3.5 mL
Red blood cells: Absent
White blood cells: 0–200/mm^3 *or* SI: 0–200 × 10^6/L
Neutrophils: 0%–25%
Protein: 3 g/dL or less *or* SI: 30 g/L or less
Uric acid: <8 mg/dL *or* SI: 476 μmol/L
Glucose (fasting): 70–110 mg/dL *or* SI: 3.9–6.1 mmol/L
Mucin string test: Formation of a long string
Culture: No growth

HOW THE TEST IS DONE

Joint

Under sterile conditions, an aspiration needle is inserted into the joint space and fluid is withdrawn. The fluid specimen is placed into one green-topped tube with heparin and two red-topped tubes.

Blood

A red-topped tube is used to obtain 10 mL of venous blood for a serum chemistry profile. If additional tests are to be performed, a second red-topped tube is filled. The blood is drawn at the same time the joint aspiration is performed.

Culture

If gonococcus is suspected, some synovial fluid is inoculated onto a plate that contains Thayer-Martin culture medium. This is carried out immediately after the arthrocentesis is completed. Other cultures are started in the laboratory.

SIGNIFICANCE OF TEST RESULTS

Abnormal Values

Rheumatoid arthritis
Rheumatic fever
Infectious arthritis
Traumatic arthritis
Osteoarthritis
Gout
Hemophilic arthritis
Systemic lupus erythematosus
Tuberculosis
Lyme disease

INTERFERING FACTORS

- Failure to maintain a nothing-by-mouth status

NURSING CARE

Pretest

- A signed consent is required and is placed in the patient's record.
- ***Patient Teaching.*** Instruct the patient to fast for 6 to 8 hours before the test. A serum glucose test will be performed on the blood sample. Also inform the patient that the procedure is performed with local anesthesia. Mild discomfort may be felt as the physician injects the anesthetic and as the needle penetrates the joint capsule.

During the Test

- The nurse assists with positioning of the extremity. The skin is cleansed with antiseptic, and the area is covered with a sterile drape. The nurse also assists with the preparation of the local anesthetic and the collection of all specimens.

Posttest

- After the physician withdraws the needle, the nurse can apply a pressure dressing to the aspiration site to prevent hematoma. An elastic binding may be applied to the joint for 8 to 24 hours to increase the stability of the joint.
- ***Patient Teaching.*** Instruct the patient to apply a cold pack to the joint for 24 to 36 hours to decrease the swelling. The extremity may be elevated on pillows. Teach the patient to avoid excessive use of the joint for 2 to 3 days. This will help prevent stiffness, pain, and swelling.

◆ Nursing Response to Complications

Infection is a possible complication of arthrocentesis or any other procedure that opens the joint capsule. The infection can be introduced from environmental contamination or from aggravation of infection already present in the joint tissues.

Infection. The nurse instructs the patient to notify the physician if the dressing becomes wet with purulent, malodorous secretions. In addition the patient usually develops a fever and the joint becomes swollen and painful.

Arthroscopy

ahr-thros-kuh-pee

SPECIMEN OR TYPE OF TEST: Endoscopy

PURPOSE OF THE TEST

Arthroscopy provides direct visualization of the interior of the joint and tissue surfaces. It is used to detect torn tendon or ligament, injured meniscus, abnormal synovial tissue, pannus formation, and damaged cartilage.

BASICS THE NURSE NEEDS TO KNOW

The arthroscope is a thin, flexible fiberoptic endoscope that provides direct visualization of the joint structures and tissues in the joint space. Special accessory instruments can be used to obtain biopsy specimens or to aspirate synovial fluid.

The joint and its interior ligaments, structures, synovial lining, and bony surfaces can develop infection, inflammation, tumor growth, or injury from trauma. When the pathologic change in the joint is not fully explained by more simple laboratory tests and diagnostic procedures, arthroscopy may be needed to confirm the diagnosis and evaluate the extent of the problem. The knee is the most common joint to be examined by arthroscopy, but the shoulder and other joints also can be examined by this method.

Diagnostic arthroscopy is performed as a same-day surgical procedure. Either local or general anesthesia may be used. Arthroscopy is an invasive procedure because surgical openings are made into the joint capsule to allow the insertion of the endoscope. After the diagnostic phase, arthroscopic surgical repair of the torn or damaged tissue may be performed.

NORMAL VALUES

No tissue or structural abnormalities of the joint space are noted.

HOW THE TEST IS DONE

The orthopedic surgeon makes two surgical incisions in the skin. A trocar is inserted into the joint capsule through one incision, followed by insertion of the arthroscope. A probe or the accessory instruments are inserted through the other incision. Additional incisions may be needed to visualize all aspects of the joint. Tissue and fluid samples may be collected for laboratory analysis. Once the fluid is drained and the instruments removed, sutures or tape strips are used to close the incisions. The total time needed for the procedure is 2 to 3 hours.

SIGNIFICANCE OF TEST RESULTS

Abnormal Values

Torn ligament or meniscus
Degenerative articular cartilage
Synovitis

Loose bodies
Subluxation, fracture, or dislocation of the bone
Chondromalacia
Osteochondritis desiccans
Arthritis
Gout
Ganglion or Baker's cyst

INTERFERING FACTORS

- Failure to maintain nothing-by-mouth status

NURSING CARE

Pretest

- Once the procedure has been explained by the physician, obtain written consent from the patient and place the consent in the patient's record. In preoperative teaching, the patient learns about the procedure, the anesthetic, the tests that will be done, the incisions, and the postoperative inflammation. Mild postoperative pain will occur, but it will be controlled with analgesics.
- ***Patient Teaching.*** Instruct the patient to discontinue all food and fluids for 8 hours before the procedure.
- ***Patient Teaching.*** Instruct the patient to have a responsible person available to provide transportation after the procedure.
- Take baseline vital signs and record the results.

During the Test

- Position the patient, including possible placement of a stabilizing support mechanism. The extremity is prepped and draped. The nurse also sets up the arthroscopy equipment and ensures that it is operational, including the irrigation system and suction unit.
- On completion of the procedure, bulky sterile dressings are applied and covered with an elastic bandage. An immobilizer may also be applied.

Posttest

- If general anesthesia was administered, monitor vital signs immediately and thereafter every 15 minutes for the first 2 hours, then every 30 minutes for 1 hour, and then every hour for 2 hours or until discharge from the postanesthesia unit. If intravenous sedation and local anesthesia were administered, monitor initial vital signs and repeat monitoring at regular intervals thereafter.
- The nurse assesses for neurovascular function in the distal extremity every 15 minutes, comparing the findings with assessment of the unaffected side. The distal pulses should be strong, and the skin should be cool to warm with satisfactory color. Movement and sensation should be present in the fingers or toes.

NURSING CARE—*cont'd*

- The nurse also assesses for pain and provides the prescribed medication for relief of pain, as needed. The elastic compression dressing is checked for any signs of excessive bleeding, constriction, or excessive swelling of the joint or distal extremity.
- ***Patient Teaching.*** For discharge instructions, remind the patient to keep the extremity elevated for 24 to 48 hours to reduce the swelling. Ice should be applied for 24 hours. The nurse instructs the patient about the prescriptions for medications to be taken at home. Pain is usually minimal and can be relieved by nonsteroidal, anti-inflammatory medications and nonnarcotic analgesics.
- ***Patient Teaching.*** With arthroscopy of the knee, remind the patient that walking is permitted, but that no exercise or excessive use of the joint should occur for 24 hours. The patient may be instructed to use crutches to keep all weight off the knee or to walk only with a partial weight-bearing gait. With arthroscopy of the shoulder, the arm is placed in a sling. Activity requirements or restrictions depend on the type of injury and any surgical repair that may have been done after the diagnostic phase of the test. Range-of-motion exercises are usually started on the second to third postoperative day, and physical therapy may be instituted to strengthen the muscles.

◆ **Nursing Response to Complications**

Infection. The complications of diagnostic arthroscopy are rare, but infection can occur. If infection occurs, the patient will develop a fever and experience increased pain in the infected joint. The dressing will become wet with drainage that has a bad odor. The nurse instructs the patient to report any sign of infection to the physician.

Aspartate Aminotransferase

as-par-tayt a-mee-noh-trans-fuhr-ays

Also called: (AST); Glutamate Oxaloacetate Transaminase, Serum

SPECIMEN OR TYPE OF TEST: Serum

PURPOSE OF THE TEST

AST is an indicator of inflammation, injury, or necrosis of the tissues that contain this transaminase enzyme. In liver disease, it is an indicator of liver damage from any cause. The AST test may also be used to monitor liver function in patients who receive medication that potentially is hepatotoxic.

BASICS THE NURSE NEEDS TO KNOW

AST is a transaminase enzyme found in high concentrations in the heart and liver tissues, and to a lesser extent in skeletal muscle, brain, kidney, pancreas, spleen, and lung tissues.

When there is mild or moderate liver inflammation, injury, or necrosis, the liver cells release AST through damaged cell membranes, resulting in rising AST levels in the blood. With severe damage, the liver cells are destroyed and greater amounts of AST are released into the blood stream. For example, in severe, acute hepatitis, the AST level can rise to a value of 20 to 100 times the normal value.

Because AST is also present in skeletal muscle tissue and other organs, the serum AST will rise when there is trauma, inflammation, or necrosis in these tissues. Generally these elevations are slight to moderate, although shock, acute pancreatitis, and infectious mononucleosis occasionally cause a severe elevation of the serum value.

AST-to-ALT Ratio

A comparison of the AST to ALT is sometimes used to differentiate among the causes of damage to liver cells. The results are expressed as a ratio of AST to ALT. Because the amounts of each enzyme are about equal, the ratio is expressed as AST = ALT, or the normal value of AST:ALT = 1.

In alcoholic hepatitis, the AST value is greater than the ALT value, or the ratio is expressed numerically. For example, AST:ALT = 3: 1 means that the AST value is three times greater than the ALT value. In viral hepatitis, the ALT value can rise to greater than the AST value, as AST:ALT = 1: 3

NORMAL VALUES	Adult: 8–33 Units/L or SI: 8–33 Units/L AST:ALT = 1
▼ **Critical Values**	An AST value that is three times the upper limit of normal An AST:ALT ratio that is greater than 1.

HOW THE TEST IS DONE

A venipuncture is performed to collect 10 mL of venous blood in a red-topped tube.

SIGNIFICANCE OF TEST RESULTS

Elevated Values

Hepatitis (viral, toxic)
Cirrhosis
Hemochromatosis
Cancer of the liver
Delirium tremens
Obstructive jaundice
Acute pancreatitis

Infectious mononucleosis
Myocardial infarction
Pericarditis
Cardiac surgery
Cardiac catheterization
Cardiac arrhythmias
Pulmonary infarction
Renal infarction
Cerebral necrosis (trauma, stroke, craniotomy)
Severe injury to the skeletal muscle tissues
Dermatomyositis
Polymyositis
Muscular dystrophy

INTERFERING FACTORS

- Hemolysis
- Failure to maintain a nothing-by-mouth status
- Intensive exercise before the test

NURSING CARE

Nursing actions are similar to those used in other venipuncture procedures (see Chapter 2), with the following additional measures.

Pretest

- ***Patient Teaching*** Instruct the patient to fast for 12 hours before the test. Advise the ambulatory patient to avoid strenuous exercise before the test.

Posttest

▼ Nursing Response to Critical Values

If the AST value is greater than three times the upper limit of the normal value or the AST:ALT ratio is greater than 1, notify the physician of this elevated result. Many commonly prescribed medications can cause hepatotoxicity (a toxic effect on liver cells). The rise above the critical value is usually an indicator to stop the particular medication that has caused liver damage.

The patient's overall condition may not appear to be changed as a result of the rise in the AST level. Measurement of the vital signs can be done to assure that shock has not occurred. The nurse should review the patient's medication list and ask the physician if any should be withheld or discontinued.

Barium Enema

B

bar-ee-um e-nuh-muh

Also called: (BE); Double-Contrast Barium Enema, (DCBE)

SPECIMEN OR TYPE OF TEST: Radiography

PURPOSE OF THE TEST

The barium enema is used to investigate and identify pathologic conditions that change the structure and function of the colon (Figure 20). It may be used as a screening test for early detection of colon cancer.

BASICS THE NURSE NEEDS TO KNOW

The barium enema is a radiographic test that is used to investigate the cause of a change in elimination patterns, melena (blood in the stool), obstruction of the colon, or the presence of an abdominal mass that has a suspected location in the colon. Barium is a contrast medium that is radiopaque, has a different density than body tissue, and can be instilled into hollow organs such as the colon. In the barium enema, the entire colon and the distal portion of the ileum can be visualized on x-ray film (Figure 21).

NORMAL VALUES No lesions, deficits, or abnormalities of the colon are noted

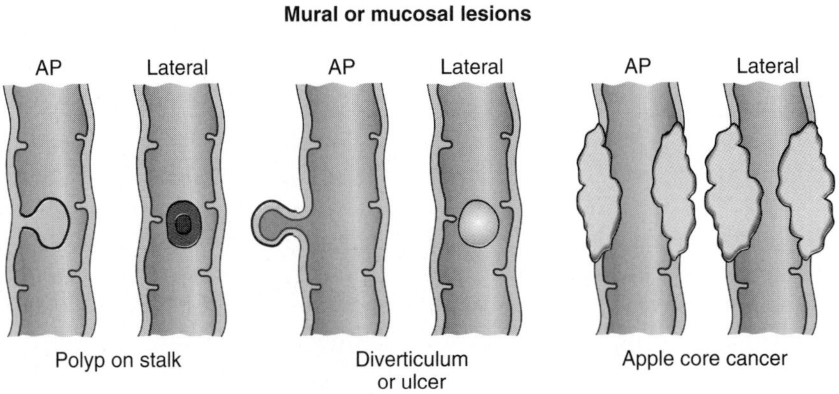

Mural or mucosal lesions

AP Lateral AP Lateral AP Lateral

Polyp on stalk

Diverticulum or ulcer

Apple core cancer

Figure 20. Schematic appearance of various gastrointestinal lesions on contrast examination. A polyp seen in profile will show a stalk. Seen end-on, it will be darkest in the center, with an ill-defined, fading edge. A diverticulum seen in tangent will project outside the lumen and, when seen end-on, will have very sharp edges. Cancer can be in one wall or, if circumferential, can leave contrast in the lumen that resembles an apple core. *(Reproduced with permission from Mettler, F. A. [1996].* Essentials of radiology *[p. 213]. Philadelphia: W. B. Saunders.)*

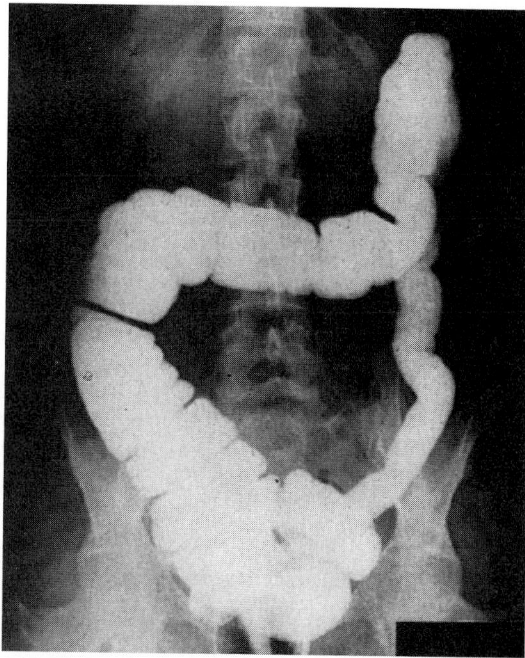

Figure 21. Barium enema. Radiopaque barium sulfate fills the colon in this lower gastrointestinal study. *(Reproduced with permission from Adler, A. M., & Carlton, R. R. [1994].* Introduction to radiography and patient care *[Vol. 1, Slide 200]. Philadelphia: W. B. Saunders.)*

HOW THE TEST IS DONE

After the colon is emptied of feces, the contrast medium enema is administered by the radiology technologist. In a double-contrast study, carbon dioxide or air is then put into the colon to dilate the lumen and provide a clearer view. The patient must retain the contrast medium in the colon during the test. The patient's positional changes, (supine, prone, lateral) are used to enhance gravity flow of the contrast medium throughout the entire colon. X-rays are taken to image the abnormal area(s). The procedure takes 45 minutes to 1 hour to complete.

SIGNIFICANCE OF TEST RESULTS

Adenocarcinoma
Diverticulitis
Sarcoma
Hirschsprung's disease
Idiopathic megacolon
Polyps of the colon

Gastroenteritis
Chronic amebic dysentery
Ulcerative colitis
Intussusception

INTERFERING FACTORS

- Upper gastrointestinal series within 3 days before the test
- Inability to retain barium
- Incomplete cleansing of the colon

NURSING CARE

- ***Health Promotion.*** The nurse can be very instrumental in health teaching, to encourage people to have scheduled colorectal screening tests and not wait until symptoms appear. Early detection leads to early intervention, with a more positive treatment outcome.
- ***Health Promotion.*** The barium enema is one method of routine screening for colorectal cancer. It has a high level of accuracy and is readily available throughout the nation. Precancerous colon polyps and cancer of the colon can be detected at a very early stage, before they cause symptoms or become invasive. Most colorectal cancers develop after age 50 and the risk increases with every succeeding decade of life. If the double contrast barium enema is used as a screening test, the recommended interval for testing is every 5 years for the patient older than 50 years and who is of average risk for colon cancer. For a variety of reasons, healthy people are reluctant to have a colorectal screening test. Currently, less than 30% of the people who should have a colorectal screening test actually have it done. Greater education efforts will increase the public's awareness of health promotion efforts.

Pretest

- Schedule the barium enema before any other barium studies. Residual barium from the upper gastrointestinal tract would obscure the images of the colon.
- The patient must sign a consent form that is then entered into the patient's record.
- For bowel preparation the goal is to eliminate all fecal matter, gas, and mucus so that visualization is clear and accurate. The exact bowel cleansing procedure is defined by the protocol of the radiologist, and variations exist. The common methods of preparation are presented here.
- ***Patient Teaching.*** Teach the patient to begin a clear liquid diet 12 to 24 hours before the test to reduce the amount of fecal matter.
- A cathartic such as castor oil, magnesium citrate, or senna extract (X-Prep) is taken on the afternoon before the test. Bisacodyl (Dulcolax) tablets are taken on the evening before the test and a bisacodyl suppository is inserted on the morning of the test. A warm tap water enema (1500 mL for adults) is given on the night

NURSING CARE—*cont'd*

before the test or at 6:00 AM on the day of the test. When all fecal matter has been removed, the enema returns will be clear.

- Extra oral fluids are taken in the pretest period to prevent dehydration or excess absorption of the barium solution from the colon. Some protocols require extra amounts of oral fluids in the afternoon and evening, but a nothing-by-mouth status is started by midnight before the test.
- For children younger than age 4, the bowel preparation is prescribed on an individualized basis. It is helpful to provide all pretest and posttest instructions in writing because the patient usually does them at home.

Posttest

- The patient is assisted to the toilet or commode to evacuate the contrast medium.
- A laxative is prescribed to eliminate the residual barium and prevent the constipation caused by the barium. Residual barium changes the color of feces to a gray or whitish color for 24 to 72 hours after the test.
- Encourage the patient to rest for the remainder of the day because this test is tiring.
- Elderly patients are vulnerable to a fall. Since they may also become mentally confused because of dehydration, instruct the patients to increase their fluid intake.

Nursing Response to Complications

Complications from the barium enema procedure are not frequent, but are very serious when they occur. Perforation can occur when the colon tears and barium spills into the peritoneal cavity. The cause can be excessive intracolonic pressure and distension, or a tear in thin, damaged colon tissue that is affected by disease. The instillation of large amounts of fluid into the colon can trigger vagus nerve stimulation, with resultant bradycardia. In addition, fluid and electrolyte imbalance and dehydration can cause cardiac arrhythmia or a heart attack, usually in patients who are elderly or have a preexisting heart condition. If complication occurs, it usually happens during the test. However, complications can progress and cause very serious illness that becomes apparent in the posttest period. The nurse monitors for complications and notifies the physician of abnormal assessment findings.

Perforation. The nurse assesses for post-procedure complaints of abdominal pain and abdominal distension. With perforation, the patient may develop shock or peritonitis, with changes in vital signs and the onset of fever. The patient may die.

Cardiac arrhythmia and heart attack. The nurse monitors the pulse for changes of rate and rhythm and assesses for complaints of chest pain as primary indicators of cardiac complications. If a heart attack occurs, there will be shock, as evidenced by a low or falling blood pressure, tachycardia, and acute dyspnea. There may be a cardiac arrhythmia. The patient can die of these complications unless there is sufficient and timely medical and nursing intervention.

B

Barium Swallow

bar-ee-um swah-loh

Also called: Videofluorographic Swallowing Study, (VFSS)

SPECIMEN OR TYPE OF TEST: Radiography

PURPOSE OF THE TEST

The barium swallow is used to identify abnormalities in the structure and function of the esophagus (Figure 22).

BASICS THE NURSE NEEDS TO KNOW

Barium Swallow

The barium swallow procedure may be performed as a separate barium study or as part of the upper gastrointestinal series. Dysphagia (difficulty swallowing) is the most common problem investigated by the barium swallow. The cause can be an obstruction in

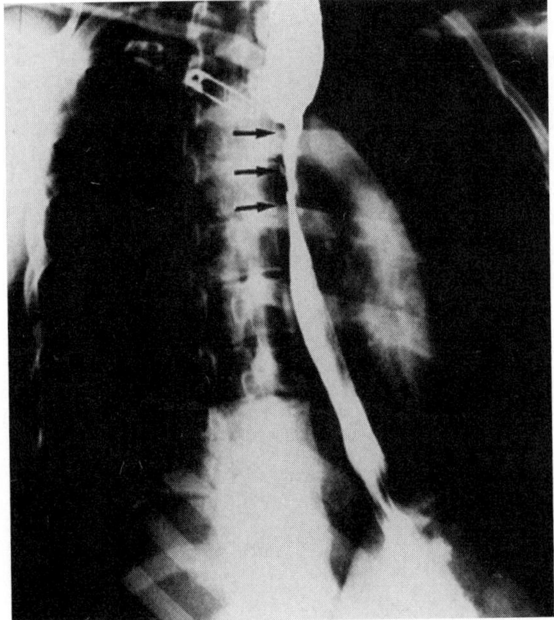

Figure 22. Benign esophageal stricture. This upper esophageal stricture (*arrows*) was the result of attempted suicide by lye ingestion. *(Reproduced with permission from Mettler, F. A. [1996].* Essentials of radiology *[p. 185]. Philadelphia: W. B. Saunders.)*

the esophagus or a neuromuscular deficit that interferes with swallowing and slows the transit time for the passage of food to the stomach. The normal transit time from the oropharynx to the stomach is 6 to 15 seconds.

Videofluorographic Swallowing Study (VFSS)

This newer procedure is very similar to the barium swallow study and is done to evaluate the mechanism of swallowing and to investigate complaints of dysphagia. It is particularly useful to investigate neuromuscular weakness or incoordination that affects swallowing. The barium is mixed with different foods and drinks and the patient sits upright to swallow the various mixtures. Fluorography images are seen on the video screen and recorded on videotape. The different textures and consistencies of foods and beverages are observed in their esophageal transit, to note which ones can be tolerated and which cause dysphagia, choking, or discomfort. The results are used to identify foods that can be swallowed safely by the patient. Some test maneuvers such as the patient turning the head toward the weak side, holding the breath before swallowing, and flexing the neck are observed during swallowing, to identify methods that push the bolus of food toward the stronger areas of muscle function to improve swallowing ability. The data of this test are used to provide for appropriate rehabilitation therapy and swallow therapy.

NORMAL VALUES **No esophageal structural or functional abnormalities are visualized.**

HOW THE TEST IS DONE

The patient takes repeated swallows of barium liquid to provide views of the passage of contrast medium during swallowing and peristaltic movement of the esophagus. Fluoroscopy, x-rays and videotape recordings are used for visualization.

SIGNIFICANCE OF TEST RESULTS

Swallowed foreign body
Achalasia (neuromuscular incoordination)
Esophageal stricture
Esophageal spasm
Hiatal hernia
Pharyngeal neuromuscular weakness
Polyps, tumor, cancer
Varices
Ulcers or peptic esophagitis

INTERFERING FACTOR

- Failure to maintain a nothing-by-mouth status

B

NURSING CARE

Pretest

- The patient signs a written consent for the test and the consent is entered into the patient's record.
- ***Patient Teaching.*** Instruct the patient to fast from all food and liquids for 12 hours before the test.
- At the radiology setting, the patient will remove all clothes, jewelry, and metallic objects. A surgical gown is worn.

Posttest

- A laxative is given to help eliminate the barium from the intestinal tract. Inform the patient that the feces will appear gray or whitish for 24 to 72 hours until all barium is expelled.

Base Excess/Deficit

See Arterial Blood Gases on p. 99.

Bence Jones Protein Test

See Protein Electrophoresis, Urinary on p. 548.

β-Amyloid(1-42)

See Lumbar Puncture and Cerebral Spinal Fluid Analysis on p. 435.

Bilirubin, Serum

bil-i-rue-bin, see-ruhm

Also called: Bilirubin: Total Bilirubin
Direct Bilirubin: Conjugated Bilirubin
Indirect Bilirubin: Unconjugated Bilirubin
Neonatal Bilirubin: Total Bilirubin, Neonatal

SPECIMEN OR TYPE OF TEST: Serum

PURPOSE OF THE TEST

Total serum bilirubin is the sum total of indirect bilirubin and direct bilirubin.

The purposes of the total bilirubin test are to evaluate liver function, diagnose jaundice, and monitor the progression of jaundice.

The purpose of direct and indirect bilirubin tests is to identify the underlying cause of the elevated bilirubin level.

In the newborn baby with jaundice, the neonatal bilirubin test is used to determine whether the infant needs treatment to prevent kernicterus (brain damage from high levels of bilirubin).

BASICS THE NURSE NEEDS TO KNOW

Most bilirubin is produced by the liver and spleen as part of the process of hemolysis (breakdown) of senescent (old) or damaged red blood cells. Once created, the bilirubin is transported in the bloodstream as indirect (unconjugated) bilirubin. The liver then converts indirect bilirubin to direct (conjugated) bilirubin. The direct bilirubin mixes with fluid and enters the bile canaliculi and hepatic ducts of the liver in the process that makes bile.

Bile, with its component direct bilirubin, flows from the hepatic ducts of the liver to the biliary ductal system. It is stored in the gall bladder and, on demand, flows through the cystic duct, the common duct, and enters the duodenum to help in the process of digestion of fats.

Jaundice

This is a clinical term that describes the yellow discoloration of the skin and sclera caused by excess bilirubin in the blood and body tissues. The jaundice becomes visible when the total serum bilirubin is elevated to greater than 2 mg/dL. An elevated level of bilirubin in the blood is called hyperbilirubinemia.

Classifications of Jaundice

One way to classify jaundice is based on the physiologic location of bilirubin manufacture, transport, and excretion (Table 6). The prehepatic classification refers to bilirubin manufacture and transport before the blood circulation reaches the liver. The hepatic classification refers to problems within the liver, due to injury to the liver cells or blockage within the intrahepatic bile ducts. The posthepatic classification refers to blockage of bile within the liver or in the gall bladder or gall bladder ducts. As seen in Table 6, pathophysiologic changes will be detected by elevated values of the indirect or direct bilirubin tests. These tests help provide information about the cause of the problem.

Neonatal Jaundice

In the first few days of life, newborns experience varying levels of elevated bilirubin. The condition is called physiologic jaundice. It is not clear why this condition occurs, but it is temporary. The indirect bilirubin rises modestly for 3 to 4 days and then declines to a normal value.

Other causes of neonatal jaundice are considered abnormal or pathologic, including ABO and Rh incompatibility. The rapid destruction of reds blood cells in hemolytic disease of the newborn causes a great increase in indirect bilirubin. The onset is usually in the first day of life. If the total bilirubin level is greater than 20 mg/dL (SI: 340 μmol/L), potential exists for bilirubin encephalopathy or kernicterus. In kernicterus, bilirubin is deposited in the brain, and permanent damage can occur.

B

TABLE 6 Classifications of Jaundice

Category of Jaundice	Type of Bilirubin Elevation	Origin of the Problem
Prehepatic	Indirect (unconjugated)	Excessive hemolysis of red blood cells Hemolytic jaundice
Hepatic	Indirect (unconjugated)	Defect in transport or conjugation in hepatocytes Physiologic jaundice
	Direct (conjugated)	Injury to or disease of hepatocytes Blockage of intrahepatic bile ducts Intrahepatic cholestasis
Posthepatic	Direct (conjugated)	Blockage in the biliary ductal system Extrahepatic cholestasis

If the infant is born with biliary atresia, the biliary drainage system is incompletely developed and there is no open passageway for bile to flow into the duodenum. Because of the blockage, a rapid, severe rise in total bilirubin and direct bilirubin will occur.

NORMAL VALUES

Total Bilirubin
Adult-child: 0.1–1.2 mg/dL *or* SI: 2–21 µmol/L
Neonate: 1.0–12 mg/dL *or* SI: 17–205 µmol/L

Direct Bilirubin
Adult: < 0.3 mg/dL *or* SI: <5 µmol/L

Indirect Bilirubin
Adult: 0.1–1.0 mg/dL *or* SI: 2–17 µmol/L

Critical Values
Term infant: >15 mg/dL *or* SI: >257 µmol/L
Premature infant: 10–15 mg/dL *or* SI: 171–257 µmol/L

HOW THE TEST IS DONE

Adult: A venipuncture is performed to collect 10 mL of venous blood in a red-topped tube.

Infant: A blue capillary tube is used to draw drops of blood from the heel that has been pricked by a sterile lancet.

SIGNIFICANCE OF TEST RESULTS

Elevated Values

TOTAL SERUM BILIRUBIN

Hepatocellular damage (toxic, infectious, or malignancy)
Obstruction in the biliary system
Neonatal jaundice
Hemolytic diseases
Familial hyperbilirubinemia
Reaction to some medications

DIRECT BILIRUBIN

Hepatotoxins that cause liver necrosis
Infection of the liver (hepatitis, bacterial infection, parasitic disease)
Cirrhosis
Cancer (liver, gall bladder, pancreas, ampulla of Vater)
Sclerosing cholangitis
Primary biliary cirrhosis
Biliary atresia
Gall stones
Lymphoma
Acute pancreatitis

INDIRECT BILIRUBIN

Inherited defects of red blood cells (sickle cell anemia, spherocytosis)
Inherited enzyme disorders
Neonatal
Reaction to some medications
Malaria
Physiologic jaundice
Rh or ABO incompatibility
Blood transfusion reaction due to incompatibility

INTERFERING FACTORS

- Sunlight
- Hemolysis
- Failure to maintain a nothing-by-mouth status (adults only)

NURSING CARE

Nursing actions are similar to those used in other venipuncture or capillary puncture procedures (see Chapter 2), with the following additional measures.

Pretest

- ***Patient Teaching.*** Instruct the patient to fast from food for 8 to 12 hours (overnight) because serum lipids will alter the results.

Continued

NURSING CARE—*cont'd*

B

Posttest

- Ensure that the vial of blood or the microcapillary tube is covered and sent to the laboratory without delay. Because bilirubin is photosensitive, the blood sample must be protected from exposure to light or a prolonged time in a lighted environment.

▼ Nursing Response to Critical Values

If the neonatal bilirubin rises to a critical value in the newborn or premature infant, notify the physician immediately. If the elevation is considered to be pathologic, rather than physiologic, the baby must be evaluated medically to determine the cause of hyperbilirubinemia. At this level, the physician will consider the treatment of phototherapy. If the level goes higher, phototherapy will be performed, and exchange transfusion may also be necessary.

The nurse observes the baby for signs of jaundice. Yellow color will appear in the skin and the sclera of the eyes. The urine may become dark brown as excess bilirubin is filtered from the blood by the kidneys.

Biopsy, Bone

bai-op-see, bohn

Also called: Bone Needle Aspiration Cytology

SPECIMEN OR TYPE OF TEST: Biopsy tissue

PURPOSE OF THE TEST

Bone biopsy is performed to examine a specimen of bone tissue for its cell type and to distinguish benign from malignant bone tumor.

BASICS THE NURSE NEEDS TO KNOW

Benign bone tumors are characterized by their uniform density and well-defined margins. The most common benign tumor is the giant cell tumor, often located in the end of a long bone near a joint.

Malignant primary bone tumors are characterized by borders that extend outward into surrounding fat or muscle tissue or inward into the marrow and medullary cavity, or both (Figure 23). The most common primary bone malignancy is osteogenic sarcoma, which is often located in the region of the knee. Malignant bone tumors may also be metastatic tumors, with the primary site located elsewhere in the body. Most bone metastases are in multiple sites, usually located in the vertebrae, ribs, sternum, or pelvis.

When bone tumor is suspected, a bone scan or computed tomographic (CT) scan is performed first. These preliminary tests are used to verify the presence of the tumor and identify the site for bone biopsy. These preliminary tests also are used to identify additional metastatic sites and to help assess the extent of growth or invasion of the tumor. Unlike biopsy, the preliminary tests cannot distinguish benign from malignant disease.

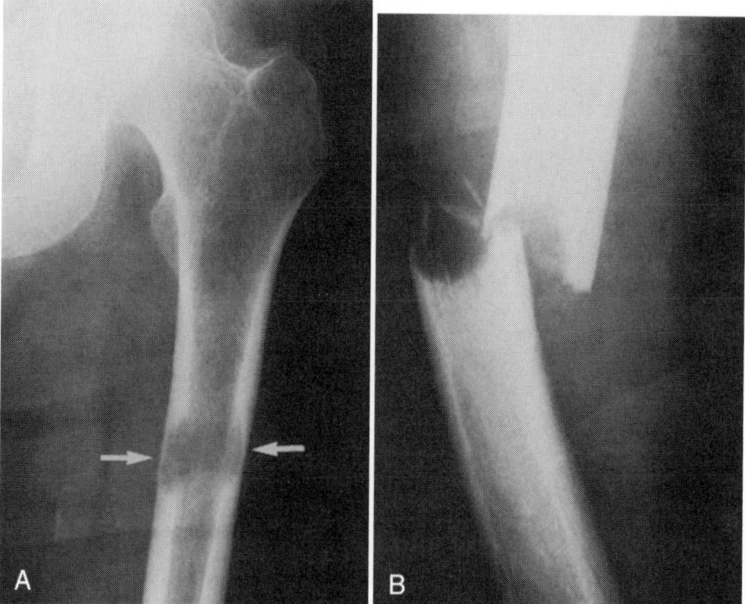

Figure 23. X-ray of bone metastasis. *A,* View of the femur in a patient with known lung cancer shows a destructive lesion expanding from the marrow space and thinning the bone cortex (*arrows*). The lesion has no defined, clear margin to distinguish it from normal bone. It is important to find lesions such as this in weight-bearing bones so that treatment can be undertaken to prevent pathologic fracture. *B,* View of the femur of the same patient who returned 2 weeks later with a pathologic fracture. *(Reproduced with permission from Mettler, F. M. [1996].* Essentials of radiology *[p. 342]. Philadelphia: W. B. Saunders.)*

NORMAL VALUES Bone tissue is normal, with no tumor cells present.

HOW THE TEST IS DONE

Using local anesthesia, the physician makes a small incision in the skin, and uses a bone biopsy needle to drill or push into the bone. Once it is in place, the biopsy needle is rotated 180 degrees to obtain a core sample of the tissue. The specimen is placed on a slide with fixative or in a specimen jar with 95% alcohol or both. The procedure takes 30 minutes or more.

SIGNIFICANCE OF TEST RESULTS

Abnormal Values

Malignant

Osteogenic sarcoma
Ewing's sarcoma

Reticulum cell sarcoma
Angiosarcoma
Multiple myeloma
Metastatic tumor

Benign

Giant cell tumor
Osteoma
Osteoid osteoma
Chondroma

INTERFERING FACTORS

- Failure to obtain an adequate sample of tissue
- Failure to send the specimen to the laboratory immediately

NURSING CARE

Pretest

- After the physician has explained the procedure to the patient, obtain written consent from the patient and place the document in the patient's record.
- ***Patient Teaching.*** The nurse instructs the patient to remove all clothing and put on a hospital gown.
- Baseline vital signs are taken and the results are recorded. The skin is shaved at the site of the biopsy location and is then cleansed with antiseptic. The nurse uses a calm, reassuring approach with the patient. The procedure and potential biopsy results can cause the patient to feel anxious.

During the Test

- Provide support to the patient as the physician anesthetizes the skin and subcutaneous tissue and inserts the biopsy needle. Despite the local anesthetic, the patient feels momentary pain as the needle penetrates the periosteum and enters the bone.
- The nurse labels all specimen containers and slides with the patient's name and the tissue source. The requisition form for a tissue cytologic study is completed, including the patient's name, age, history of carcinoma or infection, and the site of biopsy. The slides or specimen, or both, are sent to the laboratory without delay. The final preparation of the slides must be completed within 6 hours to prevent deterioration of the tissue.

Posttest

- The nurse assesses vital signs and monitors them at regular intervals until they are stable.
- Assessment findings should include observation that the pressure dressing remains clean, dry, and intact.

NURSING CARE—*cont'd*

- ***Patient Teaching.*** The nurse instructs the patient to rest quietly with an ice pack over the dressing for about 2 hours. In preparation for discharge from the ambulatory setting, instruct the patient to resume routine activity but to avoid strenuous physical activity for a few days. The pressure dressing may be changed to a small adhesive bandage on the day after the procedure, and a shower is permitted. Mild discomfort is common, and the patient can take an analgesic medication as needed.

◇ Nursing Response to Complications

Infection. Infection of bone is a possible complication. If infection occurs, the patient develops a fever and headache. He or she feels bone pain and pain on movement. The biopsy site becomes red, with purulent drainage or an abscess. The nurse instructs the patient to notify the physician if these symptoms occur.

Biopsy, Bone Marrow

bai-op-see, bohn ma-roh

Also called: Bone Marrow Aspiration

SPECIMEN OR TYPE OF TEST: Tissue, bone marrow

PURPOSE OF THE TEST

The bone marrow biopsy or aspiration with microscopic examination of the tissue is used to evaluate hematopoiesis. It diagnoses malignancy of primary and metastatic origin and determines the cause of infection. The examination of the marrow also is used to evaluate the progression of some hematologic diseases or the response of the marrow to chemotherapy treatment, such as in Hodgkin's disease and acute myelogenous leukemia.

BASICS THE NURSE NEEDS TO KNOW

The bone marrow is responsible for *hematopoiesis*—the formation of blood cells. The aspirated cells of the bone marrow are used to investigate hematologic disorders. A small sample of the cells is often representative of the whole marrow. Microscopic examination of the cells provides information about the cause, type, and extent of the abnormality. A peripheral blood smear is performed on the same day to compare and incorporate pertinent findings.

The marrow cells are examined for characteristics of the tissue including *cellularity,* the proportion of aspirate that is hematopoietic cells rather than fat cells; *distribution,* an estimate or count of the number of each type of cell found in the marrow specimen; *maturation*, the balance of cells in stages of development; and *abnormal cells,* the presence of irregular or abnormal cells in the marrow. In addition, the examination provides data about the underlying cause of abnormality in the cells of the blood.

NORMAL VALUES

Normal bone marrow

HOW THE TEST IS DONE

The physician administers a local anesthetic in the skin and performs the procedure. In bone marrow aspiration, a bone marrow needle is inserted into the medullary cavity of a bone. Fluid and marrow cells are aspirated into several syringes. When a bone marrow biopsy is required, the biopsy needle removes a core of marrow tissue. Slides are prepared and tissue specimens collected. When indicated, culture specimens are obtained.

The aspiration sites include the sternum, iliac crest, spinous process of the vertebrae, and proximal tibia (Figure 24). In adults, the posterior iliac crest is the most common site. In infants and young children, the proximal tibia is used.

SIGNIFICANCE OF TEST RESULTS

Abnormal Values

Iron deficiency anemia
Infection: histoplasmosis, miliary tuberculosis, infectious mononucleosis
Sideroblastic anemia
Anemia of chronic disease
Megaloblastic anemia
Macroglobulinemia
Agammaglobulinemia
Myelofibrosis

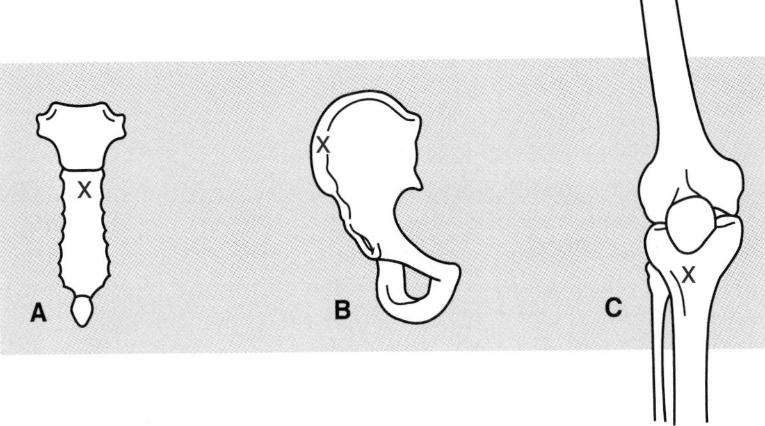

Figure 24. Anatomic sites (X) for bone marrow aspiration. *A,* The sternum between the second and third intercostal spaces. *B,* The iliac crest on the rim or upper posterior surface. *C,* The proximal tibia about 1 to 2 inches below the patella of the infant or small child.

Aplastic anemia
Leukemia
Collagen disease
Multiple myeloma
Parasitic disease: malaria, leishmaniasis
Hodgkin's disease
Lymphoma
Metastatic bone cancer

INTERFERING FACTORS

- Failure to obtain an adequate specimen

NURSING CARE

Pretest

- After the physician explains to the patient the reason for the bone marrow examination and how the procedure will be done, the patient signs consent for the procedure.
- The nurse assesses the patient for anxiety and provides a calming, supportive presence. Common sources of anxiety are fear of the procedure and fear of the possible diagnosis.

During the Test

- The nurse positions the patient according to the site that will be biopsied. For a sternal or tibial biopsy, the supine position is used. Biopsy of the iliac crest requires a lateral recumbent or prone position. Vertebral biopsy is performed with the patient in a seated position. Prepare the skin by cleansing it with an antiseptic solution.
- The nurse provides support and reassurance as the physician instills the local anesthetic. The patient feels brief discomfort as the needle and anesthetic solution penetrate the skin and infiltrate the periosteum. Caution the patient to remain immobile as the biopsy needle is inserted into the marrow. Some pain is felt as the marrow is aspirated.
- The nurse assists with the preparation and labeling of the slides. The clot and biopsy tissue are placed in a sterile specimen jar that contains fixative (formalin or Zenker's solution). Once the needle is removed, the nurse applies pressure to the site, using small sterile gauze. After bleeding has stopped, a small sterile dressing is placed over the puncture site. The patient with a low platelet count is prone to prolonged bleeding so it may take longer to stop blood from oozing out.

Posttest

- Arrange for prompt transport of the specimens and slides to the laboratory.
- Reassure the patient that for a few days, mild discomfort at the biopsy site is expected. Any signs of persistent bleeding or infection should be reported to the physician.

Biopsy, Breast

bai-op-see, brest

SPECIMEN OR TYPE OF TEST: Tissue biopsy

PURPOSE OF THE TEST

The pathology examination of the biopsy specimen is used to distinguish benign from malignant change in the tissue.

BASICS THE NURSE NEEDS TO KNOW

A suspicious palpable or nonpalpable lesion of the breast requires a biopsy to determine the cause and differentiate between benign and malignant tissue. Several methods can be used to obtain the tissue specimen. An open surgical incision may be used to remove the abnormal tissue or a wedge of the tissue. Alternatively, a fine needle aspiration, skinny needle biopsy, or mammotome suction biopsy may be used to remove a small section of tissue from the affected area.

A mammogram is often performed before the biopsy to visualize the size and location of the growth. Increasingly, stereotactic guidance is used to provide three-dimensional imaging for either surgical or needle biopsy measures. In this procedure, automated mammography and computers provide a three-dimensional view for precise localization of the abnormal tissue.

NORMAL VALUES

Normal breast tissue

HOW THE TEST IS DONE

The surgeon removes fluid or tissue from the breast lesion. In the laboratory, slides will be made of the fluid sample or thin slices of the tissue. Using a microscope, the pathologist examines and identifies, classifies, and stages the abnormal tissue. If the surgeon excised (removed) the tumor at the time of the biopsy, the pathologist examines the margins (edges) of the tissue to determine that the entire tumor has been removed completely and the margins are clear of malignant cells.

SIGNIFICANCE OF TEST RESULTS

Abnormal Values

Fibroadenoma
Carcinoma
Duct papilloma
Calcification
Abscess
Mastitis
Fat necrosis
Fibroplasia
Lipoma

Cystosarcoma
Granular cell tumor

INTERFERING FACTOR

- Inadequate tissue sample

NURSING CARE

Pretest

- After the doctor informs the patient of the procedure and the reason for it, the nurse obtains a written consent from the patient.
- Women who must undergo breast biopsy experience varying degrees of distress, depression, anxiety, and heightened emotion. The anxiety can be very high, particularly in women who have limited social support or increased stress from other causes. The emotions may be due to fear of a possible malignancy, fear of the unknown, fear of the biopsy procedure, and fear of the pain from the procedure. The nurse should provide emotional support through the personalization of care. Assist the patient in reducing her stress by listening, providing explanations, affirming feelings, or using diversions, as indicated.
- If surgical biopsy and general anesthesia are planned, instruct the patient to fast from food and fluids for 8 hours before the surgery.
- The nurse assists the patient in removing all clothes and putting on a hospital gown.
- The nurse also assesses and records the patient's vital signs, including temperature, blood pressure, pulse, and respirations.

During the Test

- Clean the breast tissue with povidone-iodine. With the surgical or fine needle biopsy approach, apply the sterile drapes over the correct breast. Assist with the preparation of the local anesthetic.
- When the procedure is to be done without general anesthesia, the nurse provides support to the patient. The patient can feel the injection of the anesthetic. Some patients can feel the push and pull of the needle, some pain, and other sensations such as stinging. They may also feel discomfort because of positioning, with the head and neck turned to the side. Assess the patient for early signs of fainting, such as lightheadedness, dizziness, pallor, and diaphoresis.
- Once the tissue is obtained, place the specimen in a sterile, dry, labeled container. Place the container on ice, and arrange for immediate transport of the specimen to the laboratory. If a frozen section can be done, the specimen may be given directly to the pathologist or technician who is waiting in the room. When microscopic slides are prepared, the aspirated material is used to prepare two to four slides. The smears are fixed immediately with 95% alcohol or a spray-on cytologic fixative. The slides are then transported to the laboratory immediately.
- Apply a dry, sterile dressing to the incision or puncture site.

Continued

B

NURSING CARE—*cont'd*

Posttest

- The nurse takes vital signs and records the results. When a general anesthetic is used, vital signs must be monitored every 15 to 30 minutes until the patient is reactive, alert, and stable.
- To help the patient cope with postoperative depression or anxiety, encourage the patient to return to normal activity as soon as possible. After a surgical procedure, however, vigorous exercise must be avoided for 2 weeks. Until the biopsy results are known, it is common for the patient to continue to experience anxiety and uncertainty in the posttest period.
- ***Patient Teaching.*** To relieve surgical pain, the nurse instructs the patient to use warm, moist compresses or a heating pad and to wear a supportive bra. The patient may shower or bathe as usual, using unscented soap for the needle puncture site. The method of cleansing of the surgical incision is prescribed by the surgeon. The patient will change the surgical dressing once a day. Advise the patient to inform the surgeon of inflammation, infection, or excessive pain in the incision.

◆ Nursing Response to Complications

The complications of incisional biopsy are hematoma and cellulitis. The needle aspiration methods can produce bruising, particularly when multiple needle insertions and aspirations occur during the procedure.

Hematoma. The assessment findings for hematoma include swelling, pain, and ecchymosis in the breast. The nurse assesses the breast, and abnormal findings include bruising, asymmetrical swelling, and leakage of fluid from the incision.

Cellulitis or infection. The nursing assessment findings of cellulitis or infection include pain, swelling, and redness in the breast tissue. In addition, the patient feels ill (malaise) and complains of a headache and elevated temperature.

Biopsy, Endomyocardial

bai-op-see, en-doh-mai-oh-kar-dee-uhl

SPECIMEN OR TYPE OF TEST: Pathology

PURPOSE OF THE TEST

An endomyocardial biopsy is usually performed to determine if a transplanted heart is being rejected. Other purposes for the biopsy are to diagnose myocarditis or doxorubicin (Adriamycin)-induced cardiomyopathy and to determine the cause of restrictive heart disease.

BASICS THE NURSE NEEDS TO KNOW

Endomyocardial biopsy is an invasive procedure requiring cardiac catheterization. It permits sampling of right or left ventricular tissue.

NORMAL VALUES Normal cardiac tissue

HOW THE TEST IS DONE

The procedure involves a cardiac catheterization (see p. 187). A catheter with a jaw-like tip is inserted under fluoroscopy, and several small tissue samples are obtained. A right or left ventricular sample may be taken. For patients at high risk, such as those with a history of left ventricular thrombus or infarction, a right ventricular biopsy may be preferred.

SIGNIFICANCE OF TEST RESULTS

Abnormal Values

Doxorubicin-induced cardiomyopathy
Cardiac amyloidosis
Cardiac fibrosis (especially radiation injury)
Chagas' cardiomyopathy
Myocarditis
Rejection of transplanted heart
Scleroderma
Toxoplasmosis
Tumor infiltrates
Vasculitis

INTERFERING FACTORS

- Bleeding disorders
- Severe thrombocytopenia
- Systemic anticoagulation
- Uncooperative patient

NURSING CARE

See section on Cardiac Catheterization.

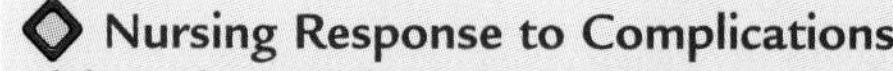

Nursing Response to Complications

Although complications of endomyocardial biopsy are rare, they include accidental biopsy of papillary muscle or chordae tendineae, cardiac perforation, and hemopericardium. Other complications can occur but are related to the catheterization rather than to the biopsy.

Accidental biopsy of papillary muscle or chordae tendineae. The nurse assesses the heart sounds of patients after an endomyocardial biopsy for new onset of a murmur. Report the existence of a new murmur to the physician, who may want to order an echocardiogram.

Hemopericardium. Bleeding into the pericardial sac will interfere with cardiac movement. The nurse will observe signs of cardiac tamponade: decrease in cardiac output, muffled heart sounds, increase in right atrial pressure and pulses paradoxus.

Continued

NURSING CARE—*cont'd*

B

Notify the physician immediately. If cardiac output is significantly compromised, anticipate need for pericardiocentesis.

Cardiac perforation. See above, plus the nurse will assess for shock, as evidenced by hypotension, tachycardia, and dyspnea.

Biopsy, Gastrointestinal Tract

See Gastrointestinal Cytologic Studies on p. 339.

Biopsy, Liver

bai-op-see, li-ver

Also called: Liver Biopsy

SPECIMEN OR TYPE OF TEST: Tissue biopsy

PURPOSE OF THE TEST

The biopsy sample is used to diagnose pathologic changes in the liver and help evaluate the extent of the disease process.

BASICS THE NURSE NEEDS TO KNOW

Unexplained, abnormal liver function tests, jaundice, and an enlarged liver or a history of cancer that commonly metastasizes to the liver are indicators for liver biopsy. A biopsy of the liver tissue is used to identify the cause and the extent of the disease. The tissue sample is obtained by fine needle biopsy, using needle aspiration or a needle-like instrument that shaves a very small core tissue sample. If the disease is diffuse and affects all parts of liver tissue, the biopsy sample may be aspirated without direct visualization of the organ. Often however, ultrasound is used to guide the placement of the needle. When a small and specific area of tissue is located more deeply into the liver tissue, ultrasound or computerized tomography (CT) provides visualization. Visualization during the procedure allows the physician to place the tip of the needle directly into the affected area.

NORMAL VALUES The liver cells are normal, with no evidence of inflammation, scarring, degeneration, infection, tumor, or other pathologic change.

HOW THE TEST IS DONE

After administration of local anesthetic, the physician places the needle between the anterior and midaxillary lines, usually at the level of the sixth or seventh intercostal space (Figure 25). While the patient holds his or her breath on expiration, the needle is inserted into the liver. Aspiration is performed with a 10 mL syringe that is connected

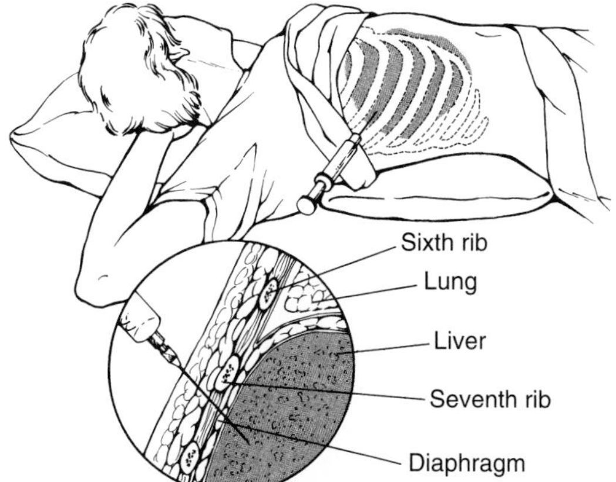

Figure 25. Liver biopsy. The patient is positioned for liver biopsy in a supine or left lateral position with the right arm abducted. *(Reproduced with permission from Burden, N. [1993].* Ambulatory surgical nursing *[p. 576]. Philadelphia: W. B. Saunders.)*

to the needle; cutting is done by rotating the needle apparatus so the cutting edge shaves off small bits of tissue. Once the needle is removed, the patient resumes breathing. The aspiration must be coordinated with breathing because during expiration, the liver and diaphragm are at their highest positions and while the patient holds his or her breath, the liver tissue is immobile. Both these factors help prevent laceration of the liver and diaphragm.

Once the tissue sample is collected, the physician prepares some slides immediately. The remainder of the tissue is placed in a sterile container filled with formalin or saline. The slides and sample are labeled and sent to the pathology laboratory for microscopic examination.

SIGNIFICANCE OF TEST RESULTS

Cirrhosis
Cancer of the liver, primary or metastatic
Cyst of the liver
Chronic hepatitis B or C
Alcoholic liver disease
Sarcoidosis
Amyloidosis
Wilson's disease
Miliary tuberculosis

INTERFERING FACTORS

- Obesity
- Infection in the right pleural cavity or right upper quadrant of the abdomen
- Uncooperative patient behavior
- Abnormal clotting ability

B

NURSING CARE

Pretest

- Once the physician has explained the procedure to the patient, the nurse obtains the patient's written consent. The form is then placed in the patient's record.
- ***Patient Teaching.*** Provide pretest teaching about positioning, breathing instructions, and posttest instructions. Patients tend to feel anxious about this test, so the nurse provides reassurance and support, as needed. The patient must discontinue all food and fluids for 8 hours before the test.
- Before the biopsy is done, the patient's clotting ability is evaluated by prothrombin time, or partial thromboplastin time, and a platelet count because liver disorders can cause impaired clotting ability. The prothrombin time should not be more than 3 seconds longer than the control time, and the platelet count should be greater than 100,000 cells/mm^3. The nurse reviews the test results and ensures that they are placed in the patient's record. If the results are abnormal, the nurse informs the physician.
- Baseline vital signs are taken and the results are entered in the patient's record.
- About 1 hour before the biopsy procedure, the nurse administers the prescribed pretest medication. Commonly, meperidine (Demerol) 50 mg or diazepam (Valium) 10 mg is injected intramuscularly to promote relaxation and analgesia.

During the Test

- The patient is positioned on the left side or supine, with the arm under the head. The skin is cleansed and draped with a sterile cloth.
- The nurse stands beside the patient to provide reassurance and help keep the patient immobile. Despite the use of local anesthesia, the patient feels some pain in the side and top of the shoulder as the needle passes through the phrenic nerves and into the liver.
- The nurse assists with the placement of the tissue in a specimen container and labels all slides and the container appropriately.
- Cover the skin at the biopsy site with a sterile bandage. Take and record vital signs and place the patient on his or her right side.

Posttest

- For 1 to 2 hours, the patient remains positioned on the right side with a pillow pressing on the waist and rib area. This helps the liver remain somewhat compressed against the rib cage to promote clotting.
- Take vital signs regularly and frequently because of the risk of hemorrhage or hypotension. Generally, the pattern is every 15 minutes for 1 hour, every 4 hours for 4 hours and every 4 hours thereafter, until the patient is stable. The nurse observes the lower right side of the rib cage for signs of bleeding. This may appear as oozing at the needle insertion site or as ecchymosis in a nearby area.
- The patient may resume food and fluid intake soon as desired. Bedrest is maintained for 12 to 24 hours. If the patient is to be discharged to the home, he or she remains on bedrest in the recovery area for 6 hours before discharge.

NURSING CARE—*cont'd*

- ***Patient Teaching.*** The nurse provides discharge instructions for the patient who is going home. The patient must avoid aspirin for 2 weeks. There must be no heavy lifting efforts until healing is complete. In 24 hours, the patient may remove the bandage and bathing can be resumed. Finally, the patient is instructed to notify the physician of any malaise, fever, pain or shortness of breath.

◇ Nursing Response to Complications

Usually, complications do not occur, but bleeding is possible. A blood vessel may have been punctured during the procedure, or impaired clotting ability may contribute to some blood loss. If excess bleeding or other abnormal assessment findings occur, the nurse notifies the physician immediately.

Bleeding. The nurse assesses for blood on or under the skin. Localized ecchymosis (bruising) would appear on the lower right lateral ribs or on the side of the abdomen just below the ribs. Signs of shock include restlessness, hypotension, tachycardia, dyspnea, pallor, and diaphoresis (cold, sweaty skin). The abdomen may be distended and painful.

Biopsy, Lung, Open

bai-op-see, lung, oh-pen

Also called: Pulmonary Biopsy, Open Lung Biopsy

SPECIMEN OR TYPE OF TEST: Pathology

PURPOSE OF THE TEST

A lung biopsy is performed to diagnose pulmonary disorders such as cancer and sarcoidosis. Lung biopsy can confirm the diagnosis of fibrosis and degenerative or inflammatory diseases of the lung.

BASICS THE NURSE NEEDS TO KNOW

A lung biopsy is performed to remove lung tissue so that the cells may be examined microscopically for pathologic features. A variety of methods are used to obtain these lung cells. Tissue samples may be obtained by bronchoscopy (see p. 158), by percutaneous or fine-needle biopsy (see p. 138), or by open biopsy.

With an open biopsy, surgery is required, with its potential risks. It involves the resection of a small portion of tissue, which is sent to the laboratory for histology examination.

NORMAL VALUES Normal tissue

HOW THE TEST IS DONE

For an open biopsy of the lung, a thoracotomy is required, which is a surgical procedure. After a small incision is made in the chest wall, the lung is exposed and tissue is excised. A chest tube or tubes are inserted to restore negative pleural pressure.

SIGNIFICANCE OF TEST RESULTS

Carcinoma
Granuloma
Infection
Sarcoidosis

INTERFERING FACTORS

- Noncompliance with dietary restrictions
- Smoking
- Obesity

NURSING CARE

Follow hospital protocol for the preoperative and postoperative care of a patient requiring open chest surgery.

◇ Nursing Response to Complications

Potential complications of an open lung biopsy are bleeding, pneumothorax, and empyema.

Bleeding. The nurse assesses for indications of bleeding: tachycardia, restlessness, hypotension, and tension pneumothorax. The nurse reports indications of bleeding immediately. Depending on the size of the hemothorax, the nurse would anticipate the need for chest tube(s) and thoracotomy tray.

Pneumothorax. Anxiety, restlessness, dyspnea, tachypnea, pallor, and decreased breath sounds are indications of pneumothorax. If a tension pneumothorax has occurred, there will be a mediastinal shift to the unaffected side. Notify the physician immediately and anticipate an order for chest x-ray to evaluate the size of the pneumothorax. Depending on the size of the pneumothorax, the nurse would anticipate the need for chest tubes and a thoracotomy tray.

Empyema. Empyema is an infection in the pleural cavity with an accumulation of pus. The patient usually presents with fever, chills, and sweating. The patient will complain of malaise, dyspnea, pain, and cough. The nurse should anticipate that the physician will order a white blood cell count and antibiotics and may want to insert chest tubes to drain the pleural cavity.

Biopsy, Lung, Percutaneous, Needle

bai-op-see, lung, per-ku-tay-nee-us, nee-duhl

Also called: PNB of the Lung; Fine-Needle Biopsy of the Lung; FNB of the Lung; Transthoracic Needle Biopsy

SPECIMEN OR TYPE OF TEST: Pathology

PURPOSE OF THE TEST

A percutaneous needle biopsy of the lung is performed to determine the pathology of a lung lesion such as cancer, granuloma, infection, and sarcoidosis. It is used for staging of malignant tumors. Percutaneous needle biopsy is also indicated for diagnosis of mediastinal masses.

BASICS THE NURSE NEEDS TO KNOW

Percutaneous needle biopsy of the lung has been made possible by the use of fluoroscopy and CT guidance. Intrathoracic lesions, especially of the lung parenchyma, can usually be visualized by biplane or C-arm fluoroscopy technique. For small intrathoracic tumors or those located in the hilar or mediastinal area, a CT scan is used to guide the biopsy.

NORMAL VALUES

Normal lung tissue

HOW THE TEST IS DONE

Under the guidance of CT scanning or fluoroscopy, a biopsy needle is inserted into a lesion and a specimen is aspirated for histology examination.

SIGNIFICANCE OF TEST RESULTS

Carcinoma
Granuloma
Infection
Sarcoidosis

NURSING CARE

Pretest

- The patient is kept on nothing-by-mouth status for 4 hours before the procedure, but may take medications (except aspirin and anticoagulants).
- The nurse takes and records baseline vital signs and ensures that an informed consent form is signed.
- The nurse assesses the patient for bleeding disorders because the needle path may be close to major vessels. The nurse also assesses the patient's history for contraindications to percutaneous needle biopsy: pulmonary hypertension, severe chronic obstructive lung disease, or arteriovenous malformation.
- ***Patient Teaching.*** Instruct the patient about the procedure and the need to remain still and not cough when instructed not to move. Practice with the patient holding breath on command.
- ***Patient Teaching.*** The nurse warns the patient that minor discomfort may be experienced during the biopsy and that multiple biopsies may be necessary.

Continued

NURSING CARE—*cont'd*

B

- Transport the patient to the CT laboratory; if fluoroscopy is planned, bring the patient to the radiology department.

During the Test

- The patient is positioned according to the location of the lesion.
- The skin is marked as a guide for needle insertion.
- The pulse oximeter is applied and baseline readings are taken and recorded. The nurse also checks vital signs. Have oxygen available in case a pneumothorax occurs during the procedure.
- Remind the patient not to cough or take deep breaths.
- Skin preparation is carried out, and the area is draped. A local anesthetic is given before the skin is nicked with a scalpel. The physician inserts the biopsy needle and tissue samples are taken. During insertion of the needle and any needle manipulation and biopsy, the patient is instructed to hold his or her breath and not move.
- A pathologist may be present to prepare slides from the aspirated specimen. If a pathologist is not present, the nurse places the tissue specimen in a sterile container, usually with a fixative. Special techniques may be required depending on studies being done. Check with the physician for desired media to use in the container. The tissue container and the requisition slip contain the appropriate patient information, the date, time, and the source of the tissue. The specimen then is sent to the laboratory.

Posttest

- The nurse records vital signs every 15 minutes during the first hour.
- Position the patient with the biopsy side down.
- Observe the patient for a minimum of 2 hours.
- Instruct the patient to avoid coughing and limit talking for 2 hours.
- A chest x-ray study is usually ordered immediately after the procedure and again 2 hours later to identify any pneumothoraces. Patients with small pneumothoraces (10% or less) are usually discharged. If a significant pneumothorax occurs, the patient is admitted to the hospital.
- ***Patient Teaching.*** The nurse instructs the patient being discharged to rest at home, to limit activities for the rest of the day, and return to the hospital if chest pain, discomfort, or shortness of breath is experienced.

◇ Nursing Response to Complications

The nurse needs to observe for indication of the complications of percutaneous needle biopsy, which are pneumothorax, hemorrhage, bile leak, and infection.

Pneumothorax. Anxiety, restlessness, dyspnea, tachypnea, pallor, and decreased breath sounds are indications of pneumothorax. If a tension pneumothorax has occurred, there will be a mediastinal shift to the unaffected side. Notify the physician immediately and anticipate an order for chest x-ray to evaluate the size of the pneumothorax.

Hemorrhage. Observe for overt or covert bleeding. Bleeding into the pleural space will cause a tension pneumothorax. The nurse will assess for tachycardia, restlessness, pallor, and hypotension. Response to bleeding will depend on the site and amount.

NURSING CARE—*cont'd*

Exert pressure if bleeding is at site of needle insertion. If large amount of bleeding has occurred into the pleural space prepare for chest tube(s) insertion.

Bile leak. Bile is very alkaline, if it leaks into the peritoneal space, the patient will complain of abdominal pain. Notify the physician. The nurse also positions the patient to maximize comfort.

Infection. Since the procedure is done under sterile technique, infection is rare. However, if indications of infection occur; such as fever, malaise, tachycardia, or elevated WBCs, the nurse informs the doctor. The nurse should anticipate that the physician will order cultures, so appropriate antibiotics may be ordered.

Biopsy, Pleural

See Thoracentesis, Pleural Fluid Analysis, and Pleural Biopsy on p. 606 or Thoracoscopy on p. 610.

Biopsy, Prostate

bai-op-see, pros-tayt

Also called: Core Biopsy of the Prostate Gland; Fine-Needle Biopsy of the Prostate; FNB of the Prostate

SPECIMEN OR TYPE OF TEST: Pathology

PURPOSE OF THE TEST

A prostate biopsy is used to determine the cause of an enlarged prostate gland or elevated PSA (prostate-specific antigen) level and to diagnose cancer of the prostate gland.

BASICS THE NURSE NEEDS TO KNOW

A biopsy of the prostate gland is indicated when a palpable nodule exists; when alteration in size, shape, or texture of the prostate gland occurs; when abnormal findings occur on ultrasound of the prostate; or when elevated levels of prostatic tumor markers exist.

Prostate cancer usually consists of multiple tumors that originate in the peripheral area of the prostate gland. The majority of these cases are adenocarcinomas. The microscopic study of the biopsy tissue confirms the diagnosis. If the tissue sample is malignant, it provides information on the tumor type, tumor grading, and local staging of the cancer.

A number of methods are used to obtain a tissue sample of the prostate. An open biopsy means that the peritoneal area is incised and a wedge of prostate tissue is surgically removed. The tissue sample also may be obtained during a transurethral resection procedure. Both these methods require general or spinal anesthesia.

Needle aspiration biopsy is another option to obtain a tissue sample. It may be performed via a transrectal or perineal approach. Ultrasound is used during a needle biopsy to guide the placement of the needle and confirm the presence of the needle in the tumor. A core biopsy procedure uses a larger needle (14- to 18-gauge) that may be attached to an automated core biopsy gun. The core biopsy needle has a higher accuracy rate in establishing a diagnosis than the fine needle biopsy, which uses a narrow, flexible prostatic aspiration needle.

NORMAL VALUE

Normal prostate tissue with no evidence of tumor or infection

HOW THE TEST IS DONE

The procedure varies dependent on whether an open or needle biopsy is done. If an open biopsy is performed, care is similar to the pre- and postoperative care of a patient with prostatic surgery. With a needle biopsy, a local anesthetic is given. Guided by ultrasound and using sterile technique, the physician inserts a needle into the prostate gland. Several samples of tissue are aspirated.

SIGNIFICANCE OF TEST RESULTS

Cancer of the prostate gland
Benign prostatic hypertrophy
Lymphoma
Prostatitis

INTERFERING FACTORS

- Failure to maintain nothing-by-mouth status
- Acute prostatitis

NURSING CARE

For an open biopsy (peritoneal or transurethral approach), the nurse carries out appropriate pre- and postoperative care of the patient with prostate gland surgery. For the needle biopsy approach, the nurse performs the following:

Pretest

- The nurse instructs the patient about the procedure.
- Ensure a signed informed consent has been obtained.
- ***Patient Teaching.*** Instruct the patient regarding bowel preparation. Usually, a disposable phosphate (Fleet) enema is ordered for the night before or in the early morning before the procedure.
- ***Patient Teaching.*** Instruct the patient that no food or fluids are permitted for 8 to 12 hours before the procedure.
- ***Patient Teaching.*** At the time of the procedure, assist the patient in removing all clothing and putting on a hospital gown. Instruct the patient to void before the procedure.
- The nurse also administers sedation as prescribed.

During the Test

- Assist patient into the lithotomy position.
- For the transperineal approach, the nurse prepares the local anesthetic for the physician. It is injected into the perineal area between the scrotum and rectum.

NURSING CARE—*cont'd*

- The nurse provides comfort and reassurance to the patient who may be anxious. Pain is felt as the anesthetic is injected. Warn patient that pain will be quickly resolved as local anesthetic takes effect.
- After it is removed, the nurse places the biopsy specimen in a sterile container with preservative. In some cases, cultures and tissue slides are prepared immediately.
- The nurse labels all specimens with the patient's name, date, and tissue source, and the specimens are sent to the laboratory immediately.
- Apply a sterile dressing to the perineal biopsy site. No dressing is needed for the transrectal approach.

Posttest

- The nurse takes vital signs and records the results.
- The nurse assesses for pain and offers pain medication as needed. The biopsy site is observed for signs of bleeding. Assess and report any patient difficulty in voiding or hematuria.
- ***Patient Teaching.*** The nurse instructs the patient to take prescribed antibiotic to prevent infection.

Nursing Response to Complications

The most common complication of this procedure is infection, especially in patients who have unknown prostatitis. It is also possible for the biopsy needle to accidentally penetrate the bladder or prostatic urethra. Bleeding, either external or within local tissue, may occur.

Infection. Fever, tachycardia, malaise, localized swelling, and pain may indicate infection after a biopsy of the prostate. The nurse anticipates the physician will order a WBC and a culture if there is any purulent discharge.

Bleeding. Observe for overt or covert bleeding in the form of rectal bleeding or hematoma formation in the perineum. The nurse will assess for tachycardia, restlessness, pallor, and hypotension. Response to bleeding will depend on the site and amount.

Biopsy, Renal

bai-op-see, ree-nuhl

Also called: Kidney Biopsy; Fine-Needle Aspiration Biopsy of the Kidney; FNB of the Kidney

SPECIMEN OR TYPE OF TEST: Tissue biopsy

PURPOSE OF THE TEST

Renal biopsy is used to determine the exact pathologic state and diagnosis of a renal disorder, monitor the progression of the renal disease, evaluate the response to treatment, and assess for rejection of a renal transplant.

B

BASICS THE NURSE NEEDS TO KNOW

Biopsy of the kidney provides specific information regarding the pathophysiologic changes in the tissue. Other laboratory tests and noninvasive procedures are performed first to obtain as much diagnostic information as possible. The broad categories of pathophysiologic conditions that require renal biopsy include acute renal failure, renal tumor, renal transplant rejection, asymptomatic hematuria, proteinuria of unknown origin, or questions regarding drug toxicity and untoward reaction to medication.

A renal biopsy may be done as a surgical procedure or more frequently by fine needle biopsy. Needle biopsy may be performed to diagnose renal cancer. It is used when computed tomography (CT) or magnetic resonance imaging (MRI) findings are inconclusive, to investigate metastatic disease or recurrence of cancer, and to diagnose type of renal tumor in the patient who is a poor surgical risk.

In renal transplant patients, the donor kidney can show signs of transplant rejection. Without biopsy, early accurate diagnosis of rejection is difficult because of other possible causes of renal dysfunction that produce the same symptoms. Fine needle aspiration biopsy is minimally invasive and can be used repeatedly on the same patient.

NORMAL VALUES

Normal renal tissue

HOW THE TEST IS DONE

After administration of local anesthesia, the physician inserts a biopsy needle percutaneously (through the skin) or through a small incision. Ultrasound or x-ray films are used to guide the exact placement and location of the biopsy needle. A syringe is used to aspirate a small core of tissue from the renal cortex. The total time needed to obtain the specimen is about 15 minutes.

SIGNIFICANCE OF TEST RESULTS

Abnormal Values

Acute or chronic glomerulonephritis
Goodpasture syndrome
Amyloid infiltration of the kidney
Systemic lupus erythematosus
Renal transplant rejection or failure
Renal cell carcinoma
Wilms' tumor

INTERFERING FACTORS

- Failure to maintain nothing-by-mouth status
- Coagulation disorder
- Urinary tract infection
- Nonfunction of one kidney

NURSING CARE

Pretest

- Ensure that written informed consent has been obtained and is entered in the patient's record. The nurse checks that all screening tests are completed and that the results are posted in the patient's chart. Coagulation studies, including prothrombin time testing, activated partial thromboplastin time testing platelet level determination, and hematocrit testing are performed to verify clotting ability. Urinalysis identifies the presence of any infection.
- The nurse takes baseline vital signs and records the results.
- The nurse administers sedation as ordered.

During the Test

- Cleanse the skin over the site with antiseptic.
- Provide reassurance to the patient to help alleviate anxiety. When the physician is about to insert the biopsy needle, instruct the patient to take a deep breath and hold it. Assist the patient in remaining still. A brief sensation of pain may occur.
- After the needle is removed, apply pressure to the puncture site for 20 minutes to help promote hemostasis. Then apply a sterile dressing and adhesive bandage to the puncture site.
- The nurse places the biopsy specimen in a sterile container with normal saline and ensures that the container is labeled with the patient's name and the tissue source of the specimen.
- Arrange for immediate transport of the specimen to the laboratory.

Posttest

- The nurse monitors vital signs every 15 minutes for 1 hour, every 30 minutes for the next hour, and at regular intervals thereafter. At frequent intervals, the nurse observes the dressing and surrounding tissue for signs of bleeding.
- For 8 hours, the nurse checks each voided specimen for hematuria. Initially, a small amount of blood may be present, but it should disappear within the 8-hour period. In some institutions, the protocol is to collect every urine specimen separately, with a notation of the time and date of voiding written on the container. Over time, progressively less blood should be present, and the urine should return to its normal color. If not contraindicated, the nurse encourages the patient to drink extra fluids to help promote urination.
- Eight hours after the test, the nurse obtains a specimen for hemoglobin and hematocrit determination. When bleeding is excessive, different time intervals and repeat testing may be necessary.
- ***Patient Teaching.*** Instruct the patient to lie flat for 12 to 24 hours. A sandbag may be used to help promote compression of the tissue. After this period of immobility, bedrest or limited activity is maintained for 24 hours to prevent the onset of fresh bleeding. The nurse also instructs the patient to avoid physical exertion, heavy lifting, and trauma to the lower back for several days.

Continued

NURSING CARE—*cont'd*

B

◇ Nursing Response to Complications

Although renal biopsy is considered safe, with a low complication rate, the procedure has some risks. These complications include retroperitoneal and urinary tract hemorrhage, pneumothorax, biopsy of other abdominal viscera, and infection.

Bleeding. The nurse observes for overt and covert bleeding. Vital signs may indicate tachycardia and hypotension. The nurse should also observe for restlessness, confusion, pallor, cool skin, and decreased urinary output. The patient may complain of dorsal, flank, or shoulder pain. The nurse immediately notifies the physician and anticipates an order for hemoglobin and hematocrit. A blood typing and cross-matching may also be ordered.

Infection. The nurse assesses site for inflammation (redness, warmth) and patient complaint of discomfort or tenderness at the site. The nurse notifies the physician and anticipates an order for a WBC.

Pneumothorax. Anxiety, restlessness, dyspnea, tachypnea, pallor, and decreased breath sounds are indications of pneumothorax. Notify the physician immediately and anticipate an order for chest x-ray to evaluate the size of the pneumothorax.

Biopsy, Skin

bai-op-see, skin

Also called: Gross and Microscopic Pathology, Skin

SPECIMEN OR TYPE OF TEST: Tissue biopsy

PURPOSE OF THE TEST

Skin biopsy is performed to differentiate a benign from a malignant growth. It is sometimes used to diagnose particular bacterial or fungal infections.

BASICS THE NURSE NEEDS TO KNOW

When a skin lesion is present and the clinical diagnosis is uncertain or must be verified, a skin biopsy is carried out to determine the cellular composition of the lesion or the presence of infection. Skin biopsy can be performed by three different types of technique, all of which cause minimal amounts of discomfort, scarring, and bleeding (Jacobs, et al, 1996). The methods are *shave biopsy, punch biopsy,* and *elliptical excision* (Figure 26).

Shave Biopsy

This procedure is used when a small, raised growth or lesion is present. The physician places the scalpel parallel to the surface of the growth, and a shallow cut is used to remove some of the superficial tissue layers.

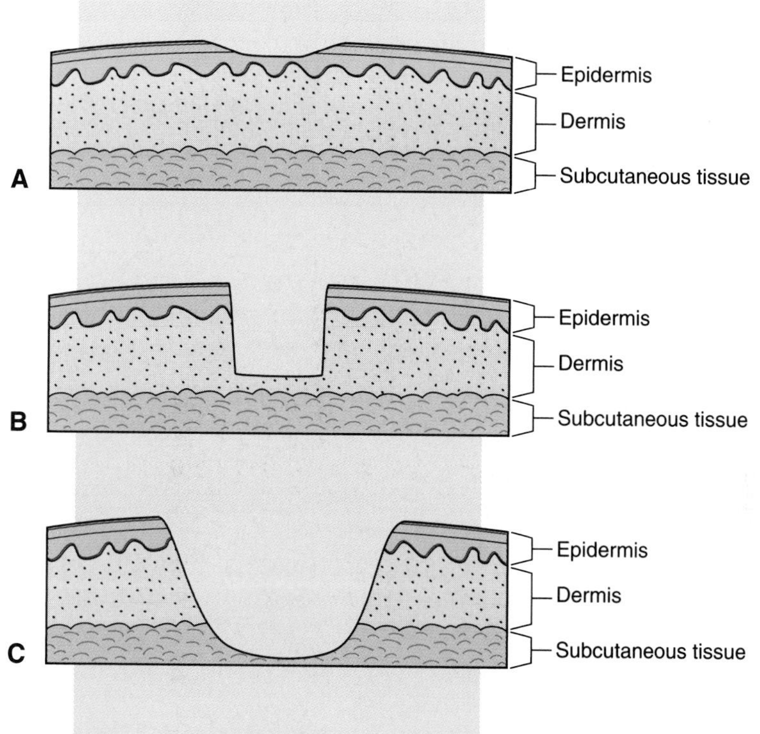

Figure 26. Skin biopsy. The depth of tissue removal for (A) shave biopsy, (B) punch biopsy, and (C) elliptical excision biopsy.

Punch Biopsy

This technique is used when the lesion extends into the middle to lower portion of the dermis. The physician places a circular cutting tool against the desired tissue and rotates with downward pressure to cut and remove a core sample of the skin. The small hole may be closed with a suture or allowed to heal by granulation.

Elliptical Excision Biopsy

This method is used when the lesion or growth is greater than 4.5 mm in diameter or is thought to extend deeper than the mid-dermis. The physician uses a scalpel to excise the tissue to a depth that includes some subcutaneous fat. The tissue defect is closed with sutures.

NORMAL VALUES Benign; no malignant cells are present. No infectious organisms are present.

HOW THE TEST IS DONE

After local anesthesia is administered, the physician removes a small sample of skin tissue surgically for histology and microbiologic examination.

SIGNIFICANCE OF TEST RESULTS

Abnormal Values

Malignant melanoma
Seborrheic dermatitis
Basal cell carcinoma
Keloid
Squamous cell carcinoma
Cyst
Neurofibroma
Bacterial infection
Dermatofibroma
Fungal infection
Mole

INTERFERING FACTORS

- Failure to identify the specimen
- Inaccurate identification of the specimen

NURSING CARE

Pretest

- After the physician has explained the procedure, the nurse obtains a written consent from the patient and places it in the patient's record.
- The nurse instructs the patient to remove the necessary clothing to expose the biopsy site. A hospital gown may be worn as needed. Vital signs are taken and the results are recorded in the patient's record. Depending on the site of the lesion, the nurse instructs the patient to sit or lie on the examining table.

During the Test

- The nurse cleanses the skin site with a surgical antiseptic. The nurse also assists with the application of the surgical drape and the preparation of the local anesthetic (lidocaine 1%).
- Once the tissue sample has been removed by the physician, it is placed in a sterile, covered container with formalin or other tissue preservative. If a tissue sample is needed for culture, place a small amount of the tissue in another sterile container *without preservative.*
- The nurse closes and labels each container accurately, including the patient's name, the date, and the tissue source. Place the same information on the requisition slip.
- After the bleeding ceases, the nurse places a small sterile dressing over the biopsy site.

NURSING CARE—*cont'd*

Posttest

- After the biopsy is completed, the nurse takes the patient's vital signs and records the results.
- The dressing is assessed for signs of bleeding. It should be clean, dry, and intact. The nurse instructs the patient to keep the dressing clean and dry as the biopsy site heals. If sutures are in place, the nurse instructs the patient to return to the physician for their removal. Facial sutures are removed in 3 to 5 days. For sites at other places on the body, the time of suture removal is 7 to 14 days.
- The nurse ensures that the specimens are transported to the laboratory promptly. Microbiologic specimens must be sent immediately, because they can dry out. The specimens in preservative are sent on a routine basis.

Biopsy, Thyroid

bai-op-see, thai-royd

SPECIMEN OR TYPE OF TEST: Pathology

PURPOSE OF THE TEST

A biopsy is performed to differentiate the cause of thyroid nodules or lumps. Thyroid nodules are more common in women and occur at any age. Thyroid cancer is rare; most nodules are benign. The biopsy will identify malignant thyroid nodules, follicular neoplasms, and benign lesions.

BASICS THE NURSE NEEDS TO KNOW

A thyroid biopsy is usually performed by fine needle aspiration (FNA). FNA has replaced surgical removal as a diagnostic technique because it avoids surgical risk and is less traumatic for the patient.

NORMAL VALUES Normal cells

HOW THE TEST IS DONE

FNA is usually carried out in the operating room to maintain sterile technique. It usually requires a local anesthetic only, which permits it to be performed on an outpatient basis. A 23- or 25-gauge biopsy needle is used to aspirate tissue from the nodule. Another method is called the capillary method, in which the needle is inserted into the nodule; with an up-and-down motion, tissue accumulates in the needle until blood is seen in the hub of the needle. The tissue is assessed by cytologic examination.

SIGNIFICANCE OF TEST RESULTS

Benign thyroid nodules
Cancer of the thyroid gland
Follicular neoplasm (cancerous or benign)

INTERFERING FACTORS

- Noncompliance with dietary restrictions
- Failure to place specimen in preservative immediately after aspiration
- Inadequate amount of tissue obtained

NURSING CARE

Pretest

- The nurse assesses the patient's level of anxiety, because fear of cancer may be significant or may interfere with the patient's ability to understand explanations.
- ***Patient Teaching.*** The nurse instructs the patient not to eat or drink for 12 hours before the test.
- Prepare the patient for the operating room according to hospital protocol.
- Ensure that a signed informed consent has been obtained.
- Administer preprocedure medication as prescribed.

During the Test

- The patient is positioned supine with a small pillow under the shoulders.
- A local anesthetic may or may not be given by the physician. General anesthesia may be required in some cases.
- The nurse encourages the patient not to move or swallow as the local anesthetic is given.
- The nurse supports the patient, who will feel pressure as the procedure is performed.
- After the needle is removed, the nurse maintains direct pressure on the site for 10 to 15 minutes.

Posttest

- The nurse reassures the patient that tenderness at the biopsy site is expected.
- Position the patient in a semi-Fowler's position with a small pillow under the head to remove stress from the site. The nurse provides an ice pack if it is ordered.
- ***Patient Teaching.*** Instruct the patient to support the head when changing position.
- ***Patient Teaching.*** The patient should keep the site clean and dry.

◆ Nursing Response to Complications

Complications of a thyroid biopsy are rare. Most patients complain only of some tenderness, but the nurse should observe for possible overt bleeding, hematoma, edema, or infection. If abnormal findings are present, the nurse notifies the physician immediately.

Bleeding. The nurse assesses for indications of bleeding: tachycardia, restlessness, hypotension, and overt bleeding at the site or at the back of the neck. The nurse reports indications of bleeding immediately.

Hematoma. Hematoma at the site of the biopsy may cause swelling, dyspnea, or stridor.

Infection. The nurse assesses site for inflammation (redness, warmth) and the patient's complaint of discomfort or tenderness at the biopsy site. The nurse anticipates an order for a WBC.

Bleeding Time

blee-ding taim

SPECIMEN OR TYPE OF TEST: Blood

PURPOSE OF THE TEST

The bleeding time test is used to screen for platelet malfunction or for a vascular defect that interferes with clotting.

BASICS THE NURSE NEEDS TO KNOW

The bleeding time test is used for the patient who is suspected of having a clotting abnormality, particularly one that involves capillaries or platelet function. The bleeding time is performed by the Mielke method. The test involves a skin puncture followed by blotting of the drops of blood until the bleeding stops. The test is measured in the time (minutes) it takes for a clot to form. The elevated level or prolonged time needed for clot formation indicates a vascular problem or disorder of platelet function. Other coagulation disorders usually result in normal values.

NORMAL VALUES	Bleeding time: Approximately 1.5–9 minutes

HOW THE TEST IS DONE

A medical technologist uses a blood pressure cuff that is applied to the arm and inflated to 40 mm Hg of pressure. This compresses the capillary circulation. Once the volar aspect of the skin is cleansed with alcohol, a template with a spring-loaded blade is used to make two cuts in the skin. Filter paper is used to blot the drops of blood every 30 seconds until the bleeding ceases (Figure 27).

SIGNIFICANCE OF TEST RESULTS

Elevated Values

Thrombocytopenia
Glanzmann's thrombasthenia
DIC
Severe metabolic acidosis
Macroglobulinemia
von Willebrand's disease
Gray platelet syndrome
Renal failure
Hereditary afibrinogenemia
Myeloproliferative diseases

INTERFERING FACTORS

- Laceration of a small vein
- Recent aspirin ingestion
- History of keloid formation
- Platelet count $<100,000$ cells/mm^3

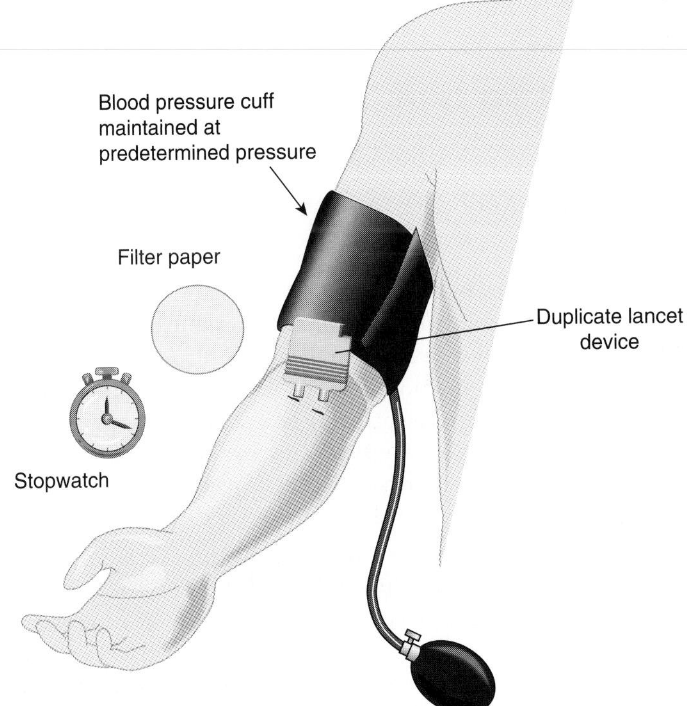

Figure 27. Bleeding time test. *(Reproduced with permission from Stevens, M. L. [1997].* Fundamentals of clinical hematology *[p. 267]. Philadelphia: W. B. Saunders.)*

NURSING CARE

Pretest

- The nurse asks the patient if he or she has taken aspirin in the past 7 days. The patient is instructed to avoid the ingestion of aspirin until the test is completed. The test cannot be scheduled until at least 7 days after the last dose of aspirin has been taken.
- The physician explains the procedure to the patient. The patient should understand that a small scar can result from the puncture or incision.
- Some laboratories require a written consent.
- The nurse or medical technologist inspects the volar aspect of the forearm for rash, infection, or skin eruption. None should be present.

Posttest

- The nurse applies a butterfly dressing to the skin site. The bandage remains in place for 24 hours.
- As it heals, the nurse or the patient inspects the skin site daily for signs of infection, as evidenced by swelling, redness, tenderness, and serous or purulent drainage.

Blood Urea Nitrogen

See Urea Nitrogen, Blood on p. 643.

Bone Mineral Density

bohn mi-ni-ruhl den-si-tee

Also called: (BMD); Bone Densitometry; Dual Energy X-Ray Absorptiometry; (DEXA, DXA)

SPECIMEN OR TYPE OF TEST: Radiography

PURPOSE OF THE TEST

Bone mineral density testing is used as a screening test to predict risk of a fracture of the bone. It also establishes the diagnosis of osteoporosis and measures the initial severity of the condition as well as the effectiveness of treatment.

BASICS THE NURSE NEEDS TO KNOW

Osteoporosis is a metabolic bone disease that causes the bones to become more porous or less dense. Because the bones become "thin" or brittle, they are at risk for fracture. Osteoporosis occurs most often in postmenopausal women older than age 65.

Bone mineral density determination can detect a decrease in bone mineral density at a very early stage, before osteoporosis or fractures occur. If the procedure is done only once, the measurement of the patient's bone mineral density is compared with the values of the general population. If the patient has follow-up procedures performed over the years, it may be possible to compare the results with previous findings and determine whether additional loss or improvement has occurred in response to therapy.

The usual method of measurement of bone mineral density is by dual energy densitometry absorptiometry (DEXA), a specialized form of x-ray examination of bones. Two other methods can be used to screen for osteoporosis. Quantitative computed tomography (CT) is very accurate in the measure of the bone density, but it uses an increased level of exposure to radiation and is more difficult to schedule for an appointment. Quantitative heel ultrasonography (QUS) is of increased interest because of its ease of measurement and availability of the equipment in small communities. The procedure uses ultrasound to measure the bone density in the calcaneus (heel bone). It is a lower cost procedure, but the test is not quite as accurate or sensitive as the DEXA bone density test.

Test Results

The patient's bone mineral density measurement is usually compared with the average test value of young normal individuals (T score). It also can be compared with the average test value of individuals who are the same sex and age (Z score). The standard deviation (SD) is a statistical measurement that represents how much the patient's value is above (+) or below (–) the average, or mean value.

A test result that is between 1.0 and 2.5 SD below the mean (written as −1.0 SD to −2.5 SD) indicates a low bone mass, or osteopenia. Osteoporosis is indicated by a test result that is −2.5 SD or more below the average value. If the level is this low and a fracture has already occurred, the osteoporosis is severe.

NORMAL VALUES

Within 1.0 SD of the average value

HOW THE TEST IS DONE

Dual x-ray beams above and below the patient scan the designated areas of bone. The usual areas are the vertebrae of the lumbar spine and the neck of the femur. From the patient's data, computer calculations measure the bone density and calculate the test results as compared with standardized normal values. The procedure is painless and takes 10 to 15 minutes to complete.

SIGNIFICANCE OF TEST RESULTS

Osteopenia
Osteoporosis
Osteomalacia

INTERFERING FACTORS

- Calcified aortic aneurysm
- Previous bone fracture
- Metal prosthetic device
- Metallic items on the clothing or the body in the imaging area

NURSING CARE

- ***Health Promotion.*** The nurse can teach women about the risks of osteoporosis and the benefits of the density scans. The goals of a screening test are early detection of osteoporosis and early treatment before there is extensive bone loss or a fracture. For women who are at increased risk for osteoporosis and fracture, the recommendation is to begin osteoporosis screening at age 60. Three established factors of increased risk for osteoporosis are low body weight, no current use of estrogen therapy, and increasing age. For women who are low risk, routine screening for osteoporosis should begin at age 65. The frequency of repeat screening for either group has not yet been established, but retesting at 2-year or somewhat longer intervals is recommended by the US Preventative Services Task Force (2003). For all postmenopausal women older than age 65, the risk of osteoporosis increases over time.

Pretest

- ***Patient Teaching.*** Instruct the patient to remove any jewelry or clothing that contains metal (buttons, belt, and clothing with a zipper) in the area to be imaged. It is not necessary to disrobe completely.

NURSING CARE—*cont'd*

- *Patient Teaching.* Explain that no noise, pain, or discomfort is associated with the procedure. Although the procedure uses radiation, the exposure and dose are minimal.

During the Test

- The patient is positioned on an imaging table. For measurement of the bone density of the vertebrae, the patient is in the supine position, with the lower legs elevated on a boxlike cushion. This aligns the pelvis and spine in a flat position on the table. For measurement of the bone density of the femoral neck, the patient is supine, with the nondominant leg braced in a position of internal rotation.

Posttest

- The patient is informed of the test results by the physician. If the patient has osteopenia or osteoporosis, medication therapy helps increase bone mineral density. The treatment lowers the risk of a bone fracture in the patient who is vulnerable. The nurse assists the patient by teaching about the prescribed medication and the specific information about when and how to take the drug.

Bone Scan

bohn skan

SPECIMEN OR TYPE OF TEST: Nuclear scan

PURPOSE OF THE TEST

The bone scan is used to detect the presence and extent of metastatic disease of the bones. In addition, it is used to monitor degenerative bone diseases, detect osteomyelitis, determine bone viability, identify bone biopsy sites, and evaluate difficult fractures or fractures in battered children.

BASICS THE NURSE NEEDS TO KNOW

Radionuclide bone studies produce sensitive, high-resolution images of the skeleton and joints. Because of the effectiveness of bone-seeking radiopharmaceuticals, the bone scan is sensitive to changes in bone.

Bone tissue is metabolically active, with a large number of nutrients exchanged in the blood vessels that supply the bones. A continual renewal of bone tissue is maintained by a balance between *osteogenesis,* the manufacture of new bone, and bone reabsorption. This renewal process is called *bone turnover.* The bone scan procedure uses the physiology of bone turnover to ensure uptake of the radiopharmaceutical into the bone where it can be detected by the scintillation camera or scanner.

Bone Imaging

The normal scan demonstrates symmetrical activity throughout the skeleton. In children, greater uptake occurs in the growth regions of the epiphyses, cranial sutures, and joints of the pelvic bones. The abnormal scan presents "hot" or "cold" spots and an asymmetrical uptake of the radiopharmaceutical. A *hot spot* is an area of increased uptake of the radiopharmaceutical that indicates increased osteogenic activity (Figure 28). The cause may be a primary or metastatic malignancy, Paget's disease, infection, healing activity in the repair of a fracture, or other conditions that accelerate osteogenesis. A *cold spot* indicates decreased uptake because of an absence of osteogenic activity. Causes of decreased or absent activity include a lack of blood supply to the area of bone or destruction of bone tissue by tumor, an inflammatory mass, or irradiation.

Joint Imaging

Because joints can be imaged, the bone scan can evaluate inflammatory joint disease. The radionuclide collects in tissues with increased blood flow, such as in the increased

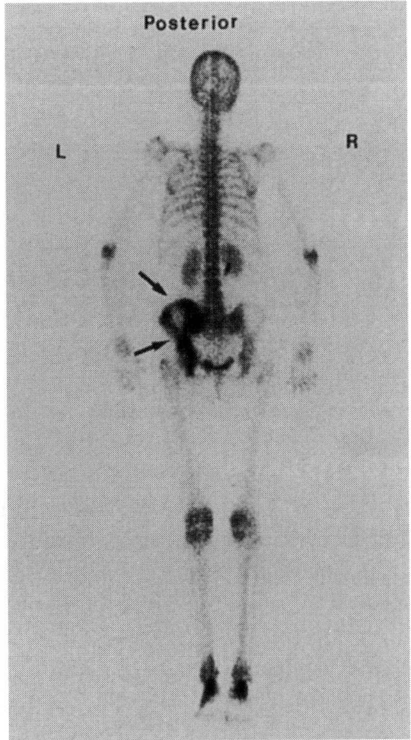

Figure 28. Bone scan of Paget's disease. This posterior view shows a darkened area *(arrows)* on the left side of the patient's iliac crest and pelvis. The increased uptake of radionuclide in the affected area is due to the markedly increased bone activity and increased blood flow that occur in Paget's disease. *(Reproduced with permission from Mettler, F. M. [1996].* Essentials of radiology *[p. 332]. Philadelphia: W. B. Saunders.)*

vascularity of synovitis or degenerative arthritis. Often, early joint inflammation is detected by radionuclide scan before it can be seen on x-ray film.

B

NORMAL VALUES Symmetry of uptake of the radionuclide, with no bone abnormalities noted

HOW THE TEST IS DONE

An intravenous injection of a technetium radiopharmaceutical is followed by scanning with a gamma camera 1 to 4 hours later. The time variable depends on the type of radiopharmaceutical used. Scans of anterior and posterior views are done. The images can be seen on the monitor and photographed for further study. The scanning process takes 1 hour to complete.

SIGNIFICANCE OF TEST RESULTS

Abnormal Values

Primary malignant bone tumor
Metastatic tumors
Osteomyelitis
Paget's disease
Fractures
Arthritis
Loose prosthesis
Soft tissue activity
Aseptic necrosis
Post radiation therapy

INTERFERING FACTORS

- Metallic objects
- Full or enlarged bladder
- Pregnancy

NURSING CARE

Pretest

- The procedure requires a signed consent from the patient that is entered into the patient's record. Ensure that the patient is not pregnant, because the radioactivity presents a potential danger to the fetus.
- ***Patient Teaching.*** Teach the patient that the radiopharmaceutical is a radioactive substance, but it is of low dosage and has a short half-life. After the test, it will be excreted rapidly in the urine so that radiation exposure is minimal. Also instruct the patient to remove all clothing and jewelry and put on a hospital gown. The bladder must be emptied before the start of the procedure, because retained urine will contain the radiopharmaceutical and prevent a clear view of the pelvis.

Continued

B

NURSING CARE—*cont'd*

During the Test

- In the radiology department, the radiopharmaceutical is injected intravenously, usually in an arm vein. After the injection but before the scanning process begins, the patient will be asked to drink several glasses of water. These extra fluids will help the patient void at the end of the procedure.

Posttest

- If disposing the patient's urine, the nurse should wear gloves and wash hands afterward. The radionuclide is excreted over a few days, although the radioactivity level is minimal after a few hours. The urine can be disposed of in the toilet.
- ***Patient Teaching.*** Instruct the patient to wash his or her hands after voiding. Reassure the patient that the amount of radioactivity in the urine is minimal, but it will remain on the hands unless they are washed.

Bronchial Provocation Test

See Pulmonary Function Studies on p. 557.

Bronchoalveolar Lavage

See Bronchoscopy, below

Bronchoscopy

bron-kos-kuh-pee

SPECIMEN OR TYPE OF TEST: Endoscopy

PURPOSE OF THE TEST

Bronchoscopy may be performed for therapeutic or diagnostic purposes. Bronchoscopy is used diagnostically to visualize possible tumors, obstructions, secretions, bleeding sites, or foreign objects in the tracheobronchial system. It permits the collection of secretions for cytologic and bacteriologic study, as well as for assessing tumors for potential resection. Tissue for lung biopsy may be obtained through the bronchoscope.

Bronchoscopy is used therapeutically to remove foreign objects from the tracheobronchial tree and to remove secretions that are obstructing the air passages. A bronchoscope may be used to fulgurate (electrodesiccate) and excise lesions.

BASICS THE NURSE NEEDS TO KNOW

Bronchoscopy is an endoscopic diagnostic procedure involving the inspection and observation of the trachea, larynx, and bronchi. Bronchoscopy is ordered when patients have unexplained pulmonary signs and symptoms or when nonspecific radiographic abnormalities exist.

A bronchoscope permits direct visualization of the tracheobronchial tree down to the subsegmental bronchi. A biopsy of lung tissue may be performed via the bronchoscope *(transbronchial lung biopsy)*. It is usually done under fluoroscopy to permit proper positioning and opening of the forceps. A *transcatheter bronchial brushing* may also be carried out to obtain a biopsy. A small brush is inserted through the bronchoscope, which is moved back and forth until cells adhere to the brush. Once the brush is removed, the cells are brushed onto slides. Most bronchoscopy is performed with a fiberoptic bronchoscope, which is flexible. To remove foreign objects lodged in the larger airways, a rigid bronchoscope is usually used.

Bronchoalveolar lavage (BAL) is an additional technique, which can be performed with a fiberoptic bronchoscope. It is used to diagnose and manage interstitial lung disease. It is also used in the diagnosis of lung cancer and pulmonary infections.

NORMAL VALUES	No abnormalities visualized No growth in culture specimen

HOW THE TEST IS DONE

A rigid (metal) or flexible fiberoptic bronchoscope may be used. The rigid bronchoscope uses a hollow metallic tube with a light at its distal end. It is useful in removing secretions, in evaluating future surgical interventions, and in dilating endobronchial strictures. The rigid bronchoscope has almost been replaced by the flexible fiberoptic bronchoscope. However, the physician may prefer the metal scope under certain circumstances, such as in the case of endobronchial tumor resection, massive hemorrhage, foreign body removal, and treatment of small children.

The bronchoscope is inserted through the nose (most common) or through the mouth. The tube is inserted as the physician observes the condition of the upper airways through the eyepiece and guides the tube to the area of the lung to be evaluated (Figure 29).

If BAL is desired, the tip of the fiberoptic catheter is inserted until it wedges in the respiratory tract. Several boluses of 20 mL of normal saline at body temperature are injected distal to the wedge catheter. After each bolus, the BAL fluid is aspirated. Usually, approximately 50% of the fluid is aspirated. Total bolus fluid should not exceed 300 mL or 3 mL/kg of patient's body weight.

SIGNIFICANCE OF TEST RESULTS

Atelectasis
Bleeding
Bronchial adenomas
Foreign objects
Infection
Lung cancer
Sarcoidosis
Secretions

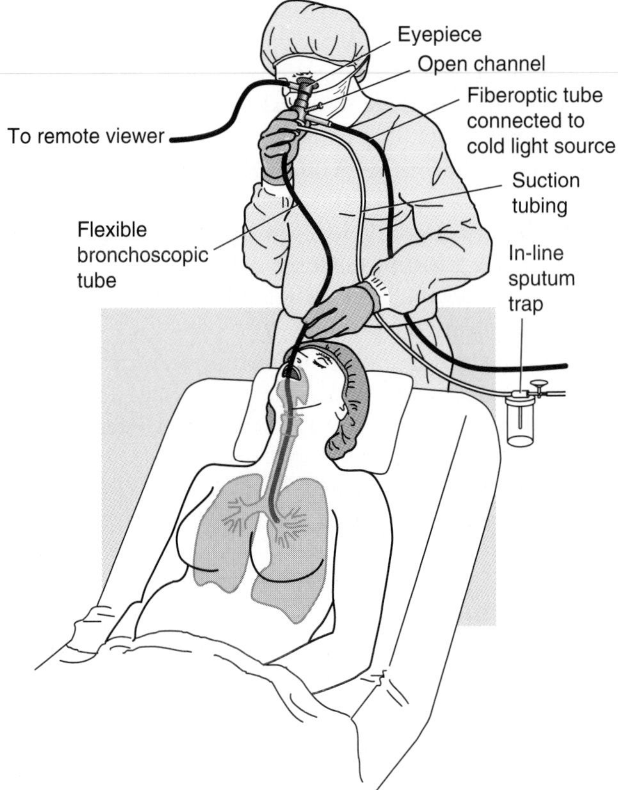

Figure 29. Flexible fiberoptic bronchoscopy.

Tuberculosis
Tumors

INTERFERING FACTORS

- Patient distress (may require general anesthesia)
- For BAL: Less than 25 mL specimen volume

NURSING CARE

Pretest

- The nurse ensures that a signed consent form has been obtained.
- The nurse assesses for and reports indications of hypoxia or history of asthma
- Obtain a medication history to determine whether the patient is receiving anticoagulant therapy or aspirin preparations. If a prothrombin time (PT), a partial thromboplastin time (PTT), and a platelet count were ordered, the nurse checks the results and reports any bleeding problems to the physician.

NURSING CARE—*cont'd*

B

- ***Patient Teaching.*** The nurse instructs the patient not to eat or drink for 4 to 6 hours before the test and explains the purpose of and procedure for the test.
- ***Patient Teaching.*** Warn the patient that the local anesthetic may taste bitter.
- ***Patient Teaching.*** Inform the patient that as the tube is inserted, it may feel like something is caught in the throat; provide reassurance that the airway is not blocked.
- The nurse evaluates and records baseline vital signs. The nurse administers atropine as prescribed to reduce tracheobronchial secretions and inhibit vagal stimulation. A sedative, such as midazolam hydrochloride (Versed), may also be ordered and given. Codeine may be ordered and administered to decrease the cough reflex.

During the Test

- The patient is positioned in the semi-Fowler or Fowler's position and the pulse oximeter is attached to the patient. The physician sprays a local anesthetic onto the pharynx, and the solution is dropped onto the vocal cords, epiglottis, and trachea to abolish the gag reflex.
- The nurse provides the patient with continuous emotional support during the procedure.
- To ensure patient comfort, a continuous infusion of diazepam is usually maintained.
- Encourage the patient to breathe through the nose or to pant.
- The nurse maintains supplemental O_2 for nonintubated patients and continuously monitors the patient's response, vital signs, and SaO_2.

Posttest

- The nurse continues to assess the patient's vital signs.
- Food and fluids are withheld until the gag reflex returns. The nurse reassures the patient that hoarseness, sore throat, and blood-streaked sputum are common. Provide throat lozenges or throat sprays as comfort measures. The nurse instructs the patient to expectorate rather than swallow saliva, because it may contain the local anesthetic.
- If a biopsy or bronchoalveolar lavage has been performed, the nurse sends the specimen to the histology laboratory and the microbiology laboratory.

◆ Nursing Response to Complications

Complications are rare but include bleeding, drug reactions, hypotension, laryngospasm, bronchospasm, hypoxia, dysrhythmia, pneumothorax, and cardiopulmonary arrest.

Bleeding. Bleeding after a bronchoscopy may vary from slight pink-tinged sputum to frank bleeding. The bleeding may also be overt or covert. The nurse assesses vital signs for tachycardia, tachypnea, and hypotension. The nurse observes for restlessness and hemoptysis. Because bleeding may occur into the pleural cavity, the nurse checks for tension pneumothorax. The nurse reports evidence of bleeding to the physician. If a tension pneumothorax is suspected, anticipate physician need for chest tube(s) and thoracotomy tray.

Hypoxia. A patient presenting with hypoxia after a bronchoscopy may complain of dyspnea, appear short of breath, will be restless or confused, and his or her skin will be pale or cyanotic. If pulse oximetry is available, a low SaO_2 will be noted. If the patient

Continued

NURSING CARE—*cont'd*

is on a cardiac monitor, assess for dysrhythmias associated with hypoxia. Notify the physician and anticipate an order for oxygen therapy.

Bronchospasm. The nurse assesses for bronchospasm by listening for breath sounds and checking for indications of hypoxia. If wheezing is heard, notify the physician. Anticipate need for respiratory therapy.

Laryngospasm. If there was difficulty in inserting the bronchoscope, the trachea may have been traumatized. If the trachea swells, there may be partial occlusion of the trachea or it may go into spasms. Partial occlusion of the upper airway will cause a high-pitched sound on inspiration, which is called *stridor*. The nurse notifies the physician, because this may interfere with the patient's oxygenation.

Pneumothorax. Nursing assessment consistent with a pneumothorax is dependent on its size. The nurse listens for decreased or absent breath sounds and observes for indications of hypoxia. Patients may complain of tightness of the chest. If a tension pneumothorax has occurred, there will be a mediastinal shift to the unaffected side. The nurse will note the trachea shifting to the unaffected side. Depending on the size of the tension pneumothorax, a thoracotomy may be needed. Anticipate physician need for chest tube(s) and thoracotomy tray.

Calcitonin

kal-si-toh-nin

Also called: (CT); Thyrocalcitonin

SPECIMEN OR TYPE OF TEST: Serum

PURPOSE OF THE TEST

A calcitonin determination is usually performed to diagnose medullary carcinoma of the thyroid gland.

BASICS THE NURSE NEEDS TO KNOW

Calcitonin is a hormone produced and secreted by the parafollicular cells (C cells) of the thyroid gland. It may also be produced and secreted by ectopic sites such as the lungs, intestines, pituitary gland, and bladder. The action of calcitonin is to inhibit bone reabsorption, inhibit calcium absorption in the gastrointestinal tract, and increase calcium and phosphate excretion from the kidneys. It is believed that calcitonin is not secreted until plasma calcium levels reach 9.3 ng/dL.

To assess familial medullary cancer in relatives of patients with the cancer, a provocation test (also called a stimulation test) may be performed. Calcium chloride is given intravenously over 10 minutes, or pentagastrin is given intravenously over 5 to 10 minutes. Patients with medullary cancer will respond to these stimulants with excessive secretion of calcitonin.

NORMAL VALUES

Adult: <150 pg/mL *or* SI: <150 ng/L
Infant (cord blood): 25–150 pg/mL *or* SI: 25–150 ng/L
Infant (7 days old): 77–293 pg/mL *or* SI: 77–293 ng/L
Calcitonin stimulation test:
Male: <190 pg/mL *or* SI: <190 ng/L
Female: <130 pg/mL *or* SI: <130 ng/L

HOW THE TEST IS DONE

Venipuncture is performed to obtain 7 mL of venous blood in a heparinized green-topped tube. Calcitonin is measured using radioimmunoassay (RIA).

SIGNIFICANCE OF TEST RESULTS

Elevated Values

Cancer of the thyroid
Chronic renal failure
Ectopic secretion by malignant tumors
Endocrine tumors of the pancreas
Pernicious anemia
Subacute Hashimoto's thyroiditis
Parathyroid adenoma or hyperplasia
Pregnancy

INTERFERING FACTORS

- Noncompliance with fasting requirement

NURSING CARE

Nursing actions are similar to those used in other venipuncture procedures (see Chapter 2), with the following additional measures.

Pretest

- Schedule isotope scans or other exposure to radioactivity after blood is drawn for this test.
- ***Patient Teaching.*** The nurse instructs the patient not to eat or drink anything except for sips of water for 8 hours before the blood is drawn.

Posttest

- Inform the laboratory personnel that a calcitonin level is being obtained, because the blood sample must be separated immediately. The blood sample must be sent to the laboratory on ice immediately after it is drawn.
- The patient may resume a normal diet.

C

Calcium, Serum

kal-see-uhm, see-ruhm

Also called: Ca^{++}; Total Serum Calcium

SPECIMEN OR TYPE OF TEST: Blood

PURPOSE OF THE TEST

The serum calcium level is measured to assist in the diagnosis of acid-base imbalance, coagulation disorders, pathologic bone disorders, endocrine disorders, cardiac arrhythmia, and muscle disorders.

BASICS THE NURSE NEEDS TO KNOW

Calcium is one of the essential mineral elements of the body. Almost all of it is concentrated in bone. The remainder is present in the cells or extracellular fluids, including the serum, in which about half the total calcium is in a free or ionized state and is physiologically active. A little less than half the total calcium is bonded to albumin and other plasma proteins. In the serum and other extracellular fluids, the normal level of calcium is maintained in homeostatic balance by the actions of the small intestine, bones, and kidneys.

Calcium is needed for the process of bone formation and is an essential element in bone structure. It is also needed for many other physiologic functions, including coagulation of the blood, excitation of cardiac and skeletal muscle, maintenance of muscle tone, conduction of neuromuscular impulses, and synthesis and regulation of the endocrine and exocrine glands. On the cellular level, calcium preserves the integrity and permeability of the cell membrane, particularly for sodium and potassium exchange.

Elevated Values

An elevated level of calcium in the blood is called *hypercalcemia*. It alters the function of most body organs and can be a life-threatening complication. Hyperparathyroidism and malignancy are the most common causes of hypercalcemia.

Decreased Values

A decreased level of calcium in the serum is called *hypocalcemia*. It causes neuromuscular hyperactivity, affecting many organs and functions. Very low calcium levels also can be life threatening. Total serum calcium is lowered in conditions that decrease plasma proteins, impair intestinal absorption, alter renal filtration and resorption functions, or decrease the amount of parathyroid hormone.

NORMAL VALUES

Adult: 8.6–10.0 mg/dL *or* SI: 2.15–2.50 mmol/L
Child: 8.8–10.8 mg/dL *or* SI: 2.20–2.70 mmol/L
Infant (0–10 days): 7.6–10.4 mg/dL *or* SI: 1.90–2.60 mmol/L

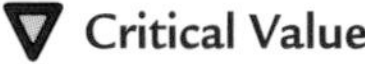

Critical Values <7.0 mg/dL (SI: 1.75 mmol/L) *or* >12 mg/dL (SI: >2.99 mmol/L)

HOW THE TEST IS DONE

Adult: A red-topped tube is used to collect 10 mL of venous blood.
Infant: A capillary pipette is used to collect capillary blood via the heelstick method.

SIGNIFICANCE OF TEST RESULTS

Elevated Values

Hyperparathyroidism
Metastatic cancer
Multiple myeloma
Vitamin D intoxication
Milk-alkali syndrome
Overuse of calcium antacids
Paget's disease
Idiopathic hypercalcemia of infancy
Polycythemia vera
Pheochromocytoma
Sarcoidosis
Adrenal insufficiency
Thyrotoxicosis
Bacteremia
Dehydration

Decreased Values

Hypoparathyroidism
Vitamin D deficiency
Alcoholism
Chronic renal failure
Hypoalbuminemia
Massive blood transfusions
Prolonged intravenous fluid therapy
Acute pancreatitis
Anterior pituitary hypofunction
Renal tubular disease
Cirrhosis of the liver
Malnutrition
Neonatal prematurity

INTERFERING FACTORS

- Upright position or prolonged activity before the test
- Prolonged storage of the blood specimen

C

NURSING CARE

Nursing actions are similar to those used in other capillary puncture or venipuncture procedures (see Chapter 2), with the following additional measures.

Pretest

- ***Patient Teaching.*** Instruct the patient to fast from food and fluids for 8 hours.
- ***Patient Teaching.*** Some medications (e.g., thiazides and other diuretics, lithium, calcium salts) cause a rise in serum value and also should be withheld during the period in which the patient fasts.
- Arrange to have the blood drawn in the early morning. This is because the calcium level normally fluctuates in a diurnal rhythm, with a lower serum calcium level in the late afternoon.

Posttest

- Arrange for prompt transport of the specimen to the laboratory. The analysis must be performed on a fresh sample to prevent a false elevation of the calcium value.

◆ Nursing Response to Critical Values

The nurse must notify the physician of any test result in the abnormal, critical value range. The nurse should also take the patient's vital signs and assess for specific manifestations that occur with calcium imbalance.

If the serum calcium level is very low, the hypocalcemia can induce depression or psychosis, laryngeal stridor, tetany, convulsions, hypotension, and decreased myocardial contractility. A severe decrease to 6 mg/dL (SI: 1.5 mmol/L) or less can be life threatening.

If the serum calcium is very elevated, the hypercalcemia can induce polyuria, anorexia, nausea, and coma. A severe elevation of 14 mg/dL (SI: 3.5 mmol/L) is more likely to induce coma and can cause death.

Calculus Analysis

kal-kyoo-luhs uh-nal-uh-sis

Also called: Kidney Stone Analysis; Renal Calculus Analysis; Nephrolithiasis Analysis

SPECIMEN OR TYPE OF TEST: Kidney stone

PURPOSE OF THE TEST

The analysis of urinary calculi is used in the work-up for nephrolithiasis. It determines the chemical composition of the stone and the metabolic factors that result in stone formation.

BASICS THE NURSE NEEDS TO KNOW

A renal *calculus* is commonly called a stone. It forms in the renal pelvis; descends through the ureter, bladder, and urethra; and exits from the body in the urine. Calculi are of various sizes, textures, colors, and chemical compositions. Common chemical compositions are: calcium, struvite, uric acid, and cystine. The composition of the stone will affect treatment to prevent reoccurrence.

Calcium stones are the most common type of renal calculi. These calculi are caused by excess calcium in the urine and consist of calcium phosphate, calcium oxalate, or a combination of the two chemical salts. These dark-colored stones are usually hard and have a rough surface. The underlying causes of calcium stone formation are thought to be increased intestinal absorption of dietary calcium, poor renal tubular resorption of calcium, a loss of calcium from bone, or any combination of these factors.

Struvite stones are sometimes called *infection stones,* because of their association with chronic urinary tract infection. It is not known whether the stone causes the infection to occur or the infection causes the stone to form. These pale stones are usually large and soft. They are also called a *staghorn calculus* because of the characteristic shape. The chemical composition of struvite stones is magnesium ammonium phosphate and carbonate apatite. Struvite stones are sometimes called *phosphate stones* based on their chemical composition.

Uric acid stones consist of uric acid and urate crystals. They are yellow-brown and moderately hard. They form in the presence of excess uric acid and concentrated acidic urine. Underlying causes include primary gout, dehydration, and some medications, including thiazide diuretics and salicylates.

Cystine stones occur rarely. They are dark yellow-brown and greasy. Their formation is caused by an autosomal recessive inborn error in metabolism that impairs the absorption of amino acids. Because of this deficit in metabolism, cystine and other amino acids are excreted in urine. The precipitate forms both crystals and stones.

NORMAL VALUES

No kidney stones are present in the urine

HOW THE TEST IS DONE

All urine is strained through a gauze strainer or a fine mesh sieve. Any stones that are recovered are placed in a glass bottle or plastic container and sent to the laboratory for qualitative analysis.

SIGNIFICANCE OF TEST RESULTS

Abnormal Values

Urolithiasis
Hypercalciuria
Hyperparathyroidism
Gout
Primary cystinuria
Dehydration
Urinary tract infection
Other infection

NURSING CARE

Pretest

- ***Patient Teaching.*** The nurse teaches the patient to use a clean container to collect the urine every time he or she voids. The first voided specimen of the morning is particularly important, because the stone may pass during the night.
- Each collected specimen is then poured through a strainer or sieve. The gauze or mesh is examined to see if a stone is present. Teach the patient to look carefully, because the stone can be extremely small. When a stone is recovered, it is washed of blood and tissue and placed in a clean, lidded container.
- ***Patient Teaching.*** The nurse instructs the patient not to wrap or place the stone on adhesive tape to secure it. The adhesive interferes with the infrared spectroscopy examination that is used to analyze the stone.

Posttest

- The nurse sends the stone to the laboratory in the labeled container. If the stone is enmeshed in the gauze, place both the stone and the gauze in the container.
- Specify on the requisition form that the source of the stone is urinary, and include the date and time that the stone was passed.

Cancer Antigen 125

Kan-suhr an-tuh-gen wun-twen-tee-faiv

Also called: CA 125

SPECIMEN OR TYPE OF TEST: Serum, body fluids

PURPOSE OF THE TEST

In patients with cancer of the ovary, this test is used to monitor response to treatment or the progression of the disease.

BASICS THE NURSE NEEDS TO KNOW

Cancer antigen 125 (CA 125) is a tumor marker for ovarian cancer. Normally, this antigen is present in small amounts in the serum. If cells are destroyed or cancer begins to grow, the rising level of the antigen can be detected in the blood. A variety of different benign and malignant disorders can cause the test value to be elevated. Because of the lack of specificity, this test cannot be used as a screening test for the general population. It is, however, a very helpful and reliable test to monitor the activity of known cancer of the ovary. A serum value greater than 35 U/mL (SI: >35 kU/L) is positive and correlates with malignancy. Further diagnostic testing is needed to verify the medical diagnosis and locate the malignancy.

A persistently rising value of cancer antigen 125 is associated with advancing malignancy, particularly advanced ovarian cancer. When the value rises after cancer treatment, the test gives early warning that the treatment is inadequate and additional or alternative medical intervention is needed. Conversely, in the patient with known ovarian cancer, a decline in the cancer antigen 125 value indicates a good response to treatment.

C

NORMAL VALUES

<35 U/mL *or* SI: <35 kU/L

HOW THE TEST IS DONE

A red-topped tube with a serum separator is used to collect 10 mL of venous blood.

SIGNIFICANCE OF TEST RESULTS

Elevated Values

Ovarian cancer
Adenocarcinoma of the cervix, endometrium, or fallopian tubes
Adenocarcinoma of the lung, colon, pancreas, or breast
Acute pelvic inflammatory disease
Endometriosis
Pregnancy

INTERFERING FACTORS

- Pregnancy
- Menstruation
- Recent radioisotope scan or abdominal surgery

NURSING CARE

Nursing actions are similar to those used in other capillary puncture or venipuncture procedures (see Chapter 2), with the following additional measures.

Pretest

- This test should be scheduled no sooner than 3 weeks after abdominal surgery to avoid a false positive result. The test should also be scheduled before or at least 7 days after any radioisotope scan so that the radioisotopes of the scan will not interfere with the test methodology.
- For the patient with a history of cancer, provide empathetic support. Her anxiety level is likely to be high because of the implications of a potentially elevated test result.

Posttest

- When the patient with a known history of ovarian cancer has a rising or elevated level of cancer antigen 125, a high probability exists that the cause is progression or recurrence of the malignancy. Before new treatment is instituted, additional diagnostic testing (including surgery, biopsy, or both) to examine abnormal tissue is indicated. Provide additional emotional support to help the patient cope during the stress of additional testing and in the decision-making that is part of the overall treatment plan.

Capillary Glucose/Sugar Monitoring

See Glucose, Capillary on p. 346.

C

Capnogram

kap-noh-gram

Also called: Exhaled Carbon Dioxide; Capnography; End-Tidal Carbon Dioxide; $ETco_2$; ($PETco_2$) Partial Pressure End Tidal CO_2

SPECIMEN OR TYPE OF TEST: Spectrometry

PURPOSE OF THE TEST

Monitoring exhaled carbon dioxide (CO_2) permits continuous evaluation of alveolar ventilation, reducing the number of ABG determinations needed. $ETco_2$ may be used to evaluate ventilator changes and weaning parameters from mechanical ventilation. It will confirm endotracheal intubation, because no capnographic waveform will occur if the tube is in the esophagus.

BASICS THE NURSE NEEDS TO KNOW

Capnography provides a CO_2 waveform, which visualizes CO_2 elimination patterns during exhalation and a total percentage of CO_2 exhaled per breath. CO_2 is measured at the end of exhalation, because at this point the exhaled CO_2 approximates arterial CO_2 levels. With normal perfusion of the lungs, arterial CO_2 will be a few millimeters higher (5 mm Hg) than end-tidal CO_2 ($ETco_2$). When perfusion is not adequate, this assumption cannot be made. Figure 30 shows a typical tracing of a capnogram.

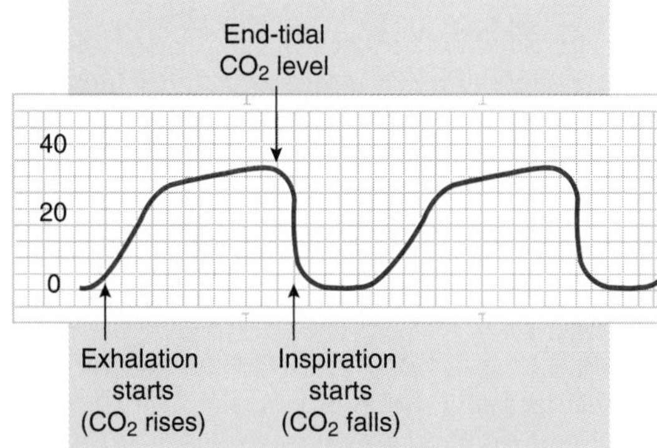

Figure 30. Capnographic tracing. On exhalation, the capnographic tracing shows a rapid rise in carbon dioxide followed by a plateau. At the end of exhalation, the end-tidal carbon dioxide level is obtained. As inspiration begins, there is a dramatic decrease in carbon dioxide.

Elevated Values

The $ETco_2$ increases in hypermetabolic states because of increased production of CO_2, and in hypoventilation because CO_2 is retained and not excreted.

Decreased Values

The $ETco_2$ decreases when the metabolic rate is reduced, as production of CO_2 decreases, and when there is reduced perfusion, causing a decrease in pulmonary blood flow.

NORMAL VALUES

35-45 mm Hg

HOW THE TEST IS DONE

Exhaled CO_2 is measured with exhaled gas analyzers. These analyzers measure the CO_2 by mass spectrometry or infrared analysis. Mass spectrometry requires aspiration of exhaled gas, whereas the infrared gas analyzer is usually attached to the exhalation tubing on a ventilator. The recorded value refers to the amount of infrared light absorbed by the exhaled breath. The higher the CO_2 level, the more infrared light is absorbed and the higher the reading.

For endotracheal tube placement, disposable colorimetric devices are available for single use.

SIGNIFICANCE OF TEST RESULTS

Elevated Values

Burns
Hypermetabolic states
Hypoventilation
Malignant hyperthermia
Multiple trauma

Decreased Values

Acute cardiac failure
Anesthesia
Bronchial spasms
Cardiac and pulmonary arrest
Dislodgment of the endotracheal tube
Hypothermia
Hypothyroidism
Hypovolemia
Mucous plug
Pulmonary edema
Pulmonary embolism

INTERFERING FACTORS

- Cardiopulmonary abnormalities
- Leak in system
- Metabolic disorders

NURSING CARE

During the Test

- Check the capnographic waveform. It should return to zero baseline on inspiration. If it does not, check the seal of the expiratory demand valve on the ventilator and the fresh gas flow in the tube.
- If the waveform disappears or drops to zero, it may indicate accidental extubation, obstruction, esophageal intubation, or cardiac arrest.

C

Carbohydrate Antigen 19-9

kar-boh-hai-drayt an-tuh-gen nain-teen-nain

Also called: CA 19-9; Cancer Antigen CA19-9

SPECIMEN OR TYPE OF TEST: Serum

PURPOSE OF THE TEST

Carbohydrate antigen 19-9 (CA 19-9) is a tumor marker that is used in preoperative staging for cancer of the pancreas. It is also used to monitor the course of pancreatic cancer, the response to treatment and to predict recurrence.

BASICS THE NURSE NEEDS TO KNOW

CA 19-9 is an antigen made by the pancreas, liver, colon, and other tissues. The antigen appears in the serum when these source tissues undergo healing or when there is a tumor growing in that organ or tissue. This tumor marker is most accurate in cases of pancreatic cancer. The serum level does not rise in an early stage of disease, but is most accurate in the late stages of cancer or during recurrence.

Malignancy causes this test result to rise dramatically. Large tumors of the pancreas can cause the serum level to rise to >1000 units/mL (SI: >1000 kU/L). Any result greater than 300 units/L (SI: 300 kU/L) is an indicator that the pancreatic cancer may be too advanced for surgical removal and in cancer of the colon the prognosis is ominous. After treatment of the cancer, CA 19-9 is used to monitor the patient's condition. A renewed elevation of CA 19-9 indicates that the cancer has returned. The serum level will rise before clinical symptoms appear.

Benign conditions of the pancreas, liver and gall bladder also can cause an elevation of CA 19-9. In benign disease, the elevation is much lower than the dramatically high elevations associated with cancer.

NORMAL VALUES Adult: <37 U/mL *or* SI: <37 kU/L

HOW THE TEST IS DONE

A red-topped tube with a serum separator is used to obtain 10 mL of venous blood.

SIGNIFICANCE OF TEST RESULTS

Elevated Values

MALIGNANCY

Cancer of the pancreas
Cancer of the stomach
Cancer of the colon
Hepatobiliary cancer
Cancer of the lung
Cancer of the head and neck
Gynecologic cancer

BENIGN CONDITIONS

Hepatobiliary disease
Acute pancreatitis

INTERFERING FACTORS

- None

NURSING CARE

Nursing actions are similar to those used in other venipuncture procedures (see Chapter 2), with the following additional measures.

Pretest

- Provide emotional support for the patient. Ongoing testing for cancer and tumor markers can be upsetting because of the implications of an elevated result.

Posttest

- When the elevated test result indicates recurrence of cancer, the patient will need emotional support. In some cases, there may be additional treatment options, but in cases of recurrent cancer of the pancreas, the prognosis is bleak. The nurse can use listening skills and empathy to allow the patient to verbalize or express emotion. As the patient becomes aware of declining health, he or she may express denial or anger, or may become depressed. Some will express hope and others will begin to make decisions regarding their future. Listening to the patient can provide the cues as to what the patient believes and how he or she wants to use the time that remains.

Carbon Dioxide, Total

kahr-buhn dai-ok-said, toh-tuhl

Also called: CO_2 Content; TCO_2

SPECIMEN OR TYPE OF TEST: Whole blood, serum, plasma

PURPOSE OF THE TEST

The total carbon dioxide (CO_2) determination is used to help evaluate acid-base balance and the bicarbonate buffer system.

BASICS THE NURSE NEEDS TO KNOW

Total CO_2 measures the combined forms of CO_2 in the blood. The largest component is bicarbonate ion, composing 90% of the total CO_2 content in the blood. The total CO_2 content provides the principal extracellular buffer system, which is called the bicarbonate carbonic acid buffer. Buffer systems are needed in the regulation of acid-base balance. The concentration of CO_2 is controlled by the lungs, and the concentration of bicarbonate is controlled by the kidneys.

Elevated Values

An elevated serum level of CO_2 is called *hypercapnia*. It often is caused by poor CO_2 excretion by the lungs or an inadequate respiratory drive.

Hypercapnia is associated with respiratory acidosis, CO_2 retention, and metabolic alkalosis.

Decreased Values

A low serum level of CO_2 is called *hypocapnia*. It is caused by excess elimination of CO_2, excess elimination of bicarbonate, excess accumulation of hydrogen ions in the blood, or a combination of these conditions. Hypocapnia is associated with respiratory alkalosis or metabolic acidosis.

NORMAL VALUES	2 years–adult (venous): 22–26 mEq/L *or* SI: 22–26 mmol/L 2 years–adult (arterial): 23–29 mEq/L *or* SI: 23–29 mmol/L Infant–2 years: 18–28 mEq/L *or* SI: 18–28 mmol/L
 Critical Values	<15 mEq/L (SI: <15mmol/L) *or* >50 mEq/L (SI: >50 mmol/L)

HOW THE TEST IS DONE

For venous or arterial blood testing, a green-topped tube with heparin is used to obtain 5 mL of blood. The rubber stopper must remain firmly in place so that the CO_2 cannot diffuse out and result in a falsely lowered value.

SIGNIFICANCE OF TEST RESULTS

Elevated Values

Respiratory acidosis
Emphysema

Pneumonia
Cystic fibrosis
Congestive heart failure
Pulmonary edema
Metabolic alkalosis
Hypokalemia
Excessive intake of antacids
Severe, prolonged vomiting
Cushing syndrome
Primary aldosteronism

Decreased Values
Respiratory alkalosis
Hyperventilation
Metabolic acidosis
Diabetes mellitus
Severe diarrhea
Renal tubular acidosis
Renal failure
Dehydration
Hypovolemia

INTERFERING FACTORS

- Exposure of the specimen to air

NURSING CARE

Nursing actions are similar to those used in other arterial or venipuncture procedures (see Chapter 2), with no additional measures.

◆ Nursing Response to Critical Values

The physician must be notified immediately if the TCO_2 reaches a critical value (either very low or very high). The blood pH and serum electrolytes also are likely to be in serious imbalance. The patient requires an immediate nursing assessment of all vital signs, with particular attention to abnormal changes in the rate and quality of respirations.

Carcinoembryonic Antigen

kahr-suh-noh-em-bree-yo-nik an-tuh-gen

Also called: (CEA)

SPECIMEN OR TYPE OF TEST: Serum, body fluid

PURPOSE OF THE TEST

Carcinoembryonic antigen (CEA) is a tumor marker used to monitor for and detect recurrence of colorectal cancer. It also may be used to help stage for cancers of the ovary, breast, stomach and pancreas (Figure 31).

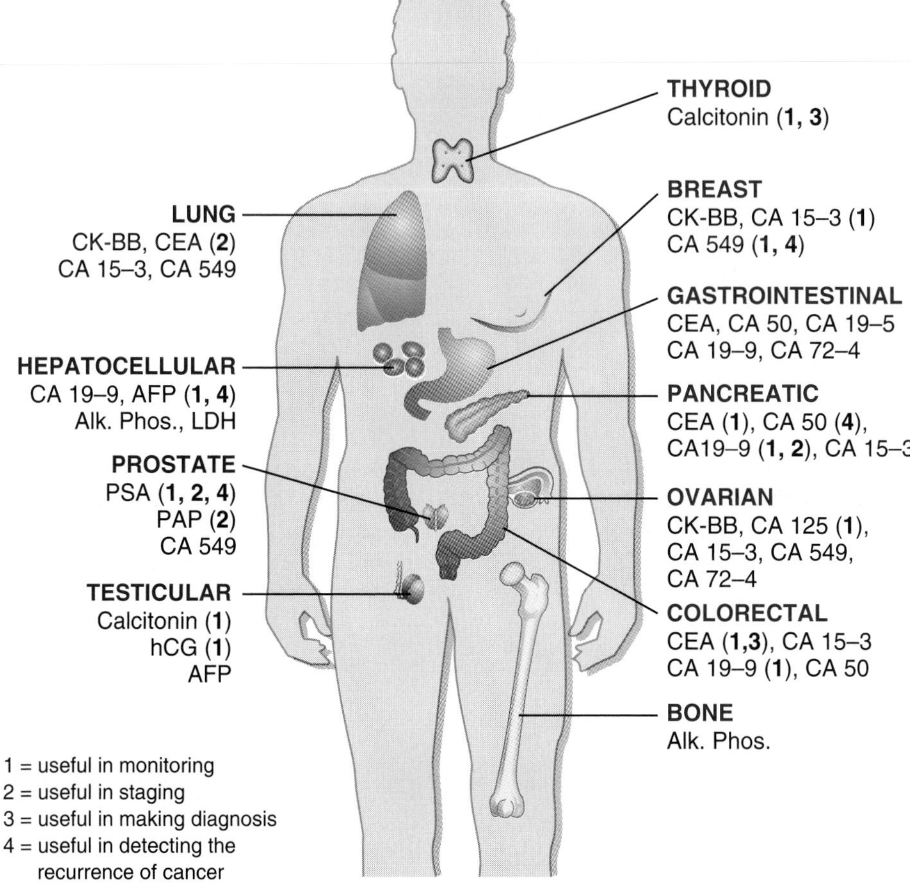

Figure 31. Tumor markers. Various tumor markers are used in the diagnosis, monitoring, staging, and detection of recurrence of cancer. *(Reproduced with permission from Lehmann, C. A. [1998].* Saunders manual of clinical laboratory science. *Philadelphia: W. B. Saunders.)*

BASICS THE NURSE NEEDS TO KNOW

In cancer, the necrosis of malignant tissue permits large amounts of antigen to leak out of the tumor and enter the blood and body (effusion) fluids. An elevated value of serum CEA indicates that there is extension or recurrence of cancer at the primary site or metastases to a distant site (often liver lung or bone). The CEA value often rises many months before other laboratory tests become abnormal and before the patient experiences symptoms.

Elevated levels can occur in benign disease, but the test values are in a lower range than those of malignancy. Smokers have a normal value that is higher than non-smokers, but do not necessarily have benign or malignant disease. A CEA value of >20 ng/mL (SI: >20 mcg/L) usually indicates cancer at a primary or metastatic site.

Interpretation of the test results is made with consideration of when the test is done. If the CEA value is normal after surgical removal of the cancer, the information means that no new cancer is growing. If the CEA value rises in the weeks, months, or years after surgical removal, it provides very early warning that cancer has recurred in the primary or metastatic site. Additional testing to locate the site of the cancer and additional cancer treatment are likely.

C

NORMAL VALUES

Adult, nonsmoker: <2.5 ng/mL *or* SI: <2.5 mcg/L
Adult, smoker: up to 5 ng/mL *or* SI: up to 5 mcg/L

HOW THE TEST IS DONE

Blood: A red-topped tube is used to obtain 10 mL of venous blood, or a lavender-topped tube is used to obtain 7 mL of venous blood. Blood specimens are generally done before surgery, 4 weeks postoperatively, and at regular intervals thereafter for 5 years.

Effusion Fluid: A sample of the effusion fluid is aspirated by the physician during a diagnostic procedure, such as a thoracentesis or paracentesis.

SIGNIFICANCE OF TEST RESULTS

Elevated Values

Malignant Conditions

Colorectal cancer
Stomach cancer
Pancreatic cancer
Breast cancer
Lung cancer
Thyroid cancer
Ovarian cancer
Cancer metastases (liver, bone, lung)

Benign Conditions

Ulcerative colitis
Crohn's disease
Hepatitis
Cirrhosis
Pulmonary infection
Radiation therapy

INTERFERING FACTORS

- Recent administration of radioisotopes
- Smoking
- Heparin
- Hemolysis

NURSING CARE

Nursing actions are similar to those used in other venipuncture procedures (see Chapter 2), with the following additional measures.

Pretest

- Schedule any nuclear scan after this test is completed. The radioisotopes of the nuclear scan would interfere with the laboratory method of analysis for CEA.

Posttest

- The nurse should be prepared to provide emotional support, as needed. Repeated CEA testing can cause the patient to experience some anxiety because it is a reminder of the uncertainty about future health. A negative or normal CEA value is "good news" regarding no recurrence of the cancer. If the CEA test becomes elevated at any time after the initial treatment, the patient's anxiety level will rise. In addition to emotional support, the nurse can provide or instill hope, because the CEA warning may occur up to 36 months before symptoms are felt. With additional treatment, there is still hope for a cure or remission of the disease.

Cardiac Markers

kahr-dee-ak mahr-kuhrs

Also called: Biochemical Cardiac Markers; Biomarkers; Cardiac Enzymes; Cardiac Isoenzymes

SPECIMEN OR TYPE OF TEST: Serum

PURPOSE OF THE TEST

Cardiac markers are used with clinical presentation and electrocardiographic studies to diagnose acute myocardial infarction (AMI). Accurate and rapid diagnosis of an MI will lead to early intervention, which will decrease mortality and infarction size. Based on clinical presentation, to rule out an acute MI, CK-MB (creatine kinase-MB) and troponin levels are usually ordered. These tests can be done at the bedside, permitting early intervention.

BASICS THE NURSE NEEDS TO KNOW

No single test currently can absolutely rule out an AMI. Based on timing (when the infarction actually occurs), there are cardiac markers with a high degree of sensitivity and specificity. The nurse needs to be aware that whereas the AMI is assumed to occur when chest pain is experienced, this is not always so. Patients may have severe chest pain from angina, before the infarction. Also, patients may experience atypical chest pain or no chest pain with an AMI.

The following is a brief discussion of the varied laboratory tests that may be ordered.

Enzymes are complex compounds, found in all tissues, that speed up the biochemical reactions of the body. Damage to body tissue causes release of the enzymes from the injured cells into the serum. Enzymes may be common to more than one type of tissue. Elevated serum levels of the enzymes reflect tissue damage, but because the enzymes are not specific, patterns of enzyme elevations are used to determine myocardial tissue damage.

Creatine kinase (CK) is an enzyme found in the heart, brain, and skeletal muscle. The individual with greater muscle mass has a higher CK level than does the average person. CK levels may be higher in African Americans. CK may be separated into three isoenzymes. *Isoenzymes* refer to the various forms of an enzyme, which can differ chemically, physically, or immunologically, but catalyze the same reaction. The CK isoenzymes include CK-MM, CK-MB, and CK-BB. With myocardial damage, the elevated fraction that rises is CK-MB. CKMB isoforms, a new cardiac marker, have even greater specificity.

Troponin is a protein found in skeletal and cardiac muscle fibers. Three forms of troponin exist, two of which are used in diagnosing cardiac disorders (cardiac troponin T [cT_nT], cardiac troponin I [cT_nI]). Normally, cardiac troponin levels are very low, but the level increases rapidly with an MI. Troponin I is found only in the cardiac muscle complex; therefore, it is very specific to cardiac injury. This is especially important if the person being evaluated for a cardiac problem has renal disease or a musculoskeletal disorder, which would make interpretation of the CK-MB difficult. Troponin levels increase earlier than CK-MB levels; thus, their evaluation may be helpful in diagnosing MI earlier than the enzymes studies. Earlier diagnosis may lead to earlier treatment and salvaging more myocardium.

Myoglobin (Mb, S-Mgb) is an oxygen-binding protein found in striated muscle. It releases oxygen at very low tensions. Any injury to skeletal muscle will cause a release of myoglobin into the blood. Because myoglobin rises and falls so rapidly, its use in diagnosing AMI is limited.

Lactate dehydrogenase (LDH) is present in almost all metabolizing cells but is especially high in the heart, kidneys, brain, red blood cells, liver, and skeletal muscles. Because LDH is present in so many tissues of the body, the origin of its release cannot be determined without the use of electrophoresis, which separates out its five isoenzymes. The LDH isoenzymes, LDH_1 and LDH_2, are used to assess myocardial damage.

C-reactive protein (CRP) is a marker for inflammation. It is produced by the liver and increases in response to tissue inflammation or injury. It lacks specificity in identifying myocardial injury. Currently, some studies have shown CRP as a better predictor for an MI than cholesterol. It is believed inflammation in the arterial walls and the body's response to inflammation may trigger a "cardiac event." Some recommend that men with a CRP higher than 0.15 mg/dL and women with a CRP higher than 0.38 mg/dL should be considered at significant risk and aggressive therapy be initiated. (Also see C-Reactive Protein, p. 241.) At this time CRP is not used to rule out an AMI.

C

NORMAL VALUES

CK
Adult male: 38–174 units/L *or* SI: 0.65–29.6 μKat/L
Adult female: 26–140 units/L *or* SI: 0.44–2.38 μKat/L
Newborn: 50–525 units/L *or* SI: 0.85–8.93 μKat/L

CK-MB
0%–6% of total CK *or* SI: 0.00%–0.06% (fraction of total CK)

Cardiac Troponin T
<0.2 mcg/L

Cardiac Troponin I
<0.35 mcg/L

Myoglobin
<90 mcg/L

LDH
Adult: 200–400 units/L
Neonate: 400–700 units/L

LDH Isoenzymes
LDH_1 14%–26% *or* SI: 0.14–0.26 (fraction of total LDH)
LDH_2 29%–39% *or* SI: 0.29–0.39 (fraction of total LDH)

HOW THE TEST IS DONE

A venipuncture is necessary to obtain 10 mL of blood in a red-topped tube.

SIGNIFICANCE OF TEST RESULTS

In diagnosing MI, a pattern of test changes *supports* the diagnosis. CK levels begin to rise 6 hours after the infarction; they peak in 18 hours, and return to normal in 2 to 3 days. CK-MB levels rise within 3 to 6 hours after an infarction, peak in 12 to 24 hours, and return to normal in 12 to 48 hours. An increase in CK-MB, expressed as a percentage of the total CK, supports the diagnosis of myocardial damage. The percentage accepted as diagnostic of an infarction varies from laboratory to laboratory. If the CK-MB level rises quickly and then drops quickly, myocardial contusion may be suspected. CK-MB levels will also drop quickly if thrombolytic therapy for an AMI has been successful.

Cardiac troponin is cardiac specific. It rises 2 to 6 hours after the onset of an AMI, peaks in 16 hours, and returns to normal in 5 to 9 days.

Myoglobin rises and falls within 2 to 6 hours of the onset of MI; therefore, timing of the specimen is crucial. If the patient delayed seeking treatment, myoglobin is not helpful in diagnosing an MI.

LDH elevations do not occur until 24 to 48 hours after an infarction. They peak in 3 to 4 days and do not return to normal levels for 10 to 14 days after an infarction. LDH_2 levels are normally greater than LDH_1 levels. A "flipped" LDH, which occurs when LDH_1 levels become greater than those of LDH_2, is indicative of an MI. The flipped LDH is especially helpful if the person delayed seeking help when chest pain occurred.

Because of their nonspecificity, other clinical problems may create changes in the cardiac markers. Common causes of these changes are as follows:

CK

Elevated Values

Amyotrophic lateral sclerosis
Biliary atresia
Burns
Some cancers
Cardiomyopathy
Central nervous system trauma, including cerebrovascular accident
Hypokalemia, severe
Hypothermia
Hypothyroidism
Infarction: cerebral, bowel, myocardial
Intramuscular injections
Muscular dystrophy
Myocarditis
Organ rejection
Pulmonary edema
Pulmonary embolism
Renal insufficiency or failure
Surgery

Decreased Values

Addison's disease
Anterior pituitary hyposecretion
Connective tissue disease
Cirrhosis, alcoholic
Metastatic cancer
Steroid administration

Troponin I

Elevated Values

Acute myocardial infarction

Troponin T

Elevated Values

Acute myocardial infarction
Angina
Renal failure
Muscle trauma
Rhabdomyolysis
Polymyositis
Dermatomyositis

Myoglobin

Elevated Values

MI
Muscle injury or breakdown
Polymyositis
Renal failure
Open heart surgery
Exhaustive exercise

LDH

Elevated Values

Alcoholism
Anemia
Burns
Cancer
Cardiomyopathy
Cerebrovascular accident
Cirrhosis
Convulsions
Delirium tremens
Hepatitis
Hypothyroidism
Infectious mononucleosis
Codeine
Lithium carbonate
Meperidine
Morphine
Niacin
Pneumonia
Pulmonary infarction
Procainamide
Propranolol
Shock
Thyroid hormones
Ulcerative colitis

Decreased Values

Radiation therapy
Oxalates

INTERFERING FACTORS

- CK: Cardioversion, drugs (alcohol, aspirin, halothane, lithium, succinylcholine), gross hemolysis of specimen, muscle trauma, recent vigorous exercise or massage, surgery
- Troponin: Hemolysis of specimen
- LDH: Pregnancy, prosthetic heart valves, recent surgery, hemolysis of specimen

- Myoglobin: Any trauma to skeletal muscle. Recent administration of radioactive material, if radioimmunoassay (RIA) is used for analysis.

NURSING CARE

Nursing actions are similar to those used in other venipuncture procedures (see Chapter 2), with the following additional measures.

Pretest

- The nurse reassures the patient, who is usually frightened and having chest pain, and may also be in denial.
- Do *not* give intramuscular injections or perform repeated venipunctures, if possible, until all the initial enzyme studies are completed.
- Instruct the patient about the need for repeat blood sampling.
- The nurse determines if alcohol or drugs that affect results have been ingested.

During the Test

- Serial specimens are taken according to hospital protocol.
- If the tourniquet is in place too long, inaccurate results may occur.

Posttest

- Nursing actions are similar to those for any venipuncture.

Catecholamines, Plasma

kat-uh-kawl-uh-meenz, plaz-muh

Also called: Catecholamine Fractionalization, Plasma

SPECIMEN OR TYPE OF TEST: Plasma

PURPOSE OF THE TEST

Plasma catecholamines are usually assessed to diagnose pheochromocytoma or to identify extra-adrenal tumors after abdominal surgery. Pheochromocytomas are tumors developing in the sympathetic nervous system. These tumors usually secrete epinephrine, norepinephrine, or both, and sometimes dopamine.

A *clonidine suppression test* may be performed to differentiate between pheochromocytoma and essential hypertension. With this test, clonidine is given 2 to 3 hours before a venous blood sample is taken. Clonidine suppresses neurogenic catecholamine release. If suppression occurs, the test result is consistent with the diagnosis of essential hypertension. If the catecholamines remain elevated, the diagnosis of pheochromocytoma is supported.

BASICS THE NURSE NEEDS TO KNOW

The catecholamines are three hormones produced and secreted by the adrenal medulla. This structure is the inner core of the adrenal glands, which lie at the superior pole of each kidney. The catecholamines are epinephrine, norepinephrine, and dopamine (a precursor of norepinephrine). The adrenal medulla secretes the catecholamines when stimulated by preganglionic neurons. The result mimics the effect of a mass discharge of the sympathetic nervous system. Their secretion is part of the "fight or flight" response. The catecholamines help maintain serum glucose levels by promoting liver glycogenolysis, by stimulating the secretion of insulin and glucagon, and by lipolysis. The catecholamines stimulate the reticular activating system, making the person more alert.

NORMAL VALUES

Epinephrine (supine): <110 pg/mL *or* SI: <650 pmol/L
Epinephrine (standing): <140 pg/mL *or* SI: <900 pmol/L
Norepinephrine (supine): <750 pg/mL *or* SI: <4431 pmol/L
Dopamine (supine): <30 pg/mL *or* SI: <178 pmol/L

HOW THE TEST IS DONE

Plasma catecholamines are measured using radioenzyme technique. A venous sampling of 10 mL of blood is drawn into a green-topped tube, once while the patient is lying down and then once with the patient standing. The normal values vary among laboratories. Results may not reveal a tumor that secretes intermittently, so the test may be ordered for when the patient is symptomatic. To localize small tumors, percutaneous venous catheterization may be needed.

SIGNIFICANCE OF TEST RESULTS

Elevated Values

Pheochromocytoma
Ganglioneuroma
Neuroblastoma

INTERFERING FACTORS

- Noncompliance with diet and relaxation requirements
- Amine-rich foods and drinks
- Anger
- Cold environment
- Medications such as amphetamines, barbiturates, decongestants, epinephrine, levodopa, phenothiazines, reserpine, sympathomimetics, and tricyclic antidepressants
- Severe anxiety

NURSING CARE

Nursing actions are similar to those used in other venipuncture procedures (see Chapter 2), with the following additional measures.

Pretest

- Since many drugs interfere with test results, the nurse should check with the physician if any medications are to be withheld.

NURSING CARE—*cont'd*

- ***Patient Teaching.*** The nurse instructs the patient to avoid amine-rich foods and drinks (e.g., avocados, bananas, beer, cheese, Chianti wine, cocoa, coffee, and tea) for 48 hours before the test.
- ***Patient Teaching.*** Instruct the patient not to smoke for 4 hours before the test.
- ***Patient Teaching.*** The nurse explains to the patient that a venous catheter (heparin lock) is inserted 24 hours before the blood sample is drawn, because venipuncture may increase catecholamine levels.
- ***Patient Teaching.*** Instruct the patient to lie down and relax for an hour before the blood is drawn.

During the Test

- The nurse carries out duties similar to those of other venipuncture procedures, except that blood is drawn through the heparin lock. If the heparin lock has been flushed with heparin, withdraw 3 mL of blood and discard it before drawing the sample.
- After the first sample is drawn, the patient may be asked to stand for 10 minutes, and a second sample is drawn.
- Include on the requisition slip the position of the patient when the blood was drawn.
- The nurse flushes the heparin lock according to hospital protocol.

Posttest

- The patient may resume pretest diet and activity. Notify the laboratory that the specimen is coming, because it must be frozen immediately.

Catecholamines, Urinary

kat-uh-kawl-uh-meenz, yur-i-ner-ee

Also called: Catecholamines; Fractionation; Free Catecholamine Fractionation

SPECIMEN OR TYPE OF TEST: Urine

PURPOSE OF THE TEST

Urinary catecholamine determinations are usually obtained as a part of the work-up to identify the cause of hypertension and to diagnose pheochromocytoma.

BASICS THE NURSE NEEDS TO KNOW

Catecholamines are excreted in the urine in conjugated and unconjugated (free) forms. Together these forms make up the total urinary catecholamines. As serum catecholamines are metabolized, several end-product metabolites are created, which are excreted in the urine (Figure 32). The primary metabolite is *vanillylmandelic acid* (VMA). Other major metabolites of epinephrine and norepinephrine are metanephrine and normetanephrine. Dopamine's metabolites are 3-methoxy-4-hydroxyphenylacetic acid (*homovanillic acid,* or HVA) and 3,4-dehydroxyphenylacetic acid ($DOPA_c$).

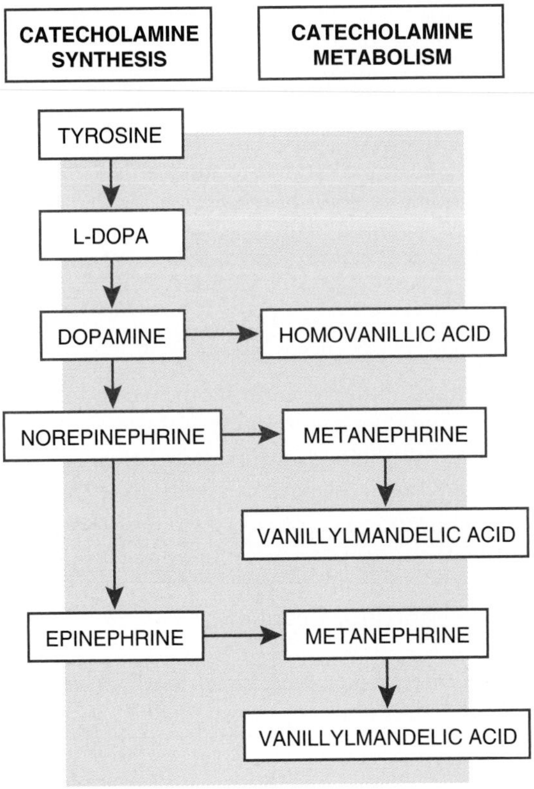

C

CATECHOLAMINE SYNTHESIS | CATECHOLAMINE METABOLISM

TYROSINE → L-DOPA → DOPAMINE → NOREPINEPHRINE → EPINEPHRINE

DOPAMINE → HOMOVANILLIC ACID

NOREPINEPHRINE → METANEPHRINE → VANILLYLMANDELIC ACID

EPINEPHRINE → METANEPHRINE → VANILLYLMANDELIC ACID

Figure 32. Catecholamine synthesis and metabolism.

NORMAL VALUES

Norepinephrine: 15–56 mcg/24 hr *or* SI: 88.6–331 nmol/24 hr
Epinephrine: <20 mcg/mL *or* SI: <109 nmol/24 hr
Dopamine: 100–400 pg/mL *or* SI: 625–2750 nmol/24 hr
Vanillylmandelic acid: 2–7 mg/24 hr *or* SI: 10–35 μmol/24 hr
Metanephrine: <1.4 mg/day *or* SI: <7.0 μmol/day
Normetanephrine: <0.4 mg/day *or* SI: <2.0 μmol/day
Homovanillic acid: <0.8 mg/day *or* SI: <44.0 μmol/day

HOW THE TEST IS DONE

A 24-hour urine specimen is collected, with a boric or acetic acid or potassium bisulfate preservative added to the container.

SIGNIFICANCE OF TEST RESULTS

Elevated Values

CATECHOLAMINES AND VANILLYLMANDELIC ACID

Pheochromocytoma
Neuroblastoma
Ganglioneuroma

Homovanillic Acid
Pheochromocytoma ruled out
Tumors of the autonomic nervous system
Ganglioblastoma

INTERFERING FACTORS

- Epinephrine: Stress
- Norepinephrine: Exercise
- Dopamine: Foods and drugs containing catecholamines, high-fluorescent compounds (e.g., tetracycline, quinidine), levodopa, or methyldopa
- Metanephrine: Catecholamines and monoamine oxidase (MAO) inhibitors
- Normetanephrine: Severe stress
- Vanillylmandelic acid: Catecholamines, foods with vanilla, levodopa, and MAO inhibitors

NURSING CARE

Nursing actions are similar to those used in other 24 hour collections of urine procedures (see Chapter 2), with the following additional measures.

Pretest

- The nurse checks with the physician to see if any medications are to be held.
- ***Patient Teaching.*** The nurse instructs the patient to avoid stress, exercise, smoking, and pain before and during the testing. The nurse also instructs the patient to avoid chocolate, coffee, bananas, foods with vanilla, and citrus fruits.

During the Test

- ***Patient Teaching.*** At the start of the test, the nurse instructs the patient to void at 8 AM and discard this urine. The collection period begins at this time, and all urine is collected for 24 hours, including the 8 AM specimen of the following morning.
- On the requisition slip and specimen label, the nurse writes the patient's name and the time and date of the start and finish of the test period.
- Keep the urine specimen refrigerated or on ice throughout the collection period.

Posttest

- Arrange for prompt transport of the cooled specimen to the laboratory.

Catheterization, Cardiac

kath-uh-ter-i-zay-shun, kahr-dee-ak

Also called: Angiocardiography; Coronary Arteriography

SPECIMEN OR TYPE OF TEST: Radiography

PURPOSE OF THE TEST

A cardiac catheterization is performed to (1) evaluate coronary artery disease with unstable, progressive, or new-onset angina or angina that is not responsive to medical therapy; (2) diagnose atypical chest pain; (3) diagnose complications of myocardial infarction such as septal rupture and refractory dysrhythmias; (4) diagnose aortic dissection; (5) evaluate the need for coronary artery surgery or angioplasty; (6) assess valvular function; and (7) determine the efficacy of a heart transplant. Rarely, a cardiac catheterization may be carried out to obtain a biopsy specimen.

BASICS THE NURSE NEEDS TO KNOW

Cardiac catheterization is an invasive procedure that permits the assessment of anatomic abnormalities of the heart, as well as the state of the coronary arteries. Cardiac catheterization may assess (1) pressures, oxygen content, and oxygen saturation in the various heart chambers; (2) cardiac output and index; (3) patency of the coronary arteries; and (4) pressure gradients across the valves.

Cardiac catheterization may be a right-sided catheterization, a left-sided catheterization, or both. A right-sided catheterization is performed today in specialized units under the category of hemodynamic monitoring; therefore, this section will focus on left-sided catheterization.

Left-heart cardiac catheterization, because it is invasive, has significant risk. Increasingly, *impedance cardiography (ICG)* is being used to obtain noninvasively many of the parameters obtained by cardiac catheterization. These measurements include cardiac output, left ventricular ejection fraction, stroke volume, left cardiac work indexes, and systemic vascular resistance. ICG obtains hemodynamic data with application of electrodes on the neck and thorax. It measures cardiac flow, not pressure. Very-low-grade electrical stimuli are emitted from electrodes on one side of the body and sensed by the electrodes on the opposite side. The wave-form created is interpreted and cardiac values are displayed. The reader may wish to review the general principles of Angiography, Vascular, p. 84.

NORMAL VALUES

Pressures

Right atrium: 2–6 mm Hg
 Neonate: 0–3 mm Hg
 Child: 1–5 mm Hg
Right ventricle: 20–30/2–8 mm Hg
 Neonate: 30–60/2–5 mm Hg
 Child: 15–30/2–5 mm Hg
Pulmonary artery pressure: 20–30/8–15 mm Hg
 Neonate: 30–60/2–10 mm Hg
 Child: 15–30/5–10 mm Hg
Pulmonary artery wedge pressure: 4–12 mm Hg
Left atrium: 4–12 mm Hg
 Neonate: 1–4 mm Hg
 Child: 5–10 mm Hg
Left ventricle: 90–140/4–12 mm Hg
 Neonate: 60–100/5–10 mm Hg
 Child: 80–130/10–20 mm Hg

Cardiac Output
4–8 L/min

Cardiac Index
2.5–4 L/min
Neonate and child: 3.5–4 L/min

Stroke Index
30–60 mL/beat/min

Ejection Fraction
55%–75%

Oxygen Saturation
75% (right side of heart); 95% (left side of heart)

Oxygen Content
14–15 volume % (right side of heart)
19 volume % (left side of heart)

Oxygen Consumption
250 mL/min

Volume
Left ventricular end-diastolic: 50–90 mL
Left ventricular end-systolic: 14–34 mL
Right ventricular end-diastolic: 70–90 mL
Left atrium: 57–79 mL

Mass
Left ventricular thickness
  Male: 12 mm
  Female: 9 mm
Left ventricular wall mass
  Male: 99 g
  Female: 76 g

Wall Motion
Normal

Valve Gradient
None

Valve Orifice Areas
Aortic valve: 0.7 cm^2
Mitral valve: 1 cm^2

HOW THE TEST IS DONE

A left-sided catheterization is performed in a cardiac catheterization laboratory. This laboratory is designed with fluoroscopy, electrocardiographic equipment, and emergency equipment and drugs (code cart). For a left-sided catheterization, the physician must thread a catheter through an artery into the left side of the heart; therefore, arterial access is necessary. Pressure measurements are obtained in the aorta and left atrium and ventricle. Samples of blood are obtained for oxygen analysis. Cardiac output, stroke volume, and ejection fractions are measured.

When a *coronary angiogram* is included in the test, dye is instilled into the heart to visualize the size of the ventricles, wall motion, and contractility and to identify valvular dysfunction.

A *coronary arteriogram* also may be obtained. The catheter is withdrawn from the left ventricle and positioned at the coronary ostia, where small boluses of dye are injected into the coronary arteries while a series of x-ray films are taken.

SIGNIFICANCE OF TEST RESULTS

Cardiac catheterization provides a significant amount of data for analysis, which may support the following diagnoses:

Coronary artery disease (CAD)
Coronary occlusions and degree of blockage
Congenital abnormalities
Septal defects
Shunting
Aneurysms
Valvular defects

INTERFERING FACTORS

- Allergic reactions to contrast medium
- Uncontrolled congestive heart failure
- Dysrhythmias
- Renal insufficiency
- Electrolyte imbalances
- Infection
- Drug toxicity

NURSING CARE

Pretest

- ***Patient Teaching.*** The nurse instructs the patient about the purpose and procedure for the study. Explain to the patient that the table rotates and that the physician may ask the patient to change positions or cough. Explain to the patient that when the dye is given, a feeling of warmth, or flushing or a metallic taste may be sensed.

NURSING CARE—*cont'd*

- The nurse verifies that an informed consent has been obtained.
- Assist with the precatheterization evaluation: blood tests, including a prothrombin time test and a partial thromboplastin time test; an electrocardiogram (ECG); and chest x-ray film if the procedure will be performed on an outpatient basis.
- Obtain patient weight and height.
- If contrast dye is going to be used, the nurse checks for allergies. Report elevated blood urea nitrogen (BUN) or creatinine levels, because these patients are at risk for renal failure.
- The nurse assesses the patient's fears and anxieties. Correct any misperceptions and reassure the patient that the nurse, physician, and technicians are there to assist during the procedure and will be continuously present.
- The patient is to have nothing by mouth after midnight, except if the catheterization is planned for late in the afternoon. In that case, a clear liquid breakfast may be taken.
- The nurse checks with the physician(s) if they want cardiac drugs held.
- The nurse prepares the catheter site according to laboratory protocol. The femoral artery is commonly used for the percutaneous insertion of the catheter. Usually both sides of the groin are prepared.
- The nurse gives the premedication as ordered, to reduce the patient's anxiety. In some catheterization laboratories, the patient also is medicated routinely to decrease the risk of allergic reaction to the contrast dye.
- Encourage the patient to wear his or her glasses to the catheterization laboratory.
- The patient is instructed to void before going to the catheterization laboratory.

During the Test

- The patient is awake. The nurse provides emotional support and reinforces explanations given about the procedure.
- Continuous cardiac monitoring is maintained. The nurse observes constantly for complications, especially dysrhythmia from catheter irritation or sensitivity to the contrast dye.
- The physician uses a local anesthetic after the insertion site is prepared and draped.
- The physician inserts the cardiac catheter under fluoroscopy.
- The patient may be asked to change position or cough during the procedure.
- Heparin usually is given during the procedure to prevent emboli. At the end of the procedure, protamine sulfate is given to reverse the effect of the heparin.

Posttest

- The nurse observes the insertion site for signs of bleeding. Palpation around the puncture site will help detect bleeding into tissue. If bleeding is present, the nurse exerts pressure just proximal to the puncture site with a gloved hand for a minimum of 15 minutes.
- The nurse checks distal pulses for arterial patency and documents findings.
- The nurse monitors vital signs and cardiac rhythm according to hospital protocol.
- Report any significant changes in vital signs, rhythm, and circulation or the occurrence of chest pain.
- Evaluate the patient's psychologic response to the procedure and its findings.

Continued

C

NURSING CARE—*cont'd*

- ***Patient Teaching.*** If cardiac catheterization is done as an outpatient procedure, instruct the patient (1) not to drive or climb stairs for 24 hours; (2) to avoid heavy lifting, sports, and strenuous housework for 3 days; and (3) to take no baths until the wound is healed. Instruct outpatients that they may shower and change the dressing after 24 hours.

Nursing Response to Complications

The nurse needs to assess for and report any observations indicating complications that may occur during or after the cardiac catheterization. Complications include dysrhythmias, asystole, vasovagal reaction, retroperitoneal bleeding, air embolism, contrast media reaction (see Angiography, Vascular, p. 84), thrombus, or hematoma formation at insertion site, cardiac tamponade, myocardial infarction, pulmonary edema, cerebral vascular accident, and infection.

Dysrhythmias. During and after the procedure, the patient is kept on a cardiac monitor. The nurse needs to monitor for dysrhythmias and respond to possible lethal dysrhythmias. Supraventricular and ventricular tachycardia and fibrillation may occur. Cardiac arrest, especially in patients with preexisting heart blocks, may also occur. Dysrhythmias may also occur because of a vasovagal response. Notify the physician and anticipate treatment based on established protocols.

Bleeding. Bleeding may occur at the access site of the catheterization. It may be overt bleeding, or a thrombus or hematoma may occur. The nurse checks the arterial puncture site frequently for overt bleeding. Assess pulses, skin temperature, and color distal to the insertion site. If retroperitoneal bleeding has occurred, there will be tachycardia, tachypnea, restlessness, hypotension, and a drop in hematocrit. The patient may also complain of lower abdominal pain or flank pain. The nurse notifies the physician immediately if bleeding is suspected. If bleeding is significant, the nurse checks to see if the patient has been typed and cross-matched for blood.

Cardiac tamponade. A feared complication of cardiac catheterization is cardiac tamponade, which occurs from bleeding into the pericardial sac. As blood accumulates into the pericardial sac, the heart is restricted. The nurse will observe a decrease in cardiac output, muffled heart sounds, increase in right atrial pressure, and pulsus paradoxus. Notify the physician immediately. If the size of the pericardial effusion is significant, emergency surgery may be necessary.

Ceruloplasmin

suh-roo-loh-plaz-min

SPECIMEN OR TYPE OF TEST: Serum

PURPOSE OF THE TEST

This test is used to evaluate chronic active hepatitis, cirrhosis, and other liver diseases. Because low levels can indicate Wilson's disease, the test is also used to help diagnose unexplained central nervous system disorders that affect coordination.

BASICS THE NURSE NEEDS TO KNOW

Ceruloplasmin is an alpha$_2$-globulin, a plasma protein made by the liver. The exact function is unknown, but in plasma, ceruloplasmin contains most of the total plasma copper.

Elevated Values

Ceruloplasmin is one of the serum proteins that are part of the body's acute phase response in conditions of extensive insult or trauma. The serum value rises in conditions of inflammation, infection, surgery, trauma, and malignancy.

Decreased Values

A low level of ceruloplasmin is associated with malabsorption, protein loss, and advanced liver disease that result in inadequate manufacture of all serum proteins. A low serum value is specifically associated with Wilson's disease, an inherited disorder that results in the deposit of copper in all body tissues including the brain and liver. A value of $<$10 mg/dL (SI: 0.63 μmol/L) indicates a diagnosis of Wilson's disease.

NORMAL VALUES

Adult: 20–40 mg/dL *or* SI: 1.26–2.52 μmol/L

HOW THE TEST IS DONE

A venipuncture is performed to collect 10 mL of venous blood in a *chilled* red-topped tube.

SIGNIFICANCE OF TEST RESULTS

Elevated Values

Leukemia
Hodgkin's disease
Cancer
Tissue necrosis
Trauma
Primary biliary cirrhosis
Systemic lupus erythematosus
Rheumatoid arthritis
Inflammation

Decreased Values

Wilson's disease
Hepatocellular disease
Malabsorption syndrome
Nephrotic syndrome

INTERFERING FACTORS

- Pregnancy
- Hemolysis
- Failure to maintain a nothing-by-mouth status

C

NURSING CARE

Nursing actions are similar to those used in other venipuncture procedures (see Chapter 2), with the following additional measures.

Pretest

- ***Patient Teaching.*** Instruct the patient to fast from food and fluids for 8 to 12 hours before the test. High levels of serum lipids will alter the test results.
- Inform the laboratory if the patient is pregnant or taking oral contraceptives because high levels of estrogen will elevate the test results.

Posttest

- Ensure that the vial of blood is placed on ice and sent to the laboratory immediately. Warming of the specimen by prolonged exposure to room temperature will result in a false lowering of the test value.

Chlamydia trachomatis Tests

kluh-mi-dee-yuh truh-ko-muh-tis tests

Also called: Lymphogranuloma Venereum Test

SPECIMEN OR TYPE OF TEST: Urine, blood, culture specimen

PURPOSE OF THE TEST

The various test methods help detect infection with *Chlamydia trachomatis,* a sexually transmitted disease (STD).

BASICS THE NURSE NEEDS TO KNOW

Chlamydia trachomatis is a bacterium that causes genital infection that is often asymptomatic. Untreated, it can ultimately result in pelvic inflammatory disease, ectopic pregnancy, and infertility in women. In pregnancy, the infected mother can transmit the infection to the newborn during vaginal delivery, resulting in severe conjunctivitis or pneumonia in the newborn infant.

Because this infection is the most common and frequently occurring STD in the United States, screening testing is recommended for the high risk, vulnerable population groups who are most frequently infected. For legal purposes, genital culture is used when sexual abuse of a child is suspected. Both test methods are highly accurate. Antibody testing may also be used to detect the infection, but the presence of antibodies to *Chlamydia trachomatis* may be from a current or past infection.

DNA Testing for *Chlamydia trachomatis*

The newest method of testing is DNA testing for *Chlamydia trachomatis* that used a first voided urine specimen of the morning. This is the sample that will have the greatest number of bacteria. As a method for screening, the specimen is easy to obtain and is a noninvasive test that delivers rapid test results.

C

NORMAL VALUES

Negative for *Chlamydia trachomatis*

HOW THE TEST IS DONE

Cell culture: Dacron swabs are used to obtain mucosal cells from the urethral meatus of the male or the cervix of the female (see also Culture, Genital, p. 251).

The swabs are placed in a sterile tube with transport medium. Depending on the patient's history, the individual also may need a cell culture sample from the anus, conjunctiva, nasopharynx, or throat.

DNA testing: A urine specimen container is used to collect a sample of a first morning specimen of urine. A specimen of cells obtained during a genital culture also may be tested for the DNA of *Chlamydia trachomatis*.

Serology (antibody) testing: A venipuncture is performed to collect 10 mL of venous blood in a red-topped tube.

SIGNIFICANCE OF TEST RESULTS

Positive Values

Chlamydia trachomatis infection

INTERFERING FACTORS

- Inadequate culture sample

NURSING CARE

Nursing actions are similar to those used in other first morning urine or venipuncture procedures (see Chapter 2), with the following additional measures.

Pretest

- The patient's history includes a sexual history, particularly for the high-risk populations of adolescents and young adults, ages 15 to 25, who are sexually active. Sexual intercourse may begin at an earlier age than the interviewer expects. A history of sexual activity that is monogamous, with a previous negative result for *Chlamydia trachomatis* is considered low risk. High-risk factors of unprotected sexual activity, inconsistent use of condoms, sexual intercourse with more than one partner, and a change in partners all place the individual at increased risk of acquiring an STD. The nurse or physician may acquire the information through interview.
- For genital culture of the female, the specimen is acquired during a pelvic examination. A specific culture test kit for *Chlamydia trachomatis* is used.

Posttest

- When the test result is positive for *Chlamydia trachomatis,* the patient is treated with tetracycline. Retesting in 6 to 12 months may be recommended because of the potential for reinfection. The infection is a reportable disease. The nurse or physician advises the patient that the sexual partner should also be tested or treated for presumptive disease.

Continued

C

NURSING CARE—*cont'd*

- ***Health Promotion.*** Routine DNA screening for *Chlamydia trachomatis* is recommended for sexually active females, ages 25 and younger. It is also recommended for those individuals who engage in high-risk sexual activity behaviors. One goal is to detect and treat this infection before it progresses to a complicated problem or affects the newborn child. The other is to reduce the overall number of infections caused by this organism.
- When working in a community or with population groups that have a high incidence of this infection, the nurse can participate with the health care team to develop a screening protocol. Communication with the local public health authorities would provide the data regarding the incidence of this infection in the nurse's local or regional area.

Chloride, Serum

klor-īd, se-rum

Also called: Cl^-

SPECIMEN OR TYPE OF TEST: Blood

PURPOSE OF THE TEST

Serum chloride measurements are obtained in the evaluation of electrolyte levels, water balance, and acid-base balance and in the measurement of the cation-anion balance (anion gap).

BASICS THE NURSE NEEDS TO KNOW

Sodium (Na^+), potassium (K^+), bicarbonate (HCO_3^-), and chloride (Cl^-) are electrolytes with positive or negative charges. In combination, the electrolytes determine the osmolarity, pH, and hydration status in intracellular and extracellular fluids. In addition, the concentration differences between intracellular and extracellular electrolytes regulate the functions of the nervous system, cardiac, respiratory, and muscle tissues. Chloride is a major electrolyte in extracellular fluid and it generally increases or decreases with the sodium level. Chloride also increases or decreases inversely with bicarbonate, meaning as the bicarbonate level increases, chloride decreases, or as bicarbonate decreases, the chloride level increases.

Elevated Values

An elevated level of chloride in the blood and extracellular fluid is called *hyperchloridemia.* It occurs during metabolic acidosis, resulting from excessive loss of bicarbonate fluids and electrolytes from the lower intestine, from renal tubular acidosis, and from mineralocorticoid deficiency. The chloride concentration may also rise with dehydration.

Decreased Values

A decreased level of chloride in the blood and extracellular fluid is called *hypochloridemia*. It occurs during a loss of hydrochloric acid from the upper gastrointestinal tract as well as from mineralocorticoid excess, salt-losing renal disease, or diabetic acidosis. The low level of chloride may also occur in conditions that cause a rise in bicarbonate or a decreased sodium concentration. Hypochloridemia may occur with overhydration.

NORMAL VALUES	Adult and child: 97–107 mEq/L *or* SI: 97–107 mmol/L Newborn: 96–106 mEq/L *or* SI: 96–106 mmol/L Premature infant: 95–110 mEq/L *or* SI: 95–110 mmol/L
▼ Critical Values	>115 mEq/L (SI: >115 mmol/L) *or* <80 mEq/L (SI: <80 mmol/L)

HOW THE TEST IS DONE

A red-topped tube is used to collect 10 mL of venous blood; or a green-topped tube is used to collect 5 mL of venous blood. In infants, a heelstick puncture and a capillary tube may be used to collect capillary blood.

SIGNIFICANCE OF TEST RESULTS

Elevated Values

Dehydration
Renal tubular acidosis
Prolonged diarrhea
Acute renal failure
Diabetes insipidus
Respiratory alkalosis
Hyperparathyroidism
Adrenocortical hyperfunction

Decreased Values

Prolonged vomiting
Nasogastric drainage
Salt-losing nephritis
Chronic renal failure
Chronic respiratory acidosis

Metabolic alkalosis
Addison's disease
Congestive heart failure
Intestinal fistula
Overhydration
Diuretic therapy

C

INTERFERING FACTORS

- Hemolysis
- Warming of the specimen

NURSING CARE

Nursing actions are similar to those used in other venipuncture procedures (see Chapter 2), with the following additional measures.

Pretest

- ***Patient Teaching.*** For a routine test, instruct the patient to discontinue all food and fluids for 8 hours before the test. This prevents the normal drop in value after eating. For tests performed on an urgent or emergency basis, the fasting status is omitted.

Posttest

- Arrange for prompt transport of the blood to the laboratory. The serum or plasma will require refrigeration until the analysis can be performed.
- If the patient receives intravenous fluids, the nurse monitors the flow of fluids and electrolyte replacement. The goal is to control the amount of fluid and the rate of flow correctly, so that the replacement is received in the prescribed time period.
- The nurse also monitors the laboratory results for alterations of other electrolytes because changes in the chloride level are usually accompanied by changes in carbon dioxide and sodium levels. Because of the patient's disease process, changes in the potassium level and the pH also may be in the abnormal range. The chloride measurement is not used as an independent test, but is interpreted together with the other electrolyte tests.
- The monitoring and recording of intake and output are important nursing measurements. Outputs include measurement of drainage (fistula, vomitus, gastric suction, urine) and inputs include recording oral and intravenous intake.

▼ Nursing Response to Critical Values

A severe elevation or loss of chloride indicates serious fluid and electrolyte imbalance. The physician must be notified immediately. Specific medical treatment and nursing intervention depend on the cause of the problem, but immediate action must be taken to restore the electrolyte balance.

Cholangiography, Percutaneous, Transhepatic

ko-lan-jee-o-gruh-fee, per-kyuh-tay-nee-uhs, tranz-huh-pa-tik

Also called: (PTC); Transhepatic Cholangiography

SPECIMEN OR TYPE OF TEST: Radiography

PURPOSE OF THE TEST

Percutaneous transhepatic cholangiography is used to demonstrate biliary anatomy in conditions of biliary tract obstruction. It may also be as the first step in procedures to drain the biliary tract of infected bile and to place a stent in the biliary tract to provide for drainage of the bile.

BASICS THE NURSE NEEDS TO KNOW

When obstructive jaundice is present and ultrasound has demonstrated dilated biliary ducts, the site of the obstruction may be in the intrahepatic or extrahepatic ducts. The usual causes of obstruction are gallstones, tumor, or parasites. If endoscopic cholangiography is incomplete or cannot be performed, this procedure can be used to visualize the biliary tract and the location of the obstruction. Contrast medium can be instilled into the biliary tree via the needle that has been inserted into the hepatic ducts of the liver. Fluoroscopy and x-ray films are used to assist the physician in the placement of the needle and in obtaining multiple views of obstruction in the biliary ductal system.

NORMAL VALUES	The biliary ducts are patent and demonstrate normal anatomic structure

HOW THE TEST IS DONE

Percutaneous transhepatic cholangiography is performed in a room equipped with fluoroscopy. The patient is placed on the fluoroscopy table and sedated with diazepam, (Valium). The skin is prepared, draped and anesthetized locally. The site of the needle insertion is at the lower right aspect of the rib cage at or near the mid axillary line.

The patient is instructed to inhale deeply, exhale fully, and hold his or her breath on expiration. At that point, the physician inserts the needle into the liver near the hepatic ducts. As the patient resumes shallow breathing, the needle is repositioned until its tip is well into one of the main hepatic ducts (Figure 33). When excess bile has dilated the ducts, the bile is removed and a specimen is sent to the laboratory for culture and cytologic analysis. Contrast medium is injected slowly into the ducts until the entire biliary tree is filled with the contrast medium. Using fluoroscopy, the physician is able to visualize the needle placement and gradual aspiration of bile and replacement with contrast medium.

A tilt table is used to take multiple x-ray films of the patient in various positions until the total biliary tree is visualized. At the end of the procedure, the biliary ducts are aspirated of the contrast medium, and the dilated ducts are decompressed. At this time, if a biliary stent is needed to relieve ongoing biliary obstruction, the physician puts the stent into place. The entire procedure takes 45 minutes to 1 hour.

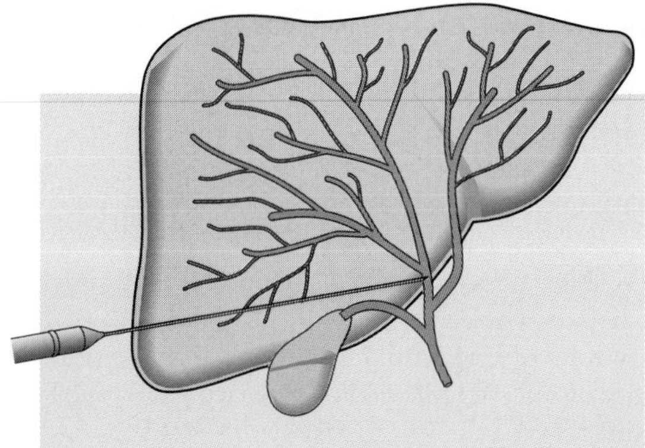

Figure 33. Percutaneous transhepatic cholangiography. The aspirating needle is passed through the patient's skin and liver tissue until the tip penetrates one of the hepatic ducts. Radiopaque medium is then instilled into the biliary tree to enhance radiographic visualization.

SIGNIFICANCE OF TEST RESULTS

Abnormal Values

Gallstones
Biliary tract obstruction
Cancer of the bile duct
Cancer of the head of the pancreas

INTERFERING FACTORS

- Obesity
- Ascites
- Gas in the intestinal tract
- Failure to maintain a nothing-by-mouth status
- Bleeding abnormalities
- Sepsis, peritonitis
- Allergy to iodine-based contrast medium

NURSING CARE

Pretest

- Question the patient about any history of allergy to iodine or seafood, or a previous reaction to iodine-based contrast medium.
- An informed consent form must be signed and present in the patient's record.
- To prevent sepsis, antibiotics are started in the pretest period and continued into the posttest period.

C

NURSING CARE—*cont'd*

- *Patient Teaching.* Instruct the patient to take a prescribed laxative on the night before the test. A cleansing enema is done on the morning of the test. The patient discontinues all food and oral fluids for 12 hours before the test. Additional pretest instructions relate to the procedure itself. The patient is reassured that pain control will be provided by intravenous medication and the local anesthetic. The breathing instructions of deep inspiration, complete expiration and holding the breath should be practiced.
- The nurse assesses and records baseline vital signs, including blood pressure, pulse and respirations and temperature. Any elevation of temperature is reported to the physician and radiologist because sepsis and peritonitis are absolute contraindications to performing the procedure.
- The nurse also ensures that recent prothrombin time and complete blood count reports are also placed in the patient's record. The prothrombin time should be no more than 3 seconds greater than the control time and the platelet count should be greater than 100,000 cells/mm^3. Poor clotting ability is an absolute contraindication to performing this procedure. Moderate to severe anemia may be a contraindication to performing the procedure. The nurse notifies the physician and radiologist of these abnormal test values.

Posttest

- Take vital signs regularly and frequently because of the risk of hemorrhage or hypotension. Generally, the pattern is every 15 minutes for 1 hour, every 4 hours for 4 hours, and every 4 hours thereafter, until the patient is stable. Take the temperature initially and every 4 hours thereafter because of the risk of sepsis and cholangitis.
- Place the patient on his or her right side, with a pillow or sandbag pressed against the lower ribs and abdomen. The gentle pressure and immobility help to promote clotting. Bed rest is maintained for 6 hours after the procedure. Because hemorrhage or biliary leakage could require surgery, nothing-by-mouth status is maintained until the patient is stable.
- The nurse observes the lower right side of the rib cage for signs of bleeding, hematoma formation, ecchymosis, or leakage of bile onto the skin. Some small leakage of blood is expected.

◇ Nursing Response to Complications

Bleeding complications can begin during or after the procedure is completed and may require emergency surgery to correct or control it. The complications of bleeding, sepsis, cholangitis, and peritonitis tend to appear within hours after completion of the procedure.

Bleeding. In the assessment for bleeding, the nurse assesses for signs of shock, including hypotension, tachycardia, dyspnea, pallor, and diaphoresis (cold, sweaty skin). The abdomen may be distended and painful. Localized ecchymosis (bruising) would appear on the lower right lateral ribs or on the side of the abdomen just below the ribs.

Continued

C

NURSING CARE—*cont'd*

Cholangitis and sepsis. Cholangitis (infection in the biliary tree) and sepsis (infection in the blood and other tissues) can cause a rapid rise of temperature, with shaking chills. In addition to monitoring the temperature vital signs, the nurse should also review posttest laboratory reports for an abnormally elevated white blood count (leukocytosis) and abnormal liver function studies (particularly, elevations of the ALT and AST values).

Peritonitis. Infected bile can leak into the peritoneal cavity and cause acute peritonitis. The nurse takes vital signs, noting pertinent changes associated with shock and infection. These include hypotension, tachycardia, dyspnea, and fever. Using the technique of light palpation, assessment reveals that the abdomen is distended and board-like. The patient also has acute abdominal pain.

Cholecystography, Oral

ko-le-sis-to-gruh-fee, ohr-uhl

Also called: Gall Bladder Series

SPECIMEN OR TYPE OF TEST: Radiography

PURPOSE OF THE TEST

The oral cholecystogram is used to visualize the gall bladder and the cystic and common ducts in an effort to identify stones and other causes of obstruction of the bile flow. It is also used to evaluate the gall bladder's ability to function in the storage and excretion of bile.

BASICS THE NURSE NEEDS TO KNOW

Stones can form in the gall bladder and lodge in the cystic or common duct (Figure 34). Most of these stones are made of bile pigment and cholesterol and some are made of calcium carbonate. Stones in the gall bladder often cause acute pain as the gall bladder contracts and squeezes down on them. Stones in the ducts will obstruct the flow of bile and cause jaundice.

The oral cholecystogram is no longer the primary test to image gallstones, obstruction, or nonfunction of the gall bladder. It is not always precise, in part because of interfering factors. In this test, the contrast medium is taken orally, and must be absorbed by the intestinal tract, taken up by the liver, and concentrated in the gall bladder. With problems of intestinal or liver function, the contrast may not reach the gall bladder to provide for accurate imaging. The test remains in use, however, particularly for the confirmation of ultrasound imaging or as an additional test when ultrasound or nuclear scan has failed to demonstrate the presence of a suspected gallstone(s).

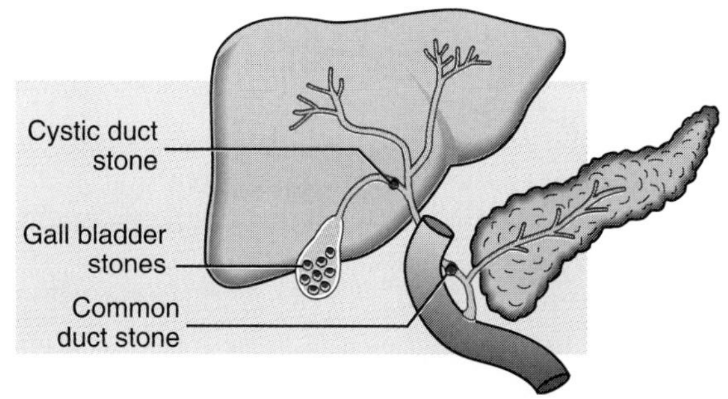

Figure 34. Common anatomic locations of gallstones.

NORMAL VALUES **The gall bladder and biliary ductal system are able to fill, concentrate, contract, and empty of contrast medium, with no evidence of stone or obstruction of bile flow.**

HOW THE TEST IS DONE

The patient takes oral, iodinated contrast tablets on the evening before the test. The next day, a series of x-rays are taken over a 45- to 60-minute period, to image the gall bladder and biliary ductal system that is filled with contrast medium, including the imaging of any stones or areas of stricture/obstruction. Then, after the patient ingests a fatty meal or synthetic fat substance, a second series of films is taken. These films image the emptying gall bladder, and the contrast medium that is now in the cystic duct, common duct, and duodenum. This second phase takes an additional 1 to 2 hours to complete.

SIGNIFICANCE OF TEST RESULTS

Gallstones
Cholestasis
Nonfunctioning gall bladder
Polyp or benign tumor of the biliary tract

INTERFERING FACTORS

- Failure to follow dietary instructions followed by nothing-by-mouth status before the test
- Failure to take all of the tablets of contrast medium
- Intestinal loss of the contrast medium
- Pregnancy, first trimester
- Retained barium in the intestine
- Impaired hepatic function
- Biliary obstruction and jaundice

C

NURSING CARE

Pretest

- Schedule this test before any barium tests, because retained barium in the intestine would block the view of the gall bladder and biliary tree.
- The nurse questions the patient about any history of allergy to iodine or seafood, or a previous reaction to iodine-based contrast medium.
- Once the physician has explained the procedure, the nurse obtains the patient's written consent form that must be signed and present in the patient's record.
- *Patient Teaching.* The nurse instructs the patient regarding pretest procedure. The patient must eat a fat-free meal the night before the test, with no further intake of food or fluids, except water. Two or three hours later, all the tablets of contrast medium are taken with water. After midnight, water intake is discontinued. A saline enema in the morning may be required. After ingestion of the contrast tablets, any vomiting or diarrhea must be reported to the radiologist because loss of part or all of the contrast medium will invalidate the test.

Posttest

- Generally, there is no specific nursing care that is required during or after the procedure, except to monitor for allergic reaction that can occur any time during or soon after the test is completed.

◆ Nursing Response to Complications

Allergy to the iodine in the contrast medium can cause an allergic reaction. It may be a mild reaction that is delayed in onset or a severe reaction with potentially catastrophic consequences. The physician must be notified about the reaction, because treatment with medication may be effective in minimizing the allergic response before it progresses in seriousness.

Mild allergic reaction. In a mild reaction, nursing assessment findings include urticaria (hives and itching), angioedema (diffuse swelling of the skin), hoarseness that results from swelling of the larynx and trachea, wheezing and coughing, and nausea and vomiting. The patient seems apprehensive.

Severe allergic reaction. Severe allergic reaction begins as a mild allergic response, but progresses rapidly to greater severity. Assess the patient's breathing ability, because swelling and bronchospasm can result in pallor, cyanosis, dyspnea, and respiratory failure. Shock can occur, as evidenced by hypotension and tachycardia. If the severe reaction cannot be reversed, the patient can develop seizures, coma, and then die.

Cholesterol, Serum

See Lipid Profile on p. 431.

Chorionic Gonadotropin, Human

ko-ree-on-ik goh-nad-uh-tro-pin, hyoo-muhn

Also called: Human Chorionic Gonadotrophin (hCG); (β-hCG)

SPECIMEN OR TYPE OF TEST: Serum, urine

PURPOSE OF THE TEST

The serum and urine tests are used to detect pregnancy and, as part of multiple marker testing, are used to identify Down syndrome in the second trimester of pregnancy. The serum test also is used to help confirm the diagnosis of a trophoblastic or germ cell tumor and to monitor the patient after the surgical removal of the tumor.

BASICS THE NURSE NEEDS TO KNOW

Human chorionic gonadotropin (hCG) is a hormone normally produced by the developing placenta. In the normal, nonpregnant person, only a trace amount of this hormone is found in the blood. In abnormal conditions, the hormone is produced by some germ cell malignancies and malignancy of other organs.

The measurement of the serum value detects a normal pregnancy within 6 to 10 days after the fertilized egg is implanted. During the early part of a normal pregnancy, the amount of hCG in the blood rises dramatically. The level generally peaks in the seventh to tenth week of gestation. Very high values suggest a multiple pregnancy. In ectopic pregnancy, however, the secretion of hCG is much lower and does not progress in the same pattern. If urine is used to identify pregnancy, the test result is positive in 6 to 10 days after conception.

The urine test may be used when a teratogenic medication or treatment such as x-ray, chemotherapy, or radiotherapy must be given to a young, sexually active female patient. The test can screen for an unknown pregnancy before treatment begins. The test also is used on an emergency basis to determine if pregnancy is the cause of pelvic pain.

Benign or malignant trophoblastic disease and germ cell tumors are usually associated with very high levels of hCG. After surgical removal of the tumor, the serum level recedes and returns to normal within 8 to 12 weeks. Because hCG is a tumor marker, the serum level continues to be monitored monthly for 1 year. A persistent or recurrent elevation of the serum value indicates an invasive malignancy with the need for additional diagnostic testing and treatment.

Multiple Marker Screening for Down Syndrome

Pregnant women can now be tested for fetal Down syndrome in the second trimester, using the triple- or quadruple-marker screening test. This blood test is offered in the fifteenth to twenty-second week of the pregnancy. The triple-marker screening test consists of alpha-fetoprotein, hCG, and unconjugated estriol. The newest, most improved method is to use the quadruple-marker screening test, consisting of the above three tests and adding a fourth test, inhibitin A.

When Down syndrome affects the fetus, the quadruple-marker screening test demonstrates characteristic changes in the second trimester of pregnancy. The alpha-fetoprotein result is 25% lower than normal, and the unconjugated estriol result is 30% lower than normal. Both hCG and inhibitin A rise to twice the normal value. Pregnancy ultrasound must be done first, to obtain an accurate gestational age. The quadruple-marker screening test detects 80% of fetal Down syndrome pregnancies, with a 5% false positive rate of error. It is a very useful test for pregnant women younger than age 35, because a high rate of Down syndrome occurs in pregnancies of younger females, and amniocentesis is not done routinely to detect the problem.

NORMAL VALUES

Serum: Negative
Male and nonpregnant female: <5 mIU/mL *or*
SI: <5 international units/L
Pregnant female (1 week of gestation): 5–50 mIU/mL *or*
SI: 5–50 international units/L
Pregnant female (6–8 weeks of gestation):
12,000–270,000 mIU/mL *or* SI: 12,000–270,000 international units/L
Urine: Negative

HOW THE TEST IS DONE

Serum: A red-topped tube is used to obtain 10 mL of venous blood.
Urine: A clean plastic container is used to collect a first voided morning specimen of urine.

SIGNIFICANCE OF TEST RESULTS

Elevated Values

Pregnancy
Hydatidiform mole
Islet cell neoplasm of the pancreas
Choriocarcinoma
Ovarian-testicular cancer
Cancer of the lung, stomach, liver, or colon

INTERFERING FACTORS

- Recent radioactive isotope scan

NURSING CARE

Nursing actions are similar to those used in other venipuncture procedures (see Chapter 2), with the following additional measures.

Pretest

Serum

- It is preferable to schedule this test for before or at least 7 days after a nuclear scan, because the radioisotopes of the scan would interfere with the laboratory method of analysis.

NURSING CARE—*cont'd*

Urine

- *Patient Teaching.* Instruct the patient to collect a single specimen of urine in the laboratory collection container. The urine should be from the first voided morning specimen, collected on arising from sleep. This urine sample is more concentrated and produces the most accurate result.

Posttest

- On the requisition slip, the nurse includes the date of the patient's last menstrual period. This information is used to help determine whether the results are within normal limits.

Chorionic Villus Sampling and Genetic Abnormality Analysis

ko-ree-on-ik vi-luhs sam-pling and juh-ne-tik ab-nohr-mal-uh-tee uh-nal-uh-sis

Also called: (CVS)

SPECIMEN OR TYPE OF TEST: Placental Tissue

PURPOSE OF THE TEST

The procedure is used to obtain a small sample of chorionic villus tissue of the placenta. The analysis of the tissue identifies genetic abnormalities of the fetus.

BASICS THE NURSE NEEDS TO KNOW

The genetic material of the placenta is exactly the same as the genetic make-up of the fetus. The genetic analysis of the placental tissue reveals genetic fetal abnormality at a very early stage of the pregnancy. When it is needed, the chorionic villus sampling is done within the tenth to twelfth week of gestation, approximately 4 to 6 weeks earlier than the more traditional procedure of amniocentesis. When information of genetic abnormality in the fetus becomes known at an early date, termination of the pregnancy in the first trimester is possible. If the decision to terminate the pregnancy is made, a first trimester abortion is safer and less traumatic emotionally for the woman.

There are several reasons why chorionic villus sampling may be helpful. Maternal age over 35 years is associated with a higher risk of Down syndrome in the fetus. In addition, the procedure is beneficial when both reproductive partners are known carriers of genetic mutations that can produce offspring with diseases including cystic fibrosis, sickle cell disease, hemophilia, or muscular dystrophy. The procedure is also useful for the couple who already had a child with an inherited genetic disorder or multiple congenital abnormalities.

NORMAL VALUES No genetic mutations of the fetal trophoblast tissue

HOW THE TEST IS DONE

Guided by ultrasound, the physician uses a catheter (transcervical approach) or spinal needle (transabdominal approach) to penetrate the placenta and aspirate a sample of placental tissue into a syringe. A special medium is in the syringe; both the tissue and medium are placed in a sterile tube or container for transport to the laboratory.

SIGNIFICANCE OF TEST RESULTS

Abnormal Findings

Genetic mutation of the fetus

INTERFERING FACTORS

- Failure to aspirate placental cells
- Contamination of the specimen

NURSING CARE

Pretest

- After the physician has explained the procedure and all other appropriate information, the patient must sign consent for the procedure and the genetic analysis of the specimen. The consent is added to the patient's record.
- The nurse provides emotional support to the patient. Often, the patient is apprehensive about the results of the genetic analysis. There may be a strong desire for a good pregnancy outcome, but it is tempered by anxiety or fear. The fetus may have a serious inherited disorder that would negatively affect its life or health.

During the Test

- Depending on the approach that is used, the nurse assists the physician with the antimicrobial cleansing of the abdomen or vaginal canal and surface of the cervix. This helps reduce bacteria that could contaminate the specimen or infect the uterine cavity.
- The specimen and the laboratory requisition form must be identified with the appropriate patient identification and the source of the tissue. The request form should also include the maternal age, gestational age (as determined by ultrasound), and relevant patient history (number of pregnancies, miscarriages). In addition, a history of recent maternal medications, viral infections, or blood transfusions is included.

Posttest

- If bleeding from the vagina or at the abdominal puncture site happens, it is likely to occur very soon after the procedure is completed. The nurse observes for this complication and notifies the physician, immediately.
- If the mother has an Rh negative blood type, she is given an injection of immune globulin (RhoGAM). This procedure can cause some mixing of the fetal and maternal blood. If the fetus is Rh positive and the mother Rh negative, a mixing of the two blood types would result in an antigen-antibody response that affects the fetal red blood cells. The maternal injection of immune globulin prevents isoimmunization (the production of the antibodies).
- The patient or the couple will return to the physician for the results of the genetic analysis of the fetus and discussion of the findings.
- ***Patient Teaching.*** In discharge teaching, the nurse instructs the patient to notify the physician of any unusual bleeding or cramping sensations, leakage of amniotic fluid, or fever.

NURSING CARE—*cont'd*

 **Nursing Response to Complications**

For this procedure, the complication rate of fetal loss is approximately 1%. The complications that can occur include bleeding, rupture of the membranes, chorioamnionitis (infection), and miscarriage.

Bleeding, ruptured membranes, infection or onset of labor. If the patient returns to the physician or specialized center with procedure-related health concerns, the nurse interviews the patient quickly and carefully to determine the nature of the problem. The nurse asks the patient to describe bleeding, spotting, or leakage of fluid, including duration and amount. If the patient has cramping or pelvic pain, the nurse asks the patient to describe the sensation, including the intensity, frequency, and duration. Vital signs, including temperature, are also taken and the physician is notified immediately of the assessment findings.

Clonidine Suppression Test

See Catecholamines, Plasma on p. 183.

Coagulation Inhibitors

ko-a-gyoo-lay-shun in-hi-bi-tohrs

Also called: Antithrombin; Protein C; Protein S

SPECIMEN OR TYPE OF TEST: Plasma

PURPOSE OF THE TEST

The three tests are used to investigate the underlying cause of a thrombus, particularly in young adults or in patients who have a family history of thrombus formation. These tests also are used to assess the cause of a hypercoagulable state and a fibrinolytic state. Antithrombin is used to evaluate the response to heparin or to investigate the cause of heparin failure.

BASICS THE NURSE NEEDS TO KNOW

The regulation or control of the coagulation cascade consists of a balance between the activation and the inhibition of coagulation factors. Antithrombin, protein C, and protein S all are natural inhibitors of coagulation. When the coagulation inhibitors neutralize the coagulation factors, the formation of a blood clot is inhibited. The patient may have deficiencies of one or more of these coagulation factors. The reference values vary according to the method of analysis that is used.

Antithrombin

Antithrombin is a primary inhibitor of thrombin and several factors in the coagulation cascade. The deficiency of antithrombin can result in the formation of recurrent or extensive thrombus formation or a thromboembolic disorder. The disorder can be hereditary or caused by illness, as disseminated intravascular coagulation (DIC) or liver disease. When the amount of antithrombin is adequate, the anticoagulant action of heparin is increased. With low or inadequate levels of antithrombin, patients can experience a resistance to heparin, but they respond to anticoagulant therapy with warfarin sodium (Coumadin).

Protein C

Protein C is synthesized by the liver and is a natural inhibitor of coagulation. Its actions delay or reduce thrombus formation and help to dissolve the thrombus that has already formed. Extensive or recurrent thrombus formation occurs with decreased levels of protein C. When the cause is hereditary, homozygous protein C deficiency usually results in death from massive clot formation in infancy. Heterozygous protein C deficiency is less severe. These patients often experience thrombus formation in adulthood in the form of a deep vein thrombosis, thrombophlebitis, pulmonary embolus, or a hypercoagulable state. Acquired deficiency is associated with the decreased synthesis of protein C in liver disease.

Protein S

Like protein C, protein S is a vitamin K–dependent coagulation protein that is synthesized by the liver. It is a cofactor of protein C, accelerating and enhancing the effect of protein C. In combination, proteins C and S inhibit the formation of a thrombus. The patient who has a deficiency of protein S also has the tendency to form recurrent thrombi in the form of a deep vein thrombosis, thrombus, embolus, or hypercoagulable state. The condition may be of hereditary or acquired origin.

NORMAL VALUES

Antithrombin
17–39 mg/dL *or* SI: 170–390 mg/L
80%–130% of normal activity *or* SI: 0.80–1.30 (fraction of normal activity)

Protein C
2.82–5.65 mcg/mL *or* SI: 2.82–5.65 mg/L
70%–140% of normal activity *or* SI: 0.70–1.40 (fraction of normal activity)

Protein S
21–42 mcg/mL *or* SI: 21–42 mg/L
70%–140% of normal concentration *or* SI: 0.67–1.40 (fraction of normal concentration)

HOW THE TEST IS DONE

Antithrombin

One blue-topped tube with sodium citrate is used to collect 4.5 mL of blood.

Protein C

One blue-topped tube with sodium citrate is used to collect 4.5 mL of venous blood.

Protein S

One blue-topped tube with sodium citrate is used to collect 4.5 mL of venous blood. As an alternative, a heelstick, earlobe, or finger puncture may be used to collect capillary blood in siliconized sodium citrate micropipettes.

For each of these specimens, the tube must be filled with blood. If too little blood is used, the proportion of sodium citrate will be greater than that of blood, and a false elevation of the test results will occur. To mix the anticoagulant with the blood, the specimen tube is tilted gently from side to side five to ten times. When multiple specimens are drawn, the coagulation inhibitor specimen is obtained last. When this is the only test specimen, a double-tube technique must be used to prevent specimen contamination with tissue thromboplastin. In the double-tube technique, a 1- to 2-mL blood sample is obtained and discarded, and the blue-topped tube is then used to collect the test sample.

SIGNIFICANCE OF TEST RESULTS

Decreased Values

Antithrombin

Congenital deficiency
DIC
Nephrotic syndrome
Pregnancy or postpartum condition
Liver transplant
Hepatectomy
Cirrhosis
Chronic liver failure

Proteins C and S

Congenital deficiency
DIC
Cirrhosis

INTERFERING FACTORS

- Hemolysis
- Coagulation of the specimen
- Warming of the specimen
- Heparin
- Time delay in analysis of the specimen

NURSING CARE

Nursing actions are similar to those used in other venipuncture procedures (see Chapter 2), with the following additional measures.

Pretest

- The nurse schedules the test 2 to 4 weeks after anticoagulation therapy has been discontinued. This is because warfarin (Coumadin) therapy lowers the patient's protein C value and may increase the antithrombin value. Heparin can cause erroneous results for the antithrombin and protein C tests.

Continued

C

NURSING CARE—*cont'd*

Pretest—*cont'd*

- If the patient is currently receiving anticoagulant therapy, the nurse includes the name and dosage of the drug on the requisition slip.

During the Test

- Do not collect the blood from the arm with an intravenous line or a saline lock device. The heparin flush procedure that is used to keep a venous catheter patent would contaminate the specimen and cause erroneous test results.

Posttest

- Place the antithrombin tube on ice immediately and arrange for prompt transport of all specimens to the laboratory. These three tests become invalid if a delay of more than 2 hours occurs before the blood is prepared for analysis. The coagulation inhibitors are more stable in cold temperatures.

Cobalamin

ko-bal-uh-min

Also called: Vitamin B_{12}; Cb1

SPECIMEN OR TYPE OF TEST: Serum

PURPOSE OF THE TEST

This test is used to identify cobalamin deficiency or to investigate the cause of hematologic and neurologic symptoms that suggest cobalamin deficiency.

BASICS THE NURSE NEEDS TO KNOW

Cobalamin, also known as vitamin B_{12}, is an essential vitamin and coenzyme needed for the formation of normal erythrocytes and other bone marrow functions. In terms of dietary intake, this vitamin is present in meat, milk, butter, cheese, fish, and eggs. The absorption of the vitamin occurs in stages. Initially, it is bound to intrinsic factor, manufactured by the gastric parietal cells. In the ileum, it is absorbed into the portal vein system, aided by intrinsic factor and pancreatic enzymes. Some will be used by the bone marrow for hematopoiesis and the remainder is stored by the liver.

Elevated Level

The vitamin B_{12} level is elevated in the blood when a disorder exists that increases the manufacture of transport substances or increases hematopoiesis.

Decreased Level

Several possible causes exist for a decreased amount of vitamin B_{12} in the blood. The most common cause is a problem with the production and function of intrinsic factor. It is estimated that 10% to 25% of the elderly have unrecognized and untreated cobalamin deficiency, probably due to hypochlorhydria, achlorhydria, or atrophic gastritis that interferes with cobalamin absorption. These individuals tend to ignore the manifestations of pernicious anemia until they experience cognitive impairment or peripheral neuropathy. Without intrinsic factor, the available vitamin B_{12} cannot enter the circulation from the intestinal tract. Defective absorption also may be the cause. Disorders that impair the absorption in the ileum also prevent the absorption of the vitamin. A lack of dietary intake of the vitamin may be the cause, but it is not a very common occurrence. Persons who are strict vegetarians are the most vulnerable.

Without sufficient cobalamin in the blood and a depletion of the vitamin reserves that were stored in the liver, the patient develops megaloblastic anemia, with erythrocytes that are too large. Because of their size, the erythrocytes have difficulty passing through the microcirculation, and they become damaged. The limited lifespan of these erythrocytes is 27 to 35 days before hemolysis occurs. Because of hemolysis, the patient's indirect bilirubin rises. In addition, the lack of this vitamin impairs the bone marrow function of white blood cells and platelets, causing thrombocytopenia (a low platelet count) and leukopenia (a low white blood count).

NORMAL VALUES

Adult: 200–900 pg/mL *or* SI: 148–666 pmol/L
Adult (60–90 years): 110–770 pg/mL *or* SI: 81–568 pmol/L
Newborn: 160–1300 pg/mL *or* SI: 118–959 pmol/L

HOW THE TEST IS DONE

A red-topped tube is used to collect 10 mL of venous blood.

SIGNIFICANCE OF TEST RESULTS

Elevated Values

Chronic leukemia
Chronic renal failure
Polycythemia vera
Liver disease
Liver metastases

Decreased Values

Pernicious anemia
Intrinsic factor antibodies
Postgastrectomy
Atrophic gastritis
Achlorhydria
Malabsorption in the ileum
Chronic pancreatitis

INTERFERING FACTORS

- Failure to maintain nothing-by-mouth status
- Radioactive isotopes
- Hemolysis
- Exposure of the specimen to sunlight

C

NURSING CARE

Nursing actions are similar to those used in other venipuncture procedures (see Chapter 2), with the following additional measures.

Pretest

- Schedule this test before a radioisotope scan, because the radioisotopes of these procedures interfere with the radioimmunoassay method of analysis for this test.
- Schedule this test before a blood transfusion is administered or a trial of vitamin B_{12} treatment is started.
- ***Patient Teaching.*** The nurse instructs the patient to fast from food for 8 hours before the test.

Posttest

- Send the specimen to the laboratory without delay. If a delay in analysis occurs, the specimen must be protected from exposure to sunlight.
- The nurse should assess the patient with cobalamin deficiency. The hematologic manifestations associated with this anemia include fatigue, weakness, pallor, and jaundice. In the inspection of the mouth, the tongue is sore and smooth because of a loss of the epithelial surface. The neurologic manifestations are more troubling to the patient because there are changes in the brain, spinal cord, and peripheral nerves. The patient complains of peripheral neuropathy, including symptoms of numbness, tingling, and a loss of vibratory sensation in the hands and feet. There is a loss of position sense and difficulty walking. Brain changes also are present, causing impairment in thinking, change in personality, irritability, and emotional instability. In pernicious anemia, the hematologic symptoms disappear with correct vitamin replacement therapy, but the neurologic damage remains. The therapy prevents additional neurologic losses and a worsening condition.
- Once the medical diagnosis is made and treatment prescribed, the nurse can assist the patient with the monthly injections of vitamin B_{12}. Because this treatment will continue for life, the nurse teaches the patient or family member to give the injections. The nurse also encourages the patient to follow through with recommended physical therapy rehabilitation and to maintain regular follow-up visits to the physician to monitor the results of the anemia treatment.

Colonoscopy

koh-loh-nos-kuh-pee

Also called: Lower Panendoscopy

SPECIMEN OR TYPE OF TEST: Endoscopy, computed tomography

PURPOSE OF THE TEST

The purposes of a colonoscopy, by endoscopic method or by computed tomography (CT), are to perform a routine screening of the colon for detection of polyps and cancer and to investigate the cause of chronic diarrhea and other gastrointestinal complaints related to the colon. The procedure may be done to further investigate an abnormal result of a fecal occult blood test, barium enema, or sigmoidoscopy. It may be used to locate and evaluate the colon pathology before surgical intervention. The purpose of lower panendoscopy is to examine the terminal ileum, particularly for sources of inflammation and bleeding.

BASICS THE NURSE NEEDS TO KNOW

Colorectal cancer is the second leading cause of cancer death in the United States. There is evidence that polyps grow slowly and some eventually become malignant. Colorectal cancer also may be present in the colon or rectal area, and it grows slowly. Early detection and removal of a precancerous or cancerous growth provides for a high rate of survival. Late detection and late-stage cancer is associated with a much lower cure rate and lower survival rate. Many major health organizations now recommend routine screening for colorectal cancer. Colonoscopy is the most thorough and accurate method for colorectal screening. Despite the benefits of screening, it is estimated that less than one third of the eligible people have screening by colonoscopy.

Endoscopy

Colonoscopy is usually performed with a flexible fiberoptic endoscope. This instrument enables the physician to insert the endoscope through the entire length of the colon, and view the walls of the lumen. The flexibility of the instrument allows it to curve around the flexed areas of the colon (sigmoid, splenic, and hepatic flexures) without interrupting the viewing or damaging the tissue of the colon walls (Figure 35). The instrument provides light, focus, flexibility for positioning, and special channels for instillation of gas or air, cautery, suctioning, removal of polyps, and the taking of biopsy specimens. The colon must be completely clean, without fecal material that would obstruct the view.

Almost all patients require conscious sedation and narcotic medications to tolerate the procedure comfortably.

Lower Panendoscopy

This procedure is the same as an endoscopic colonoscopy, but proceeds farther to enter and explore the terminal ileum. It is used primarily to explore the cause and extent of inflammatory illness of the colon and ileum. It is possible to pass the instrument tip of the colonoscope through the ileocecal valve and into the distal ileum for a distance of 8 to 10 inches (20 to 30 cm).

Virtual Colonoscopy

This is the newest method of examining the lumen of the colon. It is sometimes called computed tomography colonography (CTC) because it uses a CT scan to image the colon to screen for polyps and bowel cancer. It also may be used as part of the preoperative workup when surgery on the colon is planned.

Virtual colonoscopy is not invasive, so it has the advantage of not requiring conscious sedation of the patient. There is no risk of a complication of perforation of the bowel, a potential problem with an invasive procedure. Virtual colonoscopy can image the colon despite the presence of an obstruction that would prevent the passage of

C

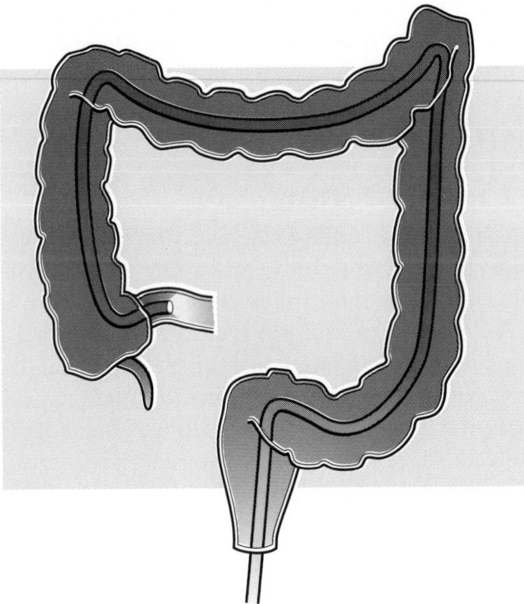

Figure 35. Colonoscopy. The endoscopic instrument is passed through the entire colon. As needed, the tip of the instrument can be passed into the distal segment of the ileum. The examination is used to identify sites of bleeding, inflammation, tissue irregularity, or abnormality, including polyps and tumor.

the endoscope. Compared to the endoscope, virtual colonoscopy is faster, painless, and easily tolerated. The patient does not lose a day of work recovering from a lengthy procedure and the sedation that is used with endoscopic examination.

The disadvantages of virtual colonoscopy are that the bowel preparation (complete evacuation of the bowel in the pretest period) is the same for virtual colonoscopy as for the endoscopic procedure. Additionally, when abnormality of colon tissue is encountered, the virtual colonoscopy does not permit the taking of biopsy specimens or removal of polyps.

NORMAL VALUES No abnormalities of colon tissue are observed

HOW THE TEST IS DONE

Colonoscopy and Lower Panendoscopy

A complete bowel preparation is done by the patient, to empty the colon of all feces. Almost all patients have the procedure done after receiving conscious sedation. Infants and small children generally require general anesthesia. Once sedated or anesthetized, the physician passes the endoscope into the rectum and advances the instrument on through the sigmoid, descending, transverse, and ascending colon. The colonoscopy procedure reaches the cecum; the lower panendoscopy procedure continues the advance of the endoscope into the terminal part of the ileum. As the instrument is withdrawn slowly, the physician examines all parts of the lumen of the colon and biopsy samples are taken, as needed.

Virtual Colonoscopy

A complete bowel preparation is done by the patient, to empty the colon of all feces.

A CT scan of the abdomen is used for imaging of the colon, without any need for pain medication or sedation.

SIGNIFICANCE OF TEST RESULTS

Polyps in the colon
Cancer
Ulcerative colitis
Colitis (radiation, ischemia, infection)
Lower intestinal bleeding
Diverticulitis
Crohn's disease

INTERFERING FACTORS

- Poor bowel preparation
- Uncooperative patient behavior
- Retained barium
- Failure to maintain pretest dietary restrictions
- Pregnancy
- Acute medical conditions as recent heart attack, toxic colitis, peritonitis, and others

NURSING CARE

- ***Health Promotion.*** The nurse can teach people to begin routine health screening for colorectal cancer. After age 50, the healthy individual is at increased risk to develop colon cancer, and that risk increases with each succeeding decade of life. Colonoscopy is one of the available methods to detect colon abnormalities. Screening offers prevention by removing polyps before they become cancerous and detecting tumors before symptoms occur. Early detection of abnormality leads to early intervention, when cure is still possible. For the average-risk individual, the recommended screening schedule is to have a colonoscopy every 10 years, starting at age 50.
- ***Health Promotion.*** There is a need for education of the public as to the benefits of regular screening tests. For many years, people were taught to observe for symptoms of disease and then seek medical advice and diagnosis. Today, the emphasis is on screening to detect abnormality before the problem is advanced enough to cause symptoms. The educational focus should include "unlearning" old information as well as learning the new and greatly improved methods of detection.

Continued

NURSING CARE—*cont'd*

Pretest

- Schedule the colonoscopy before any barium studies are performed.
- After the physician has explained the procedure, a consent form must be signed by the patient and the form is placed in the patient's record.
- ***Patient Teaching.*** Provide instructions about bowel cleansing. Because the protocol varies somewhat among institutions, the nurse follows the endoscopist's requirements. General guidelines are presented here.
- The patient is taught to begin a low residue or clear liquid diet for 24 hours before the test, to reduce the amount of feces. Starting at 5:00 PM on the afternoon before the test, the patient begins the colon lavage by drinking the PEG (polyethylene glycol) solution. Four liters of the PEG solution (GoLYTELY, Colyte, or NuLytely) are ingested over a period of 2 hours. The suggested schedule is to drink 8 oz of the preparation every 10 minutes. The bowel begins to empty of feces and watery diarrhea soon after the PEG regimen begins. The bowel is considered to be clear of feces when the patient expels clear, watery fluid. The patient may continue to drink clear fluids until midnight, but is instructed to maintain a nothing-by-mouth status thereafter.
- On the morning of the test, the nurse takes the patient's vital signs and enters the results in the patient's record.
- When colonoscopy is done for screening purposes, the patient may experience mild anxiety or feelings of embarrassment about the procedure. When the patient reports abnormal bowel symptoms or has abnormal findings from a previous colorectal screening test, fear or anxiety can be greatly increased. The nurse and physician need to support the patient emotionally before, during, and after the colonoscopy procedure.

During the Test

- For the endoscopic procedure, the patient is premedicated with intravenous meperidine (Demerol) for analgesia and relaxation. This may be followed by intravenous diazepam (Valium) or intravenous midazolam (Versed). Because these drugs can cause apnea, respiratory depression, or cardiac arrest, the doses must be administered very slowly, over a period of 5 minutes. Naloxone (Narcan) must be kept on hand to reverse the respiratory depression of meperidine, but it is ineffective against diazepam.
- Oxygen by nasal cannula increases the patient's oxygen reserves and helps prevent hypoxia from the effects of intravenous sedation. The nurse monitors the vital signs at frequent intervals throughout the procedure. Automated blood pressure, pulse oximetry, and cardiac monitoring may be used for all endoscopy patients or for selected patients who are more vulnerable, including the elderly or those with a history of cardiac disease.
- The nurse and physician also monitor for the vasovagal reflex that can occur during the procedure. Atropine sulfate is kept on hand to reverse sudden bradycardia.
- The nurse provides comfort and emotional support to help promote relaxation. As the physician insufflates and manipulates the endoscope, the patient may become uncomfortable and restless, requiring more medication.

NURSING CARE—*cont'd*

- The nurse also assists with the collection of biopsy specimens. Additional information is presented in the section on Gastrointestinal Cytologic Studies (p. 339). These specimens are sent to the laboratory as soon as the procedure is completed.

Posttest

- Vital signs are monitored every 15 minutes or the automated monitoring is continued until the patient is stable. The nurse checks the rectal area for signs of blood. As soon as the patient is more responsive, food and fluid intake can resume. On discharge from the ambulatory care setting, the patient must be accompanied by a responsible person who will take the patient home. Because of the effects of the intravenous sedation, the patient cannot drive the car for 8 to 12 hours, until thinking is clear and memory is restored.

◆ **Nursing Response to Complications**

The overall risk of complication from colonoscopy is very low. The two complications are bleeding and perforation of the colon. If complications occur, the nurse must notify the physician of abnormal assessment findings.

Bleeding. The nurse observes the rectal area for signs of bleeding. Vital signs are taken and if blood work is done, it should include a hemoglobin and hematocrit. If the blood loss is moderate, the patient will have hypotension and tachycardia. Additionally, the hemoglobin and hematocrit values would decrease, but generally, these laboratory values do not decline until hours later, depending on the amount and rapidity of the blood loss.

Perforation. If the colon is perforated, the patient would complain of malaise and persistent abdominal pain. On palpation of the abdomen, the nurse's findings would include distension and tenderness. An elevated temperature and elevated white blood count are early signs of infection in the peritoneal cavity.

Colposcopy

kol-pos-kuh-pee

SPECIMEN OR TYPE OF TEST: Endoscopy, Biopsy

PURPOSE OF THE TEST

Colposcopy is performed to further evaluate an abnormal Pap smear, to monitor for precancerous abnormalities, or to evaluate a lesion of the vagina or cervix.

BASICS THE NURSE NEEDS TO KNOW

The colposcopy procedure is done because the results of the Papanicolaou (Pap) smear were abnormal. As a follow-up examination, colposcopy allows for more precise examination of the cervix and vagina for cellular and vascular changes. Endocervical curettage is used to scrape the tissue and obtain cell samples of the endocervical canal, and a biopsy forceps is used to nip small samples of tissue from the cervix. After a biopsy, bleeding is controlled with an application of silver nitrate, pressure, or sutures.

NORMAL VALUES

No abnormalities of the vaginal or cervical tissue are noted.

HOW THE TEST IS DONE

A colposcope is inserted into the vagina to provide magnification and illumination of vaginal and cervical tissue. A tissue biopsy is performed.

SIGNIFICANCE OF TEST RESULTS

Abnormal Values

Atrophic cellular changes
Cervical intraepithelial neoplasia
Papilloma
Condyloma
Infection, inflammation
Cervical erosion
Invasive carcinoma

INTERFERING FACTORS

- Vaginal creams
- Menstruation

NURSING CARE

Pretest

- After the physician informs the patient about the procedure, obtain written consent from the patient.
- The patient is likely to become concerned when told that the Pap smear is abnormal and that follow-up colposcopy is needed. Some women do not know what a colposcopy is, why it is needed, or what the findings could indicate. Because of fear and anxiety, some may fail to keep the appointment for the colposcopy. For some, there is a total lack of information, and for others, fear of the possibility of tumor or cancer already exists. The patient may be nervous and frightened. Before the examination, the patient may desire more information about the test and its implications. The nurse can provide information and education about the test, particularly for the woman who is scheduled for colposcopy. The information should include what the test is, why it is needed, and what the patient will feel as the test is performed. The anticipatory teaching can help reduce anxiety.
- Schedule the procedure for the early part of the menstrual cycle, preferably between days 8 and 12. In this period, the cervical mucus is clear and thin and allows maximum visibility.
- ***Patient Teaching.*** The nurse instructs the patient to refrain from the application of any creams or vaginal medications before the test because they obscure the view of the cervix.

NURSING CARE—*cont'd*

During the Test

- The nurse assists the patient to change into a hospital gown. The patient is then assisted to lithotomy position on the examination table, with the patient's legs placed in stirrups.
- As the physician inserts the speculum and colposcope, the nurse instructs the patient to breathe through the mouth to help relax the muscles. As the physician performs endocervical curettage of the specimen, the patient can feel a "pinch" or a brief cramping sensation. Also, she can hear the snipping sound when the clamp closes as a small piece of biopsy tissue is obtained.
- Once the glass slides are prepared with cell scrapings, the nurse can apply the fixative to prevent drying of the cells. If biopsy specimens are taken, place the tissue on hard brown paper or on nonstick gauze (Telfa). Each sample is placed in a separate specimen jar that contains fixative.

Posttest

- The nurse ensures that all specimens are labeled appropriately and that the requisition slip also identifies the source of the tissue.
- ***Patient Teaching.*** When a cervical biopsy is performed as part of the colposcopy procedure, the nurse instructs the patient to refrain from sexual intercourse and to avoid the insertion of anything into the vagina until the lesion is healed. Arrange for a follow-up appointment to evaluate the healing process.

Complement, Total

kom-pluh-ment, toh-tuhl

Also called: C_{50}

SPECIMEN OR TYPE OF TEST: Serum

PURPOSE OF THE TEST

Total complement is used to evaluate or monitor systemic lupus erythematosus and its response to therapy. The test is also used to diagnose complement deficiency and to detect disease caused by the immune complex.

BASICS THE NURSE NEEDS TO KNOW

Complement is a system of 25 plasma proteins and cell-membrane–associated proteins that circulate in inactive forms in the blood. When activated, they serve to work with the defense system and protect against infection. In supporting the work of antibodies, the complement cells facilitate phagocytosis, eliminate antigen-antibody complexes, and puncture the cell membranes of bacteria. These complexes penetrate the walls of the bacteria and cause lysis of the cells. In an active form, complement induces an inflammatory response. Total complement proteins increase in an acute response to inflammation or infection and are decreased or absent in autoimmune disease, hereditary deficiency, and excess use of the complexes in active disease.

NORMAL VALUES 25–110 CH_{50} units/mL

HOW THE TEST IS DONE

A red-topped tube is used to collect 10 mL of venous blood.

SIGNIFICANCE OF TEST RESULTS

Elevated Values

Chronic infection
Rheumatoid arthritis
Acute rheumatic fever
Ulcerative colitis
Diabetes mellitus
Thyroiditis

Decreased Values

Systemic lupus erythematosus
Lupus nephritis
Multiple myeloma
Acute post-streptococcal glomerulonephritis
Hypogammaglobulinemia
Advanced cirrhosis of the liver
Acute vasculitis

INTERFERING FACTORS

- None

NURSING CARE

Nursing actions are similar to those used in other venipuncture procedures (see Chapter 2), with no additional nursing measures needed.

Complete Blood Count

kuhm-pleet blud kount

Also called: (CBC)

SPECIMEN OR TYPE OF TEST: Whole blood

PURPOSE OF THE TEST

The CBC is used to assess the patient for anemia, infection, inflammation, polycythemia, hemolytic disease, and the effects of ABO incompatibility, leukemia, and dehydration status. It is also used to identify the cellular characteristics of the peripheral blood and manage chemotherapy or radiation treatment for cancer.

BASICS THE NURSE NEEDS TO KNOW

The complete blood count (CBC) is a series of different tests used to evaluate the blood and the cellular components of red blood cells, white blood cells and platelets. Automated analyzers vary somewhat in the selection of tests that comprise the CBC. In most laboratories, the CBC consists of hemoglobin, hematocrit, red blood cell count, red blood cell indices, white blood cell count, platelet count, and reticulocyte count. These tests may also be prescribed singly. The white blood cell differential count is no longer a part of a routine CBC, but may be ordered separately. In this text, the White Blood Cell Differential Count is presented separately under its own heading (p. 679).

Hemoglobin (Hgb) is used to measure the severity of anemia, which is characterized by a low hemoglobin value, or polycythemia, which is characterized by a high hemoglobin value. It also is used to monitor the results of medical or nutritional treatment for the condition. An elevated hemoglobin value often is the result of excess production of red blood cells, but it also may be the result of dehydration, which causes the concentration of red blood cells in a smaller volume of plasma. A decreased value of hemoglobin can be caused by a low red blood cell count, by a lack of hemoglobin in the erythrocytes, or by fluid retention, which causes a normal number of red cells to disperse in a larger than normal volume of plasma. The patient is considered anemic when the hemoglobin for the male is less than 13 g/dL (SI: <130 g/L) and for the female is less than 11 g/dL (SI: <110 g/L).

Hematocrit (Hct) is used to evaluate blood loss, anemia, polycythemia, and dehydration. The Hct value is elevated when the number of red blood cells increases or when the volume of plasma is reduced. The Hct value falls when there is excessive loss of red blood cells, as in anemia or after excessive blood loss. It can also decrease because of fluid overload that dilutes the concentration of red blood cells. In hemorrhage, the Hct value drops several hours after the bleeding episode. The severity of the drop in value correlates directly with the amount of blood lost.

Red blood cell count, or erythrocyte count, is used to evaluate polycythemia and anemia. An elevated red cell count may be the result of hyperactivity of the bone marrow in the manufacture of the erythrocytes or an increase of erythropoietin from renal disease. In dehydration, there is a relative increase of red blood cells, meaning that there are a normal number of erythrocytes, but they are concentrated in decreased plasma volume. A decreased red cell count can occur from excessive loss of the cells, as in hemorrhage, or excessive destruction of red cells, as in hemolytic anemia. The decreased count also may be caused by impaired bone marrow production of the blood cells, such as in bone marrow damage from radiation therapy or chemotherapy in the treatment of cancer.

C

Red cell indices are used to help diagnose, classify, and evaluate the different types of anemia. The tests measure the size and weight of the average erythrocyte, the amount of hemoglobin in the average erythrocyte, and the average hemoglobin concentration. The tests include the mean corpuscular volume (MCV), mean corpuscular hemoglobin (MCH), the mean corpuscular hemoglobin concentration (MCHC), and the red cell distribution width (RDW). Additional information related to changes in the characteristics of red blood cells can be done by examination of the peripheral blood smear. In this text, this information is presented in the test for Red Blood Cell Morphology (p. 568).

Mean corpuscular volume calculates the average erythrocyte size. If the MCV value is elevated, the erythrocytes are large, or *macrocytic*. If the MCV value is decreased, the erythrocytes are small, or microcytic.

Mean corpuscular hemoglobin calculates the weight of the hemoglobin in the average erythrocyte. The MCH value is elevated when the erythrocyte is macrocytic and decreased when the erythrocyte is microcytic.

Mean corpuscular hemoglobin concentration measures the average concentration or percentage of hemoglobin in the average erythrocyte. When the MCHC value is elevated, a high concentration of hemoglobin exists in the erythrocyte, and the cell is hyperchromic. When the value is in a normal range, the red cell is normochromic. When the MCHC value is decreased, a lower concentration of hemoglobin exists, and the erythrocyte is hypochromic.

Red cell distribution width is a numeric calculation of the widths of the erythrocytes. When the RDW value is elevated, the laboratory personnel review the peripheral blood smear for *anisocytosis*, a variation in the size of erythrocytes. The presence and amount of anisocytosis is used to estimate the severity of anemia and to differentiate among the microcytic anemias. Some of the microcytic anemias cause an RDW elevation and others cause minimal or no change in this laboratory value.

White blood cell, or leukocyte, count is the total number of the five types of leukocytes present in 1 mm^3 of blood. The leukocyte count is a general indicator of infection, tissue necrosis, inflammation, or bone marrow activity. More specific diagnostic information is obtained by the differential count that identifies the numbers of each type of white blood cell. *Leukocytosis* is an elevated number of white blood cells. The elevated value occurs in response to infection and is usually directly proportionate to the degree of bacterial invasion. The elevated value also may be caused by necrosis of tissue or malignancy of the bone marrow. A white blood cell count of 11,000 to 17,000 cells (11 to $17 \times 10^3/\mu L$ *or* SI: 11 to $17 \times 10^9/L$) is considered to be a mild to moderate leukocytosis. When the white blood cell count falls to less than normal limits, it is called *leukopenia*. Mild leukopenia is indicated by a white blood cell count of 3000 to 5000 cells (3 to $5 \times 10^3/\mu L$ *or* SI: 3 to $5 \times 10^9/L$). Any significant decrease is usually in neutrophils, although all five forms of leukocytes may be decreased. Decreases in the leukocyte count usually are a result of bone marrow depression or particular infection that has exhausted the supply of neutrophils and bone marrow reserves.

Platelet count is used to assess the ability of the bone marrow to produce platelets and to identify the destruction or loss of platelets in the circulation. It also is used to evaluate the untoward effects of chemotherapy or radiation treatment. Platelets function to initiate the process of coagulation. When there is a nick or opening in a blood vessel, platelets quickly aggregate, adhere to the endothelial surface of the blood vessel, and plug the opening. As additional platelets and clotting factors arrive, the clot becomes firm and seals off the opening effectively.

Thrombocytosis is an excess number of platelets (>400,000 cells/μL *or* SI: >400 × 10^9/L) in the blood. The condition may occur when platelets are produced at a fast rate in response to injury. This condition rarely causes symptoms and is self-limiting. The level of platelets returns to a normal value as the underlying condition is corrected. Thrombocytosis also may be a symptom of myeloproliferative disease, such as chronic myelocytic leukemia. The platelet count rises severely, and potential exists for hemorrhage or thrombosis. Bleeding probably results from defects in the platelets and the inability to form a clot. Thrombosis in either veins or arteries can occur as platelets aggregate and trap erythrocytes in the microcirculation. Common sites of vascular occlusion include the splenic, hepatic, and pulmonary veins; the mesenteric and axillary arteries; and the fingers and toes.

Thrombocytopenia is a decreased number of platelets (<100,000 cells/μL *or* SI: <100 × 10^9/L) in the blood. This condition causes a prolonged bleeding time because the patient's clotting ability is seriously compromised. With inadequate numbers of platelets, the patient is vulnerable to bleeding, particularly into the skin. The decrease in platelets is caused by three possibilities: (1) deficient platelet production; (2) rapid platelet destruction; and (3) abnormal pooling of the platelets. The most common cause is the rapid destruction of platelets.

Reticulocyte count is used to evaluate erythropoiesis, distinguish among different types of anemia, assess the severity of blood loss, and evaluate the bone marrow response to treatment of anemia. Reticulocytes are immature erythrocytes. The normal reticulocyte count is expressed as a percentage of the erythrocyte count and, normally, few reticulocytes exist in the circulation in proportion to the number of erythrocytes.

An increase in reticulocytes indicates the ability of the bone marrow to produce erythrocytes. The elevated value is considered a healthy response after a loss of erythrocytes from hemorrhage or hemolysis. It also is a healthy response to anemia or to a reduced amount of hemoglobin in the red blood cells. The reticulocyte count may also rise after treatment for anemia. A decreased reticulocyte count indicates that erythropoiesis is diminished in the bone marrow. The cause may be a lack of stimulation by erythropoietin, a disease that affects the bone marrow cells, or a faulty maturation process in the bone marrow.

NORMAL VALUES

Hemoglobin
Male: 14.0–17.5 g/dL *or* SI: 140–175 g/L
Female: 12.3–15.3 g/dL *or* SI: 123–153 g/L

Hematocrit
Male: 41.5%–50.4% *or* SI: 0.415–0.504 (volume fraction)
Female: 35.9%–44.6% *or* SI: 0.359–0.446 (volume fraction)

Red Blood Cell Count
Male: 4.5–5.9 × 10^6/μL *or* SI: 4.5–5.9 × 10^{12}/L
Female: 4.5–5.1 × 10^6/μL *or* SI: 4.5–5.1 × 10^{12}/L

Red Cell Indices
MCV: 80–96 μm^3 *or* SI: 80–96 fL
MCH: 27.5–33.2 pg *or* SI: 27.5–33.2 pg
MCHC: 33.4%–35.5% *or* SI: 0.334–0.355 (concentration fraction)
RDW-CV: 11.7%–14.2% *or* SI: 0.117–0.142 (number fraction)

White Blood Cell Count
4.4–11 × 10^3/μL *or* SI: 4.4–11 × 10^9/L

Platelet Count
150,000–450,000 cells/μL *or* SI: 150–450 × 10^9/L

Reticulocyte Count
Adult: Percentage of cells: 0.5%–1.5% *or* SI: 0.005–0.015 (number fraction)
Cell count: 25,000–75,000 cells/μL *or* SI: 25–75 × 10^9/L
Newborn: Percentage of cells: 3.0%–7.0% *or* SI: 0.03–0.07 (number fraction)

▼ Critical Values

Hemoglobin: <6.0 g/dL *or* >18.0 g/dL *or* SI: <60 g/L *or* >180 g/L
Hematocrit: <18% *or* >54% *or* SI: <0.18 *or* >0.54 (number fraction)
WBC: <2.5 × 10^3/μL *or* >30 × 10^3/μL *or* SI: 2.5 ×10^9/L *or* >30 × 10^9/L
Platelets: <20,000 cells/μL *or* >1,000,000 cells/μL *or* SI: <20 cells × 10^9/L *or* >1000 cells × 10^9/L

HOW THE TEST IS DONE

A purple-topped tube with ethylenediaminetetraacetic acid (EDTA) anticoagulant is used to collect 7 mL of venous blood. As an alternative, two purple-tipped capillary tubes can be used to collect blood from a heelstick, earlobe, or finger puncture.

SIGNIFICANCE OF TEST RESULTS

Elevated Values

Hemoglobin

Polycythemia
Dehydration

C

Hematocrit
Polycythemia
Dehydration
Red Blood Cell Count
Polycythemia
Renal tumor
Dehydration
Red Blood Cell Indices
MCV: Pernicious anemia, deficiency of vitamin B_{12}, folic acid deficiency
MCH: Hereditary spherocytosis
MCHC: Hereditary spherocytosis
RDW: Iron deficiency anemia, pernicious anemia, deficiency of vitamin B_{12}, folate, beta thalassemia major
White Blood Cell Count
Infection
Inflammation
Leukemia
Platelets
Myeloproliferative diseases
Multiple myeloma
Iron deficiency anemia
Postsplenectomy response
Hodgkin's disease
Lymphomas
Renal disease
Infection or inflammation
Reticulocytes
Treatment for iron deficiency anemia and pernicious anemia
Hemolytic anemia
Hemorrhage
Chronic blood loss

Decreased Values
Hemoglobin
Hemorrhage
Anemia
Hemolysis of erythrocytes
Fluid overload
Hematocrit
Hemorrhage
Anemia
Hemolysis of erythrocytes
Fluid overload
Red Blood Cells
Hemorrhage
Fluid overload

Anemia
Aplastic anemia
Bone marrow depression
Hemolysis of erythrocytes

Red Blood Cell Indices

MCV: Iron deficiency anemia, chronic inflammation
MCH: Iron deficiency anemia
MCHC: Iron deficiency anemia

White Blood Cells

Aplastic anemia
Bone marrow depression
Pernicious anemia
Some infectious or parasitic diseases

Platelets

Idiopathic thrombocytopenic purpura
Aplastic anemia
Anemias
Malignancy of the spleen
Disseminated intravascular coagulation
Bone marrow depression
Systemic lupus erythematosus
Uremia
Liver disease

Reticulocytes

Aplastic anemia
Iron deficiency anemia
Anemia of chronic disease
Sideroblastic anemia
Pernicious anemia
Renal disease
Endocrine disease

INTERFERING FACTORS

- Hemolysis
- Coagulation of the specimen
- Hemodilution

NURSING CARE

Nursing actions are similar to those used in other venipuncture procedures (see Chapter 2), with the following additional measures.

Pretest

- No special measures are needed.

NURSING CARE—*cont'd*

During the Test

- Ensure that the blood is not taken from the hand or arm that has an intravenous line. Hemodilution with intravenous fluids causes a false decrease in the values of some tests.

Posttest

- Assess the puncture site for signs of bleeding or bruising (ecchymosis) of the skin. If the platelet count is decreased, clotting will be slow to occur. To promote clotting, the nurse can use sterile gauze to apply pressure to the site or raise the arm above the head while maintaining pressure on the site.
- Arrange for prompt transport of the specimen. If there is an anticipated delay, refrigerate the specimen.

▼ Nursing Response to Critical Values

If the test result is in the range of the critical values or worse, the nurse notifies the physician immediately. When the change develops slowly or gradually, the patient may not have immediate abnormal assessment findings. When the result occurs rapidly or is severely abnormal, assessment findings are more likely to be abnormal. Further medical investigation is needed to determine the cause of the abnormal value.

Hemoglobin, hematocrit, and red blood cell count. When the hemoglobin, hematocrit, and red blood cell count are severely altered, abnormal findings of the nursing assessment may include fatigue, pallor, tachycardia, rapid respirations, dyspnea on exertion, and a low blood pressure.

White blood count. For a severely low white blood count (leukopenia), the patient is at risk to develop an infection that can become life threatening. The patient has too few white blood cells to protect against infection or combat one that occurs. The nurse prepares to implement measures that will help protect the patient from acquiring an infection. A severely elevated white blood count (hyperleukocytosis) is a potential emergency situation. Hyperleukocytosis is usually the result of leukemia in the crisis stage. The patient may have a fatal hemorrhage in the lung or brain as leukocytes clump or aggregate in small blood vessels. The nurse assesses for any change in vital signs, dyspnea, or levels of consciousness and for other signs of a stroke.

Platelets. When the platelet value shows a severe depletion, the patient is at risk to develop a spontaneous hemorrhage. There are too few platelets to start the clotting process. The nurse assesses for bruising or bleeding in the skin, as evidenced by petechiae or ecchymosis, or bleeding from the nose or gums of the mouth (gingivae). More seriously, a hemorrhage in the brain can occur, causing a stroke. The nurse assesses for any change in the patient's level of consciousness or loss of speech, motor, or sensory function. When the platelet count rises severely, the patient is at risk to develop a thrombosis (clot) that can form anywhere, including in the blood vessels of the heart, brain, fingers, toes, or abdominal organs. The nurse assesses for change in vital signs and levels of consciousness, changes in the circulation to the extremities, or the patient's complaint of pain.

Computed Tomography

kohm-pyoo-ted tuh-mo-gruh-fee

Also called: CT Scan, Computerized Axial Tomography, CAT Scan

SPECIMEN OR TYPE OF TEST: Radiography

PURPOSE OF THE TEST

The computed tomography (CT) scan provides precise visualization of the structure, size, shape, and density of soft tissue, bone, major blood vessels, and organs of the head and torso. It distinguishes between benign and malignant tissue and is used in the staging of cancerous tumors. It also can be used to analyze the bone mineral content of the vertebrae in the assessment of osteoporosis.

BASICS THE NURSE NEEDS TO KNOW

Computed tomography uses radiation energy, a scanner, and specialized computer software to produce detailed images of the internal organs and tissues. The views are cross-sectional images of the anatomic structures and each image is called a *tomographic slice* or *axial slice*. In the CT scanning process, as the patient passes through the ring of x-ray beams, cross-sectional images of the targeted tissue are taken every few centimeters or millimeters. The photons pass through the body and are received by detectors on the opposite side of the scanner. After computerized treatment of the data, the CT scan provides clear and very detailed digital images (Figure 36, *A* and *B*). The CT image is reviewed, identifying the size, shape, and structure of the organs, including the positions and spatial relationships to the other nearby tissues.

Conventional CT

The different tissues of the body have different densities. Those tissues and objects that are very dense or solid, such as bone, metallic implant, calcium deposit, or thrombus absorb most of the photons. Other tissues are less dense, or radiolucent, and allow more photons to pass through the tissue and reach the detectors. Fat tissue and hollow organs that contain air permit the passage of almost all photons. In combination, the different tissue densities provide detailed images in shades of white, gray, and black that correlate to the size, shape, and density of the tissues that are scanned.

Helical (Spiral) CT

The newer CT technology is used particularly for scanning the body because the imaging is more rapid and continuous. The speed of the examination is particularly helpful when the patient requires a CT scan and has a critical illness. In helical scanning, the x-ray tube traces a helical or spiral pattern over the patient's body surface as the imaging is done (Figure 37). Hundreds of images can be obtained in less than 1 minute, and the entire scan can be completed rapidly. With this faster imaging and the specialized computer applications, the patient's motion from respiration or bowel peristalsis no longer interferes with the clarity of the images within the torso.

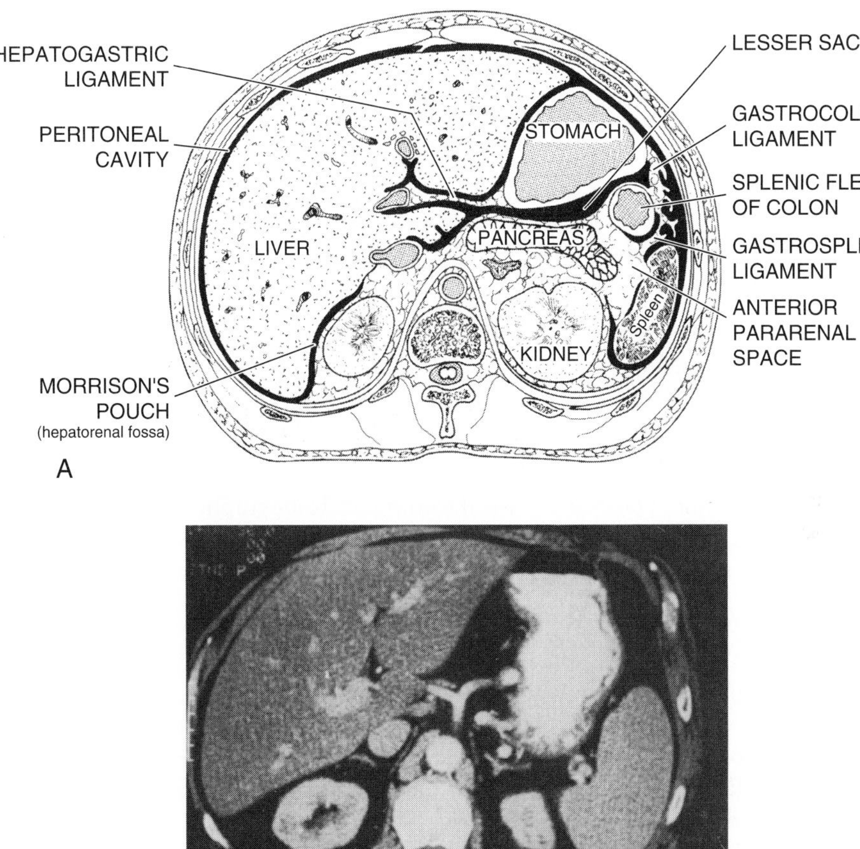

Figure 36. Cross-sectional views of the abdomen. *A*, Diagram of a transverse section of the upper abdomen showing the relationship of the organs and structures. *B*, A transverse computed tomographic (CT) image of the abdomen. *(A, Reproduced with permission from Moss, A. A., Gansu, G., & Genant, H. K. [1992].* Computed tomography of the body with magnetic resonance imaging *[2nd ed., Vol. 3 p. 1140]. Philadelphia: W. B. Saunders. B, Reproduced with permission from Thompson, M. A., Hall, J. D., Hattaway, M. P., & Dowd, S. B. [1994].* Principles of imaging science and protection *[Vol. 2, Slide 390]. Philadelphia: W. B. Saunders.)*

The helical CT scan can produce transaxial slice images, similar to the conventional CT scan. In addition, helical CT can provide three-dimensional (3-D) images from the data, producing a different view and additional information for the physician or surgeon. For example, 3-D images of vascular abnormalities such as aneurysm, stricture, or stenosis are readily visible, and the size of the abnormality is measurable. The 3-D images of a bone can reveal greater detail about a fracture, tumor, or metastasis.

C

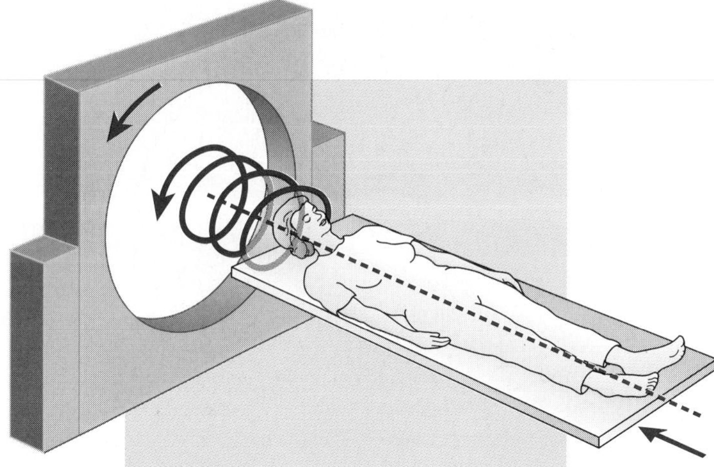

Figure 37. The scanning process in helical Computed Tomography (CT). The patient is moved on a table through the scanner. As the x-ray and detector system rotate, a helix or spiral of data is obtained. *(Reproduced with permission from Brink, J. A. [1995]. Technical aspects of helical [spiral] CT.* Radiologic Clinics of North America, *33[5], 826.)*

CT uses a high level of ionizing radiation. The exposure to radiation can be up from 6 to 50 times higher than that which is needed for a plain x-ray. The increased exposure is of particular concern with children because their organs are more radiation sensitive than those of adults. For children, the risk is that excess exposure in childhood can cause radiation-induced cancer at a later stage of life.

CT Scan of the Head

The imaging of the head can be done with or without contrast medium. When contrast is used, the brain tissue is more clearly imaged. The CT of the head is often needed in cases of trauma or head injury. A fracture of the skull can be identified and the CT can demonstrate hematoma, swelling, or bleeding within the brain or space between brain and skull. Because the helical CT examination is so rapid, treatment of life-threatening injury can begin at a much earlier time.

CT Scan of the Eye Orbits

The CT scan with intravenous iodinated contrast medium is the primary imaging procedure used to examine the eye orbits and their contents. It provides visual information about the eyes and the bones and soft tissues surrounding the eyes. The use of tomographic slices and different visual planes allows the assessment of the parts in a complex anatomic area.

In imaging the bones of the orbits, the CT scan identifies abnormalities caused by abscess, calcification, fracture, trauma, and metastatic lesion (Figure 38). In the assessment of the orbital contents, the CT scan can image the globe, lens, ocular muscles, and optic nerve. Abnormalities that are clearly defined include retinoblastoma, menin-

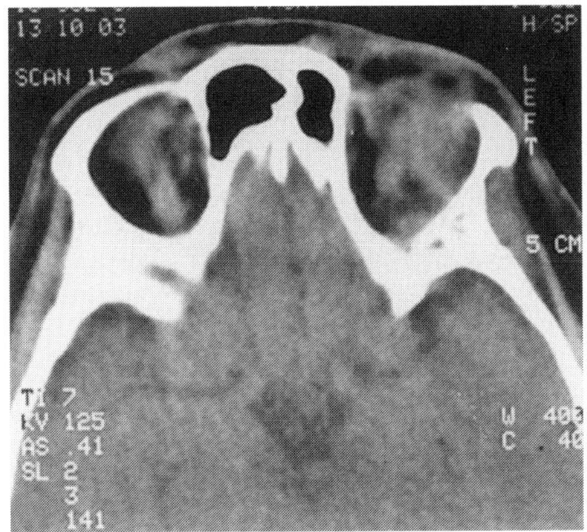

Figure 38. Orbital metastasis. Transverse computed tomographic (CT) section showing a tumor mass in the left orbit of the eye. The enlarged size and irregular shape of the bone of the left orbit are the result of metastasis from ovarian cancer. *(Reproduced with permission from Bomanji, J., Glaholm, J., Hungerford, J. L., Mather, S. J., Granowska, M., Britton, K. E., & Whitelock, R. [1990]. Radioimmunoscintigraphy of orbital metastases from ovarian carcinoma.* Clinics in Nuclear Medicine, *15, 825–827.)*

C

gioma, granuloma, penetrating foreign bodies, orbital hematoma, some vascular lesions, and the muscle changes associated with the exophthalmos of Graves' disease.

CT of the Brain and Spinal Cord

The CT scan can investigate intracerebral, extracerebral, and spinal lesions. The abnormalities may be congenital, degenerative, inflammatory, vascular, or tumor in origin. Because the scan produces tomographic axial slices for viewing, the precise location, size, and characteristics of the abnormality can be seen. The procedure is performed with or without the use of contrast material.

Intracranial lesions that are identified by CT are hydrocephalus and aqueduct stenosis, cerebral atrophy, hemorrhage, hematoma, infarction, and edema of the brain. Tumors within the cranium may be (1) intracerebral and often malignant or (2) extracerebral and probably benign. Extracerebral tumors include meningiomas, acoustic neuromas, epidermoid tumors, dermoid tumors, craniopharyngiomas, and pituitary tumors. CT arteriography uses contrast medium to visualize better the lumens of the intracranial arteries. Helical CT provides very sharp, clear images of cerebral blood vessels and their structural abnormalities, including stenosis, aneurysm, and arteriovascular malformation.

In imaging the spinal cord, the CT scan demonstrates the bony and soft tissue abnormalities that compress the cord and nerve roots. It images a bulge in a disc, a degenerative change, the alignment and structure of the vertebrae, spinal infection, and hypertrophy of the ligaments. Also the diameter of the spinal cord can be measured. CT is often used to confirm spinal stenosis as a cause of spinal cord disorder.

C

CT of the Chest

The CT scan can be used to diagnose benign or cancerous pulmonary lesions. With some bronchogenic cancers, the CT scan can be used to determine the invasive extent of the cancer into the chest wall, diaphragm, and mediastinum, as well as extrathoracic metastasis.

The CT scan is used to plan radiation therapy for the patient with cancer of the lung. It may also be useful in the diagnosis of silicosis, asbestosis, lung abscess, and empyema.

Vascular CT

With the use in intravenous iodinated contrast medium, vascular problems such as aneurysm, arteriovenous malformation, central pulmonary embolus, and septic embolus may be identified (Figure 39). With the use of orally ingested contrast medium, esophageal lesions can be evaluated.

CT of the Abdomen

This procedure provides a view of the bowel wall, mesentery, peritoneum, and organs adjacent to the gastrointestinal tract. CT is used to detect intra-abdominal masses, including abscess, tumor, infarct, perforation, obstruction, inflammation, and diverticulitis. It is also useful in detection of metastases and in the staging of abdominal malignancy. Intravenous contrast medium is used to image the vascular structure within the abdomen. Barium and air are used as contrast media to improve the visualization of the lumen of the intestinal tract.

With or without intravenous iodinated contrast, CT of the abdomen can be useful in identifying changes in the pancreas. The CT scan is useful to visualize benign or malignant tumors of the pancreas, diagnose acute or chronic pancreatitis, and locate a pancreatic abscess.

CT of the Pelvis

In the evaluation of the female pelvis, CT with intravenous contrast material produces clear, cross-sectional images of the pelvic tissues and organs. The pelvic CT scan is often used to determine the extent of malignancy or the source of infection. For these purposes, the scan usually includes the abdomen and the pelvis so that nearby organs, structures, and blood vessels are visualized. Oral and rectal barium contrast material may be administered to opacify the bowel loops. If a pelvic tumor or abscess is located, the CT scan is used to guide the placement of a needle in a percutaneous aspiration biopsy or in percutaneous needle drainage of the purulence.

CT of Bones and Joints

In orthopedics, the CT scan is particularly useful because the bone tissue is dense and absorbs many of the x-ray photons. Thus, the image of the bones appears white or bright on the film. The scan gives accurate definition of the structure of the bones and demonstrates subtle pathologic changes, such as the small linear fracture, stenosis of a bony canal, erosion of the bone, or degenerative changes from osteoporosis. It also

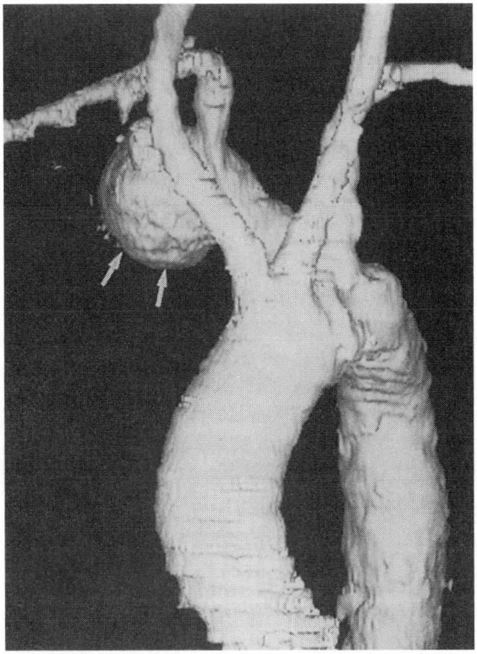

Figure 39. Helical (spiral) CT three-dimensional image of an artery. The image of the aneurysm of the subclavian artery *(arrows)* is generated from the data of a helical computed tomographic (CT) scan. The vascular image clearly shows the external surface of the artery and documents the abnormality. *(Reproduced with permission from Touliopoulos, P., & Costello, P. [1995]. Helical [spiral] CT of the thorax.* Radiologic Clinics of North America, *33[5], 848.)*

images problems of subluxation, dislocation, calcification, and cancer of the bone (Figure 40).

Traditional CT also may be used to assess the spinal column, confirming the presence of bony or soft tissue changes that affect the vertebrae or spinal canal. CT detects congenital malformation, bony overgrowth, bone spurs, lumbar stenosis, cervical spondylosis, scoliosis, degenerative changes, a bulging disc, and ligament hypertrophy.

The helical CT scan is particularly useful in cases of cervical spine trauma with a suspected fracture, subluxation, or dislocation that could result in compression of the spinal cord. It also is very useful in cases of massive or multiple fractures, such as trauma to the pelvis involving the pelvic and hip bones. Helical CT also is used to identify abnormality in the bone due to neoplasm, infection, degenerative disease of the spine, and postsurgical difficulty with a spinal repair of the lumbar spine.

NORMAL VALUES No structural or anatomic abnormalities are noted

C

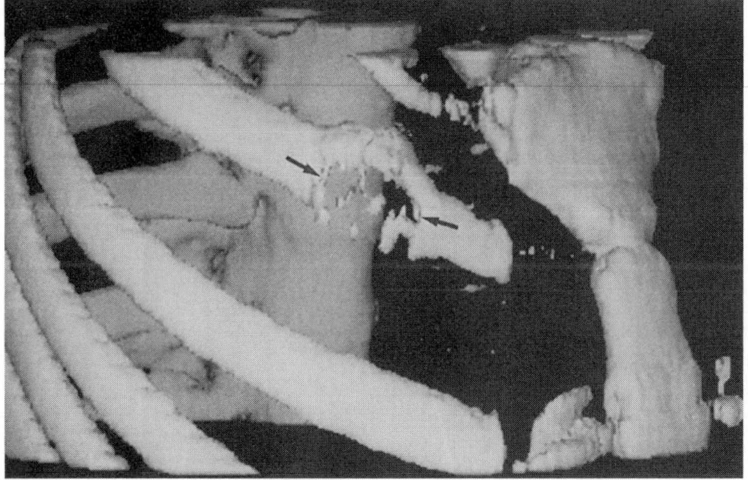

Figure 40. Helical (spiral) CT three-dimensional image of a rib. The 3-D image shows the extent of a cancer metastasis *(arrows)* to the right fifth anterior rib from a primary synovial sarcoma. *(Reproduced with permission from Touliopoulos, P., & Costello, P. [1995]. Helical (spiral) CT of the thorax.* Radiologic Clinics of North America, *33[5], 858.)*

HOW THE TEST IS DONE

With or without the use of a contrast medium, the patient moves through a scanner ring, and multiple x-ray beams pass through the tissue. As the x-ray photons fall on the detectors, data are collected. Computerized treatment of the data produces two- or three-dimensional images of the internal tissues.

SIGNIFICANCE OF TEST RESULTS

Abnormal Values

Tumor
Malignancy
Cyst
Stenosis
Thrombus
Embolus
Arteriosclerotic plaque
Calcification
Congenital malformation
Abscess
Calculus
Inflammation
Fluid collection
Bleeding or hemorrhage
Organ atrophy
Bone fracture

INTERFERING FACTORS

- Jewelry or metal in the CT field
- Uncooperative behavior
- Pregnancy
- Failure to maintain nothing-by-mouth status (as indicated)
- Allergy to iodine (with the use of intravenous contrast medium)
- Severe liver or kidney disease (with the use of intravenous contrast medium)

NURSING CARE

Pretest

- In preparation for the CT scan, the nurse recognizes that the patient may experience some apprehension related to the procedure and equipment or anxiety related to a potential diagnosis. Listening to the patient will provide guidance as to how to lessen the anxiety and what information to provide. With an explanation of the procedure, the patient will have less apprehension about the unknown. In addition, the information helps the patient to cooperate during the procedure, so that the best possible images are obtained.
- The nurse explains that the patient will be positioned on a moveable table and restrained to prevent movement. The table will move the patient into the scanner, which has a small, air-conditioned chamber, equipped with a microphone. The patient can communicate with the technologist at all times. To help the patient remain motionless during scans of the abdomen or chest, the technologist will instruct the patient to hold his or her breath at intervals. While the scanning is performed, the patient will hear the quiet whirring of the machine and feel the table move further into the chamber, or tilt to achieve different angles of imaging. When no contrast is used, the scanning procedure is painless.
- To help the patient control anxiety or a mild feeling of claustrophobia, the nurse can suggest various diversionary or relaxation techniques. The patient may already have a preferred way to help control anxiety or remain calm. Suggestions can include visual imagery, muscle relaxation, meditation, and prayer.
- ***Patient Teaching.*** The nurse inquires if the patient has any history of allergy to iodine or shellfish or of allergic reaction to dye or contrast material used in a previous x-ray study. When it is used, iodinated contrast medium is injected by bolus or slow intravenous drip. The nurse or technologist should explain that the patient may feel a sensation of warmth, a salty taste, headache, or nausea as the agent is injected. These are temporary sensations that will disappear in a few minutes.
- ***Patient Teaching.*** If intravenous contrast medium is to be used, instruct the patient to discontinue all food and fluids for 4 to 8 hours before the test. In gastrointestinal CT imaging, instruct the patient to drink prescribed amounts of liquid contrast on the night before the test and again at timed intervals in the hours before the scan. If the colon is to be imaged by a CT scan, pretest bowel preparation will be required to cleanse the organ and remove the feces. Just before the scan, a barium enema or air will be instilled in the colon as the contrast medium.

Continued

C

NURSING CARE—*cont'd*

- ***Patient Teaching.*** Instruct the patient to remove all clothes, jewelry, and other metal objects. For the procedure, a hospital gown is worn.
- Sedatives are usually used for the infant or child younger than age 3, particularly when the scan requires an extended period of immobility. For these patients, general anesthesia may also be used and requires sedation before the administration of the anesthesia.

During the Test

- Instruct the patient to remain motionless while in the scanner and to hold his or her breath when instructed to do so. Keep an emesis basin in a nearby area in case the patient vomits after receiving the contrast medium.

Posttest

- If sedatives were administered, the nurse monitors the vital signs on a regular basis until the patient is responsive and awake.
- If barium was used in a gastrointestinal scan, the nurse explains that the barium will appear as gray material in the feces. It will be eliminated from the body within a day or two. Intravenous contrast medium is excreted in the urine within a few hours, with no noticeable change or impact on the patient.

Coronary Arteriography

See Catheterization, Cardiac on p. 187.

Corticotropin

See Adrenocorticotropic Hormone, Plasma on p. 46.

Cortisol, Total

kohr-tuh-sohl, toh-tuhl

Also called: Hydrocortisone, Serum

SPECIMEN OR TYPE OF TEST: Plasma, serum

PURPOSE OF THE TEST

Cortisol levels are used to diagnose Cushing syndrome, Cushing's disease, and primary and secondary adrenal insufficiency. Primary adrenal insufficiency is called Addison's disease.

BASICS THE NURSE NEEDS TO KNOW

The adrenal cortex produces a group of hormones called *glucocorticoids.* The primary glucocorticoid is cortisol. Secretion of cortisol is regulated by ACTH, which is secreted by the anterior pituitary gland. When secreted, most of the cortisol in the plasma binds with corticosteroid-binding globulin (CBG). The free cortisol is the biologically active form, whereas the bound hormone acts as a storehouse to replace the free cortisol.

The actions of cortisol and the other glucocorticoids are multiple and relate to their plasma concentrations. At normal plasma levels, glucocorticoids, as the name implies, maintain glucose levels by promoting hepatic gluconeogenesis and glycogenolysis, prevent fatigue by making tissues more responsive to glucagon and catecholamines, reduce the secretion of antidiuretic hormone (ADH), increase glomerular filtration rates, and make the distal tubules of the kidneys more permeable to water reabsorption.

Elevated Values

At elevated levels, for example, in times of stress or in pharmacologic doses, the glucocorticoids have an immunosuppressive and an anti-inflammatory effect.

Cushing syndrome includes excessive secretion of the adrenal cortex hormones resulting from a primary adrenal dysfunction. When a pituitary or hypothalamic disorder causes an increase in the production of glucocorticoids, including cortisol, it is called Cushing's disease. The high cortisol levels may be dangerous for the individual, because the inflammatory response is suppressed. The inflammatory response is necessary to destroy invading microorganisms, to wall off infected areas, and to initiate normal wound healing.

NORMAL VALUES

Adult: 8–10 AM: 5–23 mcg/dL *or* SI: 138–635 nmol/L
4–6 PM: 3–16 mcg/dL *or* SI: 83–441 nmol/L
Newborn: 8–10 AM: 0.1–3.4 mcg/dl *or* SI: 28–938 nmol/L
4–6 PM: 0.1–8.0 mcg/dl *or* SI: 28–288 nmol/L

HOW THE TEST IS DONE

Venipuncture is performed to obtain 5 mL of blood in a green-topped tube.

If a serum level is desired instead of a plasma level, 5 mL of blood is collected in a red-topped tube. Varied methods are used to measure cortisol, including radioimmunoassay (RIA), competitive protein-binding assay, fluorometric assay, and high-performance liquid chromatography.

For newborns, instead of performing a heelstick or venipuncture when doing cortisol levels, saliva may be used to test for cortisol. If a saliva specimen is used, no milk should be present in the infant's mouth.

SIGNIFICANCE OF TEST RESULTS

Elevated Values

Cushing syndrome
Cushing's disease
Stress
Acute illness
Surgery
Trauma
Excessive exogenous glucocorticoids
Exogenous estrogen

Anxiety
Starvation
Anorexia nervosa
Alcoholism
Chronic renal failure
Adrenal hyperfunction
Excessive ACTH (pituitary or ectopic production)

Decreased Values
Addison's disease
Pituitary destruction or failure
Hypophysectomy
Postpartum pituitary necrosis
Pregnancy
Hepatitis
Cirrhosis of the liver

INTERFERING FACTORS

- Noncompliance with dietary or activity restrictions
- With RIA: Androgens, estrogens, phenytoin, hepatic dysfunction, and renal failure
- With competitive protein-binding assay: Prednisolone and 6-alpha-methylprednisolone
- With fluorometric assays: Jaundice, renal failure, and medications (niacin, quinacrine, quinidine, spironolactone)
- With high-performance liquid chromatography: Prednisone, prednisolone

NURSING CARE

Nursing actions are similar to those used in other venipuncture procedures (see Chapter 2), with the following additional measures.

Pretest

- The nurse obtains a medication history and asks the physician if any interfering drugs should be withheld. The nurse also inquires and notes on the requisition slip if the patient is pregnant, because this may affect test results.
- ***Patient Teaching.*** The nurse explains to the patient the need to obtain two specimens of blood, one in the early morning and one in the evening to obtain peak and low secretion times. Instruct the patient to ingest nothing by mouth for 12 hours before the test. Some physicians recommend a low-carbohydrate diet for 2 days before the test. The nurse also instructs the patient to limit physical activity for 12 hours before the test and to lie down for 30 minutes before the blood is drawn.

Cortrosyn Stimulation Test

See Adrenocorticotropic Hormone Stimulation Test on p. 49.

Cosyntropin Test

See Adrenocorticotropic Hormone Stimulation Test on p. 49.

C-Reactive Protein

see-ree-ak-tiv proh-teen

Also called: (CRP), hs-CRP

SPECIMEN OR TYPE OF TEST: Serum

PURPOSE OF THE TEST

C-reactive protein is used as a nonspecific indicator of infection or inflammation and also is used to monitor the response to antibiotic or anti-inflammatory medication. It is commonly used to help with the diagnosis of rheumatoid arthritis and rheumatic fever; particularly when the erythrocyte sedimentation rate (ESR) and other test results are inconclusive. It is also under investigation as a possible risk factor or marker of cardiovascular disease.

BASICS THE NURSE NEEDS TO KNOW

C-reactive protein is a serum protein. Normally, it is absent from the blood, except when tissue necrosis, trauma, inflammation, or infection exists. The older method, called standard CRP, is not sensitive at the lower range of positive serum values. The new method, called high sensitivity CRP (hs-CRP) is much more accurate in measurement of CRP values. The normal values are different for each of these test methods.

The serum level of C-reactive protein rises rapidly in response to bacterial infection and acute inflammation. The progressive rise in value reflects increasing infection, inflammation, or tissue damage. Equally, the progressive fall in the serum value indicates healing or the effectiveness of antibiotic or anti-inflammatory medication. In a normal postoperative course, the CRP rises sharply by the third postoperative day. If no bacterial infection is present, the value will fall to a normal level by the seventh day.

Serial testing for C-reactive protein may be used to monitor bacterial infection. A rising or persistently high C-reactive protein level may indicate antibiotic treatment failure or the onset of a postoperative infection. Because the protein level does not rise in the presence of viral infection, the test may be used to differentiate between viral and bacterial sources of infection.

High-Sensitivity C-Reactive Protein (hs-CRP)

Recent research has identified that a high normal value of hs-CRP is a possible marker or risk factor for coronary artery disease and potential acute myocardial infarction. In addition, a rising level of the hs-CRP together with a low-density lipoprotein (LDL) elevated cholesterol level predicts a much greater risk for a heart attack. If an acute myocardial infarction occurs, the CRP level will rise dramatically, even to five times the upper limit of the normal value, or higher. More research is needed to clarify the role of CRP as a marker or a risk factor and to determine the best use of the test results in treatment to prevent a heart attack (See also Cardiac Markers, p. 178).

NORMAL VALUES

Standard CRP: 0.08–3.1 mg/dL *or* SI: 0.8–31 mg/L
High-sensitivity CRP (hs-CRP): 0.02–8 mg/dL *or* SI: 0.2–80 mg/L

HOW THE TEST IS DONE

A red-topped tube is used to collect 10 mL of venous blood.

SIGNIFICANCE OF TEST RESULTS

Elevated Values

Rheumatoid arthritis
Rheumatic fever
Systemic lupus erythematosus
Bacterial sepsis
Tuberculosis
Pneumococcal pneumonia
Crohn's disease
Myocardial infarction

INTERFERING FACTORS

- Oral contraceptives
- Serum lipidemia
- Hemolysis

NURSING CARE

Nursing actions are similar to those used in other venipuncture procedures (see Chapter 2), with the following additional measures.

Pretest

- ***Patient Teaching.*** Instruct the patient to fast from food for 4 to 8 hours before the test. Fluids are permitted. Fasting is necessary because it is desirable to have the level of serum lipids as low as possible. Serum lipids cause a false positive result.

NURSING CARE—*cont'd*

Posttest

- The nurse monitors the CRP results of the patient as one of the indicators that infection or inflammation is increasing or decreasing, particularly in response to medication. Inflammatory disorders may be arthritic, affecting joints or involving specific organs. If the heart tissue is inflamed, the nurse monitors the pulse for an elevated rate and altered rhythm. If CRP is used as a predictor of coronary artery disease, the nurse monitors for a sudden onset of chest pain and altered vital signs. In detecting sepsis and estimating its severity, CRP monitoring is more accurate than the leukocyte (WBC) count and the body temperature.

Creatine Kinase

See Cardiac Markers on p. 178.

Creatine Kinase Isoenzymes

See Cardiac Markers on p. 178.

Creatinine Clearance

kree-a-tuh-neen kleer-uhns

Also called: (Ccre)

SPECIMEN OR TYPE OF TEST: Urine, blood

PURPOSE OF THE TEST

A creatinine clearance is done to measure glomerular filtration rates. Almost all the creatinine produced by protein metabolism is filtered by the glomeruli. Creatinine clearance is often done to evaluate the progression of renal insufficiency. It is sometimes done to ensure adequate filtration and removal of medications from the blood.

BASICS THE NURSE NEEDS TO KNOW

Creatinine clearance is the total amount of creatinine excreted in the urine within a designated time period. Creatinine is an amino acid waste product that is derived from muscle creatinine, a product of protein metabolism. It is distributed throughout body fluids and is excreted by the kidneys. In the process of urinary elimination, creatinine is almost totally filtered by the glomeruli. Age affects the creatinine clearance value. After age 40, creatinine clearance decreases every 10 years by almost 10%.

Elevated Values

Creatinine clearance increases after intense exercise, with infection, diabetes mellitus, and after eating a meat meal.

Decreased Values

Urinary creatinine decreases with acute and advanced chronic renal failure because the glomeruli are impaired or unable to remove the creatinine from the blood. In these conditions, the serum creatinine level rises, but the urinary creatinine and creatinine clearance rate decreases.

NORMAL VALUES	Adults: 75–125 mL/min/1.73 m^2 *or* SI: 1.25–2.08 mL/s/1.73 m^2 Children: 70–140 mL/min/1.73 m^2 *or* SI: 1.17–2.33 mL/s/1.73m^2
Critical Values	<30 mL/min/1.73 m^2 *or* SI: <0.02 mL/s/1.73 m^2

HOW THE TEST IS DONE

Blood: A red-topped tube is used to collect 10 mL of venous blood. For infants and small children, a heelstick puncture is used to fill a capillary pipette. The blood is collected at the midpoint of the time of the urine collection period.

Urine: Urine is collected for a 4-, 12-, or 24-hour period.

Creatinine clearance is a calculated value obtained by using the urine and plasma creatinine levels, urinary volume, and the patient's body surface area.

SIGNIFICANCE OF TEST RESULTS

Increased Values

Pregnancy
Burns
High-protein diet
Hypothyroidism
Diabetes mellitus

Decreased Values

Renal insufficiency or failure
Glomerulonephritis
Nephrotic syndrome
Pyelonephritis
Shock
Congestive heart failure
Hyperthyroidism

INTERFERING FACTORS

- Exercise
- Ingestion of meat
- Ketosis
- Many medications

NURSING CARE

Nursing actions are similar to those used in other venipuncture and timed urine collection procedures (see Chapter 2), with the following additional measures.

Pretest

- The nurse asks the physician if any medications are to be withheld during the test. Generally, medications including cephalosporins are withheld because they alter the test result.
- The patient's height, weight, and age are recorded in the patient's record and on the laboratory requisition slip. The data are used in the calculation of the creatinine clearance.
- ***Patient Teaching.*** The nurse instructs the patient to discard the first urine of the morning at 8 AM and then begin the urine collection. All urine for the timed period is to be placed in a special collection container, including the last voided specimen at the end of the collection period. The container with the urine is kept on ice. The patient is instructed to maintain fluid intake before and throughout the collection period.

During the Test

- The nurse writes the date and time of the start and finish of the collection period on the collection container and the requisition slip.

Posttest

- The nurse arranges to send the urine to the laboratory, promptly.

▼ Nursing Response to Critical Values

A creatinine clearance value at the critical value level or worse occurs in advanced renal failure. The nurse assesses the patient's intake and output of fluids, vital signs, and mental status. In advanced renal failure, the patient has decreased urinary output, or *oliguria*, that is, a urine output or 100 to 400 mL per day, or *anuria*, a urine output of 100 mL or less per day. When the kidneys cannot filter and remove water, the patient develops edema in body tissues. The patient develops hypertension and tachypnea and may be somnolent (excessively drowsy). The nurse notifies the physician of the creatinine clearance result and the assessment findings, including the patient's intake and output.

Creatinine, Serum, Plasma

kree-a-tuh-neen, see-ruhm, plaz-muh

Also called: (pCR); Plasma Creatinine

SPECIMEN OR TYPE OF TEST: Serum, plasma

PURPOSE OF THE TEST

Serum creatinine determination is the most common laboratory test used to evaluate renal function and to estimate the effectiveness of glomerular filtration.

C

BASICS THE NURSE NEEDS TO KNOW

Creatinine is an amino acid and waste product of protein metabolism. It is derived from creatine, which is synthesized in the liver, kidneys, and pancreas, and stored in muscle tissue. As creatine is metabolized in the muscle, creatinine is produced. Creatinine is released into the extracellular fluid and excreted through the kidneys.

In the kidneys, creatinine is filtered by the glomeruli and is usually not resorbed. Additional creatinine is secreted by the renal tubules. When the kidneys are functional, they maintain the serum creatinine level at a minimal, low level.

Elevated Values

When renal function is impaired, the creatinine level increases.

Decreased Values

The serum levels of creatinine decrease in conditions that cause decrease in muscle mass, including old age and muscle-wasting diseases. In these conditions, there is less creatine synthesis and storage, and therefore less creatinine production.

NORMAL VALUES	Adult male: 0.7–1.3 mg/dL *or* SI: 62–115 µmol/L Adult female: 0.6–1.1 mg/dL *or* SI: 53–97 µmol/L Adolescent: 0.5–1 mg/dL *or* SI: 44–88 µmol/L Child: 0.3–0.7 mg/dL *or* SI: 27–62 µmol/L Infant: 0.2–0.4 mg/mL *or* SI: 18–35 µmol/L Newborn: 0.3–1 mg/dL *or* SI: 27–88 µmol/L
▼ Critical Values	Renal insufficiency: 1.5–3.0 mg/mL Renal failure: >3.0 mg/mL

HOW THE TEST IS DONE

A red-topped tube is used to collect 10 mL of venous blood. For infants and small children, a heelstick puncture is used to fill a capillary pipette.

SIGNIFICANCE OF TEST RESULTS

Elevated Values

Acute or chronic renal insufficiency/failure
Uremia or azotemia
Renal artery stenosis
Congestive heart failure
Shock
Dehydration
Rhabdomyolysis
Acromegaly

Decreased Values

Advanced liver disease
Long-term corticosteroid therapy

Hyperthyroidism
Muscular dystrophy
Paralysis
Dermatomyositis
Polymyositis

INTERFERING FACTORS

- Hemolysis
- Warming of the specimen
- Lipemia
- Recent ingestion of meat

NURSING CARE

Nursing actions are similar to those used in other venipuncture procedures (see Chapter 2), with the following additional measures.

Pretest

- ***Patient Teaching.*** When indicated by the laboratory protocol, the nurse instructs the patient to fast from food and fluids for 8 hours before the test.

Posttest

- Arrange for prompt transport of the specimen to the laboratory. Prolonged delay causes ammonia to form in the specimen. Warming will cause a falsely elevated test result.

▼ Nursing Response to Critical Values

When the serum creatinine elevates to the critical value level or higher, the finding indicates acute or severe chronic renal insufficiency or renal failure. The glomeruli are unable to filter the blood and remove the accumulating creatinine. The nurse assesses the patient for signs of renal failure, including hypertension, tachypnea, edema, and somnolence (drowsiness). The urine output may be *oliguric*, with an output of 100 to 400 mL per day, or *anuric*, with a volume of 100 mL per day, or less. The nurse notifies the physician of the elevated serum creatinine level and of the assessment findings.

Creatinine, Urine

kree-a-tuh-neen, yur-in

Also called: Urinary Cre

SPECIMEN OR TYPE OF TEST: 12- or 24-hour urine

PURPOSE OF THE TEST

The urine creatinine test is performed to assess renal function. It usually is not assessed alone, but is done as part of the Creatinine Clearance Test (see p. 243).

BASICS THE NURSE NEEDS TO KNOW

Creatinine is an amino acid waste product that is derived from muscle creatine, a product of protein metabolism. It is distributed throughout body fluids and is excreted by the kidneys. In the process of urinary elimination, creatinine is almost totally filtered by the glomeruli.

NORMAL VALUES

Adult male: 1–2 g/day *or* SI: 8.8–17.7 mmol/day
Adult female: 0.8–1.8 g/day *or* SI: 7.1–15.9 mmol/day
Child: 6–30 mg/kg/day *or* SI: 53–264 µmol/kg/day

HOW THE TEST IS DONE

The test usually requires urine collection for 24 hours, but collection periods of 12 hours are sometimes prescribed.

SIGNIFICANCE OF TEST RESULTS

Elevated Values

Muscular dystrophy
Polymyositis
Paralysis
Muscular inflammatory disease
Hyperthyroidism
Anemia
Leukemia

Decreased Values

Glomerulonephritis
Congestive heart failure
Acute tubular necrosis
Advanced pyelonephritis
Shock
Polycystic kidney disease
Renal malignancy
Dehydration
Bilateral ureteral obstruction
Nephrosclerosis

INTERFERING FACTORS

- Excessive exercise during the test period
- Failure to collect all the urine
- Failure to time the test accurately
- Warming of the urine specimen
- High protein intake before the test

NURSING CARE

Nursing actions are similar to those used in other timed urine collection procedures (see Chapter 2), with the following additional measures.

Pretest

- ***Patient Teaching.*** The nurse instructs the patient to avoid excessive intake of meat on the day before the test. The patient is taught to collect all urine for the 24-hour period of the test, storing the container in the refrigerator or on ice. The nurse encourages the patient to maintain adequate hydration before and during the test and to omit coffee and tea during the test.

During the Test

- ***Patient Teaching.*** At 8 AM, instruct the patient to void and discard the urine. The test begins at this time, and all subsequent urine specimens are collected for 24 hours, including the 8 AM specimen of the next morning. Advise the patient to avoid vigorous exercise during the test period.
- ***Patient Teaching.*** The nurse ensures that the patient's name and the time and date of the start and finish of the test are written on the label and requisition slip.

Posttest

- Arrange for prompt transportation of the refrigerated specimen to the laboratory.

Culture, Blood

kul-chur, blud

SPECIMEN OR TYPE OF TEST: Blood

PURPOSE OF THE TEST

The blood culture identifies the organism that is causing infection in the bloodstream. Susceptibility testing measures the sensitivity of the pathogen to various antibiotics.

BASICS THE NURSE NEEDS TO KNOW

Septicemia, an infection of the blood, can be caused by almost any bacterial organism. In sepsis, the bacteria are often present in the blood on an intermittent basis only. Specimen collection is timed to try to obtain the blood when the bacteria are present. The best time to collect the specimen is just before a chill or temperature spike, with two additional specimens taken at hourly intervals thereafter. It can take several blood culture attempts before the bacteria are identified.

There are variations in the timing of specimen collection to help isolate the elusive organism. The maximum total number of specimens, however, is four. Each blood culture specimen must be collected at a different vascular site with a separate venipuncture. There must be at least a 1-hour interval between collections of specimens. These guidelines help to obtain at least one successful culture, and they prevent blood loss that results from excessive specimen collection.

Susceptibility Testing

When bacteria are identified, susceptibility testing may be done. In the presence of antibiotic or antimicrobial medication, bacteria are described as susceptible, intermediate, or resistant. Susceptible means that the bacteria can be treated effectively with the particular medication. Intermediate means that the bacteria can be treated effectively with a higher dosage of the medication or with medication that concentrates in a particular body site where the bacteria are located. Resistance means that the bacteria will not be killed or eliminated by the particular medication.

NORMAL VALUES

Negative; no growth of organisms

HOW THE TEST IS DONE

For the adult, a needle and syringe, a transfer set, or a special set of blood tubes with culture media is used to collect 20 mL of venous blood.

For infants and small children, the procedure is the same, but 1 to 5 mL of blood may be obtained from pediatric patients.

For the neonate, 0.5 to 1 mL of blood is sufficient for each specimen. The heelstick method and capillary tube blood sample are used only as a last resort because of the problem of contamination.

SIGNIFICANCE OF TEST RESULTS

Positive Values

Bacterial endocarditis
Bacterial meningitis
Septic arthritis
Typhoid fever
Brucellosis
Sepsis or septicemia
Osteomyelitis
Bacterial pneumonia
Toxic shock syndrome

INTERFERING FACTORS

- Contamination of the specimen
- Antibiotic therapy

NURSING CARE

Nursing actions are similar to those used in other venipuncture procedures (see Chapter 2), with the following additional measures.

Pretest

- Schedule the tests before antibiotic therapy is administered.
- The nurse informs the patient about the procedure, including the series of blood specimens and the skin asepsis. The patient is asked about any history of skin sensitivity to iodine.

NURSING CARE—*cont'd*

- To assist with the timing of the blood sampling, the nurse monitors the patient's temperature, pulse, respiration, and blood pressure at frequent and regular intervals. The results are recorded in the patient's chart.

During the Test

- The nurse assists the physician or lab technician as needed. The skin of the venipuncture site is scrubbed in concentric circles in an outward direction with 80% to 95% alcohol and then allowed to dry. The second scrub is done in the same pattern, using povidone-iodine solution. This solution remains on the skin for at least 1 minute. If the patient is sensitive to iodine, green soap may be substituted or the alcohol preparation alone can be used.
- The tops of the culture bottles or tubes are cleansed with alcohol or povidone-iodine before the blood is injected into them. If a blood collection system is used, only alcohol may be applied to clean the stoppers.
- Using sterile gloves and aseptic technique, the blood is drawn from the vein. The blood is then divided among the different bottles or tubes. If an *intravenous* catheter is in place, the specimen is obtained from a venous site *distal* to the catheter or from the opposite extremity. This prevents hemodilution with intravenous fluids. Blood is never drawn from the intravenous line or the heparin-lock device because of the risk of external contamination.

Posttest

- Ensure that each requisition slip and all collection containers or tubes are correctly identified. The time, date, and venous site are included. In the patient's chart, the nurse documents each blood culture specimen collection, the time, date, and venous site. These data help keep track of the number and timing of the blood culture specimens and ensure that alternative venous sites are used.
- The nurse continues to assess the septic patient who is very ill. Common findings include fever, a rapid or changing pulse rate, hypotension, and sometimes shaking chills. The patient's history may include intermittent or persistent fever. The nurse also should assess the patient's heart, particularly listening for a murmur that would indicate bacterial endocarditis.
- The physician must be notified immediately of a positive blood culture result. Septicemia is very serious, and effective antibiotic treatment should be started promptly.

Culture, Genital

kul-chur, jen-i-tuhl

Also called: Genitourinary Culture, Cervical Culture, Endocervical Culture, Prostatic Fluid Culture, Vaginal Culture

SPECIMEN OR TYPE OF TEST: Secretions

PURPOSE OF THE TEST

The genital culture is used to identify the pathogenic organism that causes abnormal discharge and inflammation of the vagina or urethra.

BASICS THE NURSE NEEDS TO KNOW

A genital infection in the female is indicated by inflammation of the vagina and vulva, with the presence of vaginal secretions. In the male, it is indicated by inflammation of the urethra and urethral discharge. The infection may be caused by a sexually transmitted disease, or it may be the result of other causes that are not related to sexual contact. Numerous pathogens may be responsible for a sexually transmitted disease. The culture of the secretions or tissue scrapings is used to identify the causative organism.

Susceptibility Testing

When bacteria are identified, susceptibility testing may be done. In the presence of antibiotic or antimicrobial medication, bacteria are described as susceptible, intermediate, or resistant. Susceptible means that the bacteria can be treated effectively with the particular medication. Intermediate means that the bacteria can be treated effectively with a higher dosage of the medication or with medication that concentrates in a particular body site where the bacteria are located. Resistance means that the bacteria will not be killed or eliminated by the particular medication.

NORMAL VALUES

Negative; normal flora present

HOW THE TEST IS DONE

For any of the following procedures, a sterile culture tube is used to receive the specimen of cell scrapings or fluid aspirate:

Male

A sterile cotton swab is used to collect secretions from the penile discharge. The physician may insert a wire loop into the urethra to obtain cell scrapings or a swab to obtain urethral secretions (Figure 41, *A*).

Female

With the assistance of a speculum, a sterile swab or wire loop is inserted into the cervical canal to obtain secretions or endocervical cell scrapings (Figure 41, *B*).

Chancroid

The base of the genital ulcer is irrigated with saline. The fluid is aspirated with a sterile pipette or a moist, sterile cotton swab.

Herpes Simplex

A sterile cotton swab is used to remove epithelial cells from the base of fresh lesions. Fluid from vesicles may also be obtained by aspiration with a sterile pipette.

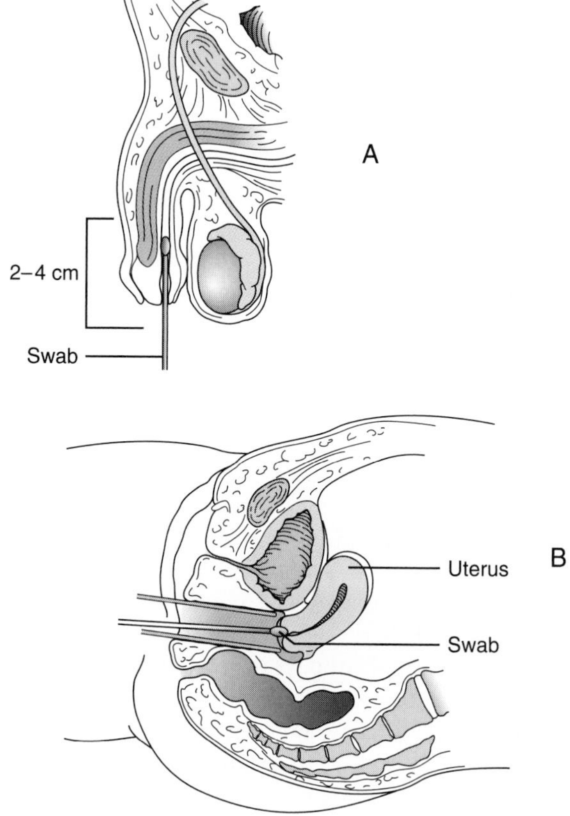

Figure 41. Specimen collection for genital culture. *A*, Sterile swab in male urethra. *B*, Sterile swab in female endocervical canal. *(Reproduced with permission from Stepp, C. A., & Woods, M. A. [1998].* Laboratory procedures for medical office personnel *[p. 364]. Philadelphia: W. B. Saunders.)*

SIGNIFICANCE OF TEST RESULTS

Positive Values

Neisseria gonorrhoeae
Candida albicans
Staphylococcus aureus
Group B streptococcus
Gardnerella vaginalis
Giardia lamblia
Herpes simplex virus
Trichomonas vaginalis
Chlamydia trachomatis
Human papillomavirus
Haemophilus ducreyi

C

INTERFERING FACTORS

- Recent urination
- Recent douching
- Improper collection technique
- Contamination of the specimen
- Antibiotic administration

NURSING CARE

Pretest

- ***Patient Teaching.*** Instruct the patient about pretest conditions as follows:
  Male: Do not urinate within 1 hour of the test, because there will be fewer organisms available for culture.
  Female: Do not douche for 24 hours before the test, because douching results in fewer organisms available for culture.
- The nurse inquires about any current use of antibiotics. The culture should be performed before any antibiotic therapy is started.

During the Test

- Place the male in the supine position. The female is placed in the lithotomy position, as for gynecologic examination.
- The nurse provides emotional support to the patient during the collection of the specimen. For the female, the procedure may produce mild apprehension or discomfort, but it is not painful. The male may experience nausea, sweating, fainting, or weakness as the wire loop or swab is inserted into the urethra. These discomforts are temporary.
- The requisition slip should include information regarding the source of the specimen, the patient's name and age, the clinical diagnosis, the time and date of the specimen collection, and any current antibiotic therapy.

Posttest

- ***Patient Teaching.*** Instruct the patient to abstain from sexual contact until any infection is identified, treated, and cured. With gonorrheal infection, instruct the patient to have the culture repeated 1 week after the completion of antibiotic therapy.
- ***Patient Teaching.*** When the culture is positive for a sexually transmitted disease, counsel the patient to inform all sexual partners of the test results. Sexual contacts are advised to undergo testing.
- ***Patient Teaching.*** As part of follow-up nursing care for a sexually transmitted disease, the nurse discusses ways to reduce risk for a repeat infection. From the patient's sexual history, the nurse can identify the individual's practices that resulted in infection and make suggestions for the future. The best protection from sexually transmitted disease is achieved through abstinence, a long-term monogamous relationship, or the use of condoms.

Culture, Nasopharyngeal

kul-chur, na-soh-fuh-rin-jee-uhl

SPECIMEN OR TYPE OF TEST: Secretions

PURPOSE OF THE TEST

The nasopharyngeal culture is performed to identify the bacteria that cause upper respiratory tract infection.

BASICS THE NURSE NEEDS TO KNOW

A variety of normal flora exists in the nose and nasopharynx. These normal organisms may multiply and cause illness, particularly in children, the elderly, immunocompromised individuals, or individuals in a weakened condition. A nose culture positive for one of these organisms may indicate infection in the nasopharynx, sinuses, oropharynx, or tonsils. Infection can also occur elsewhere in the body, with the source of the infection being in the nose or throat.

Staphylococcus aureus

The anterior nasal cavity is a major reservoir of *S. aureus*. In drug addicts with bacterial endocarditis, or in renal dialysis patients with septicemia, the nasal passageway may be the source of infection. This bacterium is also implicated in postoperative wound infection and in bacterial infection of the skin (furunculosis). As asymptomatic carriers, individuals may harbor *S. aureus* and the incidence is higher in hospital personnel and hospitalized patients. When an outbreak of this infection occurs, the nasopharyngeal culture may be performed as a screening test to identify asymptomatic carriers.

Bordetella pertussis

Bordetella pertussis and *Bordetella parapertussis* are the organisms that cause pertussis or whooping cough. This respiratory tract infection usually occurs in infants who are not vaccinated or who are incompletely vaccinated and are in close contact with an infected individual. The nasopharyngeal culture is a very important test when this infection is suspected.

Severe Acute Respiratory Syndrome (SARS)

SARS is a respiratory infection that causes severe pneumonia from a newly recognized corona virus. The virus may be detected in the respiratory tract within a period of 72 hours after symptoms begin. When SARS is suspected, the patient must be placed in isolation. Contact and respiratory droplet precautions are maintained.

The nasopharyngeal swab or aspirate is an early part of the diagnostic testing that is done when this lung infection is suspected. Each swab or aspirate sample of the secretions is placed in separate culturette tubes with viral transport medium. The specimens of mucus and cells are tested by polymerase chain reaction (PCR) technology to identify the DNA of the virus. If the nurse assists the physician with collection of diagnostic samples from the patient suspected to have SARS, the nurse, physician, and all other personnel must use protective equipment and adhere to the procedures of droplet precautions. This includes gown, a respirator mask, and goggles or face mask. Before specimen collection begins, the departments of epidemiology and the laboratory should be consulted (see also Severe Acute Respiratory Syndrome Tests, p. 581).

Susceptibility Testing

When bacteria are identified, susceptibility testing may be done. In the presence of antibiotic or antimicrobial medication, bacteria are described as susceptible, intermediate, or resistant. Susceptible means that the bacteria can be treated effectively with the particular medication. Intermediate means that the bacteria can be treated effectively with higher dosage of the medication or with medication that concentrates in a particular body site where the bacteria are located. Resistance means that the bacteria will not be killed or eliminated by the particular medication.

NORMAL VALUES

Normal nasopharyngeal flora

HOW THE TEST IS DONE

A special sterile, flexible nasopharyngeal wire swab or Dacron swab is used to collect a specimen from the posterior nasopharynx. For the pertussis culture, the swab is placed near the septum and floor of the nose. The swab is carefully rotated and then withdrawn. Once collected, the swab is placed in the culture tube. The specific culture medium is designated by the laboratory.

SIGNIFICANCE OF TEST RESULTS

Positive Values

Pharyngitis
Scarlet fever
Diphtheria
Thrush
Pertussis
Asymptomatic carrier of bacteria
SARS

INTERFERING FACTORS

- Antibiotic therapy
- Improper technique in specimen collection

NURSING CARE

Pretest

- If possible, the nurse ensures that the specimen is obtained before antibiotics are started.
- ***Patient Teaching.*** Inform the patient that the sterile wire swab will be put into the back of the nose and throat. Any mild discomfort disappears after the swab is removed. Instruct the patient to cough before the swab is inserted.

During the Test

- Help the patient sit up and tilt the head back. Use a light or sterile nasal speculum, or both, to visualize the posterior nasal passage and nasopharynx.

Nasopharyngeal culture. Insert the sterile wire through the nasal passage into the nasopharynx. Allow the wire to remain for about 15 to 30 seconds. The wire may trigger the patient's gag reflex.

Pertussis culture. Insert the sterile wire 1 inch into the nares and rotate it against the nasal mucosa.

Posttest

- Place the swab or wire in the sterile culture tube.
- On the requisition slip, write the time, date, specific site used to obtain the culture specimen, and patient's name and age. Include the suspected clinical diagnosis and any current antibiotic therapy.

Culture, Sputum

kul-chur, spyoo-tuhm

SPECIMEN OR TYPE OF TEST: Sputum

PURPOSE OF THE TEST

Sputum culture is performed to identify the pathogenic organism responsible for the lower respiratory tract infection, particularly pneumonia. Susceptibility testing determines the selection of appropriate antibiotic therapy.

BASICS THE NURSE NEEDS TO KNOW

Sputum is a product of the lower respiratory tract, not a product of the oropharynx, such as saliva. Sputum cultures are obtained to identify pathogenic organisms in patients with suspected pulmonary infection. If bacteria are present, microscopic examination of a *Gram stain* of the specimen identifies the bacteria as gram positive or gram negative. This knowledge may be used to initiate appropriate antibiotic therapy until the bacterial culture and susceptibility testing is completed. A stat (immediate) Gram stain result is available in 15 to 30 minutes. Identification of the specific organism growing in the culture medium requires about 48 hours.

C

Susceptibility Testing

When bacteria are grown in the culture and identified, susceptibility testing is usually done. In the presence of antibiotic or antimicrobial medication, bacteria are described as susceptible, intermediate, or resistant. Susceptible means that the bacteria can be treated effectively with the particular medication. Intermediate means that the bacteria can be treated effectively with higher dosage of the medication or with medication that concentrates in a particular body site where the bacteria are located. Resistance means that the bacteria will not be killed or eliminated by the particular medication.

Severe Acute Respiratory Syndrome

Severe Acute Respiratory Syndrome (SARS) is a respiratory infection that causes severe pneumonia from a newly recognized corona virus. The virus may be detected in the respiratory tract within a period of 72 hours after symptoms begin. When SARS is suspected, the patient must be placed in isolation. Contact and respiratory droplet precautions are maintained.

The sputum specimen or bronchial aspirates are part of the diagnostic testing that is done when this lung infection is suspected. Collected by the patient's ability to cough productively or by aspiration or bronchial suction methods, each sputum sample is placed in separate culturette tubes with viral transport medium. The specimens of mucus and cells are tested by PCR technology to identify the DNA of the virus.

If the nurse assists the physician with collection of diagnostic samples from the patient suspected to have SARS, the nurse, physician, and all other personnel must use protective equipment and adhere to the procedures of droplet precautions. This includes gown, a respirator mask, and goggles or face mask. The departments of epidemiology and the laboratory should be consulted before specimen collection begins (see also Severe Acute Respiratory Syndrome Tests, p. 581).

NORMAL VALUES No growth

HOW THE TEST IS DONE

Expectoration Method

A sputum specimen may be obtained by the patient's coughing up the sputum into a wide-mouthed sterile container with a cap.

Aspiration Method

A bronchial sputum specimen may be obtained by aspiration. If a bronchial specimen is needed, suctioning equipment and a sterile sputum trap are used.

Bronchoscopy or Transtracheal Method

A sputum specimen may also be obtained during a bronchoscopy or via transtracheal aspiration. The nurse may assist with these procedures but does not perform them.

SIGNIFICANCE OF TEST RESULTS

Positive Values

Pneumonia
Influenza
Gonorrhea
Diphtheria
Tuberculosis
Parasitic infection of the lungs
SARS

INTERFERING FACTORS

- Contamination of the specimen
- Antibiotic therapy

NURSING CARE

Pretest

- The nurse has the patient complete this test before antibiotic therapy is started. This timing helps prevent a false-negative result. The nurse also assesses the patient's ability to follow instructions in coughing up the sputum as well as his or her ability to expectorate.
- Provide a sterile container with a cap.
- ***Patient Teaching.*** Instruct the patient to do the following:
  1. Collect the specimen on arising in the morning before eating or drinking. Dentures should be removed. A rinse of the mouth with water is done before collecting the sputum.
  2. Take several deep breaths.
  3. Cough up the sputum from deep within the lungs.
  4. Expectorate into the sterile container.

  The nurse teaches the procedure to help the patient avoid contamination of the container and lid during the collection procedure. A major problem with the expectoration method is contamination of the specimen by the normal flora, the microorganisms found in the mouth and throat.

During the Test

Expectoration Method

- Support and encourage the patient's attempts to produce sputum. If it is not contraindicated, postural drainage, clapping, and vibration of the back may assist in raising the sputum. If the sputum is very tenacious, aerosol therapy may be necessary.
- Approximately 1 tsp of sputum is necessary for a sputum culture and sensitivity test. When the patient is unable to produce this amount in one attempt, the container should be capped between attempts to expectorate.

Continued

C

NURSING CARE—*cont'd*

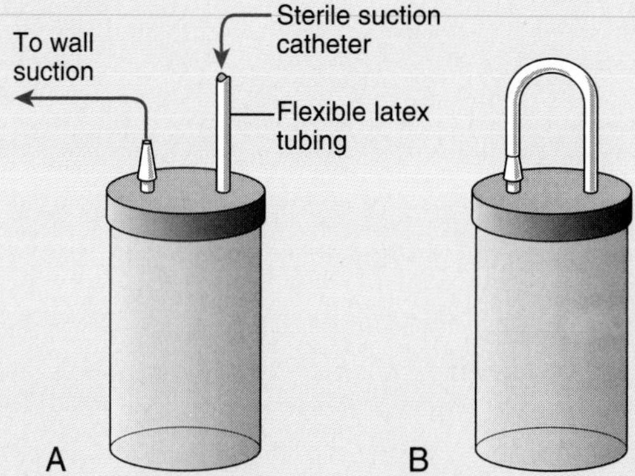

Figure 42. Sputum aspiration. *A*, Sputum trap. *B*, Closed sputum trap.

- If the patient is extubated, a sputum trap is used to obtain the specimen (Figure 42). In this case, suctioning is performed as usual, except that the sputum trap is inserted between the sterile suction catheter and the suction tubing attached to the wall suction regulator.

Aspiration Method

- Use the sputum trap as follows:
  1. Tighten the cap to obtain an airtight seal.
  2. Attach the wall suction tubing to the plastic "chimney" on the cap.
  3. Connect the distal end of the sterile container to the latex tubing.
  4. Suction as usual, but do not flush the catheter while the trap is in place.
  5. After suctioning, disconnect the suction tubing and catheter.
  6. Connect the latex tubing to the chimney of the cap.

Posttest

- Ensure that the lid is tightly sealed and that the container is labeled correctly.
- Send the specimen to the laboratory as soon as possible. Do not refrigerate the specimen.
- No complications result from the sputum collection procedure. The nurse should be aware, however, of the complications that can result from endotracheal suctioning, if that method is used to obtain the specimen.

Culture, Stool

kul-chur, stool

Also called: Stool Culture for Enteric Pathogens

SPECIMEN OR TYPE OF TEST: Feces

PURPOSE OF THE TEST

The stool culture is used to identify the bacterial organism that caused intestinal infection.

BASICS THE NURSE NEEDS TO KNOW

Stool culture may be used when the patient experiences severe, persistent, or recurrent bloody diarrhea with fever and tenesmus (painful, ineffectual straining at stool). The patient may have a history of travel to a developing country, a recent dietary intake of seafood, or exposure to a known bacterial agent.

Susceptibility Testing

When bacteria are identified, susceptibility testing may be done. In the presence of antibiotic or antimicrobial medication, bacteria are described as susceptible, intermediate, or resistant. Susceptible means that the bacteria can be treated effectively with the particular medication. Intermediate means that the bacteria can be treated effectively with a higher dosage of the medication or with medication that concentrates in a particular body site where the bacteria are located. Resistance means that the bacteria will not be killed or eliminated by the particular medication.

NORMAL VALUES

Negative for *Campylobacter, Salmonella,* and *Shigella*

HOW THE TEST IS DONE

Random Stool Method

A small amount of freshly passed feces is placed directly into a clean, dry container.

Rectal Swab Method

The swab is inserted past the anal sphincter and into the rectum. The swab is gently rotated around the canal. To attain maximum absorption, the swab is kept in place for 15 to 20 seconds before it is withdrawn. Once the swab is placed in the special culture tube, the media compartment is crushed to moisten the specimen.

SIGNIFICANCE OF TEST RESULTS

Positive Values

Shigellosis
Salmonella infection
Cholera
Bacillary dysentery
Infant botulism
Enteric fever
Acute gastroenteritis
Typhoid fever
Food poisoning

C

INTERFERING FACTORS

- Contamination of the specimen with urine, detergent, or soap
- Improper technique of specimen collection
- Antibiotic therapy

NURSING CARE

Pretest

- ***Patient Teaching.*** The nurse instructs the patient to evacuate a small amount of feces directly into the container. If a bedpan is used, it must be rinsed with water and dried thoroughly before use. No urine can be mixed with the feces. The reason that these guidelines are used is because urine, soap, detergent, and drying of the specimen act to destroy the bacteria before they can be cultured. (Additional information on fecal collection procedures is presented in Chapter 2.)
- The nurse obtains the specimen before any antibiotic therapy is started.

Posttest

- The nurse uses gloves to handle the open container or culturette until it is sealed. Hands are washed thoroughly after the gloves are removed. These bacteria are highly transmissible via a fecal-oral route.
- The nurse arranges for direct transport of the specimen to the laboratory without delay. If a delay of more than 2 to 3 hours is anticipated, the specimen should be placed in a laboratory-determined type of transport medium to maintain a moist environment.

Culture, Throat

kul-chur, throht

Also called: Oropharyngeal Culture

SPECIMEN OR TYPE OF TEST: Secretions

PURPOSE OF THE TEST

The throat culture identifies the bacteria that cause infection of the oropharynx, pharynx, and tonsils. It is also used to screen for an asymptomatic carrier of the infection.

BASICS THE NURSE NEEDS TO KNOW

A variety of flora is found in the normal oropharynx. These organisms do not cause respiratory illness unless some change occurs in the patient's health. When acute pharyngitis occurs, or when a clinical illness indicates an oropharyngeal source of infection, a throat culture may be indicated. Untreated, group A beta-hemolytic streptococcal throat infection can develop into complications of rheumatic fever, scarlet fever, glomerulonephritis, wound infection, and sepsis. With early identification of the bacteria and effective antibiotic therapy, the potential for development of a serious complication is diminished or eliminated.

Other serious organisms of an abnormal throat culture include *Corynebacterium diphtheriae,* the cause of diphtheria, and *Neisseria gonorrhoeae,* the gonorrheal cause of an infected oropharynx. Diphtheria infects the tonsils, oropharynx, nasopharynx, larynx, and trachea. Generally, a routine throat culture and a nasopharyngeal culture are performed simultaneously. When gonorrhea infection is in the throat, the infection may be asymptomatic or may cause tonsillitis and acute pharyngitis. The throat is a primary site of sexually transmitted infection in homosexual males. Often, cultures of the genitalia and anal canal are performed at the same time. In children, a throat culture positive for this pathogen is indicative of child sexual abuse.

Severe Acute Respiratory Syndrome (SARS)

SARS is a respiratory infection that causes severe pneumonia from a newly recognized corona virus. The virus may be detected in the respiratory tract within 72 hours after symptoms begin. When SARS is suspected, the patient must be placed in isolation. Contact and respiratory droplet precautions are maintained.

The throat culture is an early part of the diagnostic testing done when this lung infection is suspected. Each swab sample of the secretions is placed in separate culturette tubes with viral transport medium. The specimens of mucus and cells are tested by polymerase chain reaction (PCR) technology to identify the DNA of the virus.

If the nurse assists the physician with collection of diagnostic samples from the patient suspected to have SARS, the nurse, physician, and all other personnel must use protective equipment and adhere to the procedures for droplet precautions. This includes gown, a respirator mask, and goggles or face mask. The departments of epidemiology and the laboratory should be consulted before specimen collection begins (see also Severe Acute Respiratory Syndrome Tests, p. 581).

Susceptibility Testing

When bacteria are identified, susceptibility testing may be done. In the presence of antibiotic or antimicrobial medication, bacteria are described as susceptible, intermediate, or resistant. Susceptible means that the bacteria can be treated effectively with the particular medication. Intermediate means that the bacteria can be treated effectively with a higher dosage of the medication or with medication that concentrates in a particular body site where the bacteria are located. Resistance means that the bacteria will not be killed or eliminated by the particular medication.

NORMAL VALUES Negative; normal organisms in the oropharynx

HOW THE TEST IS DONE

Two sterile Dacron swabs are used to obtain a specimen of exudates from the throat. The swab is then placed in a culture tube and capped tightly.

SIGNIFICANCE OF TEST RESULTS

Abnormal Values

Group A beta-hemolytic streptococcus throat infection
Scarlet fever
Pertussis
Pharyngitis
Thrush
Diphtheria
Gonococcal infection
Severe acute respiratory syndrome (SARS)

INTERFERING FACTORS

- Antibiotic therapy
- Contamination of the specimen

NURSING CARE

Pretest

- Obtain the culture specimen before antibiotic therapy is started. Inform the patient that the test involves swabbing the throat. The swabbing may cause a brief gagging sensation. The discomfort disappears as soon as the procedure is finished.
- In cases of acute epiglottitis or suspected diphtheria, the nurse does not perform the throat culture, but would assist the physician. The test should not be performed until preparation has been made to establish an alternate airway, as needed. If diphtheria is suspected, the nurse notifies the laboratory in advance so that a special isolation medium can be prepared.

During the Test

- Instruct the patient to tip the head back. Use a tongue blade to depress the tongue.
- The two sterile swabs are used together to rub the inflamed sites and areas of exudate in the oropharynx and tonsils (Figure 43). During the swabbing of the throat, ensure that the tongue, cheeks, and uvula are not touched. These tissues commonly have many organisms present and poor technique will cause a false-positive result.
- The swabs from a routine culture are placed in a regular culture tube. Throat culture for suspected diphtheria or gonococcal infection requires a special swab and culture-transport medium.

Posttest

- Ensure that the specimen is placed in the sterile culture tube or transport medium as appropriate for the specific test.
- On the requisition slip, identify the source of the specimen, the name and age of the patient, the clinical diagnosis, and any antibiotic therapy that the patient is currently undergoing.

◆ Nursing Response to Complications

There are no complications from a routine throat culture. In cases of acute epiglottitis or suspected diphtheria, the patient may experience a laryngospasm immediately after the specimen is obtained.

NURSING CARE—*cont'd*

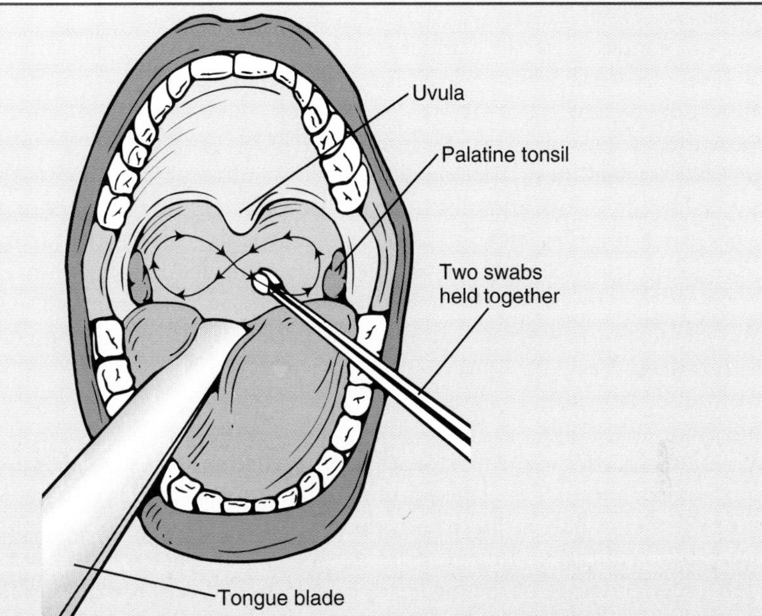

Figure 43. Technique for obtaining a throat culture. *(Reproduced with permission from Stepp, C. A., & Woods, M. A. [1998].* Laboratory procedures for medical office personnel *[Fig. 25–12, p. 339]. Philadelphia: W. B. Saunders.)*

Laryngospasm. The nurse assesses for signs of respiratory obstruction, including dyspnea and stridor (a high pitched, crowing sound) and increased respiratory effort. The nurse records the results of the respiratory assessment in the patient's chart. If laryngospasm and respiratory obstruction begins, the nurse prepares to support oxygenation and assist the physician with the establishment of an airway, as needed.

Culture, Urine

kul-chur, yur-in

Also called: Midstream Urine Culture; Urine Culture, Midvoid Specimen; Urine Culture, Clean Catch; Urine Culture, Indwelling Catheter

SPECIMEN OR TYPE OF TEST: Urine

PURPOSE OF THE TEST

Culture of the urine is used to diagnose a urinary tract infection and to monitor the number of microorganisms in the urine. Sensitivity testing identifies the appropriate antibiotics and antimicrobials that are effective.

C

BASICS THE NURSE NEEDS TO KNOW

Bacteriuria is the presence of bacteria in the urine. A lower urinary tract infection consists of an infection in the bladder or urethra, or both. An upper urinary tract infection involves the renal pelvis or renal interstitial tissues, or both. Any bacterial or fungal organism can cause a urinary tract infection, but the most common pathogens are those that are present in normal feces.

A bacterial count of 10,000 colony-forming units per milliliter (CFU/mL) or more is considered positive and indicates significant bacteriuria. The count of the organism is evaluated together with the patient's symptoms, predisposing factors, and the type of organism(s) isolated. In the female patient, the test may be repeated once or twice to ensure the accuracy of the diagnosis, because contamination of the specimen could cause a false-positive result. In the male patient, only one specimen is needed for a correct diagnosis.

Susceptibility Testing

When bacteria are identified, susceptibility testing may be done. In the presence of antibiotic or antimicrobial medication, bacteria are described as susceptible, intermediate, or resistant. Susceptible means that the bacteria can be treated effectively with the particular medication. Intermediate means that the bacteria can be treated effectively with a higher dosage of the medication or with medication that concentrates in a particular body site where the bacteria are located. Resistance means that the bacteria will not be killed or eliminated by the particular medication.

NORMAL VALUES No growth

HOW THE TEST IS DONE

Midstream catch: A clean-voided midstream technique is used to obtain 15 mL or more of urine in a sterile container. A first voided specimen of the day is used, because it has the highest colony count after an overnight incubation period.

Indwelling catheter: A sterile needle and syringe are used to obtain 4 mL or more of urine from the urine sample port of the catheter. The urine is then placed in a sterile container.

Suprapubic puncture: Occasionally, suprapubic puncture is used to obtain the specimen. Using sterile technique, a needle is inserted into a full bladder and the urine is aspirated with a syringe. The nurse may assist with this procedure but does not perform a suprapubic aspiration.

SIGNIFICANCE OF TEST RESULTS

Abnormal Values

Escherichia coli
Enterobacter spp.
Klebsiella spp.
Staphylococcus aureus
Mycobacterium spp.

Proteus spp.
Pseudomonas
Streptococcus faecalis
Candida albicans

INTERFERING FACTORS

- Contamination of the specimen
- Antimicrobial therapy
- Inadequate volume of urine

NURSING CARE

Pretest

- ***Patient Teaching.*** The nurse instructs the patient regarding the proper procedure for collection of a clean-catch midstream urine sample. The patient must wash his or her hands with soap before the specimen is collected. As described later, the perineum and urinary meatus must be cleansed carefully. The procedure for cleansing is very important because contamination of the specimen from the external genitalia, hair, vagina, or rectum would introduce microbes into the urine sample and cause a false-positive result.

During the Test

Midstream or Clean-Catch Method

Cleansing procedure. *Female:* Instruct the female patient that after spreading the labia, the perineum, vulva, and urinary meatus are cleansed with three soapy sponges, using one downward stroke for each sponge. Each sponge is used only once and is discarded, and then a sponge with water is used to remove the soap. The same single downward stroke is used, and the sponge is discarded. After the cleansing is completed, the labia must be maintained in that separated position until after the urine is collected.

- *Male:* Instruct the male patient to cleanse the urethral meatus with the three soapy sponges and then rinse with the water sponge. Each sponge is used once and discarded. If the patient is uncircumcised, the prepuce must be retracted and the glans cleansed.

Collection procedure. Instruct the patient to begin the urinary stream and void about 1 oz and then, as the urine flow continues, collect the urine by catching it midstream into the container. The first and last parts of the urinary stream are not used for the collection of the specimen. During the collection process, the container must not touch the perineal skin or hair. Once the specimen is obtained, the patient places the lid on the container without touching the inner surfaces.

Indwelling Catheter Method

- When the urinary catheter is already in place, the nurse removes the urine from the catheter port. The nurse clamps the tubing below the urine collection port for 10 minutes. Cleanse the port with an alcohol sponge. A sterile needle and syringe are

Continued

NURSING CARE—*cont'd*

used to collect the urine sample through this port. The urine is then placed in a sterile container and the catheter tubing is unclamped.

- Urine must not be collected from the drainage bag, because bacteria can be present on the outside of the bag. Additionally, the urine is not fresh, and bacteria have had an opportunity to colonize while the specimen remained at room temperature. Lastly, the Foley catheter must not be separated from the collecting tube to obtain the specimen. If the closed drainage system is opened, bacteria will enter the tubing and cause infection in the bladder.

Posttest

- The specimen and requisition slip are labeled, including the patient's name, the time of collection, and the date. On the requisition slip, include the method of collection and any antibiotic therapy that may have been initiated already.

Culture, Wound

kul-chur, woond

Also called: Bacterial Culture, Wound

SPECIMEN OR TYPE OF TEST: Secretions, cell scrapings

PURPOSE OF THE TEST

The wound culture is used to determine the presence of infection and to identify the causative organism.

BASICS THE NURSE NEEDS TO KNOW

Soft-tissue infections affect various depths of tissue layers, including the epidermis, dermis, subdermis, fascial planes, and muscle tissue. The infectious organism may be enclosed, such as in an abscess. The pathogens also may be in an open, ulcerated, or necrotic wound or fistulous tract that is exposed to the external environment.

One of the problems in culturing the infected wound is that many normal flora grow in an open, draining wound, fistula, or opened abscess. In the case of an ulcerated or necrotic infection, the wound must be cleansed and débrided to remove dead tissue and many of the surface bacterial flora. After exploring the wound, the culture is performed on the underlying tissue or sinus tract at the base of the wound.

Susceptibility Testing

When bacteria are identified, susceptibility testing may be done. In the presence of antibiotic or antimicrobial medication, bacteria are described as susceptible, intermediate, or resistant. Susceptible means that the bacteria can be treated effectively with the particular medication. Intermediate means that the bacteria can be treated effectively with a higher dosage of the medication or with medication that concentrates in a particular body site where the bacteria are located. Resistance means that the bacteria will not be killed or eliminated by the particular medication.

NORMAL VALUES

No growth

HOW THE TEST IS DONE

The physician may use a syringe and needle to aspirate purulent material from a wound. The liquid can be placed in a sterile tube. Tissue samples from a biopsy or scraping of the wound may also be obtained. For transport, the tissue sample is protected from drying by the addition of a small amount of sterile saline.

Swabs and a culture tube can be used, but this is not the best choice because the swab often fails to absorb sufficient material from the wound. If this method is used, two swabs are needed, one for culture and one for a smear.

SIGNIFICANCE OF TEST RESULTS

Positive Values

Staphylococcus aureus
Streptococcus pyogenes
Staphylococcus epidermidis
Escherichia coli
Proteus spp.
Pseudomonas spp.
Bacteroides spp.
Clostridium spp.
Group D streptococci
Klebsiella spp.

INTERFERING FACTORS

- Antibiotic therapy
- Contamination of the specimen

NURSING CARE

Pretest

- If possible, schedule this procedure before antibiotic therapy is started.
- Explain that only minor discomfort occurs as an open wound is swabbed. If the physician must open an abscessed area surgically or perform a tissue biopsy, debridement, or scraping, a local anesthetic may be used. A written consent is needed for these surgical procedures.

During the Test

- Prior to obtaining the specimen from an open wound, the wound must be thoroughly cleansed with surgical soap and then alcohol. The goal is to culture the infecting organism and avoid contamination by flora and colonizing organisms. The contamination of the specimen with surface organisms produces invalid results.

Posttest

- Ensure that the requisition slip indicates the patient's name and age, specific culture site, time, date, clinical diagnosis, and any current antibiotic therapy.

Cystoscopy

sis-tos-kuh-pee

C

SPECIMEN OR TYPE OF TEST: Endoscopy

PURPOSE OF THE TEST

Cystoscopy is used to diagnose and evaluate structural and functional changes of the urinary bladder.

BASICS THE NURSE NEEDS TO KNOW

Cystoscopy provides direct visualization of the urinary bladder. When the urethra also is examined, the procedure is called *cystourethroscopy*. The examination is performed with a cystoscope—a thin, lighted tube with a telescopic lens. The procedure may be performed in the urologist's office or in the operating room with local, spinal, or general anesthesia. Following the diagnostic component, treatment may include dilation of stricture, cauterization of bleeding spots, removal of superficial tissue, implantation of radium seeds, and placement of a ureteral stent or catheter.

Cystoscopy is used to investigate the cause of painless hematuria, particularly when cancer of the epithelial lining is suspected. It also is part of the investigation into the cause of urinary incontinence or retention.

NORMAL VALUES	No anatomic or structural abnormalities are present

HOW THE TEST IS DONE

With the patient under anesthesia, the cystoscope is inserted through the urethra into the urinary bladder. Once the bladder is filled with saline for irrigation, all aspects of the bladder walls are examined. Biopsy samples for tissue examination and cell washings for cytologic analysis may be carried out. Urine samples may be collected from the bladder or from each ureter. The procedure takes approximately 30 to 45 minutes.

SIGNIFICANCE OF TEST RESULTS

Abnormal Values

Cancer of the bladder
Polyps
Diverticulum of the bladder
Bladder fistula
Bladder stones
Bladder neck stricture
Congenital anomaly
Benign prostatic hypertrophy
Cancer of the prostate gland

INTERFERING FACTORS

- Failure to maintain nothing-by-mouth status
- Acute infection of the bladder, urethra, or prostate gland

NURSING CARE

Pretest

- The nurse ensures that written informed consent is obtained from the patient or the person legally designated to make health care decisions for the patient.
- ***Patient Teaching.*** When bowel emptying is part of the protocol, instruct the patient to administer a cathartic or enema, as ordered, the night before or the morning of the test.
- ***Patient Teaching.*** For general or spinal anesthesia preparation, the nurse instructs the patient to fast from food and fluids for 8 hours before the procedure. For local anesthesia, fasting from food is required, but clear liquids on the morning of the test are permitted.
- On the morning of the procedure, the nurse obtains baseline vital signs and records the results. The nurse also administers preoperative sedatives or antispasmodics as prescribed.

During the Test

- The nurse provides reassurance to the patient who may be awake during the procedure. The instillation of the local anesthetic into the urethra is mildly painful until the tissue becomes numb. When the bladder is filled with saline, discomfort and the urge to void are normal sensations.
- The biopsy tissue is placed in a sterile glass container with formalin preservative. For the cytologic study, 50 to 75 mL of bladder irrigation fluid is placed in a sterile jar with 50% alcohol as a preservative.
- The nurse assists with the collection of urine specimens and on the container and requisition slip, writes the source of the tissue (bladder, right ureter, left ureter).

Posttest

- The nurse takes vital signs and records the results. For patients who have undergone general anesthesia, the nurse continues to monitor the vital signs every 15 to 30 minutes until the patient is stable.
- The nurse assesses for pain or bladder spasms and administers prescribed medication as needed.
- ***Patient Teaching.*** The nurse encourages extra oral fluids to promote adequate hydration and the voiding of urine. Instruct the patient to void within 8 hours after the test. The nurse notifies the physician if the patient is unable to void within this time. Reassure the patient that it is normal to have a burning sensation on voiding and to see a small amount of blood or pink-tinged urine. These problems usually disappear after the third voiding.

Continued

D

NURSING CARE—*cont'd*

- ***Patient Teaching.*** At home, warm tub baths can help alleviate the patient's discomfort or pain of bladder spasms. Instruct the patient to avoid alcohol for 48 hours because of its irritant effect on the bladder mucosa. To prevent infection, the nurse instructs the patient to take the prescribed antibiotic

◆ Nursing Response to Complications

The most common complications of cystoscopy are persistent bleeding, infection, and urinary retention. Because the patient usually goes home soon after the test, a review of abnormal problems should be provided, and the patient should be advised to notify the urologist when these problems occur.

Bleeding. After a cystoscopy, bleeding may be evident by persistent, painless hematuria, bright red urine, or the passage of blood clots. Notify the urologist or instruct patient who has been discharged to call the urologist to report any of these findings.

Urinary obstruction. The urologist should be informed if the patient is unable to urinate within 8 hours of the procedure. The nurse palpates the bladder and reports the level where it is felt. The nurse also reports the patient's sensation of needing to void. The nurse anticipates the physician's need for a Foley catheter and catheterization tray.

Infection. The nurse assesses for infection and instructs the patient being discharged to report signs of infection, including fever, chills, flank or abdominal pain, or cloudy urine.

Darkfield Examination, Syphilis

dahrk-feeld eg-za-mi-nay-shun, si-fuh-lis

SPECIMEN OR TYPE OF TEST: Cell scrapings

PURPOSE OF THE TEST

This test is used to diagnose syphilis infection.

BASICS THE NURSE NEEDS TO KNOW

Treponema pallidum is the spirochete that causes the sexually transmitted infection of syphilis. During the primary stage of infection, an ulcerated lesion called a chancre appears on a mucosal or tissue surface. The spirochete is present in the cell scrapings and in the moist exudate (serous drainage) at the base of the lesion. In the secondary stage of disease, it is also present in enlarged lymph nodes. Using darkfield microscopy, the slides of the cells and secretions reveal the absence or presence of the syphilis spirochete and provide visualization of the characteristic movements. *T. pallidum* is a corkscrew-shaped organism that has rapid bending, flexing, and rotational movements.

NORMAL VALUES Negative

HOW THE TEST IS DONE

Pipette Method

The physician cleans surface of the chancre with a saline-moistened swab and then uses a sterile pipette to aspirate cells and exudate from the base of the ulcer. The secretions are placed on a sterile glass slide.

Slide Method

The physician cleans the surface of the chancre with a saline-moistened swab and then presses a sterile glass slide directly on the ulcerated lesion.

With either method, a coverslip is placed over the slide to prevent drying of the secretions and cells.

SIGNIFICANCE OF TEST RESULTS

Positive Values

T. pallidum infection

INTERFERING FACTORS

- Contamination of the specimen
- Drying of the specimen
- Antibiotic therapy
- Healed lesion
- Ointment on the lesion

NURSING CARE

Pretest

- The nurse schedules this test before antibiotic therapy is started.
- *Patient Teaching.* The nurse instructs the patient to avoid placing lotions or creams on the lesion before the test is performed. These applications would interfere with the microscopic examination of the specimen.

During the Test

- The nurse should wear gloves during the test and when handling the specimen slide. If the test result is positive, the lesion and secretions are contaminated and are transmitted by skin to skin contact.

Posttest

- The nurse ensures immediate transport of the specimen to the laboratory. The microscopic examination of the slide must be performed within 15 minutes of collection. The secretions must not become dry before the examination is completed.
- When the test is positive for syphilis, counsel the patient to inform all sexual partners of the test results. Sexual contacts are advised to undergo testing. Instruct the patient to refrain from sexual contact until the infection is treated and cured. Positive test results for syphilis are reported to the state health department.

Continued

NURSING CARE—*cont'd*

- As part of follow-up nursing care of the patient with a sexually transmitted disease, the nurse discusses ways to reduce risk for a repeat infection. From the patient's sexual history, the nurse can identify the individual's practices that resulted in infection and make suggestions for the future. The best protection from syphilis is achieved through abstinence, a long-term monogamous relationship, or the use of condoms.

D-dimer and Fibrin Degradation Products

dee-dai-muhr and fai-brin de-gruh-day-shun pro-duhkts

Also called: (FDP); Fibrin Breakdown Product (FBP)

SPECIMEN OR TYPE OF TEST: Blood

PURPOSE OF THE TEST

The D-dimer test helps determine whether a clot is present in the diagnosis of deep vein thrombosis, disseminated intravascular coagulation (DIC), or an acute myocardial infarction. It is also used in the diagnosis of hypercoagulable conditions that cause recurrent thrombosis.

BASICS THE NURSE NEEDS TO KNOW

D-dimers are fragments of fibrin that appear in the blood when a thrombus (clot) undergoes degradation or dissolution. In fibrinolysis, the fibers of fibrin in the clot are dissolved and the clot undergoes lysis or breakdown. Fibrin degradation products, including D-dimers, are end products of the dissolving clot and can be detected in the blood. The test is a highly specific method used for emergency screening to exclude the presence of a deep vein thrombus. When the results are in the normal range or negative, no thrombus is present. Elevated test results or the presence of D-dimer fragments is evidence that thrombus formation occurred and lysis of the thrombus is occurring. The combination of elevated levels of fibrin degradation products and D-dimer fragments is highly predictive of DIC.

DIC Screen

D-dimer and fibrin degradation products may be part of the panel of tests to assess for DIC. The additional tests in this group include Prothrombin Time (see p. 555), Partial Thromboplastin Time (see p. 503), Platelet Count (see p. 523), and Fibrinogen (see p. 325). DIC is a common and often severe coagulation disorder commonly precipitated by sepsis, severe tissue injury, or some complications of pregnancy. When the anticoagulation and fibrinolytic systems are overwhelmed by the underlying disorder, DIC can result. In DIC, the patient develops systemic microvascular thrombi and, as platelets and natural anticoagulant factors are depleted, the patient begins to bleed. In laboratory testing, DIC may cause the values of D-dimer and fibrin degradation products to be elevated because of the lysis (break up) of thrombi. The loss of platelets and anticoagulants cause the prothrombin time to be prolonged and the platelet count and fibrinogen value to decrease.

NORMAL VALUES

D-dimers: <0.5 mcg/mL *or* SI: <500 mcg/L
FDP: <0.5 mcg/mL *or* SI: <500 mcg/L

HOW THE TEST IS DONE

A plastic syringe and a blue-topped tube are used to collect 4.5 mL of venous blood.

SIGNIFICANCE OF TEST RESULTS

Elevated Values

Thrombotic disease
Deep vein thrombosis
Pulmonary embolism
Arterial thromboembolism
Thrombolytic-defibrination therapy
DIC
Sickle cell anemia crisis
Pregnancy (postpartum phase)
Malignancy
Surgery (postoperatively)

INTERFERING FACTORS

- None

NURSING CARE

Nursing actions are similar to those used in other venipuncture procedures (see Chapter 2), with the following additional measures.

Posttest

- When the laboratory result of the D-dimer or FDP test is elevated, the nurse notifies the physician immediately. The nurse recognizes that the patient may have a thrombus or embolus. Nursing assessment should include identification of the location of impaired circulation. A deep vein thrombosis, particularly in the calf of the leg, may produce a positive Homan sign. The patient's legs should be assessed, observing for swelling, redness, and pain in one leg. The patient may already have manifestations of a pulmonary embolus that resulted from the thrombus, with signs of shock, chest pain and dyspnea.
- When the DIC panel shows the characteristic abnormal coagulation values associated with this illness, the nurse would immediately notify the physician. The nurse should assess the patient for signs of bleeding, including petechiae (multiple red hemorrhagic spots) or ecchymosis (bruising) of the skin, hematoma, or oozing of blood from a wound or venipuncture site. There may be hematuria, blood in the

Continued

NURSING CARE—*cont'd*

Posttest—*cont'd*

feces, or blood in nasogastric drainage. The nurse assesses vital signs often because of the potential for shock. The patient may develop oliguria (scanty urine output) or anuria (no urinary output). Neurologic manifestations include severe headache, lethargy, or coma, and other alterations of neurologic status. The overt signs of bleeding are serious, but the more significant damage is to organs, which develop microthrombi, leading to ischemia and permanent tissue damage. The assessment findings vary with the severity of the condition but tend to worsen over a short time.

Dexamethasone Suppression Test

dek-suh-meth-uh-zohn suh-pre-shun test

SPECIMEN OR TYPE OF TEST: Serum, urine

PURPOSE OF THE TEST

The dexamethasone suppression test assesses the hypothalamic-pituitary-adrenal axis. It usually is performed to identify Cushing syndrome. With the dexamethasone test, Cushing's disease and ectopic production of adrenocorticotropic hormone (ACTH) and adrenal tumors can be differentiated.

BASICS THE NURSE NEEDS TO KNOW

Dexamethasone (Decadron) is a potent glucocorticoid. It will normally suppress ACTH secretion by the pituitary gland via the normal hormonal feedback mechanism. With the suppression of ACTH, the stimulation for cortisol secretion is suppressed in the adrenal cortex, resulting in a decrease in plasma cortisol and urinary corticosteroid levels.

High-dose dexamethasone testing can be helpful in distinguishing Cushing's disease (pituitary hypersecretion of ACTH) from adrenal tumors or ectopic secretion of ACTH. With high-dose dexamethasone, pituitary secretion of ACTH can be suppressed, with a resulting decrease in plasma cortisol levels. No change will occur with adrenal tumors or ectopic ACTH production.

NORMAL VALUES

Serum cortisol: <5 mcg/dL *or* SI: <138 nmol/L
Urine 17-hydroxycorticosteroid (17-OHCS): <4 ng/24 hr
Urine for free cortisol: <25 mcg/24 hr

HOW THE TEST IS DONE

A variety of dexamethasone procedures are possible. Low-dose dexamethasone testing may be carried out overnight or over 2 days. Overnight testing requires the oral administration of dexamethasone at night (10 PM to 11 PM). The next morning, a plasma cortisol level is determined. With the 2-day method, dexamethasone is given orally every 6 hours for 2 days. A 24-hour urine specimen is obtained before and after administration (see discussion of 17-Hydroxycorticosteriods, p. 400), and a plasma cortisol test is performed 6 hours after the last dose of dexamethasone.

High-dose dexamethasone testing begins with a baseline plasma cortisol level being obtained, then dexamethasone given orally at night, and the next morning another plasma cortisol level being obtained.

SIGNIFICANCE OF TEST RESULTS

Elevated Values
Ectopic corticotropin syndrome

Unchanged Values
Cushing syndrome

Decreased Values
Cushing's disease

INTERFERING FACTORS

- Review discussions of 17-Hydroxycorticosteriods (p. 400), Free Cortisol (p. 331), and Cortisol, Total (p. 238).

NURSING CARE

Nursing actions are similar to those used in other venipuncture and urine collection procedures (see Chapter 2). Also, review discussions of 17-Hydroxycorticosteroids (p. 400), Free Cortisol (p. 331), and Cortisol, Total (p. 238).

Dipyramidamole Scan

See Stress Testing, Cardiac on p. 596.

Disseminated Coagulation Screen

See D-dimer and Fibrin Degradation Products on p. 274.

Dopamine

See Catecholamines, Plasma on p. 183.

Drugs of Abuse

drugz uv uh-byoos

Also called: (DAU); Pre-employment Drug Screen

SPECIMEN OR TYPE OF TEST: Urine

PURPOSE OF THE TEST

This urine test is used to screen for the presence of drugs of abuse, often as a condition of pre-employment or in cases of suspected overdose.

BASICS THE NURSE NEEDS TO KNOW

This test screens for the most commonly used drug substances or classes of drugs. The panel screen for 10 drugs includes amphetamines, barbiturates, benzodiazepines, cannabinoids, cocaine, methadone, methaqualone, opiates, phencyclidine, and propoxyphene. Positive test results identify the presence of one or more of these drugs, but do not measure the amount or identify the specific drug. When the drug test is positive, as measured by one method of laboratory analysis, a second test is done on the specimen, using a different and more sensitive method of analysis.

NORMAL VALUES

Negative

HOW THE TEST IS DONE

A random specimen of urine is collected in a clean container with a lid.

SIGNIFICANCE OF TEST RESULTS

Positive Value

Use of a drug of abuse

INTERFERING FACTORS

- Dilution of the specimen
- Alteration of the specimen

NURSING CARE

Pretest

- When this test is needed for forensic purposes or for pre-employment requirements, the nurse institutes the protocol and paperwork for chain-of-custody. The individual providing the specimen should be observed voiding and collecting the urine, as per the protocol. Once the specimen is collected, the container is sealed with tape and identified by a special patient number. Because individuals have been known to tamper with their specimen in hopes of passing the test, the nurse follows the protocol guidelines to prevent tampering. Common methods of tampering with the specimen include dilution with water from the sink or toilet bowl and adding a chemical to the specimen to interfere with the analysis. The laboratory will test for evidence of tampering.

Posttest

- If the voided specimen has an unusual color, odor, or appearance, the nurse records the description in the individual's record and on the form. For forensic testing, signatures are required by all those who have custody of the specimen (nurse, transporter, laboratory personnel), as described by the chain-of-custody protocol.

d-Xylose Absorption

dee-ek-suh-lohs ab-sohrp-shun

Also called: Xylose Tolerance Test; Xylose Absorption Test

SPECIMEN OR TYPE OF TEST: Serum, urine

PURPOSE OF THE TEST

This test is used to investigate the cause of steatorrhea (fat in the stool), to diagnose malabsorption syndrome, and to evaluate the ability of the duodenum and jejunum to absorb carbohydrates.

BASICS THE NURSE NEEDS TO KNOW

One of the causes of steatorrhea is a defect in the mucosal lining of the duodenum and jejunum that prevents or limits carbohydrate absorption. If unabsorbed, the carbohydrate passes through the intestinal tract. The concentration of sugar pulls fluid into the intestinal lumen by osmosis. This osmotic effect causes the patient to experience persistent steatorrhea, diarrhea, and abdominal cramping and discomfort.

In this test, the patient ingests a prescribed amount of liquid d-xylose, a pentose sugar. If the intestinal tract is able to absorb the sugar, there will be a measured rise in blood glucose and a later rise in urinary glucose as the kidneys clear the glucose from the blood.

If there is a defect in the intestinal mucosa, the d-xylose will not be absorbed and the glucose levels in the blood sample and urine collection will have lower than normal values. Low blood and urine values are indications of malabsorption. Further diagnostic testing may be needed to determine the exact cause of the malabsorption.

NORMAL VALUES

Whole Blood: Adult (2 hours, 25-g dose): >25 mg/dL *or* SI: >1.67 mmol/L
Adult (2 hours, 5-g dose): >20 mg/dL *or* SI: >1.33 mmol/L
Child (1 hour): >30 mg/dL *or* SI: >2.0 mmol/L

Urine: Adult (25-g dose): >4 g/5 hours *or* SI: 26.64 mmol/L/5 hr
Adult (5-g dose): 1.2 g/5 hours *or* SI: 8.00 mmol/L/5 hrs
Child: 16%–33% of ingested dose/5 hr *or* SI: 0.16–0.33 (fraction of ingested dose)

HOW THE TEST IS DONE

To verify adequate renal function, blood specimens for blood urea nitrogen and creatinine determinations are drawn and a urinalysis is obtained in the early morning before the d-xylose test begins.

The recommended dose of d-xylose is 25 g. For adults, the full dose is preferred because it will detect less severe conditions. For children younger than age 12-, the recommended dose is 5 g of d-xylose.

A red-topped tube used to obtain 10 mL of venous blood for each specimen. In most institutions, a single blood sample is collected 1 hour after the d-xylose is ingested. In some institutions several blood samples are obtained at timed intervals.

For adults and children older than age 12, all urine is collected for 5 hours.

For geriatric patients, patients with some renal insufficiency, and infants and children younger than age 12, the test may be limited to a single blood sample after 1 hour, with no urine collection.

SIGNIFICANCE OF TEST RESULTS

Nontropical sprue (celiac disease, gluten-sensitive enteropathy)
Tropical sprue
Lymphoma
Parasitic disease
Whipple's disease
Gastroenteritis
Amyloidosis
Zollinger-Ellison syndrome
Scleroderma
Radiation enteritis
Small bowel ischemia

INTERFERING FACTORS

- Failure to maintain pretest dietary restrictions
- Physical activity during the test
- Poor renal function
- Vomiting or diarrhea
- Rapid or delayed gastric emptying
- Hypermotility or stasis of the intestine
- Dehydration and hypovolemia

NURSING CARE

Nursing actions are similar to those used in other venipuncture and timed urine collection procedures (see Chapter 2), with the following additional measures.

Pretest

- ***Patient Teaching.*** Instruct the patient on the following preparation for the test:
- For 24 hours before the test, the patient should omit all intake of foods that contain pentose sugar (fruits, jams, jellies, and fruit tarts). The pentose in these fruits and fruit-based foods would increase the dose used by the test. If possible, the patient should discontinue all medications for 24 hours before the test, because some of the medications alter intestinal motility. Adults should refrain from food intake for 8 hours before the test and children should fast for 4 hours. Water intake is permitted and encouraged.
- The nurse ensures that the early morning laboratory test results are entered in the patient's record. The physician is notified of any abnormal values because impaired renal function would alter the urine phase of the test.

NURSING CARE—*cont'd*

During the Test

- At 8 AM, the patient drinks the prescribed dose of pentose mixed with 250 mL of water. This is followed by another 250 mL of water. At 9 AM, 250 mL of water is taken a third time, with water, as desired, thereafter. After ingestion of the d-xylose, the nurse observes the patient for vomiting or diarrhea. These problems would invalidate the test. If the test is to be rescheduled, a lower dose of d-xylose would be used.
- The patient voids at 8 AM and this specimen is discarded. For the next 5 hours, all urine is collected and refrigerated, using a brown or dark container.
- The patient is instructed to remain lying down throughout the test, as physical activity will increase intestinal motility and alter the test results.

Posttest

- Blood specimens are labeled, including the time and date of each specimen. The urine sample is also labeled, including the time and date of the start and finish of the collection period. The specimens are sent to the lab immediately to prevent warming by the temperature of the room.

Echocardiogram

e-koh-kahr-dee-oh-gram

Also called: (ECH); Heart Sonogram; Transthoracic Echocardiogram

SPECIMEN OR TYPE OF TEST: Ultrasound

PURPOSE OF THE TEST

An echocardiogram is performed for a variety of diagnostic reasons, such as to evaluate abnormal heart sounds; to evaluate heart size, chamber size, and valvular function; and to detect tumors, pericardial effusion, septal defects, and wall motion abnormalities.

BASICS THE NURSE NEEDS TO KNOW

An echocardiogram is a noninvasive test that uses ultrasound techniques to detect enlargement of the cardiac chambers or variations in chamber size during the cardiac cycle. When echocardiography has been integrated into stress testing, it is called *stress echocardiography* or *exercise echocardiography* (see Stress Testing, Cardiac p. 596). Stress echocardiography is similar to stress testing, but with an echocardiogram done at baseline and at each progressive level of exertion. It is especially helpful as a screening tool for women and for persons with a left bundle-branch block. If the patient is unable to use the treadmill or bicycle, stress can be induced with dobutamine or dipyridamole. Sometimes atropine is needed to reach the desired heart rate. *Dobutamine stress echocardiography (DSE)* is frequently used to assess "stunned" or "hibernating" myocardium.

NORMAL VALUES No anatomic or functional abnormalities

HOW THE TEST IS DONE

An echocardiogram may be carried out at the bedside, in a special laboratory, in a clinic, or in a doctor's office. A transducer is placed over the third and fourth intercostal spaces to the left of the sternum. The transducer emits ultrasonic beams of high-frequency sound waves that are inaudible to the human ear. The transducer then picks up the echoes created by the deflection of the beams off the various heart structures. This creates a picture on the oscilloscope. The picture is created because the echo varies in intensity based on the differing densities of the structures.

SIGNIFICANCE OF TEST RESULTS

Abnormal Values

Abnormal heart valves
Aneurysm
Cardiomyopathy
Congenital heart disorders
Congestive heart failure
Idiopathic hypertrophic subaortic stenosis
Mural thrombi
Myocardial infarction
Pericardial effusion
Restrictive pericarditis
Tumor of the heart

INTERFERING FACTORS

- Chest wall abnormalities
- Excessive movement
- Improper placement of transducer

NURSING CARE

Pretest

- ***Patient Teaching.*** The nurse informs the patient that the test is noninvasive. The patient is awake during the test and is usually in a recumbent position. The nurse informs the patient that an electromechanical transducer will be positioned on the chest. The patient will sense only the conduction jelly and the movement of the transducer. No pain or risk is involved.

During the Test

- The patient may be asked to breathe slowly or to hold the breath.

Posttest

- The nurse evaluates the patient's response to the procedure. The nurse cleanses the chest of conduction gel.

Ejection Fraction, Cardiac

See Catheterization, Cardiac on p. 187.

Electrocardiogram

e-lek-tro-kar-dee-oh-gram

Also called: (ECG); (EKG); 12-lead ECG or EKG; 15-lead ECG or EKG; 18-lead ECG or EKG

SPECIMEN OR TYPE OF TEST: Electrophysiology

PURPOSE OF THE TEST

The purpose of the 12-, 15-, and 18-lead ECG is to diagnose myocardial infarction, injury, and ischemia. It also assists in identifying hypertrophy, axis deviations, and electrolyte abnormalities, and distinguishes between ventricular and supraventricular tachycardia. Left versus right hypertrophy can be distinguished by comparing the morphologic characteristics of the QRS complex in leads V_1 and V_6, by determining axis deviation, and by interpreting the P-wave.

BASICS THE NURSE NEEDS TO KNOW

The electrocardiogram (ECG) is an invaluable tool in the assessment of the heart. It records the heart's electric activity. Several lead systems are available for the measurement of the electric activity of the heart: 12-, 15-, and 18-lead ECG. The electrochemical physiology characteristics are the same for each of these systems; that is, each uses electrodes on the body surface, amplifies changes in electric potentials, and provides a graphic recording. This is made possible by the body's fluid system, which acts as a conductor of electric forces. The 12-lead ECG is the system used most commonly; it presents a graphic recording of 12 electric planes of the heart. By manipulating the skin electrodes, 12 various views of the heart's electric activity are seen.

In a 12-lead ECG, leads I, II, and III are limb leads. In lead I, the negative electrode of the electrocardiograph is connected to the right arm, and the positive electrode is attached to the left arm. In lead II, the negative electrode is placed on the right arm, and the positive electrode is placed on the left leg. In lead III, the negative electrode is placed on the left arm, and the positive electrode is placed on the left leg. Leads I, II, and III form a triangle, which is called Einthoven's triangle (Figure 44).

The second set of three leads recorded by the electrocardiograph machine are called augmented limb leads. In these leads, two limbs are attached to negative electrodes, and a third limb is attached to a positive electrode. If the positive electrode is placed on the right arm, the lead is called aVR (augmented voltage right arm). If the positive electrode is on the left arm, it is called aVL (augmented voltage left arm). When the positive electrode is on the left foot, it is called aVF (augmented voltage foot) (Figure 45).

The limb leads and augmented leads are called the standard leads. If one takes the three sides of Einthoven's triangle and moves them to the center, they form three

E

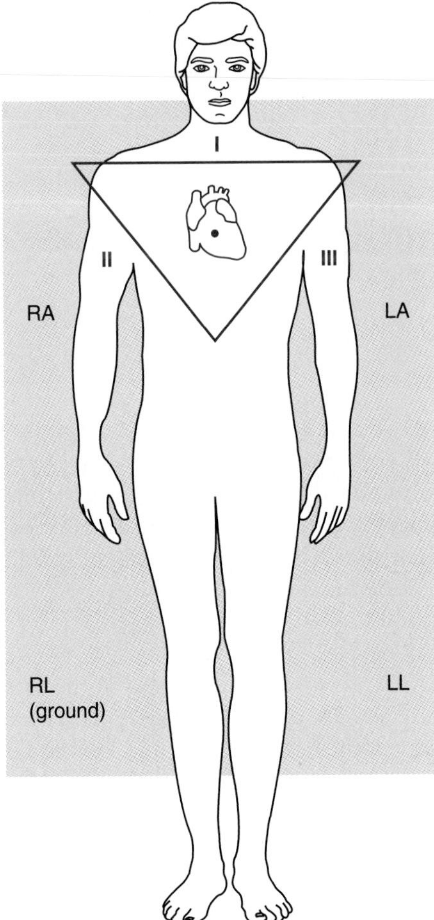

Figure 44. Einthoven's triangle.

intersecting lines of reference (Figure 46, *A*). If one superimposes the augmented limb leads, the lines of reference and the six limb leads form six intersecting lines (one every 30 degrees). Each limb and augmented lead records a different angle and, therefore, a different view of the same electric activity (Figure 46, *B*).

For the precordial, or chest, leads, the positive electrodes are applied to the person's chest and the negative electrode is applied to the limbs.

Usually, six chest leads are recorded. This is carried out by placing the positive electrodes at six different positions across the chest. The chest leads are identified as V_1 through V_6. The chest leads give various views of the horizontal plane of the left ventricle. The precordial leads can be visualized as spokes of a wheel, the center being the atrioventricular (AV) node (Figure 47).

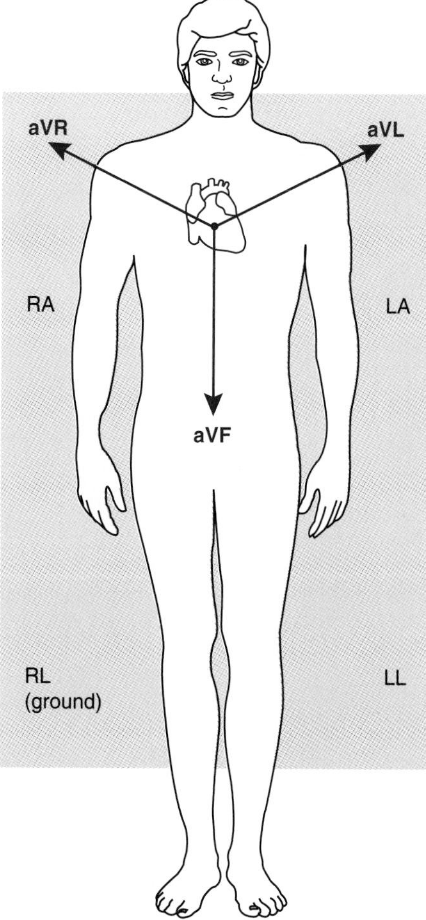

Figure 45. Augmented limb leads.

15-Lead ECG

With growing recognition of right ventricular infarction, right-sided ECGs are increasing in frequency. Right ventricular infarctions present with ST elevations of at least 1 mm in the right precordial leads V_{4r} and V_{5r}. Because the right coronary artery serves both the left ventricular inferior wall and the right ventricle, it is recommended that a right-sided or 15-lead ECG be done on any patient presenting with an inferior wall myocardial infarction.

18-Lead ECG

In the past, posterior wall infarctions were diagnosed by reciprocal changes seen on the 12-lead ECG. Now, when a posterior wall infarction is suspected (an inferior wall myocardial infarction has occurred), three additional leads may be done with the 15-lead ECG. These are the posterior leads V_7, V_8, and V_9.

E

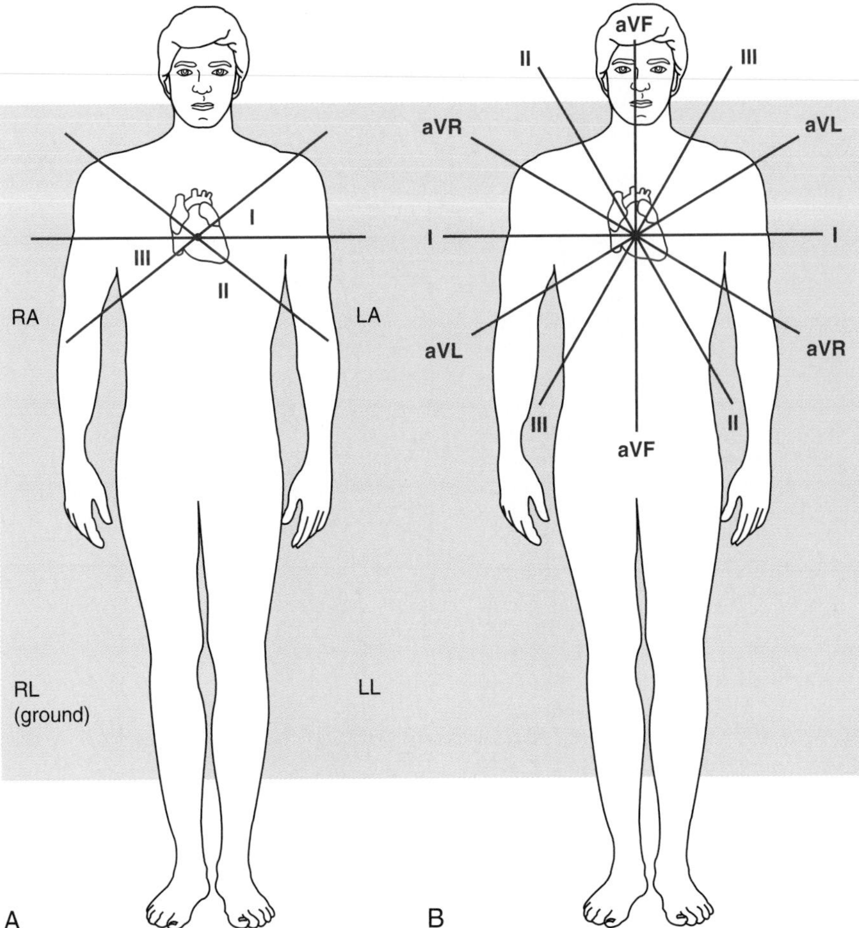

Figure 46. *A*, Intersecting limb leads. *B*, Intersecting limb and augmented leads.

NORMAL VALUES Normal rate and rhythm with no abnormalities noted

HOW THE TEST IS DONE

For a 12-lead ECG, the technician, the physician, or the nurse places the patient in a supine position. Conduction jelly is placed on the electrodes (disposable electrodes already have jelly on the electrode), and the electrodes are applied. The electrocardiograph's electrode wires are marked and color coded. It is essential that the chest leads be positioned correctly for accurate interpretation.

The chest leads are applied as follows:

V_1: Fourth intercostal space (ICS) at the right sternal border

V_2: Fourth ICS at the left sternal border

V_3: Midway between V_2 and V_4

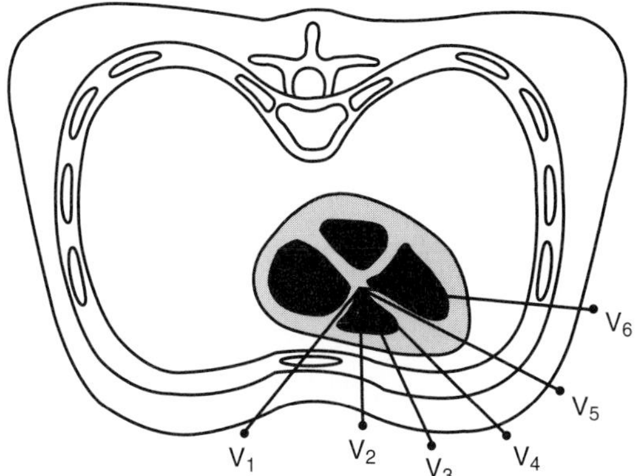

Figure 47. Precordial leads (V_1 to V_6).

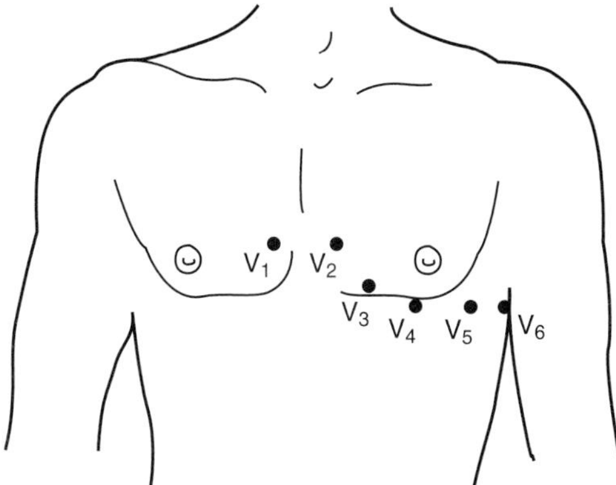

Figure 48. Chest lead placement.

V_4: Fifth ICS at the left midclavicular line
V_5: Fifth ICS at the anterior axillary line
V_6: Fifth ICS at the midaxillary line (Figure 48)

Electrocardiographs vary. Older machines record one lead at a time. Newer machines simultaneously record the 12 leads and automatically mark them.

Leads for right ventricular assessment are placed at the right fifth intercostal space at the midclavicular line (V_{4r}), at the right intercostal space at the anterior axillary line (V_{5r}), and at the right fifth intercostal space at the midaxillary line (V_{6r}).

With the 18-lead ECG, a 15-lead ECG is taken, and then three chest electrodes are placed on the line level with the fifth ICS at the posterior axillary line (V_7). The next electrode is placed at the fifth ICS at the posterior mid-clavicular line (V_8), and the last electrode is placed at the fifth ICS, left of the spinal column (V_9).

SIGNIFICANCE OF TEST RESULTS

Axis deviations (right or left)
Conduction disturbances
Dysrhythmias
Hypertrophy of the ventricles
Electrolyte imbalances
Pericarditis
Pulmonary infarctions
Therapeutic drug effects or toxicity, or both
Myocardial ischemia
Myocardial infarction

Myocardial Infarction

As a myocardial infarction evolves, a sequence of electrocardiographic changes occurs. First, the ST segment changes. Elevation of an ST segment indicates myocardial injury. ST depression occurs as a reciprocal change in the ventricular wall opposite the infarction. The ST segment will return to normal within days or weeks after the infarction.

Within hours or days of the infarction, the T-wave inverts. It reflects ischemic changes in the heart. The T-wave will revert back to normal within weeks or months of the infarction.

Lastly, an abnormal Q-wave appears in the leads directly over the transmural myocardial infarction. An abnormal Q-wave is a Q-wave in a lead in which a Q-wave is not normally seen or one that is wider than 0.04 seconds or a third of the height of the QRS complex. A non–Q-wave infarction occurs in the setting of a subendocardial infarction. A Q-wave indicates myocardial necrosis and may remain for years after the infarction.

Table 7 summarizes which leads reflect which walls of the left ventricle. Note that because leads usually are not placed over the posterior wall of the heart, posterior infarctions are diagnosed by reciprocal changes. Right ventricular infarctions are assessed by performing a right-sided ECG.

INTERFERING FACTORS

- Patient movement, poor grounding, and poor skin contact can interfere with a clear recording of the ECG.
- Improper placement of the leads.

TABLE 7 Electrocardiographic Changes with Acute Myocardial Infarction

	Lead Changes	Reciprocal Changes
Inferior wall	II, III, aVF	I, aVL
Lateral wall	I, aVL, V_5, V_6	V_1, V_2, V_3
Anterior wall	V_2, V_3, V_4	II, III, aVF
Anteroseptal	V_1, V_2, V_3, V_4	II, III, aVF
Posterior wall	V_7, V_8, V_9	V_1, V_2
Right ventricular	V_{4R}, V_{5R}	

NURSING CARE

Pretest

- ***Patient Teaching.*** The nurse explains to the patient the purpose and procedure for the ECG. No risk is involved. No pretest restrictions are required.
- Because electrodes are applied to the four extremities and the chest, clothing should permit easy access. If the male patient's chest is excessively hairy, the sites may need to be shaved.

During the Test

- Establish a relaxed environment.
- Place the patient in a supine position.
- Conduction jelly is placed on the electrodes, and the electrodes are applied.
- The recording is made.
- If a 15- or 18-lead ECG is done, clearly identify the lead placement on the ECG recording.

Posttest

- Remove electrodes and the conduction jelly.
- Help the patient to a comfortable position.

Electrocardiogram, Signal-Averaged

e-lek-tro-kar-dee-oh-gram, sig-nuhl–a-vuh-rijd

Also called: (SAECG)

SPECIMEN OR TYPE OF TEST: Electrophysiology

PURPOSE OF THE TEST

The cardiologist assesses the printout of the signal-averaged electrocardiogram (ECG) for late potentials, which place the patient at risk for sustained ventricular tachycardia (VT). A late potential is seen as a QRS complex that extends 20 to 60 msec into the ST segment.

BASICS THE NURSE NEEDS TO KNOW

Signal-averaged electrocardiography (ECG) is a technique used to detect conduction defects that may precede VT. It is a noninvasive bedside test similar to a 12-lead ECG. With a signal-averaged ECG, the recording is obtained for 15 to 30 minutes, and the electric current from the heart is amplified 1000 times. The machine then integrates all these signals and removes extraneous electric signals.

NORMAL VALUES Normal cardiac rhythm and conduction times; normal Q-T interval

HOW THE TEST IS DONE

The procedure is similar to the 12-lead ECG, except that no limb electrodes are necessary and the six chest electrodes and ground lead are positioned differently on the chest.

SIGNIFICANCE OF TEST RESULTS

Late potentials

INTERFERING FACTORS

- Because the signal-averaged ECG averages the cardiac cycle of the patient, a relatively regular rhythm is needed during the test. *Frequent* premature atrial contractions or premature ventricular contractions will interfere with the results.
- Signal-averaged ECG is also unable to detect late potentials in patients with right or left bundle branch block.

NURSING CARE

The nursing actions are similar to those for Electrocardiogram (ECG) (p. 283). In addition, review the following.

Pretest

- The nurse checks with the physician regarding discontinuing or administering the patient's antiarrhythmic medication.

During the Test

- Keep the environment quiet.
- The nurse instructs others to stay out of the patient's room.

Electroencephalography

e-lek-tro-en-se-fuh-lah-gruh-fee

Also called: (EEG); Electroencephalogram

SPECIMEN OR TYPE OF TEST: Electrophysiology

PURPOSE OF THE TEST

The major applications of electroencephalography (EEG) are in the diagnosis of epilepsy and the determination of the type of epilepsy. It also may be used to help diagnose metabolic encephalopathy and detect brain injury.

BASICS THE NURSE NEEDS TO KNOW

Electroencephalography (EEG) records the spontaneous brain activity that originates from brain cells on the surface of the brain. The fluctuations of electric activity from the larger cortical areas of the brain pass through the cranial bones and the scalp. The voltage is detected by the electrodes. Once the impulses are amplified, they can be recorded.

The older method records the brain waves on paper tracings. This is being replaced gradually by computerized tracings that are displayed on a monitor. In the process of *electric brain mapping,* the computer demonstrates trends in particular areas of brain activity. Another alternative methodology uses the *video electroencephalography monitor.* It combines the recording of the EEG waveforms with videotaping to correlate the behavioral events with electroencephalographic seizure activity. *Ambulatory monitoring* is a methodology that uses a small portable cassette recording device. It is useful for small children who have seizures in school. *Evoked potential (EP)* produces brain activity in response to a specific sensory stimulus such as a clicking noise, a mild electrical shock or a strobe light. The brain response to the stimulus is recorded by the EEG.

The rhythms of the electroencephalographic recording are identified as delta (the slowest), theta, alpha, and beta (the fastest). The interpretation of the EEG considers the frequency of the predominant rhythm, the amplitude, any abnormal waves or wave groups, and the asymmetry between the right and left hemispheres.

NORMAL VALUES

Normal patterns of electric brain activity are seen

HOW THE TEST IS DONE

Recording needle electrodes are applied to the scalp in particular groupings, using a paste that promotes conduction. The electrode wires are connected to the electroencephalograph recorder. The EEG procedure usually takes 30 to 90 minutes, but the sleep EEG is recorded all night.

SIGNIFICANCE OF TEST RESULTS

Abnormal Values

Epilepsy (grand mal, focal, temporal lobe, myoclonal, petit mal)
Intracranial hemorrhage
Mental retardation
Hypoxic, ischemic encephalopathy
Cerebral infarct
Hypocalcemia
Hypoglycemia
Meningitis
Brain tumor
Drug withdrawal
Toxoplasmosis, rubella, cytomegalovirus, herpes simplex (TORCH) infection

INTERFERING FACTORS

- Caffeine and alcohol
- Movements of the hands, body, or tongue
- Muscle contractions
- Drug intoxication (heroin, cocaine, marijuana, crack cocaine, lysergic acid diethylamide [LSD])
- Particular medications (narcotics, sedatives, tranquilizers, monoamine oxidase inhibitors, anticonvulsants, antihistamines)

NURSING CARE

Pretest

- ***Patient Teaching.*** Instruct the patient to avoid caffeine and alcohol for 12 hours before the test, because stimulants alter the electroencephalographic activity. A light meal and fluid intake are encouraged, because a low blood glucose level also can alter the electroencephalographic results. No other food or beverage restrictions are needed. Instruct the patient to wash his or her hair thoroughly before the test. Hair spray, creams, or oils must be removed because they interfere with the recording of results.
- The nurse provides information about the test and offers support to the patient and family member, as applicable. The purpose is to reduce anxiety and fear of the unknown because variables such as tense neck muscles, anxiety, and fear would alter the brain wave patterns.
- If a sleep-deprived EEG is performed to evaluate sleep disorder or seizures that occur during sleep, advise the patient not to sleep on the night before the test. At the time of the test, a sedative may be given to promote sleep. If this form of EEG is used, the nurse advises the patient to have a responsible person available to drive him or her home after the test is completed.
- Because anticonvulsant, stimulant, and tranquilizer medications alter the electric activity of the brain, these medications may be withheld for 24 to 48 hours before the test begins, as determined by the physician. If the medications cannot be withheld because of the seriousness of the patient's seizure disorder, all medications taken in the 24- to 48-hour pretest period are documented on the requisition slip.

During the Test

- Help the patient to relax in the reclining chair or on the bed. Inform the patient that the electrodes are attached to the scalp with a sticky paste. Reassure the patient that the electrodes and wires will not cause a shock or harm the patient.
- Instruct the patient not to move the head or body and not to talk during the test. These muscle movements alter the electroencephalographic readings. For the neonate, place the head in a midline alignment. Children often are more relaxed and quiet if the parent remains in the room.
- Reassure the patient that the nurse is nearby with full visibility of the patient during the procedure. If a seizure occurs, the nurse is prepared to provide care during the episode.

Posttest

- Observe the patient for seizure activity.
- Remove the electrodes. The electrode paste is cleaned from the hair and scalp with acetone and cotton balls.
- Anticonvulsant medications that were withheld for the test are not automatically restarted at the same dosage. The previous orders are reviewed by the physician, and a new set of orders are written.

Electrolyte Gap

See Anion Gap on p. 92.

Electrolytes, 24-Hour Urine

e-lek-tro-laits, twen-tee-fohr-our yur-in

Also called: Sodium, Urine; Chloride, Urine; Potassium, Urine; Calcium, Urine; Magnesium, Urine

SPECIMEN OR TYPE OF TEST: Urine

PURPOSE OF THE TEST

Urine electrolytes are used to help monitor renal function, fluid and electrolyte balance, and acid-base balance. The urinary calcium level is used to evaluate bone disease, parathyroid disorders, nephrolithiasis, calcium metabolism, and idiopathic hypercalciuria.

BASICS THE NURSE NEEDS TO KNOW

Normally, the daily intake of foods includes a renewing supply of electrolytes. The glomeruli filter the electrolytes from the blood, and the renal tubules resorb most of them for recirculation and redistribution as needed. Electrolyte excesses are not resorbed and are excreted in the urine.

The normal urinary excretion of electrolytes is dependent on the amount of intake, the serum level of the electrolytes, and the state of hydration of the body. The equilibrium of water and electrolytes is controlled by renal and multiple endocrine functions. Any condition that causes a decrease in perfusion to the kidney will cause a decrease in electrolytes excreted in the urine.

NORMAL VALUES

Sodium

Adult: 40–220 mEq/24 hr *or* SI: 40–220 mmol/24 hr

Male child (6–10 years): 41–115 mEq/24 hr *or* SI: 41–115 mmol/24 hr

Female child (6–10 years): 20–69 mEq/24 hr *or* SI: 20–69 mmol/24 hr

Male child (10–14 years): 63–117 mEq/24 hr *or* SI: 63–117 mmol/24 hr

Female child (10–14 years): 48–168 mEq/24 hr *or* SI: 48–168 mmol/24 hr

Chloride

Adult (<60 years): 110–250 mEq/24 hr *or* SI: 110–250 mmol/24 hr

Adult (>60 years): 95–195 mEq/24 hr *or* SI: 95–195 mmol/24 hr

E

Child (<6 years): 15–40 mEq/24 hr *or* SI: 15–40 mmol/24 hr
Male child (6–10 years): 36–110 mEq/24 hr *or* SI: 36–110 mmol/24 hr
Female child (6–10 years): 18–74 mEq/24 hr *or* SI: 18–74 mmol/24 hr
Male child (10–14 years): 64–176 mEq/24 hr *or* SI: 64–176 mmol/24 hr
Female child (10–14 years): 36–173 mEq/24 hr *or* SI: 36–173 mmol/24 hr
Infant: 2–10 mEq/24 hr *or* SI: 2–10 mmol/24 hr

Potassium
Adult: 25–125 mEq/24 hr *or* SI: 25–125 mmol/24 hr
Male child (6–10 years): 17–54 mEq/24 hr *or* SI: 17–54 mmol/24 hr
Female child (6–10 years): 8–37 mEq/24 hr *or* SI: 8–37 mmol/24 hr
Male child (10–14 years): 22–57 mEq/24 hr *or* SI: 22–57 mmol/24 hr
Female child (10v14 years): 18–58 mEq/24 hr *or* SI: 18–58 mmol/24 hr
Infant: 4.1–5.3 mEq/24 hr *or* SI: 4.1–5.3 mmol/24 hr

Calcium
Adult (normal calcium intake): 100–300 mg/day *or* SI: 2.5–7.5 mmol/day
Adult (low calcium intake): 50–100 mg/day *or* SI: 1.25–3.75 mmol/day
Adult (calcium-free diet): 5–40 mg/day *or* SI: 0.13–1 mmol/day
Infant and child: <6 mg/kg/day *or* SI: <0.15 mmol/kg/day

Magnesium
7.3–12.2 mg/dL *or* SI: 3–5 mmol/day

HOW THE TEST IS DONE

A 24-hour urine specimen is collected in a large, clean urine collection container. Urine is kept refrigerated or on ice during the collection period. Alternative methods include a 12-hour urine collection or a single random urine sample for electrolyte testing. If a 24-hour urine test for protein or creatinine clearance is also ordered, these tests can be performed simultaneously with the urine electrolyte test, using the same specimen.

SIGNIFICANCE OF TEST RESULTS

Elevated Values

Sodium and Chloride

Increased sodium chloride intake
Adrenal failure
Addison's disease
Nephritis (salt-wasting)
Renal tubular acidosis
Syndrome of inappropriate antidiuretic hormone
Alkalosis
Diuretic therapy
Acute or chronic renal failure

Potassium

Increased potassium intake
Cushing syndrome
Aldosteronism
Renal tubular disease
Metabolic acidosis
Adrenocorticotropic hormone or cortisone treatment
Salicylate poisoning

Calcium

Hyperparathyroidism
Vitamin D toxicity
Malignancy of bone
Renal tubular acidosis
Sarcoma
Nephrolithiasis
Multiple myeloma
Thyrotoxicosis
Paget's disease
Sarcoidosis
Osteoporosis
Schistosomiasis
Skeletal immobility
Degenerative liver disease
Cushing's disease
Diabetes mellitus

Magnesium

Chronic renal disease
Addison's disease
Chronic alcoholism
Bartter syndrome
Ingestion of excess magnesium

Cisplatin therapy
Diuretic therapy

Decreased Values

Sodium and Chloride

Decreased sodium chloride intake
Cushing syndrome
Cirrhosis (with ascites)
Congestive heart failure
Nephrotic syndrome
Prerenal azotemia
Vomiting, diarrhea
Intestinal fistula
Severe burns
Excessive sweating
Metabolic acidosis

Potassium

Addison's disease
Acute glomerulonephritis
Pyelonephritis
Nephrosclerosis
Malabsorption syndrome
Metabolic alkalosis

Calcium

Hypoparathyroidism
Hypothyroidism
Pseudohypoparathyroidism
Celiac disease
Nephrosis
Steatorrhea
Acute nephritis
Hypocalciuric hypercalcemia
Renal osteodystrophy
Vitamin D–resistant rickets
Vitamin D deficiency

Magnesium

Advanced kidney failure
Acute or chronic diarrhea
Diabetic acidosis
Starvation
Pancreatitis
Dehydration
Primary aldosteronism
Malabsorption

INTERFERING FACTORS

- Failure to collect all the urine during the 24-hour collection period
- Failure to refrigerate the specimen
- For magnesium testing: Contact with a metal bedpan or urinal

NURSING CARE

Pretest

- Obtain a urine collection container from the laboratory for the collection of all urine in the 24-hour (or 12-hour, if ordered) test period.
- ***Patient Teaching.*** If the test is used to evaluate nephrolithiasis, the nurse instructs the patient to eat the usual diet for 3 days before the test. If the patient is already receiving a calcium-restricted diet as part of the calcium stone prevention treatment, instruct the patient to maintain the dietary restriction before and during the test period.
- ***Patient Teaching.*** If thiazide diuretics are used to prevent formation of calcium stones, the nurse instructs the patient to continue the medication before and during the test. Thiazides are effective in lowering the urine calcium levels, and the benefits of the medication can be evaluated.

During the Test

- ***Patient Teaching.*** Instruct the patient to void at 8 AM and discard the specimen. The test begins immediately thereafter, and all urine is collected for the next 24 hours, including the 8 AM specimen of the next morning. The nurse needs to remind the patient periodically that all urine must be collected.
- Keep the urine in the refrigerator or on ice throughout the collection period.
- Instruct the patient to use the special laboratory container to collect the urine. If a bedpan or urinal is used for voiding, it must be made of plastic, not metal.
- Ensure that the patient's name and the date and time of the start and finish of the test are written on the label and the requisition slip.

Posttest

- Arrange for prompt transport of the chilled specimen to the laboratory.

Electromyography and Nerve Conduction Studies

e-lek-tro-mai-yo-gruh-fee and nurv cuhn-duk-shun stu-deez

Also called: (EMG); (NCS); Electrodiagnostic Studies

SPECIMEN OR TYPE OF TEST: Electrophysiology

PURPOSE OF THE TEST

These tests help distinguish among the causes of weakness and paralysis, differentiating nerve involvement from a muscle disorder. The tests also are used to identify the particular nerve or muscle group that is involved, to localize the site of the abnormality, to evaluate the severity, and to distinguish a sensorimotor nerve disorder from a pure motor disorder.

BASICS THE NURSE NEEDS TO KNOW

When a patient complains of muscle weakness, muscle spasms, or paralysis, the cause may be disease of the muscle or nervous system or a problem with neuromuscular transmission at the junction between the nerves and the muscle fibers. Electromyography (EMG) and nerve conduction studies are two diagnostic tests that help identify the physiologic location of the problem.

Electromyography

This procedure records the electric potential of various muscles in a resting state and during voluntary contraction of the muscles. The normal tracings of muscle potential demonstrate characteristic patterns at rest and during a strong voluntary muscle contraction. The recordings are examined for amplitude, duration, form, and abundance. Characteristic abnormal patterns are seen when the problem is neurologic in origin, such as denervation, or muscular in origin, such as muscle inflammation.

Nerve Conduction Studies

These studies measure motor conduction velocity and sensory conduction. Motor conduction velocity is the timed measurement of conduction along a nerve between two points, as measured by the stimulating and recording electrodes that are applied on the nerve's pathway. Sensory conduction measures the voltage or strength of the nerve stimulus in sensory nerve endings, as measured by recording electrodes applied to a distal area of tissue.

The electrodiagnostic tests are somewhat painful, and they provoke some patient anxiety. The discomfort is sharp, but it is brief and temporary. The pain is caused by the needle insertions and the electric stimuli and is increased with anxiety. Sedation is not recommended because it interferes with voluntary muscle activity.

NORMAL VALUES

The muscle shows minimal activity at rest
Nerve conduction time is within normal limits

HOW THE TEST IS DONE

Needle electrodes are inserted into muscles and connected to stimulator and recorder devices. As the electric stimulus is initiated, the results appear on an oscilloscope or video screen or are photographed. Linear tracings of the electromyography are made by the electromyographic equipment.

SIGNIFICANCE OF TEST RESULTS

Abnormal Findings

Amyotrophic lateral sclerosis
Muscular dystrophy
Herniated lumbar disc

Myasthenia gravis
Guillain-Barré syndrome
Poliomyelitis
Carpal tunnel syndrome
Inflammatory myositis
Brachial plexus injury
Myopathy (endocrine, metabolic, toxic, congenital)
Lumbosacral plexus injury
Nerve trauma
Glycogen storage disease
Hypothyroidism

INTERFERING FACTORS

- Smoking
- Caffeine
- Acute anxiety

NURSING CARE

Pretest

- After the physician explains the procedure, obtain written consent from the patient and enter it into the patient's record.
- ***Patient Teaching.*** Instruct the patient to refrain from smoking for 24 hours before the test and to avoid caffeine (coffee, tea, and cola) for 2 to 3 hours before the test.
- ***Patient Teaching.*** Inform the patient that the insertion of the needles can be painful and that the small shocks also are painful. Reassure the patient that these sensations are brief and temporary and can be tolerated. If possible, encourage the parent of a child patient to comfort the child during the procedure.

During the Test

- The examiner cleanses the skin with antiseptic before inserting the electrodes.
- As the electrodes are inserted, to help reduce anxiety the patient should be reassured that the pain will be brief and minimal.
- For grounding, place a metal plate under the patient's body. At appropriate intervals during EMG, the patient is asked to perform various voluntary muscle contractions.

Posttest

- To avoid additional pain, the needle electrodes are removed gently and slowly.
- If pain persists at the puncture sites, the nurse instructs the patient to apply warm compresses.

Electrophysiologic Studies, Cardiac

e-lek-tro-fi-zee-oh-lo-jik stu-deez, kar-dee-ak

Also called: (EPS)

SPECIMEN OR TYPE OF TEST: Radiography

E

PURPOSE OF THE TEST

Electrophysiologic studies are performed to diagnose dysrhythmias, to identify causes of ectopy and reentry phenomenon, and to determine a person's risk for lethal ventricular dysrhythmias. They are used to determine appropriate therapy for patients who have not obtained the desired effect from usual therapies and in whom noninvasive evaluation techniques have not provided the information necessary to determine which therapy or combination of therapies will be effective.

BASICS THE NURSE NEEDS TO KNOW

Electrophysiologic studies are invasive procedures performed in special laboratories or in cardiac catheterization laboratories. These studies require the insertion of catheters into the right and sometimes the left side of the heart. Several procedures are included: atrial stimulation, ventricular stimulation, His' bundle studies, and ventricular mapping.

NORMAL VALUES Normal cardiac rhythm; normal conduction, refractory, and interval times

HOW THE TEST IS DONE

Several procedures are included in the category of electrophysiologic studies. The patient may have one or all the studies performed based on the clinical state. During the test, three or four multipolar pacing catheters are inserted percutaneously. One is positioned high in the atrium, one in the low-septal right atrium, one in the coronary sinus, and one in the right ventricle.

Conduction intervals are measured to locate conduction delays by *programmed electrical stimulation (PES)*. Atrial pacing is carried out to assess sinoatrial node response, atrioventricular node response, and His' bundle and Purkinje conduction. If indicated, *atrial extrastimulus testing (AEST)* is performed. With this test, a premature atrial stimulus is initiated to assess atrial and atrioventricular node response. Atrial flutter or atrial fibrillation may be initiated. The focus or reentry pathway may then be identified. In some patients, *His' bundle electrographic studies* are performed to evaluate His' bundle conduction.

Ventricular extrastimulus testing (VEST) is performed to assess ventricular dysrhythmias. Ventricular tachycardia (VT) may be induced. If a right ventricular stimulus does not induce VT, a left-sided stimulation may be carried out. This requires the insertion of a multipolar pacing catheter through an artery. When VT is induced, its response to overdrive pacing or drugs, or both, can be evaluated. If the patient has recurrent VT, *ventricular endocardial mapping* may be performed to localize the origin of the dysrhythmia.

If ventricular mapping is performed, VT is induced, and the ectopic focus is delineated by multiple intracardiac tracings.

If the electrophysiologic studies involve evaluation of drug responses, the test must be repeated, because only one drug or combination of drugs can be assessed at a time. If this is necessary, catheters are left in place between testings.

SIGNIFICANCE OF TEST RESULTS

Electrophysiologic studies may identify dysrhythmias, conduction abnormalities, and appropriate treatment for these disturbances.

INTERFERING FACTORS

- Inability to produce arrhythmia
- Altered autonomic tone from supine position

NURSING CARE

Pretest

- Verify that an informed consent has been obtained.
- The nurse assists with the precatheterization evaluation: blood tests, including prothrombin time test and a partial thromboplastin time test; an electrocardiogram (ECG); and chest x-ray if the procedure will be performed on an outpatient basis.
- The nurse assesses the patient's fears and anxieties. Correct any misperceptions and reassure the patient that the nurses and physician will be continuously present during the procedure.
- ***Patient Teaching.*** The nurse instructs the patient about the purpose and procedure for the study. Inform the patient to report any chest pain, dizziness or shortness of breath. The patient is instructed to take nothing by mouth after midnight, except if the EPS study is planned for the late afternoon. In that case, a clear liquid breakfast may be taken.
- The nurse checks with the physician if cardiac drugs are to be withheld. Usually antiarrhythmic medications are withheld for at least twenty-four hours.
- The nurse prepares the site of catheter access according to laboratory protocols. The femoral vein is commonly used for the percutaneous insertion of the electrode catheters. Usually both sides of the groin are prepared.
- Instruct the patient to void before going to the catheterization laboratory.
- To reduce the anxiety, the nurse premedicates the patient as prescribed.
- Encourage the patient to wear his or her glasses to the catheterization laboratory.

During the Test

- The patient is awake. The nurse provides emotional support and reinforces explanations given about the procedure.
- Continuous cardiac monitoring is maintained.
- A local anesthetic is given by the physician, after the insertion site (usually the right side of the groin) is prepared and draped. The physician inserts the electrode catheters using fluoroscopy visualization.

Continued

NURSING CARE—*cont'd*

During the Test—*cont'd*

- The patient may be asked to cough during the procedure.
- When tachyarrhythmias are produced, the nurse assesses the patient's responses and reports any indication of hemodynamic instability.

Posttest

- The nurse monitors the patient's vital signs and cardiac rhythm according to hospital protocol.
- Observe the insertion site for signs of bleeding. If bleeding is present, the nurse exerts pressure just proximal to the puncture site with a gloved hand for a minimum of 15 minutes.
- The nurse evaluates the patient's psychological response to the procedure and its findings.
- ***Patient Teaching.*** If the study is done as an outpatient procedure, instruct the patient to (1) not drive for 24 hours; (2) avoid heavy lifting, sports, and strenuous housework for 3 days; and (3) avoid baths until the wound is healed. Instruct the patient that after 24 hours, he or she may shower and change the dressing.

◆ Nursing Response to Complications

The nurse needs to assess for and report any observations indicating complications, which may occur during and after the EPS study. Complications include dysrhythmias, vasovagal reaction and pericardial effusion.

Dysrhythmias. The purpose of the EPS studies includes the production of dysrhythmias; however, other nondiagnostically produced dysrhythmias may occur especially during the insertion and removal of the electrode catheters. The nurse continuously monitors the cardiac rhythm during the procedure. Notify the physician and anticipate treatment based on established protocols.

Vasovagal response. A vasovagal response may occur due to the insertion or withdrawal of the electrode catheters. The patient may experience diaphoresis, pallor, nausea, vomiting, bradycardia and hypotension. The nurse takes frequent vital signs and informs the physician of patient status.

Pericardial effusion. Because of the insertion of catheters, a small ventricular puncture may occur, causing a pericardial effusion. Small leaks usually seal themselves. Very rarely, the ventricular leak may lead to cardiac tamponade. Cardiac tamponade is an emergency. As blood accumulates in the pericardial sac, the heart is restricted. The nurse will observe signs of a decrease in cardiac output and muffled heart sounds. Notify the physician immediately. The blood in the pericardial sac must be aspirated to restore an adequate cardiac output.

Endoscopic Retrograde Cholangiopancreatography and Pancreatic Endoscopy, Cytology

en-duh-sko-pik re-troh-grayd koh-lan-jee-oh-pan-kree-uh-to-gruh-fee and pan-kree-a-tik en-dos-kuh-pee, sai-to-luh-jee

Also called: (ERCP)

SPECIMEN OR TYPE OF TEST: Endoscopy

PURPOSE OF THE TEST

Endoscopic retrograde cholangiopancreatography (ERCP) is used to investigate the cause of obstructive jaundice, persistent abdominal pain, or both, associated with biliary or pancreatic disorder. Pancreatic cytology identifies the cell type of the pancreatic biopsy specimen.

BASICS THE NURSE NEEDS TO KNOW

Bile from the liver and gall bladder and secretions from the pancreas drain through the common bile duct into the small intestine. If there is obstruction in the biliary ducts, cystic duct, or common duct or at the ampulla of Vater, the bile flow into the intestine is impeded and the patient develops obstructive jaundice. If there is blockage of the flow of pancreatic secretions, inflammation of the pancreas occurs. Because these organs and ducts are very closely located, endoscopic visualization and radiography of the biliary and pancreatic ducts are needed to determine the cause of the problem and its precise location.

NORMAL VALUES

ERCP: The anatomy of the common duct and pancreatic duct are normal, with no evidence of obstruction from stone, stricture, or tumor

Pancreatic cytology: Normal; no malignant pancreatic cells are present

HOW THE TEST IS DONE

ERCP

A gastroenterologist passes a fiberoptic endoscope through the mouth, esophagus, and stomach and into the duodenum. An intravenous dose of glucagon may be given to relax the intestine and sphincter of Oddi. At the ampulla of Vater, a small cannula (a special tube on the end of the endoscope) is inserted into the ampulla and then, in turn, into the common duct and the pancreatic duct (Figure 49). Fluoroscopy (a type of x-ray) is used to guide the placement of the instrument. Once the cannula is in the common duct, radiopaque contrast is instilled and multiple x-rays are taken. To help with the gravity flow of the contrast medium, the patient is assisted in changing positions, and the table is tilted so that all branches of the biliary tree are filled and visible. Once

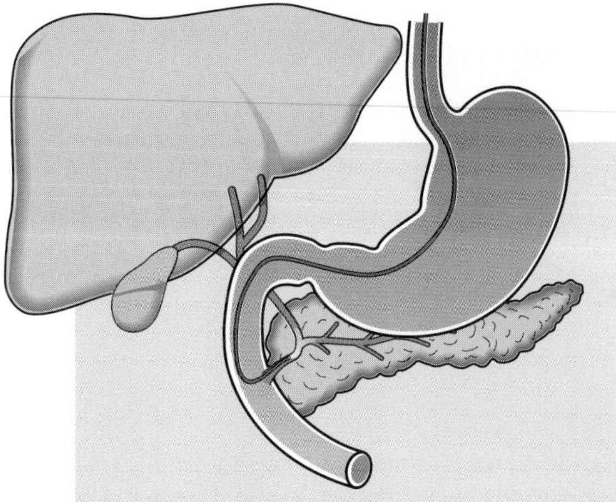

Figure 49. Endoscopic retrograde cholangiopancreatography. At the level of the duodenum, the papilla is located and the cannula is inserted through it. The cannula is passed first into the common bile duct (endoscopic retrograde cholangiography) and then into the pancreatic duct (endoscopic retrograde pancreatography).

the biliary duct examination is completed, the physician relocates the cannula into the pancreatic duct and the x-ray procedure is repeated.

Pancreatic Cytology

When cytology (a study of the cells and their pathology) examination of the pancreatic secretions is indicated, the specimen is collected when the cannula is in the pancreatic duct. The patient is given an intravenous bolus (concentrated dose) of secretin to stimulate the flow of pancreatic secretions. The endoscope is used to aspirate a sample of the secretions.

SIGNIFICANCE OF TEST RESULTS

Abnormal Biliary Findings

Biliary stone
Stenosis of the papilla
Fibrosis or stricture
Cancer of the gall bladder
Primary biliary cirrhosis
Sclerosing cholangitis
Lymphoma
Liver metastases

Abnormal Pancreatic Findings

Acute pancreatitis
Chronic pancreatitis

Pancreatic pseudocyst
Cancer
Fistula
Abscess

INTERFERING FACTORS

- The patient who cannot cooperate or relax during the examination
- Severe, acute pancreatitis
- Acute biliary obstruction
- Septic cholangitis (unless the physician performs biliary drainage)
- Acute myocardial infarction
- Pancreatic pseudocyst
- Esophageal or gastric outlet obstruction
- Hepatitis B infection

NURSING CARE

Pretest

- ***Patient Teaching.*** Provide preprocedure teaching so that the patient can relax during the 1-hour examination. Because ERCP is uncomfortable, intravenous medication will be given to promote relaxation and relief of pain. The patient will be aware enough to assist with the changing from lateral to prone position and to remain immobile during the viewing process. The nurse also instructs the patient to discontinue all food and fluids for 12 hours before the test.
- Once the physician has explained the procedure, the patient must sign a written consent. The nurse places the consent in the patient's record.
- The nurse assesses vital signs and documents the baseline values. Question the patient regarding any history of allergy to iodine, seafood, or iodine-based dye used during a previous x-ray study. Inform the physician of any positive history and record the assessment findings related to allergy.
- Before the procedure begins, the endoscopy nurse tests all equipment for correct mechanical function and proper illumination.
- One hour before the start of the procedure, an intravenous infusion is started in the patient's arm or hand. When infection in the gall bladder is suspected, systemic antibiotics are started and continued into the postprocedure period.
- Intravenous diazepam (Valium), meperidine (Demerol), and atropine are given to the patient to provide relaxation, pain relief, and reduced motility (movement) of the intestinal tract. Alternatively, a bolus (concentrated) dose of midazolam (Versed) may be ordered. Midazolam exerts a powerful, rapid enhancement of the narcotic and provides sedation and anesthesia.
- The side effects of diazepam (Valium) and midazolam (Versed) are central nervous system and respiratory depression. To prevent respiratory depression and/or cardiac arrest, the intravenous analgesics are given very slowly over a 1- to 2-minute period. Naloxone (Narcan) is kept on hand to reverse the respiratory depressive effect of

Continued

NURSING CARE—*cont'd*

Pretest—*cont'd*

meperidine, but it is ineffective against diazepam. Once the administration of medication begins, the nurse monitors the vital signs and respiratory status frequently. In many endoscopy units, automated blood pressure, pulse oximetry, and cardiac monitors are used. Because the risk of apnea exists, resuscitation equipment must be readily available.

- Before inserting the endoscope, the physician anesthetizes the patient's mouth and throat with topical anesthetic spray. The patient's tongue will then feel thick and it will be difficult to swallow. An oral brace is inserted into the mouth to keep it open and a suction catheter is inserted to remove the saliva.
- The patient wears a lead shield over the thyroid gland. The nurse and physician wear lead body shields and thyroid shields because of their repeated exposure to radiation during the procedure.

During the Test

- The nurse continues to monitor the patient's cardiac and respiratory status frequently. Oxygen administered by nasal cannula helps prevent hypoxemia (a low oxygen level in the blood). As the endoscope is manipulated by the physician, the patient may experience a vasovagal reflex, as indicated by sudden bradycardia (a slow heartbeat, less than 60 beats per minute). Atropine sulfate medication is kept on hand to overcome the effects of the bradycardia.
- The nurse assists the patient with turning, positioning, and relaxation.
- For pancreatic cytology, two vials of pancreatic secretions are collected. The first tube is discarded because the secretions contain contrast medium. The nurse labels and identifies the second specimen of fluid. This specimen is packed on ice and sent to the laboratory quickly. This cooling process and prompt delivery minimizes the deterioration of any cells in the fluid.

Posttest

- Until the patient is stable, the nurse monitors the cardiovascular and respiratory status every 15 minutes.
- The patient ingests nothing by mouth until the gag reflex and swallowing ability return, at which point clear liquids are started; a light meal can follow shortly thereafter. In the first hour or so, colicky abdominal pain can occur because of the air that was inserted in the intestinal tract during the procedure. It will disappear as food intake returns.
- ***Patient Teaching.*** For discharge teaching, the nurse instructs the patient to notify the physician of any severe or prolonged symptoms of abdominal pain, fever, nausea or vomiting.

◇ Nursing Response to Complications

Because of the tissue manipulation during the procedure and the already compromised state of the patient's health, complications can occur. The complications can begin within 1 hour or up to 2 days later. Abnormal assessment findings, should they appear, are indications of a serious problem that requires medical intervention. The nurse notifies the physician of abnormal findings and records the data in the patient's record.

NURSING CARE—*cont'd*

Sepsis. Sepsis (the presence of microorganisms and their toxins in the blood and other tissues), is the most frequent and serious complication of this procedure. The nurse's assessment findings would include moderate abdominal pain, fever, chills, and jaundice. When infection is suspected, the nurse should check the recent laboratory results for leukocytosis (an elevated white blood cell count) and abnormal liver values.

Pancreatitis. Pancreatitis (inflammation of the pancreas) is the second most frequent complication of ERCP. Assessment findings include acute epigastric pain, abdominal distension, a "board-like" abdomen, nausea, and vomiting. The serum amylase value is often elevated after the ERCP procedure and is not significant by itself. The presence of clinical symptoms in addition to an elevated serum amylase is significant of complication.

End-Tidal Carbon Dioxide

See Capnogram on p. 170.

Epinephrine

See Catecholamines, Plasma on p. 183.

Epstein-Barr Virus Serology

ep-steen–bar vai-ruhs seer-o-luh-jee

Also called: Epstein-Barr titer

SPECIMEN OR TYPE OF TEST: Serum

PURPOSE OF THE TEST

These serologic tests are used to diagnose Epstein-Barr viral infection in patients with infectious mononucleosis in whom heterophil antibody titers are negative.

BASICS THE NURSE NEEDS TO KNOW

As presented in Table 8, the Epstein-Barr virus is a herpesvirus that is responsible for most cases of infectious mononucleosis. Infectious mononucleosis causes fever, swollen lymph glands, and an inflamed oropharynx. In the blood, an increase in the number of B lymphocytes and a transient rise in the heterophil antibodies occur. The virus is transmitted via infected saliva.

The Epstein-Barr virus infects the B lymphocytes and stimulates DNA synthesis to form several new antigens. These antigens include viral capsid antigen (VCA), Epstein-Barr nuclear antigen (EBNA), and early antigen (EA). As the body develops its immunologic response to combat the infection, antibodies are formed against the specific antigens.

TABLE 8 Herpes Group of Viruses

Virus Type	Infection
Herpes simplex type 1	"Cold sores"; infection of the mouth, lips, eyes, or skin; encephalitis (adult)
Herpes simplex type 2	Genital herpes, neonatal infection, encephalitis (newborn)
Epstein-Barr virus	Infectious mononucleosis, Burkitt's lymphoma, nasopharyngeal carcinoma
Cytomegalovirus	Cytomegalovirus, infectious mononucleosis, congenital infection In immunocompromised patients: interstitial pneumonia, gastroenteritis, retinitis
Varicella-zoster virus	Chickenpox (varicella), shingles (herpes zoster)

Antibody Formation

The antibody VCA immunoglobulin M (IgM) appears in the blood before and during the acute phase of illness. It remains in the blood for 1 to 2 months and then disappears. The antibody VCA-IgG also elevates and peaks in the blood at an early stage of illness. In the convalescent stage, it declines but then persists for life at a lower, positive value. This antibody is the most often used test and is reported as the standard Epstein-Barr virus titer. It is the marker for current or prior infection.

The anti-EA antibody appears a few weeks after the onset of symptoms and then gradually disappears from the blood. The IgG type, however, may persist for several years after an acute infection.

The anti-EBNA antibody appears in the blood several weeks after the onset of symptoms of infection. It remains elevated for life.

Several of the Epstein-Barr antibody titers also are elevated in certain malignant disorders, but a tissue biopsy must confirm the presence of malignancy.

NORMAL VALUES

Antibodies to viral capsid antigen (IgM anti-VCA): <1:10; (IgG anti-VCA): <1:10
Antibody to Epstein-Barr nuclear antigen (anti-EBNA): <1:5
Antibodies to early antigen (anti-EA): <1:10

HOW THE TEST IS DONE

A red-topped tube is used to collect 10 mL of venous blood.

SIGNIFICANCE OF TEST RESULTS

Elevated Values

Infectious mononucleosis
Burkitt's lymphoma
Nasopharyngeal cancer
Hodgkin's disease

INTERFERING FACTORS

- None

NURSING CARE

Nursing measures include care of the venipuncture site as presented in Chapter 2, with the following additional measures.

Pretest

- Schedule this test to be performed at the onset of illness and again after 2 to 3 weeks. This scheduling provides data during the acute and convalescent phases of illness.

Posttest

- On the requisition slip, write the date of the onset of illness. Arrange for prompt transport of the specimen to the lab.

Ergonovine Provocation Test

uhr-guh-noh-veen pro-vuh-kay-shun test

SPECIMEN OR TYPE OF TEST: Radiography

PURPOSE OF THE TEST

Ergonovine provocation testing is indicated for patients with atypical angina in whom coronary artery spasm is *suspected.*

BASICS THE NURSE NEEDS TO KNOW

Ergonovine provocation testing is used to diagnose coronary artery spasm and vasospastic angina. Accurate diagnosis of coronary artery spasm is necessary, because treatment varies. Because of its risk, ergonovine provocation testing is limited to carefully selected patients.

NORMAL VALUES

No ST segment changes

HOW THE TEST IS DONE

The ergonovine provocation test is usually performed as part of a cardiac catheterization. First, the cardiac catheterization must rule out severe coronary artery obstruction. A pacing wire is then inserted. Intravenous ergonovine maleate (ergotrate maleate) is given, which usually will stimulate a spasm within 3 to 6 minutes. Its effect lasts 10 to 15 minutes. If a positive response occurs, the spasm is reversed by administering nitroglycerin intravenously.

Bedside ergonovine provocation testing can be performed in the coronary care unit in patients who have had a cardiac catheterization to verify that the coronary arteries are not severely obstructed. Ergonovine is given intravenously every 5 minutes, up to seven times. The ergonovine is stopped when ST segment changes are seen on the monitor, whether the patient has pain or not. Nitroglycerin is given to reverse the spasm.

SIGNIFICANCE OF TEST RESULTS

A positive response to ergonovine includes chest pain with ST segment abnormalities (rarely, chest pain does not occur), spasms visible on the arteriogram, serious dysrhythmias, or a combination of these responses.

INTERFERING FACTORS

- Severe obstruction of a coronary artery or multivessel obstructive cardiac disease
- Severe congestive heart failure
- Uncontrolled hypertension
- Pregnancy
- Acute myocardial infarction
- Possible cerebral hemorrhage
- A history of hypersensitivity to ergonovine

E

NURSING CARE

See section on Catheterization, Cardiac (p. 187). In addition, review the following.

Pretest

- ***Patient Teaching.*** Warn the patient that chest pain is expected but will be treated immediately.
- Check with the physician to determine if vasoactive medications are to be held. Usual vasoactive medications held are: nitrates for 4 hours before the test, calcium channel blockers for 24 hours before the test, and beta-blockers for 48 hours before the test.

During the Test

- Continuous cardiac monitoring is performed. If major adverse effects are noted, the physician is informed and the ergonovine is stopped.

Posttest

- Assess the patient for chest pain with or without ST segment changes, as spasms may recur after the nitroglycerin is stopped.
- The nurse maintains cardiac monitoring of and bedrest for the patient for 1 to 2 hours.

◆ Nursing Response to Complications

A variety of complications may occur with ergonovine provocation testing. Close observation of the patient as well as assessment of subjective data is essential. The complications range from nausea, vomiting, and headache to atypical chest pain, myocardial infarction, dysrhythmias, bronchospasms, and hyper- or hypotension.

The physician must be notified if these problems occur.

Erythrocyte Sedimentation Rate

i-rith-roh-sait sed-i-men-ta-shun rayt

Also called: (ESR); Sed Rate

SPECIMEN OR TYPE OF TEST: Blood

PURPOSE OF THE TEST

The erythrocyte sedimentation test is useful in identifying and monitoring disease activity in infectious and inflammatory conditions. It is especially useful in rheumatic and collagen diseases.

BASICS THE NURSE NEEDS TO KNOW

The erythrocyte sedimentation rate (ESR) test is a nonspecific measurement of infection or inflammation in the body. When venous blood is placed in a vertical tube, the erythrocytes act like sediment; over time, they fall to the bottom of the tube. In normal conditions, as the erythrocytes settle, they exhibit a characteristic *rouleau formation,* meaning that they form a stack.

Elevated Values

In inflammatory or infectious conditions, the rouleau formation is greater, the sedimentation rate is faster, and the ESR is elevated. In rheumatic disorders, such as rheumatoid arthritis and systemic lupus erythematosus, the severity or rise in the ESR is usually reflective of the severity in the inflammatory condition. Anemia also increases the ESR, because fewer erythrocytes are present in the plasma.

Decreased Values

Microcytes (abnormally small red blood cells) have a slower sedimentation rate than normal. Additionally, erythrocytes with irregularities or abnormal shape exhibit less rouleau formation. When a low plasma fibrinogen level exists, the ESR value is proportionately lower. These conditions demonstrate less erythrocyte sedimentation and a lower ESR value.

NORMAL VALUES

Adult <50 years
- Male: 0–15 mm/hr
- Female: 0–20 mm/hr

Adult >50 years: 0–30 mm/hr

HOW THE TEST IS DONE

A lavender-topped tube is used to collect 7 mL of venous blood.

SIGNIFICANCE OF TEST RESULTS

Elevated Values

Rheumatoid arthritis
Multiple myeloma
Rheumatic fever
Waldenström's macroglobulinemia
Inflammation
Anemia
Polymyalgia rheumatica

Decreased Values
Sickle cell anemia
Polycythemia
Spherocytosis
Hypofibrinogenemia

INTERFERING FACTORS

- None

NURSING CARE

Nursing actions are similar to those used in other venipuncture procedures (see Chapter 2), with the following additional measures.

Pretest

- Because many medications, including salicylate, can alter lab values, list all medications taken by the patient on the requisition slip. In some cases, the medication may be withheld until after the test.

Posttest

- Ensure that the specimen is sent promptly to the lab. The specimen must be analyzed within 4 hours of collection.

Erythropoietin

i-rith-roh-pohy-e-tin

Also called: (EP)

SPECIMEN OR TYPE OF TEST: Serum

PURPOSE OF THE TEST

Measurement of erythropoietin is performed to investigate some anemias and the anemia of end-stage renal disease. It also may be used to differentiate between primary and secondary polycythemia vera or to detect the recurrence of an erythropoietin-producing tumor.

BASICS THE NURSE NEEDS TO KNOW

Erythropoietin is a hormone manufactured primarily by the kidneys. Its action is to regulate erythropoiesis, meaning that it stimulates or promotes the proliferation, differentiation, and maturation of erythrocyte precursor cells of the bone marrow. In normal kidneys, the stimuli to produce erythropoietin are hypoxia and decreased renal oxygenation.

Elevated Values

In chronic iron deficiency anemia and other types of anemia and after a moderate blood loss, the erythropoietin level is elevated as the kidneys respond to the need for more red blood cells and oxygen. The erythropoietin level rises dramatically in pregnancy and with erythropoietin-producing tumors.

Decreased Values

In cases of end-stage renal disease or after bilateral nephrectomy, erythropoietin is greatly reduced, and erythropoiesis by the bone marrow is limited. Anemia results from the impaired function of the bone marrow.

NORMAL VALUES

Adults: 5–36 mIU/mL *or* SI: 5–36 international units/L
Children and adolescents: 1.0–21.0 mIU/ml *or* SI: 1.0–21.0 international units/L

HOW THE TEST IS DONE

A red-topped tube is used to collect 7 mL of venous blood.

SIGNIFICANCE OF TEST RESULTS

Elevated Values

Anemias
Secondary polycythemia
Pulmonary fibrosis
Chronic obstructive pulmonary disease
Erythropoietin-producing tumor
Cerebellar hemangioblastoma
Renal tumor
Hepatoma
Pheochromocytoma
Polycystic kidney disease
Early renal transplant rejection

Decreased Values

End-stage renal failure
Primary polycythemia (polycythemia vera)

INTERFERING FACTORS

- Pregnancy

NURSING CARE

Nursing actions are similar to those used in other venipuncture procedures (see Chapter 2). No specific patient instruction or intervention is needed.

Esophageal Function Tests

e-so-fuh-je-uhl funk-shun tests

Also called: Esophageal Manometry; Esophageal pH; Acid Perfusion Test

SPECIMEN OR TYPE OF TEST: Manometry

E

PURPOSE OF THE TEST

Esophageal manometry is used to diagnose and evaluate esophageal motor disorders, including the evaluation of dysphagia. It also is used to evaluate pre- or postoperative esophageal surgery that improves motility and prevents reflux.

Esophageal pH is used to document gastroesophageal reflux disease (GERD).

The acid perfusion test (Bernstein test) is used to determine that the heartburn is of esophageal rather than cardiac origin.

BASICS THE NURSE NEEDS TO KNOW

When the patient swallows food, the esophagus propels the bolus to the stomach by peristalsis. The lower esophageal segment (LES) is a sphincter muscle that relaxes to allow the food into the stomach and then contracts to prevent gastric acids from reflux (regurgitation back into the esophagus). At rest, the pressure of the LES is higher than the pressure in the stomach, and high esophageal pressure prevents gastric acid from reflux into the esophagus.

Esophageal Manometry

The pressure within various segments of the esophagus can be measured at rest and during swallowing to evaluate esophageal motor function. The patients who require this test have a history of unexplained dysphagia or chronic heartburn. Among the possible causes are progressive systemic sclerosis, neuromuscular disorder that weakens esophageal motor function, tumor, stricture, spasm, and hiatal hernia. The test can also rule out angina and other cardiac problems that can be the source of chest pain.

Esophageal pH

During manometry testing, the esophageal pH can be measured to detect regurgitation of gastric acid into the esophagus. When detected, the disorder is called GERD and is caused by an incompetent lower esophageal sphincter. The normal pH of the esophagus is 6 or higher, an alkaline environment. The normal pH of the stomach is 1 to 3, an acidic reading. An esophageal pH reading of <4 is diagnostic of gastric acid reflux. Acidity in the esophagus results in a burning sensation, pain in the chest, and inflammation of the esophagus.

Ambulatory Esophageal pH Monitoring

This is a new technique that can be done separately, rather than as part of manometry testing. It is the preferred test to document GERD. For 24 hours, the patient has a pH probe inserted into the esophagus via nasal intubation. The electrode and its catheter are attached to a monitoring device that records pH readings during periods of activity, rest, and meals. Any pH values >4 are diagnostic of GERD.

Acid Perfusion Test

During esophageal manometry testing, this procedure may be performed to identify the patient's subjective response to heartburn pain in the presence of instilled, diluted hydrochloric acid. In a positive response, the esophagus is identified as the source of the heartburn because it is sensitive to the gastric acid. If there is no pain, esophagitis has been ruled out.

NORMAL VALUES

Esophageal Manometry
LES pressure: Mean value: 19.2 ± 6.9 mm Hg
% LES relaxation: 96% ± 10%

Esophageal Acidity Test
Alkaline (esophageal pH of 6 or higher)

Acid Perfusion Test
Negative

HOW THE TEST IS DONE

Using a nasal and throat anesthetic spray, the physician passes a triple lumen catheter into the esophagus via the mouth or nose. The patient is placed in a supine position with a swallowing sensor attached at the neck.

Esophageal Manometry

The catheter (manometer) records pressures in the esophagus during a series of wet swallows (5 mL of water delivered by syringe) and dry swallows. The readings give data about LES relaxation, peristalsis, and spontaneous contractions of the esophagus.

Esophageal Acidity

The pH probe on the tip of the catheter records the pH value in the esophagus and stomach. Readings from the esophagus are taken after the patient swallows and performs the Valsalva maneuver, straight leg raising, and abdominal compressions.

Provocative Testing

This test may be performed to identify the cause of dysphagia. The cholinergic drug edrophonium (Tensilon) is given intravenously and the pressure readings are repeated.

Acid Perfusion Test

In the Bernstein test, the examiner instills very dilute hydrochloric acid through the catheter until the patient complains of heartburn or until 30 minutes have passed without pain. The acid solution is alternated with saline to confirm that the heartburn occurs in the presence of hydrochloric acid and disappears in the presence of normal saline.

Ambulatory pH Testing

In this test, the physician passes a catheter through the nose and down into the esophagus. At the tip, there is an electronic probe that records pH readings in continuous monitoring for 24 hours. A portable recorder is worn by the patient attached to the belt or a shoulder strap. The patient maintains a normal lifestyle, activity level, and diet. The patient pushes buttons on the recorder to indicate the time that meals, sleep, and heartburn occur. Acid measurements are computer-analyzed in relationship to the patient's circadian cycle, activities, and symptoms throughout a 24-hour period.

Future ambulatory measurements may be done by a temporarily implanted electrode that is catheter-free.

SIGNIFICANCE OF TEST RESULTS

Disorders of esophageal motility
Esophageal spasm
Progressive systemic sclerosis (scleroderma)
Gastroesophageal reflux disease
Hiatal hernia

INTERFERING FACTORS

- Unstable cardiac status
- Uncooperative patient behavior

NURSING CARE

Pretest

- After the nurse has explained the test to the patient, the patient must sign a consent form. The nurse places the document in the patient's record.
- ***Patient Teaching.*** In the pretest assessment, the nurse can ask the patient pertinent questions that will provide important information about the swallowing problems. "What types of foods cause difficulties in swallowing?" "Does the food stop or become stuck after swallowing?" "Can you swallow liquids?" "Is the swallowing difficulty intermittent or continual and getting worse?" "Do you experience heartburn?"
- ***Patient Teaching.*** In ambulatory pH testing, encourage the patient to complete the 24 hours of the test and to maintain a normal lifestyle during the test period. The nasal catheter is uncomfortable and may be embarrassing to the patient because it is so visible. With these feelings present, the patient may alter his or her lifestyle during the test and therefore alter the test findings.
- ***Patient Teaching.*** The nurse instructs the patient to maintain a fasting state and to abstain from smoking for 8 hours before the test. Medications that alter the acidity of the stomach should be withheld for 24 hours. These include anticholinergics, steroids, cimetidine, antacids, and reserpine. If the physician wants the medications to be taken continuously, the nurse lists them on the requisition slip. For the ambulatory pH testing, the patient is taught how to use the recorder device to identify events such as eating, sleeping, and episodes of heartburn.

NURSING CARE—*cont'd*

During the Test

- Monitor and record the patient's vital signs at intervals during the test. Observe for signs of respiratory and cardiac change.

Posttest

- Once the gag and swallow reflexes have returned, the patient may resume his or her medication schedule and resume oral intake.

◆ Nursing Response to Complications

During the test, a vasovagal response can occur because of stimulation of the vagus nerve. If edrophonium (Tensilon) is given to stimulate the neuromuscular function of the esophagus, side effects can occur also. To counteract the bradycardia in both complications, atropine sulfate must be kept on hand, ready for use.

Vasovagal response. The nurse assesses for sudden bradycardia, a pulse lower than 60. The blood pressure drops into hypotension and the patient's skin becomes cold and clammy.

Side effects of edrophonium (Tensilon). When edrophonium (Tensilon) has been used, the nurse assesses for side effects of sudden bradycardia, a pulse rate lower than 60. The patient complains of dizziness, nausea, and muscle cramps. Vomiting may occur and the patient's skin becomes flushed, warm, and diaphoretic (sweaty).

Esophagogastroduodenoscopy

e-so-fuh-goh-gas-troh-doo-o-den-os-koh-pee

Also called: (EGD)

SPECIMEN OR TYPE OF TEST: Endoscopy

PURPOSE OF THE TEST

The purposes of this upper gastrointestinal endoscopy procedure include: (1) identification and biopsy of abnormal tissue, (2) determination of the exact site and cause of upper gastrointestinal bleeding, (3) evaluation of the healing of gastric ulcers, (4) evaluation of the stomach and duodenum after gastric surgery, and (5) investigation of the cause of dysphagia (difficulty swallowing), dyspepsia (epigastric discomfort after meals), gastric outlet obstruction, or epigastric pain.

BASICS THE NURSE NEEDS TO KNOW

In esophagogastroduodenoscopy (EGD), the fiberoptic endoscope provides direct visualization of the lumen and mucosal lining of the esophagus, stomach, and duodenum in all surface areas. Tissue abnormalities are observed for their location, size, shape, appearance, and position (Figure 50). Tissue or secretion samples are obtained by biopsy, scrapings, or aspiration, and are sent for lab analysis.

E

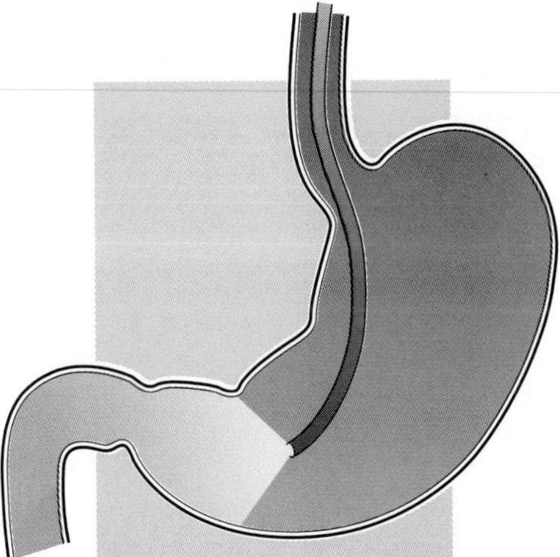

Figure 50. Endoscopic visualization of the upper gastrointestinal tract. The flexible tube, fiberoptic filaments, and a light are used to examine the mucosal surface of the esophagus, stomach, and duodenum for inflammation, erosion, ulceration, bleeding sites, stricture, and abnormal tissue.

NORMAL VALUES No abnormal structures or tissues are observed in the esophagus, stomach or duodenum

HOW THE TEST IS DONE

Virtually all adult patients receive conscious sedation and a local anesthetic throat spray to help them tolerate the procedure and cooperate during the examination. Infants and small children usually require general anesthesia.

The physician passes the endoscope through the mouth, into the esophagus, and proceeds distally through the stomach, pylorus. As the endoscope is positioned, the tip is flexed and rotated in all directions. This allows for the examination of the entire surface of the upper gastrointestinal tract. Biopsy and fluid samples are taken, as needed. The viewing continues as the endoscope is gradually withdrawn (Figure 51).

SIGNIFICANCE OF TEST RESULTS

Gastric or duodenal ulcer
Tumor, benign or malignant
Stenosis, esophageal or pyloric
Hiatal hernia
Inflammation (esophagitis, gastritis)
Mallory-Weiss tear of esophagus
Varices, esophageal or gastric

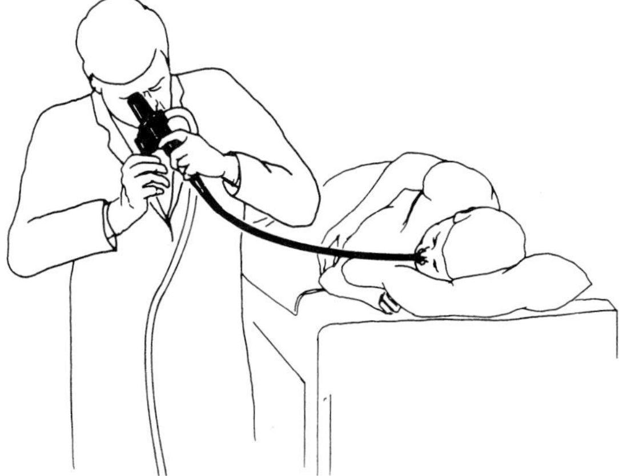

Figure 51. Esophagogastroduodenoscopy. Once the endoscope is inserted, the tube is moved around and the tip is rotated to obtain visualization of the lumen of the upper intestine. *(Reproduced with permission from Sivak, M. V. [1987].* Gastrologic endoscopy. *Philadelphia: W. B. Saunders.)*

INTERFERING FACTORS

- Failure to maintain nothing-by-mouth status
- Unstable or life-threatening cardiac or pulmonary status
- Known or suspected perforation of the stomach or intestine
- Shock
- Recent heart attack

NURSING CARE

Pretest

- Schedule this test at least 2 days after an upper gastrointestinal series so that residual barium will not interfere with the visual examination.
- A signed consent is needed and the document is entered in the patient's record.
- ***Patient Teaching.*** The nurse instructs the patient to maintain a nothing-by-mouth status for 6 to 8 hours before the test. Advise the patient to have a responsible adult accompany him or her to the location of the test and provide transportation after discharge. During pretest teaching, review the written posttest instructions with the patient. This timing is best because the conscious sedation will disrupt comprehension and memory for a short period after the test is over.
- The nurse obtains the pretest coagulation profile test results, which include prothrombin time, partial thromboplastin time, bleeding time, and platelet count. The lab results are placed in the patient's record and the nurse informs the physician of

Continued

NURSING CARE—*cont'd*

Pretest—*cont'd*

any abnormal results. The patient must have normal coagulation ability to avoid a bleeding complication during the procedure. On the morning of the test, the nurse takes vital signs, including temperature, pulse respirations and blood pressure. The results are entered in the patient's record.

- Assist the patient to remove and store eyeglasses, dentures, jewelry, and clothing. Provide a surgical gown for the patient to wear.

During the Test

- Before the procedure begins, the endoscopy nurse tests all equipment for correct mechanical function and proper illumination.
- Intravenous diazepam (Valium), meperidine (Demerol), and atropine are given to the patient to provide relaxation, pain relief, and reduced motility (movement) of the intestinal tract. Alternatively, a bolus (concentrated) dose of midazolam (Versed) may be ordered. Midazolam (Versed) exerts a powerful, rapid enhancement of the narcotic and provides sedation and anesthesia.
- The side effects of diazepam and midazolam are central nervous system and respiratory depression. To prevent respiratory depression or cardiac arrest, the intravenous analgesics are given very slowly over a 1 to 2-minute period. Naloxone (Narcan) is kept on hand to reverse the respiratory depressive effect of meperidine, but it is ineffective against diazepam. Once the administration of medication begins, the nurse monitors the vital signs and respiratory status frequently. In many endoscopy units, automated blood pressure, pulse oximetry, and cardiac monitors are used. Because the risk of apnea exists, resuscitation equipment must be readily available.
- The nurse assists the patient into a left lateral recumbent position. Oxygen may be delivered by nasal cannula to help prevent hypoxia from the respiratory depression associated with conscious sedation.
- Before inserting the endoscope, the physician anesthetizes the patient's mouth and throat with topical anesthetic spray. The patient's tongue will then feel thick and it will be difficult to swallow. An oral brace is inserted into the mouth to keep it open and a suction catheter is inserted to remove the saliva.
- The nurse assists with the collection of tissue specimens (see also Gastrointestinal Cytologic Studies, p. 339). Tissue samples are placed in sterile collection jars with preservative. They are labeled with the patient's name and the source of the tissue specimen (e.g., gastric biopsy tissue). The requisition slip includes the patient's identification data, source of the tissue, procedure, and date.

Posttest

- Until the patient is stable, the nurse monitors the cardiovascular and respiratory status and the level of alertness of the patient every 15 minutes.
- The patient ingests nothing by mouth until the gag reflex and swallowing ability return.
- Oral fluids can then be started.

NURSING CARE—*cont'd*

- ***Patient Teaching.*** For discharge teaching, the nurse reviews the protocol with the patient, as follows: Use throat lozenges or saline gargle to relieve any discomfort in the throat, no driving for 12 hours, and full resumption of food and fluids, as desired.

◆ Nursing Response to Complications

The incidence of complication during or after an EGD procedure is quite rare. During the procedure, the patient may experience respiratory depression or cardiac arrhythmia. The hypoxia and low respiratory rate usually occurs because of the conscious sedation medications, and the arrhythmia may occur as a result of the hypoxia. Perforation may also occur, usually in the esophagus, as the endoscope is passed through a narrow space. Bleeding can occur from the perforation or from a biopsy site. Although these complications occur during the test, the patient may not experience symptoms until later. With signs of complication, the nurse performs a careful assessment and notifies the physician of abnormal results.

Respiratory depression. When assessing for respiratory depression, abnormal findings include a respiratory rate <12 breaths/minute, tachycardia (a pulse rate >120 beats per minute). The patient breathes shallowly, and the color of the skin turns pale or cyanotic.

Cardiac arrhythmia. When assessing for a cardiac arrhythmia, the abnormal findings include an irregular pulse (premature atrial or ventricular contractions or atrial fibrillation).

Perforation and bleeding. In the event of perforation or bleeding, abnormal assessment findings include hematemesis (usually bright red color blood in the vomitus), persistent pain on swallowing and breathing, pain in the mediastinum or epigastric area, and fever. The nurse should pay particular attention to the patient's description of the pain and dysphagia, including the location and the severity of the complaint.

Estriol, Unconjugated, Pregnancy

es-tree-uhl, uhn-kon-juh-gay-ted, preg-nuhn-see

Also called: E_3; uE_3

SPECIMEN OR TYPE OF TEST: Blood

PURPOSE OF THE TEST

In the later stages of pregnancy, the results of the serial estriol test may be used to evaluate fetal well-being and placental function, especially in the high-risk pregnancy. It also is used as part of the multiple marker screening test to detect Down syndrome.

BASICS THE NURSE NEEDS TO KNOW

During pregnancy, estriol is the predominant estrogen present in the serum. Because this hormone is synthesized by the placenta, the serum value is considered a measure of the integrity and well-being of the fetal-placental-maternal unit. The serum level rises progressively during a normal pregnancy. Therefore, the number of weeks of gestation is a necessary consideration in the interpretation of the test result. When the test results are declining or at a lower-than-normal level, the fetus is considered to be in danger. Immediate further investigation of the status of fetal health is indicated.

Multiple Marker Screening for Down Syndrome

Pregnant women can now be tested for fetal Down syndrome in the second trimester, using the triple or quadruple marker screening test. This blood test is offered in the 15th to 22nd week of the pregnancy. The triple marker screening test consists of alpha fetoprotein, human chorionic gonadotrophin, and unconjugated estriol. The newest, improved method is to use the quadruple marker screening test, consisting of the above three tests as well as a fourth, inhibitin A.

When Down syndrome affects the fetus, the quadruple marker screening test demonstrates characteristic changes in the second trimester of pregnancy. The alpha fetoprotein result is 25% lower than normal and the unconjugated estriol result is 30% lower than normal. Both human chorionic gonadotrophin and inhibitin A rise to twice the normal value. Pregnancy ultrasound must be done first, to obtain an accurate gestational age. The quadruple marker screening test detects 80% of fetal Down syndrome pregnancies, with a 5% false positive rate of error. It is a very useful test for pregnant women younger than age 35. A high rate of Down syndrome occurs in pregnancies of younger females and amniocentesis is not done routinely to detect the problem.

NORMAL VALUES

25 weeks of gestation: 3.5–10.0 0 mcg/L *or* SI: 12–15 nmol/L
30 weeks of gestation: 4.5–14.0 mcg/L *or* SI: 16–40 nmol/L
38 weeks of gestation: 9.0–32.0 mcg/L *or* SI: 31–111 nmol/L
40 weeks of gestation: 5–40 0 mcg/L *or* SI: 17–139 nmol/L

HOW THE TEST IS DONE

A red-topped tube is used to obtain 10 mL of venous blood.

SIGNIFICANCE OF TEST RESULTS

Decreased Values

Diabetes mellitus
Fetal growth retardation
Fetal encephalopathy
Preeclampsia
Fetal adrenal abnormality
Intrauterine death
Down syndrome
Fetal chromosomal disorder

INTERFERING FACTOR

- Recent radioisotope scan

NURSING CARE

Nursing actions are similar to those used in other venipuncture procedures (see Chapter 2), with the following additional measures.

Pretest

- Schedule this test before or 7 days after any radioisotope scan. When serial tests are done, the blood should be drawn at the same time of day for each visit.
- On the lab requisition form, include the patient's information, including maternal age, gestation age as calculated by ultrasound, diabetic status, and maternal weight.

Exercise Challenge Test

See Pulmonary Function Studies on p. 557.

Fasting Blood Sugar

See Glucose, Fasting on p. 350.

Fasting Plasma Glucose

See Glucose, Fasting on p. 350.

Fasting Plasma Sugar

See Glucose, Fasting on p. 350.

Fecal Fat

fee-kuhl fat

Also called: Quantitative Fecal Fat; 72-Hour Collection

SPECIMEN OR TYPE OF TEST: Feces

PURPOSE OF THE TEST

This test identifies steatorrhea (fat in the fecal matter). It does not identify the cause of the problem, but rather evaluates the patient's ability to digest fat from dietary intake. Abnormal results support evidence of hepatobiliary, pancreatic, or small intestinal disease.

BASICS THE NURSE NEEDS TO KNOW

Dietary fats undergo digestion and absorption in the small intestine. The fat content is acted upon by bile acids, bile salts, and pancreatic enzymes until the end products can be absorbed by the small intestine. In normal digestion, almost all dietary fat is absorbed and the patient excretes only a small amount of fat in feces.

When malabsorption of fat occurs, the fat is not digested or absorbed fully. A high level of fat is eliminated in the feces and can be measured to determine the amount. The possible causes of steatorrhea are: (1) a lack of bile flow into the intestine, (2) pancreatic enzyme insufficiency, and (3) damage to the mucosa of the small intestine.

NORMAL VALUES Adult: 2–7 g/24 hours *or* SI: 2–7 g/day

HOW THE TEST IS DONE

For 3 days preceding the test and during the 3 days of specimen collection, the patient eats a standard high-fat diet (100 g of fat per day). The 72-hour collection period is performed on days 4, 5, and 6 of the diet. All fecal matter in the 72-hour period is collected in a clean, heavy plastic, screw-capped container. The specimen is kept cool in the refrigerator during the collection period.

SIGNIFICANCE OF TEST RESULTS

Elevated Values

Pancreatic obstruction
Pancreatic insufficiency
Chronic pancreatitis
Cystic fibrosis
Biliary tract obstruction
Liver cirrhosis
Impaired hepatic function
Lymphomas
Celiac disease
Tropical sprue
Radiation enteritis
Regional enteritis
Gastroduodenal fistula
Extensive small bowel resection

INTERFERING FACTORS

- Use of improper collection container
- Contamination of the specimen
- Failure to follow the dietary prescription
- Incomplete collection—omission of any specimen
- Alcohol ingestion before or during the test
- Ingestion of mineral oil before or during the test

NURSING CARE

Additional information regarding collection procedures for feces is presented in Chapter 2.

Pretest

- ***Patient Teaching.*** Instruct the patient to follow the prescribed diet for 3 days before and 3 days during the test. Ingestion of alcohol is omitted for the 72-hour test period. The nurse also instructs the patient about the correct procedure for collection of the stool specimen, including the correct container. Improper collection containers include coffee cans, paper cartons, waxed containers, or plastic bags. The specimen must be free of urine, toilet paper, tongue depressors, and plastic spoons.

During the Test

- Ensure that the specimen is refrigerated for the entire collection period and until it is transported to the lab.

Posttest

- Write the name and date for the start and finish of the collection period on the container label and on the requisition slip.

Ferritin

See Iron Studies on p. 411.

Fibrinogen

fai-brin-noh-jin

Also called: Factor I; Fibrinogen Level

SPECIMEN OR TYPE OF TEST: Blood

PURPOSE OF THE TEST

The fibrinogen test is used to help diagnose bleeding disorders, including afibrinogenemia, disseminated intravascular coagulation (DIC), and fibrinolysis.

BASICS THE NURSE NEEDS TO KNOW

Fibrinogen is a coagulation protein that is a vital contributor to the meshwork that binds platelets to form a clot. When vascular or tissue injury occurs, fibrinogen levels increase in the early phase of coagulation. Within 24 hours of the injury, the fibrinogen level rises dramatically. At the site of vascular disruption, adhesive proteins and fibrinogen bind the platelets together and plug the break in the vascular wall. As the clotting process progresses, fibrinogen converts to fibrin. The fibrin threads provide stability for the clot.

Elevated levels of fibrinogen normally occur during acute injury and in pregnancy. In abnormal conditions, the fibrinogen level rises, and an unwanted thrombus or embolus can occur. With decreased levels of fibrinogen, excess bleeding occurs because of a slower process of clot formation. This test may be performed as part of a DIC panel of coagulation tests. In DIC, the fibrinogen level is severely decreased (see also DIC Screen, pp. 274 to 275).

NORMAL VALUES

Adult: 150–400 mg/dL *or* SI: 1.5–4 g/L

HOW THE TEST IS DONE

A blue-topped tube with sodium citrate is used to obtain 4.5 mL of venous blood. As an alternative, a heelstick, earlobe, or finger puncture may be used to collect capillary blood in siliconized sodium citrate micropipettes.

F

SIGNIFICANCE OF TEST RESULTS

Elevated Values

Sepsis, infection
Inflammation
Malignancy
Traumatic injury

Decreased Values

Hereditary afibrinogenemia
Hypofibrinogenemia
Severe liver disease
DIC

INTERFERING FACTORS

- Heparinization
- Pregnancy (third trimester)
- Recent surgery
- Inadequate amount of specimen

NURSING CARE

Nursing actions are similar to those used in other venipuncture procedures (see Chapter 2), with the following additional measures.

Pretest

- For the patient who receives intermittent doses of heparin, schedule this test at least 1 hour after the medication is administered. In some methods of analysis, a recent heparin dose alters the test result.

During the Test

- When drawing the blood, the intravenous catheter line with a heparin lock should not be used, because the heparin flush procedure and residual heparin would invalidate the result of this test.

NURSING CARE—*cont'd*

Posttest

- For the patient with a suspected bleeding disorder, assess the venipuncture site for signs of bleeding or ecchymosis. To promote clotting, the nurse uses sterile gauze to apply pressure to the site, or raises the patient's arm above the head while maintaining pressure on the site.
- The nurse must notify the physician of a decreased value in the abnormal range because the patient is at risk for bleeding. The nurse assesses the patient for signs of abnormal bleeding, including petechiae (small red hemorrhagic spots in the skin), ecchymosis (bruising), hematuria, blood in the feces, or bleeding in the oral cavity. Baseline vital signs should be taken.

Fibrin Breakdown Products

See D-dimer and Fibrin Breakdown Products on p. 274.

Fibronectin, Fetal

fi-broh-nek-tin, fee-tul

Also called: (fFN); Fetal Fibronectin

SPECIMEN OR TYPE OF TEST: Cervicovaginal secretions

PURPOSE OF THE TEST

This test is used to determine the risk of a preterm (early) delivery in symptomatic and asymptomatic pregnant women.

BASICS THE NURSE NEEDS TO KNOW

Fibronectin is a glycoprotein that is present in various tissues, including the placenta and amniotic fluid. In normal processes, fetal fibronectin is present in cervicovaginal secretions of the pregnant woman before 21 weeks of gestation. It then disappears from the fluid and reappears at 37 weeks' gestation. In this late phase, the fibronectin leaks into the secretions, heralding the onset of labor.

If fetal fibronectin is present in the cervicovaginal secretions between the 21st and 37th week of gestation, the test value is positive (abnormal) and the patient is at high risk to have a preterm delivery in the next 7 days. The predictive accuracy of the test provides valuable information to the physician. With early warning of preterm labor and possible delivery of a premature infant, medical intervention can help delay labor and allow the fetus more time to mature. When fetal lungs have time to mature fully, the complication of respiratory distress syndrome (RDS) is prevented.

NORMAL VALUES Negative

HOW THE TEST IS DONE

After a dry speculum is inserted in the vagina, a special swab is rotated across the cervix and posterior fornix to collect cervicovaginal secretions. The swab is placed into a special tube with buffer solution and sealed closed with a special cap.

SIGNIFICANCE OF TEST RESULTS

Positive Value

Preterm labor within 7 days

INTERFERING FACTORS

- Sexual intercourse within the past 24 hours
- Lubricants
- Soap
- Disinfectants
- Creams
- Placenta previa
- Placental abruption
- Vaginal bleeding

NURSING CARE

Pretest

- When this test is to be performed, ensure that it is done before a digital examination or cervical ultrasound procedure. Any use of a lubricant, cream, soap, or disinfectant would interfere with the lab method of analysis, and tissue manipulation would alter the accuracy of the results. Ask the patient if she had sexual intercourse within the past 24 hours, for this activity would also manipulate the cervix and cause a false positive result.

During the Test

- After the secretions are collected and the swab is placed in the collection tube, the shaft of the swab must be broken at the scored line even with the top of the tube. The cap is pushed into the tube with the top of the shaft aligned with the hole in the center of the cap.

Posttest

- If the fetal fibronectin test result is negative, the patient is not in labor.
- If the test result is positive, and premature labor is predicted, the patient will be observed and will undergo additional assessment, including the monitoring for fetal contractions. The nurse will assist with the physician's vaginal examination and other diagnostic measures, such as testing for vaginal infection. Vital signs, including the maternal temperature and the fetal heart rate, are monitored and the results are recorded. Tocolytic medication may be prescribed to suppress the onset of labor, and antenatal corticosteroids may be prescribed to help the fetal lungs mature.

NURSING CARE—*cont'd*

- ***Patient Teaching.*** When the patient is to be discharged home, the nurse implements a plan for discharge teaching. This includes instruction to the patient to continue with prenatal visits to her health care provider. Guidelines regarding the patient's activity are individualized and reviewed with the patient. The patient also is taught to recognize the signs of preterm labor and what to do if it occurs.

Fine-Needle Biopsy of the Lung

See Biopsy, Lung, Percutaneous, Needle on p. 138.

Folic Acid, Serum

foh-lik a-sid, see-ruhm

Also called: Folate

SPECIMEN OR TYPE OF TEST: Serum

PURPOSE OF THE TEST

This test is used to detect folic acid deficiency and monitor replacement therapy. It is also used to investigate the cause of megaloblastic anemia.

BASICS THE NURSE NEEDS TO KNOW

Folic acid, also called folate, is one of the B vitamins important in the synthesis of protein and in the maintenance of a normal level of mature red blood cells in the blood. It is a necessary ingredient for DNA synthesis in the bone marrow and in other rapidly dividing cells, such as the lining of the intestinal tract and the neurologic system of the developing fetus. The natural intake of folate is from dietary sources. Foods that are rich in folate include Brewer's yeast, liver, green leafy vegetables, legumes, and citrus fruits or juices. The body's demand for folate is greatest in adolescence, the first trimester of pregnancy, and during lactation. To assist in overcoming the dietary deficiencies, the US government regulations now require that grain products be fortified with folate.

Decreased Values

The deficiency of folic acid affects DNA synthesis in the bone marrow. Fewer new red blood cells are produced and they are defective. If the problem is uncorrected, the patient develops anemia. In the mouth, the patient develops painful glossitis, or a loss of surface epithelium of the tongue. The loss of epithelium in the intestinal tract can cause gastritis, nausea, and constipation. There is new evidence that folate deficiency can cause neurologic symptoms, including depression, psychosis, and peripheral neuropathy. In the pregnant female, the deficiency is correlated with neural tube defect in the fetus, including anencephaly, spinal bifida, and others. This defect occurs in the first trimester of pregnancy. The US Department of Health and Human Services (2000) states that only 21% of pregnant women in the first trimester of pregnancy consume the optimum amount of folic acid in their diet.

Folate deficiency is usually due to a problem with dietary intake. The population groups who are most vulnerable to develop the deficiency include people who are poor and live in urban settings, elderly people, and pregnant women. Other causes include malabsorption syndrome or intestinal inflammation that interferes with absorption of this vitamin. Some medications cause folate deficiency, including anticonvulsants, methotrexate and other chemotherapy drugs, and oral contraceptives. Alcoholism will also cause folate deficiency.

NORMAL VALUES 3–20 ng/mL *or* SI: 7–45 nmol/L

HOW THE TEST IS DONE

A red-topped tube is used to obtain 10 mL of venous blood.

SIGNIFICANCE OF TEST RESULTS

Decreased Values

Megaloblastic anemia
Malnutrition
Pregnancy
Adult celiac disease
Regional enteritis
Malabsorption
Alcoholism

INTERFERING FACTORS

- Hemolysis
- Exposure to sunlight

NURSING CARE

Nursing actions are similar to those used in other venipuncture procedures (see Chapter 2), with the following additional measures.

Pretest

- The nurse should ensure that this test is done before blood transfusion is given or folate replacement is started. These factors would elevate the patient's serum value.
- If the patient takes medications, they should be listed on the lab requisition slip.
- ***Patient Teaching.*** The nurse instructs the patient to fast from food for 8 hours.

Posttest

- When folate deficiency is detected, additional data are needed to determine the cause of the deficiency and the existence of megaloblastic anemia before specific

NURSING CARE—*cont'd*

interventions are selected. Other blood tests to evaluate the problem include the complete blood count (CBC), hemoglobin, hematocrit, and mean corpuscular volume (MCV).

- The nurse assesses for signs of anemia that include pallor and fatigue or lethargy and shortness of breath. Glossitis, a reddened, sore tongue, is visible in examination of the oral cavity. The nurse can also do a nutritional assessment, especially for those patients who are pregnant, have cancer, receive chemotherapy treatment, or who are maintained on phenytoin (Dilantin), as well as those who are in the vulnerable age and economic groups.
- ***Health Promotion.*** Women who are trying to become pregnant or who just became pregnant are encouraged to take extra folic acid. The ideal time is 1 month before conception to the end of the first trimester. This is likely to be very important to prevent neural tube defect in the developing fetus. The daily requirement of folic acid is 400 mcg for nonpregnant women and 600 mcg during pregnancy. This amount can be obtained by taking one multivitamin tablet daily. The patient should be taught to eat folate-rich foods, but this intervention is insufficient to replace depleted folate stores and correct the anemia that has already occurred.

Free Cortisol

free kohr-ti-sol

SPECIMEN OR TYPE OF TEST: Urine

PURPOSE OF THE TEST

Free cortisol is evaluated to determine excessive production of glucocorticoids by the adrenal cortex.

BASICS THE NURSE NEEDS TO KNOW

When secreted by the adrenal cortex, cortisol binds with corticosteroid-binding globulin (CBG) and, to a much lesser degree, albumin. Only a small amount of cortisol circulates unbound or in the free state, which is the biologically active form. Free cortisol is normally excreted in the urine in small amounts.

If excessive secretion of cortisol occurs, the CBG-binding sites are filled, causing an increase in free cortisol; therefore, the urinary excretion increases. Because of this, an increased secretion of urinary free cortisol is helpful in diagnosing Cushing syndrome. It is not helpful in diagnosing adrenal insufficiency, because it is not sensitive at low levels, and low levels are relatively common in healthy individuals.

CBG is produced by the liver. Liver failure will affect CBG and, therefore, free cortisol levels. CBG is influenced by other factors. CBG levels increase in hyperthyroidism, diabetes, and high-estrogen states such as pregnancy. Genetic disorders may cause an increase or decrease in CBG. Hypothyroidism, protein deficiency, and renal failure may cause a decrease in CBG and influence free cortisol levels.

NORMAL VALUES 20–90 mcg/24 hr *or* SI: 55–248 nmol/24 hr

HOW THE TEST IS DONE

A 24-hour urine specimen is collected and assessed by radioimmunoassay (RIA) or by competitive protein-binding assay.

SIGNIFICANCE OF TEST RESULTS

Elevated Values

Cushing syndrome
Adrenal or pituitary tumor
Ectopic adrenocorticotropic hormone (ACTH) production

F

INTERFERING FACTORS

- Stress
- Physical activity
- Failure to collect all the urine during the 24-hour period
- Failure to store urine on ice or in a refrigerator
- Medications such as amphetamines, morphine sulfate, phenothiazines, reserpine, and steroids

NURSING CARE

Nursing actions are similar to those used in other timed urine collections (see Chapter 2), with the following additional measures.

Pretest

- ***Patient Teaching.*** The nurse instructs the patient to avoid strenuous physical activity. The patient is also taught the method to collect the specimen.

During the Test

- At the start of the test, the nurse instructs the patient to void at 8 AM and discard this urine. The collection period starts at this time, and all urine is collected for 24 hours, including the 8 AM specimen of the following morning.
- Keep the urine refrigerated or on ice throughout the collection period.

Posttest

- On the requisition slip and specimen label, write the patient's name and the time and date of the start and finish of the test period. Arrange for prompt transport of the cooled specimen to the lab.

Free Thyroxine

free thai-rok-sin

Also called: FT_4; Free T_4; Unbound T_4

SPECIMEN OR TYPE OF TEST: Serum

PURPOSE OF THE TEST

Free thyroxine is used to diagnose hyper- and hypothyroidism. It is especially helpful when abnormal thyroxine-binding globulin levels exist.

BASICS THE NURSE NEEDS TO KNOW

The majority of thyroxine (see section on Thyroxine, Total, p. 616) is carried by thyroid-binding globulin, albumin, and prealbumin. It is free thyroxine (FT_4), which is not bound, that is biologically active and converts to triiodothyronine (T_3) in the peripheral circulation. The ability to measure free thyroxine has replaced a classic test called *protein-bound iodine*.

Frequently, because of the expense of an FT_4 test, free thyroxine may be evaluated by the *free thyroxine index* (FT_4I), which is an estimated value. The FT_4I is calculated by multiplying the total T_4 by the thyroid hormone-binding ratio (THBR). The normal value for an adult is 4.2 to 13.0 (no units of value).

NORMAL VALUES

Adults: 0.9–2.7 ng/dL *or* SI: 11.5–35 pmol/L
Newborns: 2.6–6.3 ng/dL *or* SI: 33.5–81.3 pmol/L

HOW THE TEST IS DONE

Venipuncture is performed to collect 5 mL of blood in a red-topped tube.

SIGNIFICANCE OF TEST RESULTS

Elevated Values

Acute psychiatric disorders
Hyperthyroidism

Decreased Values

Anorexia nervosa
Hypothyroidism

INTERFERING FACTORS

- Medications such as carbamazepine, exogenous thyroid therapy, heparin, phenytoin, salicylates, and radioisotopes

NURSING CARE

Nursing actions are similar to those used in other venipuncture procedures (see Chapter 2), with the following additional measures.

Pretest

- The nurse checks with the lab. Depending on the lab methodology used, radionuclide scans may need to be scheduled after the blood is drawn for this test.
- The nurse checks with the physician if a serum albumin level is desired at the same time.

Free Triiodothyronine

free trai-ai-oh-doh-thai-roh-neen

Also called: FT_3; Free T_3

SPECIMEN OR TYPE OF TEST: Serum

PURPOSE OF THE TEST

Free triiodothyronine is used to diagnose hyper- and hypothyroidism.

BASICS THE NURSE NEEDS TO KNOW

Triiodothyronine is a hormone secreted by the thyroid gland. Most of the hormone is bound to thyroid-binding globulin. Some triiodothyronine is in the free state, that is, unbound. The unbound or free triiodothyronine is the biologically active form of the hormone.

NORMAL VALUES 260–480 pg/dL *or* SI: 4.0–7.4 pmol/L

HOW THE TEST IS DONE

Venipuncture is performed to collect a specimen in a red-topped tube.

SIGNIFICANCE OF TEST RESULTS

Elevated Values

Hyperthyroidism

Decreased Values

Hypothyroidism

INTERFERING FACTORS

- Exogenous thyroid therapy
- Radioisotopes within 7 days

NURSING CARE

Nursing actions resemble those of other venipuncture procedures, as presented in Chapter 2, with the following additional measures.

Pretest

- The nurse checks with the lab. Depending on the lab methodology used, radionuclide scans may need to be scheduled after the blood is drawn for this test.
- The nurse checks with the physician if a serum albumin level is desired at the same time.

Gamma-Glutamyltransferase

gam-uh-gloo-tuh-mil-trans-fuh-rays

Also called: (GGT)

SPECIMEN OR TYPE OF TEST: Serum

PURPOSE OF THE TEST

The gamma-glutamyltransferase test is used to detect hepatobiliary disease.

BASICS THE NURSE NEEDS TO KNOW

Gamma-glutamyltransferase (GGT) is an enzyme that is amply present in liver tissue. When there is damage to those hepatocytes that manufacture bile, the enzyme will release through the cell membranes and be absorbed into the blood. In addition, with cholestasis (stasis or obstruction of the flow of bile) within the liver or biliary system, the GGT level in the blood will rise early in the course of illness and remain elevated for as long as the dysfunction persists. In cases of biliary duct obstruction, the GGT value may rise from 5 to 50 times the upper limit of the normal value. In cases of hepatitis, the rise is more moderate and may be 5 times the upper limit of normal.

In the range of normal values, there are differences related to gender, age, and ethnicity. Newborn babies have values that are higher than children who are 6 months of age or older. The values for adult males are 25% higher than adult females. People of African ancestry have normal values that are double the values of those who are white, for all age groups.

G

NORMAL VALUES

Adult: 5–40 μkat(microkatal)/L *or* SI: 5–40 units/L
Male child >6 months: 2–30 units/L *or* SI: 0.03–0.51 μkat (microkatal)/L
Female child >6 months: 1–24 units/L *or* SI: 0.002–0.41 μkat (microkatal)/L

HOW THE TEST IS DONE

A venipuncture is performed to collect 10 mL of venous blood in a red-topped tube.

SIGNIFICANCE OF TEST RESULTS

Cancer of the liver (primary, metastatic)
Intrahepatic cholestasis
Hepatitis, infectious, alcoholic
Cirrhosis
Cholestasis
Biliary tract obstruction
Biliary cirrhosis
Cancer of the pancreas

INTERFERING FACTORS

- Alcohol ingested within 60 hours before the test
- Use of medications such as barbiturates, phenytoin, and acetaminophen

NURSING CARE

Nursing actions are similar to those used in other venipuncture procedures (see Chapter 2), with the following additional measures.

Pretest

- ***Patient Teaching.*** Instruct the patient to abstain from alcohol intake for 72 hours before the test. The patient should also fast from food for 8 hours before the test. The food and alcoholic intake would elevate the test result.
- If the patient takes medications that interfere with the accuracy of the test, the nurse should inform the physician or lab. Patients who must take these medications should not suspend the dosage schedule. An alternative test such as leucine aminopeptidase or 5′-nucleotidase may be preferable.

G

Gastric Analysis

gas-trik uh-nal-uh-sis

SPECIMEN OR TYPE OF TEST: Gastric secretions

PURPOSE OF THE TEST

Gastric analysis assists in the diagnosis of Zollinger-Ellison syndrome (gastrinoma) and other conditions associated with hypersecretion of gastric acid. It evaluates the ability of the stomach to produce acid secretions in a resting state.

BASICS THE NURSE NEEDS TO KNOW

Gastric analysis is a lab measurement of the volume of gastric secretions and the pH (concentration of hydrogen ions) of the gastric secretions. The basal acid output (BAO) is the analysis of the volume of gastric secretions that are aspirated via a nasogastric tube while the patient is in a resting (basal) state.

In the past, a separate phase of this test involved the use of histamine or pentagastrin stimulation to obtain the maximal acid output (MAO). In the United States, these gastric stimulants are no longer available; the gastric stimulation phase of the test cannot be done. In recent years, fiberoptic endoscopy with gastric tissue biopsy and serum gastrin have become the preferred tests to evaluate hyperacidity and gastric ulcers.

Patients who have marginal ulcers or duodenal ulcers tend to have higher-than-normal gastric acid output. Patients who have gastric cancer or gastric ulcers tend to have lower-than-normal gastric acid output. In Zollinger-Ellison syndrome, massive acid hypersecretion exists, usually >15 mEq/hr (SI: >15 mmol/hr).

Gastric pH is used to measure the concentration of the hydrogen ions and acidity. If the pH is in an alkaline range, the lack of acidity of the secretions is described as anacidity or achlorhydria, as characteristic in pernicious anemia.

NORMAL VALUES

Gastric pH
1.5–3.5 *or* SI: 1.5–3.5

BAO
Male: 0–10.5 mEq/hr *or* SI: 0–10.5 mmol/hr
Female: 0–5.6 mEq/hr *or* SI: 0–5.6 mmol/hr

HOW THE TEST IS DONE

A nasogastric tube with a radiopaque tip is passed into the patient's stomach until the tip is in the most dependent part of the stomach. Fluoroscopy or x-ray is used to confirm the location of the tip. The stomach is emptied of all secretions before the test begins and this gastric acid collection is discarded because it has been in the stomach for a while.

BAO. As the test begins, fresh secretions are removed during four consecutive 15-minute periods, using intestinal suction or manual suction with a large syringe. The secretions from each period are placed in separate containers, marked "BAO 1," "BAO 2," and so on. The test ends after 1 hour, with the collection of four specimens.

SIGNIFICANCE OF TEST RESULTS

Elevated Values

Zollinger-Ellison syndrome
Vagal hyperfunction
G cell hyperplasia
Systemic mastocytosis
Duodenal ulcers
Basophilic leukemia

Decreased Values

Pernicious anemia
Gastric ulcer
Cancer of the stomach
Chronic gastritis
Postsurgical antrectomy or vagotomy

INTERFERING FACTORS

- Failure to maintain a nothing-by-mouth status
- Failure to collect a complete amount of secretions
- Esophageal disease or aortic aneurysm
- Gastric bleeding

NURSING CARE

Pretest

- ***Patient Teaching.*** The nurse explains what will happen during the test and what the patient will feel, so that anxiety or apprehension will be minimized. Instruct the patient that for the 24 hours before the test, the patient must abstain from tobacco and alcohol. Apprehension, alcohol, and tobacco increase gastric acid secretions and would alter test results. With the physician's approval, instruct the patient to discontinue any medications that affect acid secretion and gastric motility, including antacids, H_2-receptor antagonists, tricyclic antidepressants, anticholinergics, and reserpine. Lastly, the client is instructed to discontinue food for 12 hours before the test.

During the Test

- Until the test is completed, the sight and smell of food is avoided. Psychologic, physiologic, and environmental stimuli regarding food are reduced to avoid gastric acid stimulation. This improves the reliability of the test results. The patient rests quietly in a seated position during the test. The patient is instructed to expectorate all saliva into a basin.

Posttest

- The nurse removes the nasogastric tube and the patient may resume eating. The nurse also ensures that each specimen container has a lid and that the container is appropriately labeled.

G

Gastrin

gas-trin

SPECIMEN OR TYPE OF TEST: Serum

PURPOSE OF THE TEST

Serum gastrin is a test used to help diagnose Zollinger-Ellison syndrome and pernicious anemia.

BASICS THE NURSE NEEDS TO KNOW

Gastrin is a hormone manufactured by specific cells in the gastric mucosa. Gastrin functions to stimulate the production of gastric acid and intrinsic factor and stimulates gastric motility and pancreatic secretions.

Elevated Values

A gastrinoma is a pancreatic or duodenal endocrine tumor. It produces large amounts of gastrin and the serum value can rise to >1000 pg/mL (SI: 1000 ng/L). This can cause increased gastric acid production and multiple peptic ulcers. When all three of these factors are present, the diagnosis of Zollinger-Ellison syndrome is made. In disorders with low or absent gastric acid production such as pernicious anemia, postsurgical vagotomy, and atrophic gastritis, the normal physiologic response is to increase the production of gastrin.

NORMAL VALUES	Adult (16–60 years): 25–90 pg/mL *or* SI: 25–90 ng/L Child: <10–125 pg/mL *or* SI: < 10–125 ng/L Infant (0–4 days) 120–183 pg/mL *or* SI: 120–183 ng/L

HOW THE TEST IS DONE

A red-topped tube is used to obtain 10 mL of venous blood.

SIGNIFICANCE OF TEST RESULTS

Zollinger-Ellison syndrome
Chronic atrophic gastritis
Pernicious anemia
Gastric ulcer
G cell hyperplasia
Vagotomy without gastric resection
Pyloric obstruction
Gastric cancer

INTERFERING FACTORS

- Recent radioisotope scan
- Failure to maintain a nothing-by-mouth status
- Recent gastroscopy

NURSING CARE

Nursing actions are similar to those used in other venipuncture procedures (see Chapter 2), with the following additional measures.

Pretest

- Schedule this test before gastroscopy and any nuclear scan. The gastroscopy can irritate the gastric mucosa and the radioisotopes would interfere with the lab method of analysis of the blood.
- ***Patient Teaching.*** Instruct the patient to fast from food for at least 12 hours before the test. This is because any recent intake of protein causes an elevation of the serum gastrin level.

Posttest

- Ensure that the specimen is sent to the lab without delay. Gastrin is unstable at room temperature and delay would invalidate the test result.

Gastrointestinal Cytology Studies

gas-troh-in-tes-tin-uhl sai-tol-oh-jee stu-deez

SPECIMEN OR TYPE OF TEST: Cytology, tissue culture

PURPOSE OF THE TEST

Cytologic examination identifies benign or malignant tissue. Tissue culture identifies the bacteria or virus that has caused tissue abnormality.

BASICS THE NURSE NEEDS TO KNOW

Specimens of abnormal tissue from the gastrointestinal tract are usually obtained from an endoscopy procedure, including esophagogastroduodenoscopy (EGD), endoscopic retrograde cholangiopancreatography (ERCP), colonoscopy, and endoscopic sigmoidoscopy. Once the tissue biopsy or aspiration of cells is completed, slides are prepared for microscopic study. The analysis of the tissue provides information about cellular change. If a microbiology tissue culture is required, some biopsy tissue is used to prepare a culture. After a few days of incubation, there is microbial growth in the culture medium. The bacteria, virus, or other pathogen that caused change in the tissue can be identified.

NORMAL VALUES

Within normal limits; no evidence of abnormal cells or infectious organisms

HOW THE TEST IS DONE

During the endoscopic examination, the tissue specimen is obtained by biopsy technique, brush technique, or washing technique.

Biopsy Technique

The physician passes a forceps through the endoscope and obtains several small samples of suspicious tissue. The tissue samples are placed on a filter paper, and the paper is placed in a jar with fixative solution.

Brush Technique

This technique involves using a disposable brush that is passed down the endoscopic instrument channel and passed over the suspicious tissue to obtain a sample of cells. The brush, with the cells and exudates are placed in a jar of fixative solution. As an alternative, the brush is passed over a slide that is moistened with saline. The slide is then placed in preservative in a jar, or it is sprayed with fixative.

Washing Technique

The physician uses the endoscope to inject 25 mL of normal saline on the lesion. The fluid, cells, and exudates are then aspirated and placed into a specimen container. This container must be placed on ice and sent to the lab immediately. There is no use of fixative, so warmth and time delay will cause lysis of the cells.

SIGNIFICANCE OF TEST RESULTS

Abnormal Values

ESOPHAGUS

Herpes simplex virus
Candida albicans
Cytomegalovirus
Esophageal cancer
Large cell malignant lymphoma

Stomach
Candida albicans
Large cell malignant lymphoma
Gastric cancer
Colon
Cytomegalovirus
Herpes simplex virus
Colon cancer
Premalignant polyps
Infectious colitis

INTERFERING FACTORS

- Barium study within 2 to 3 days before the endoscopy procedure
- Failure to properly label or transport the specimen
- Food or particulate matter near the specimen

NURSING CARE

The nursing care of the patient is fully presented in the section for the particular endoscopy procedure.

Posttest

- The endoscopy nurse must avoid confusion from mislabeling of the specimen.
- The lab requisition slip, the slides, and the specimen containers must all include the patient's name and the source of the tissue.

Gated Blood Pool Studies

gay-ted blud pool stu-deez

Also called: Technetium 99 Ventriculography; (MUGA); Multiple Gated Acquisition Angiography

SPECIMEN OR TYPE OF TEST: Radionuclide imaging

PURPOSE OF THE TEST

A gated blood pool study is performed to assess ventricular function by evaluating wall motion and determining ejection fractions.

BASICS THE NURSE NEEDS TO KNOW

A gated blood pool study is a noninvasive method of assessing myocardial function, particularly wall motion of the left ventricle. It also permits evaluation of left ventricular ejection without invasive catheterization.

NORMAL VALUES

Normal wall motion
Ejection fraction: 55%–75%
Response to exercise: Increase in ejection fraction greater than 5%

HOW THE TEST IS DONE

The procedure for the gated blood pool study is similar to that for myocardial imaging. The red blood cells are tagged with technetium 99m pyrophosphate, a gamma-emitting radionuclide. Because the bound technetium cannot diffuse through cell membranes, it remains in the blood. Its emissions are more concentrated in body cavities with large blood volumes, including the heart chambers.

During the procedure, the patient is monitored with a cardiac monitor, and the ECG is synchronized with the imaging equipment. Multiple images can be obtained. Results usually report the "first pass," which analyzes the radiotracing during the initial flow through the heart. In addition, a "gated" analysis is performed, which reports cardiac chamber responses of 200 to 300 cardiac cycles. Because left ventricular size can be measured at the end of diastole and systole, the ventricular ejection fraction can be measured. After a gated analysis, the patient may be reassessed with exercise stress testing.

SIGNIFICANCE OF TEST RESULTS

Hypokinesis (slightly diminished wall motion)
Akinesis (absence of wall motion)
Dyskinesia (paradoxical wall motion or bulging)
Decreased ejection fraction

INTERFERING FACTORS

- Uncooperative patient
- Failure to follow dietary restrictions

NURSING CARE

Pretest

- ***Patient Teaching.*** The nurse instructs the patient about the purpose and the procedure of the test. Explain to the patient that only a slight amount of radioactive substance is necessary, which will be excreted within hours. Patient needs to know to follow instructions regarding position changes. If an exercise stress test is included, explain procedure. The nurse also instructs the patient to wear comfortable, loose clothes and to avoid any heavy meals for 3 to 4 hours before the test.
- Check with the physician, but cardiac medications are usually continued.
- If the gated blood pool study is being done with a stress test, assess for contraindications. These include chest pain, hypertension; thrombophlebitis, second or third degree heart block, serious dysrhythmia, severe heart failure, and neurological, musculoskeletal, or vascular problems that would impede mobility.
- ***Patient Teaching.*** Ask the patient to inform the staff if he or she experiences any chest pain, shortness of breath, or nausea during the testing procedure.

During the Test

- Patient is maintained on a cardiac monitor. A blood pressure cuff is applied for periodic assessment.
- The patient is placed in the supine position and instructed to remain still. The camera is positioned close to the patient's chest.

NURSING CARE—*cont'd*

- A peripheral intravenous line is established. One or two doses of a tracer material are injected by the physician.

Posttest

- Evaluate the patient's physical and emotional response to the testing.
- The patient may resume normal diet and medications.
- Tracer elements will be excreted within hours. To handle patient's urine, the nurse will use Standard Precautions, wearing gloves and washing his or her hands afterward.
- See section on Stress Testing, Cardiac (p. 596) for Nursing Responses to Complications.

Genetic Testing for Cystic Fibrosis

je-ne-tik tes-ting fohr sis-tik fai-broh-sis

Also called: Cystic Fibrosis; DNA Detection

SPECIMEN OR TYPE OF TEST: Blood, buccal mucosal cells, amniotic fluid, chorionic villus cells

PURPOSE OF THE TEST

This test screens for the genetic mutation of cystic fibrosis that reveals carrier or disease status.

BASICS THE NURSE NEEDS TO KNOW

Cystic fibrosis is an inherited autosomal-recessive genetic disorder. In the heterozygous (carrier) form, the individual has one mutated gene for cystic fibrosis, but does not have the disease or symptoms of the disease. In the homozygous form, the individual inherits two mutated cystic fibrosis genes, one from each carrier parent. This individual inherits cystic fibrosis disease. When both reproductive partners have the heterozygous form of the genetic mutation, each pregnancy has a one in four chance (25% risk) of conceiving a child with cystic fibrosis disease. Cystic fibrosis most commonly affects the white, non-Hispanic population. This incidence of cystic fibrosis is somewhat higher in the white subgroup of Ashkenazi Jewish people and is relatively rare in all other ethnic groups.

As a disease, cystic fibrosis is a progressive disorder with a major impact on the health of the individual. Abnormal assessment findings begin in the newborn baby. The severity and manifestations vary among affected individuals, depending on the extent of the mutation of the affected genes. Commonly, however, the health problems include severe respiratory problems and recurrent respiratory infections due to the continuous production of thick, tenacious mucus that cannot be expectorated. In addition, the affected individual cannot secrete enough pancreatic enzymes to digest proteins and fats. Specific medical, nursing, and respiratory interventions are implemented in a life-long approach to manage symptoms and prolong life, but an earlier than normal death usually occurs from respiratory and cardiac failure.

To identify the carriers of this genetic mutation, the lab screening process is offered to the female prior to conception or early in the pregnancy. If she is positive for this mutation, she is given the information and genetic counseling. Her reproductive partner is then offered testing. Alternatively, both partners may be tested simultaneously. If the partner tests positive, both are given genetic counseling. They receive a thorough explanation of cystic fibrosis and their risk of transmitting the disease or the genetic carrier status to their offspring.

If the fetus is to be tested genetically for the disease, chorionic villus sampling is done at 10 to 13 weeks' gestation or amniocentesis is done at 15 to 20 weeks' gestation. If the fetus tests positive and has the homozygous genetic mutation of cystic fibrosis disease, the couple is given the information and counseling by their physician. They have a choice to terminate the pregnancy or carry the baby to term and prepare for the delivery of a child who will have many health care needs.

NORMAL VALUES

No detected genetic mutation

HOW THE TEST IS DONE

Blood: A lavender-topped (EDTA) tube or a yellow-topped (ACD) tube is used to collect 3 to 5 mL of blood.

Cell sample: Within the mouth, a sample of buccal cells from the inner surface of the cheek is collected, using a swab, scoop, or mouth rinse. The specimen is placed in a sterile container.

SIGNIFICANCE OF TEST RESULTS

Heterozygous mutation for the cystic fibrosis gene (carrier)
Homozygous mutation for the cystic fibrosis gene (disease)

INTERFERING FACTORS

- None

NURSING CARE

Nursing actions are similar to those used in other venipuncture procedures (see Chapter 2), with the following additional measures.

Pretest

- After the physician has explained this genetic screening test and its significance to the patient, a signed patient's consent is needed to perform the genetic testing.
- If the patient expresses apprehension or anxiety about the possible results of the genetic testing, the nurse can listen with empathy and support. It is important to know one's health status or risk so that potential decisions are based on fact and information. Four percent of white individuals do have one gene mutation, meaning that they are heterozygous or a carrier of the altered gene. The incidence of births of babies with cystic fibrosis disease among white individuals is 1 in every 2500 births. The risk to have a child with cystic fibrosis disease is much greater when there is a family history of cystic fibrosis or when one or both reproductive partners is a carrier.

NURSING CARE—*cont'd*

During the Test

- The lab requisition form should state additional information including the patient's ethnicity and pertinent family history.

Posttest

- ***Health Promotion.*** Screening for the genetic mutation of the cystic fibrosis gene is now recommended for all pregnant women, regardless of ethnicity. The nurse should teach women of childbearing age to have the test done early in the prenatal period. Some women and their partners may choose to have the test done when they are planning a pregnancy. If the test result is positive for the genetic mutation, it is hoped that the individual will inform the other family members so that they may decide to be tested and know their genetic status regarding this mutation.

Glucagon

gloo-kuh-gon

SPECIMEN OR TYPE OF TEST: Plasma

PURPOSE OF THE TEST

Glucagon levels are assessed in suspected pancreatic tumors, chronic pancreatitis, and familial hyperglucagonemia.

BASICS THE NURSE NEEDS TO KNOW

Glucagon is produced and secreted by the alpha cells of the islets of Langerhans of the pancreas. Glucagon stimulates the breakdown of stored glycogen and maintains gluconeogenesis. Glucagon is secreted in response to hypoglycemia, helping to meet glucose needs of tissues between intakes of food.

NORMAL VALUES

Adult: 20–100 pg/mL *or* SI: 20–100 ng/L
Child: 0–148 pg/mL *or* SI: 0–148 ng/L
Infant: 0–1750 pg/mL *or* SI: 0–1750 ng/L

HOW THE TEST IS DONE

Venipuncture is performed to obtain 7 mL of blood in a chilled lavender-topped tube. The specimen is placed on ice and sent to the lab immediately to be centrifuged.

SIGNIFICANCE OF TEST RESULTS

Elevated Values

Acute pancreatitis
Cirrhosis
Diabetic ketoacidosis
Glucagonoma
Hypoglycemia

Parasympathetic stimulation
Pheochromocytoma
Renal failure, chronic
Stress, high levels
Sympathetic stimulation

Decreased Values
Chronic pancreatitis
High fatty acid levels
Hyperglycemia
Insulinoma
Pancreatic tumors

INTERFERING FACTORS

- Stress
- Prolonged fasting
- Radioactive scan within 2 days
- Medications such as catecholamines, insulin, and glucocorticoids

NURSING CARE

The nurse takes actions similar to those used in other venipuncture procedures as described in Chapter 2, with the following additional measures.

Pretest

- ***Patient Teaching.*** The nurse instructs the patient to fast for 10 to 12 hours before the blood is drawn.

Explain to the patient the need to rest for 30 minutes before the test.

- The nurse takes a medication history and determines if any interfering drugs should be withheld until after the blood is drawn.
- Schedule any radioactive scans for after the glucagon determination is obtained.

Posttest

- Place the specimen on ice and send it to the lab immediately. (Not all laboratories require the specimen to be placed on ice.) The patient can resume a normal diet and medication regimen.

Glucose, Capillary

gloo-kohs, ka-pi-le-ree

Also called: (SBGM): Self-Blood Glucose Monitoring; (CBGM); Capillary Bedside Glucose Monitoring; Capillary Sugar Monitoring

SPECIMEN OR TYPE OF TEST: Blood

PURPOSE OF THE TEST

Capillary glucose monitoring is carried out to assess and manage patients with diabetes mellitus. It may be used in hospitals to monitor other hyperglycemic patients, such as those on hyperalimentation or high-dose glucocorticoid therapy. Capillary glucose evaluation is *not* used to diagnose diabetes mellitus, but it may indicate a need to assess plasma glucose levels. It is usually used as part of aggressive treatment for diabetes. The American Diabetes Association recommends that patients with type 1 diabetes mellitus check their capillary glucose levels three to four times a day. It is not clear how often patients with type 2 diabetes should check their capillary glucose levels; however, SBGM can help identify hypoglycemia in patients on sulfonylurea and other hypoglycemic agents. Controlling the blood glucose level in diabetes very strictly has been shown to lower the complications of the disease.

BASICS THE NURSE NEEDS TO KNOW

Capillary glucose monitoring has revolutionized the management of patients with insulin-dependent diabetes mellitus (IDDM). Capillary glucose monitoring determines the glucose level of whole blood (which is lower than serum or plasma levels). It evaluates current status, permitting more accurate management and therapy. It has replaced urine glucose testing as the preferred technique to determine insulin replacement requirements in hospitals and in the home.

To perform capillary glucose monitoring, a drop of capillary blood is dropped onto a reagent strip, and the glucose level is determined by the color changes on the strip. The color change can be compared to a color chart or assessed by a glucose meter. Because the visual method is subjective and some diabetics have visual impairment, glucose meters are preferable. Newer meters are relatively affordable (less than $50). For the diabetic who is blind, "talking" meters are available, but they are more expensive.

Non-insulin-dependent diabetics may find the use of capillary glucose monitoring helpful in managing their diabetes. These patients can check their glucose level 2 hours after they eat to see how specific foods affect it and modify their intake by an objective measurement.

For insulin-dependent and non-insulin-dependent diabetics, regular capillary glucose testing will produce greater control, with more effective long-term treatment. Capillary glucose testing can help the diabetic maintain control during periods of stress, for example, illness, pregnancy, and surgery. Usually, the patient with IDDM will monitor the capillary glucose level before each meal and at bedtime. The patient with non-insulin-dependent diabetes (NIDDM) usually monitors the capillary glucose twice a day—before breakfast and 2 hours after dinner.

Nurses need to teach their patients how to monitor capillary glucose, including how to use and care for the glucose meter and reagent strips and how to check the reliability of the meter. This information needs to be reinforced periodically.

NORMAL VALUES 60–110 mg/dL *or* SI: 3.3–6.1 mmol/L

HOW THE TEST IS DONE

A fingerstick is performed with a lancet, and a drop of blood is placed on a reagent strip. The intensity of the color change is proportional to the amount of glucose in the blood. The darker the color, the higher the glucose concentration. The color change is assessed, either visually by comparing it to a color chart or by the blood glucose meter. The meter may read the strip by the process of refractance photometry or by electrochemical technology. Either method will provide a digital readout of the glucose level.

SIGNIFICANCE OF TEST RESULTS

Elevated Values

Acromegaly
Chronic pancreatitis
Cushing syndrome
Diabetes mellitus
Hyperthyroidism
Hyperosmolar coma
Pheochromocytoma
Stress

Decreased Values

Addison's disease
Advanced liver disease
Alcohol intake when fasting
Excessive exogenous insulin
Islet cell adenoma
Leucine sensitivity
Malnutrition

INTERFERING FACTORS

- Failure to follow the manufacturer's guidelines

NURSING CARE

Many different glucose meters are on the market. It is *essential* to follow the manufacturers' guidelines for their use. In addition, a number of lancing devices are available.

Pretest

- Glucose meters should be checked daily in hospitals and once a week or when opening a new vial of strips at home, using quality control solution containing a known amount of dissolved glucose in water. The meter should also be tested if it is dropped or if the meter reading does not correlate with clinical assessments.
- When a fasting blood glucose determination is obtained, a capillary glucose level also can be obtained and the two measures compared. A variance of less than 15% is acceptable. Since plasma glucose levels are higher than whole blood levels, the nurse

NURSING CARE—*cont'd*

and patient need to know whether the glucose monitor used by the patient provides whole or plasma glucose measures.

- If the battery in the meter has worn out, recalibrate the meter with the plastic calibration strip provided in the reagent vial according to the manufacturer's guidelines.
- Check the code numbers on the glucose meter and on the reagent strip to ensure that they are the same. Check the expiration date on the reagent strip container and discard outdated strips.
- The nurse wears gloves for this procedure, because blood contact is possible.

During the Test

- Instruct the patient to wash his or her hands in warm water and soap. The warm water will help dilate the vessels.
- Hospital protocol may require the patient's finger to be wiped with an alcohol swab (this is usually not done in the home). If alcohol is used, it must be allowed to dry out or it will affect the results and increase the painfulness of the procedure.
- Have the reagent strip on hand, and puncture the skin. The puncture site should be on the side of the fingertip. The middle of the fingertip is more sensitive to pain, and the side has more capillaries. Instruct the patient to rotate sites.
- Let the drop of blood fall on the reagent strip so that the entire pad at the tip is covered with blood. Do not smear the blood or try to add another drop.
- Time the wiping of the strip, if required, and the insertion of the strip into the meter according to the manufacturer's guidelines. Timing is essential for accurate measurement. Some manufacturers require that a cotton ball be used to wipe the reagent strip.
- Insert the strip into the meter (Figure 52). Read and document the results.
- Instruct the patient on how to dispose of the lancet in a heavy plastic container, for example, an empty detergent bottle.

Posttest

- Administer insulin as ordered.
- ***Patient Teaching.*** Instruct the patient to keep an accurate record of the glucose level and insulin replacement. This record should be brought to the physician, diabetic nurse specialist, or clinic on the next visit.
- New, more sophisticated meters will keep a record of glucose values, which can be accessed by the health care provider.
- ***Patient Teaching.*** The procedure for teaching the capillary glucose testing to the patient in the home is the same as that for capillary bedside monitoring. The above nursing implementation integrates the teaching required. Emphasis must be placed on the patient's having an opportunity to practice self-blood glucose monitoring.
- ***Patient Teaching.*** Tell the patient to follow the manufacturer's instructions exactly. Unfortunately, the hospital glucometer may not be the same as the one the patient will use at home. The community health nurse needs to assess the patient's ability to apply hospital learning to the home environment. Reinforce learning. Periodically,

Continued

G

NURSING CARE—*cont'd*

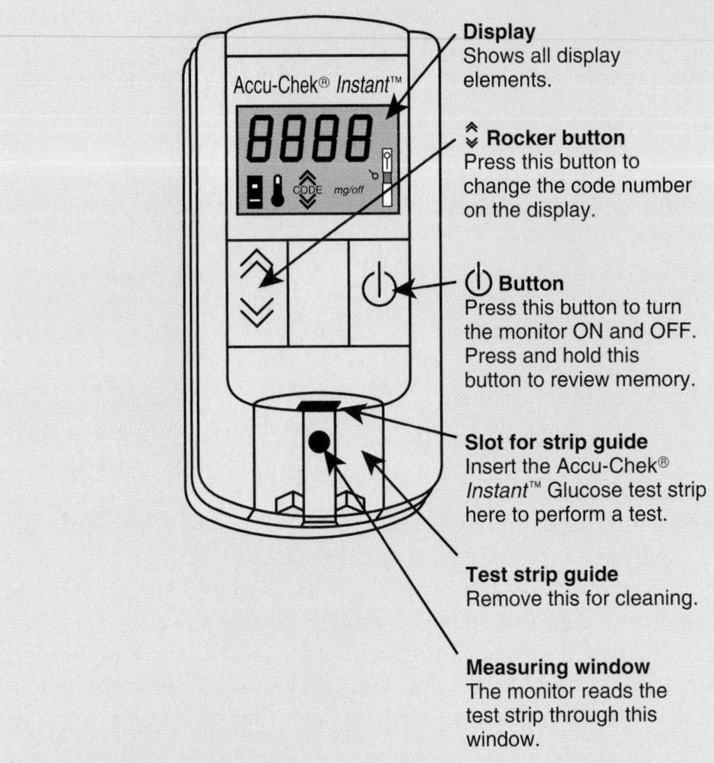
Accu-Chek® Instant™
8888
CODE
mg/off
Display
Shows all display elements.
Rocker button
Press this button to change the code number on the display.
Button
Press this button to turn the monitor ON and OFF. Press and hold this button to review memory.
Slot for strip guide
Insert the Accu-Chek® Instant™ Glucose test strip here to perform a test.
Test strip guide
Remove this for cleaning.
Measuring window
The monitor reads the test strip through this window.

Figure 52. Glucometer. *(Reproduced with permission from Stepp, C. A., & Woods, M. A. [1998]. Laboratory procedures for medical office personnel [p. 217]. Philadelphia: W. B. Saunders.)*

the community health nurse needs to observe the patient's technique to ensure accurate test results. If the patient is using a color chart to determine glucose levels, periodic visual evaluation is appropriate. Instruct the patient to document test results and any insulin administered based on the results and bring the record to the physician, nurse practitioner, or diabetic clinic on each visit.

Glucose, Fasting

gloo-kohs, fas-ting

Also called: (FBS); Fasting Blood Sugar; (FPS); Fasting Plasma Sugar

SPECIMEN OR TYPE OF TEST: Whole blood, serum, plasma

PURPOSE OF THE TEST

Fasting glucose is evaluated to diagnose and manage patients with diabetes mellitus. The fasting glucose level also is obtained as supportive data in many diagnoses, because metabolic factors will influence glucose use and storage. Certain therapies may be evaluated by checking the fasting blood glucose level, (e.g., hyperalimentation and exogenous glucocorticoid therapy).

BASICS THE NURSE NEEDS TO KNOW

To meet cellular needs, the body has developed complex mechanisms to take in, use, and store nutrients. A serum glucose level determination reflects the ability of the body to perform its metabolic tasks. Glucose levels are not static; they vary after eating, so a fasting blood glucose (FBS) level determination is desirable. Many factors influence blood glucose, but testing is most frequently used to diagnose and manage diabetes mellitus.

With age, the norms for blood and plasma glucose levels are adjusted by 1 mg/dL per year of life after age 60.

A single elevated fasting plasma glucose test is not considered diagnostic when symptoms are not present, but the test should be repeated. If the second fasting blood glucose level test result is elevated (>126 mg/dL *or* SI: 6.99 mmol/L), it supports the diagnosis of diabetes mellitus.

NORMAL VALUES	**Children 2 years to adult** Whole blood: 60–110 mg/dL *or* SI: 3.3–6.1 mmol/L Plasma or serum: 70–110 mg/dL *or* SI: 3.9–6.1 mmol/L **Elderly individuals** 80–150 mg/dL *or* SI: 4.4–8.3 mmol/L **Children <2 years** 60–100 mg/dL *or* SI: 3.3–5.6 mmol/L **Infant** 40–90 mg/dL *or* SI: 2.2–5.0 mmol/L **Neonate** 30–60 mg/dL *or* SI: 1.7–3.3 mmol/L
▼ Critical Values	<60 mg/dL or >400 mg/dL or, in neonates, <30 mg or >300 mg/dL

HOW THE TEST IS DONE

After a 12-hour fast, venipuncture is performed to obtain 5 mL of blood in a red-topped tube. Usually a plasma sampling is performed, because it reflects glucose levels in interstitial tissue and is not affected by the hematocrit.

SIGNIFICANCE OF TEST RESULTS

Elevated Values

Acromegaly
Chronic pancreatitis
Cushing syndrome
Diabetes mellitus
Hyperthyroidism
Hyperosmolar coma
Pheochromocytoma
Stress

Decreased Values

Addison's disease
Advanced liver disease
Alcohol intake when fasting
Excessive exogenous insulin
Islet cell adenoma
Leucine sensitivity
Malnutrition

INTERFERING FACTORS

- Noncompliance with fasting
- Vigorous exercise
- Stress
- Medications such as acetaminophen, arginine, benzodiazepines, beta blockers, epinephrine, ethacrynic acid, furosemide, glucocorticoids, glucose, hypoglycemic agents, insulin, lithium, MAO inhibitors, oral contraceptives, phenothiazines, phenytoin, and thiazide diuretics

NURSING CARE

Nursing actions are similar to those used in other venipuncture procedures (see Chapter 2), with the following additional measures.

Pretest

- ***Patient Teaching.*** The nurse instructs the patient to fast for 12 hours before the blood is drawn. Instruct the patient who is taking insulin or hypoglycemic agents to withhold the medication until after the blood is drawn.
- The nurse observes the patient for clinical manifestations of hypoglycemia.

Posttest

- The nurse ensures that the patient receives food and medications that were withheld.
- Send blood to the lab, because it needs to be centrifuged within 30 minutes for serum and plasma levels.

NURSING CARE—*cont'd*

- ***Health Promotion.*** The American Diabetes Association recommends that the Fasting Plasma Glucose (FPG) be used to evaluate patients. It also recommends that women at risk for gestational diabetes mellitus (obesity, history of GDM, or a family history of diabetes) should have FPG at her first prenatal visit.

Nursing Response to Critical Values

A low fasting plasma sugar (FPS) result indicates hypoglycemia. Notify the physician. If the patient is alert and not in danger of aspiration, give glucose by mouth. If the patient is unconscious, or if aspiration is likely, prepare to give 50% glucose intravenously as ordered.

High FPS indicates hyperglycemia, usually related to diabetes ketoacidosis or hyperosmolar coma. Notify the physician. Change any glucose-containing infusion the patient is receiving to a nonglucose solution. Prepare to give short-acting insulin as ordered. Assess ketone levels.

Nursing Response to Complications

Because a fasting glucose determination requires that the patient maintain a nothing-by-mouth status, hypoglycemia may occur.

Hypoglycemia. Indications of hypoglycemia are: pallor, diaphoresis, tachycardia, palpitations, hunger, paresthesia, vagueness, confusion, slurred speech, somnolence, convulsions and coma. If signs of hypoglycemia occur, the nurse should check the patient's capillary glucose level and obtain a specimen for a plasma glucose level. If the patient is awake and able to swallow, glucose is given orally. Notify the physician.

Glucose Loading Test

See Growth Hormone Suppression Test on p. 365.

Glucose, Postprandial

gloo-kohs, pohst-pran-dee-uhl

Also called: 2-Hour Postprandial Blood Sugar

SPECIMEN OR TYPE OF TEST: Plasma

PURPOSE OF THE TEST

The 2-hour postprandial glucose test is performed to support the diagnosis of diabetes mellitus and to evaluate the management of a patient with diabetes mellitus.

BASICS THE NURSE NEEDS TO KNOW

In healthy individuals, the ingestion of food raises the blood glucose level, which is a potent stimulant for insulin release. The insulin level peaks in less than an hour. Normally, within 1½ to 2 hours, the glucose level will return to baseline. It may take slightly longer in older individuals for the value to return to a baseline level. The 2-hour

G

postprandial glucose test evaluates whether the individual has an adequate insulin response to intake. A diabetic is considered in good control if the 2-hour postprandial glucose level is less than 130 mg/dL. In an undiagnosed case, a 2-hour postprandial glucose level greater than 140 mg/dL indicates that an oral glucose tolerance test (OGTT) should be performed.

NORMAL VALUES Fasting plasma glucose: <126 mg/dL *or* SI: <6.993 mmol/L
Values may be slightly elevated in elderly patients

HOW THE TEST IS DONE

Two hours after a meal is ingested, venipuncture is performed to obtain 5 mL of blood in a red-topped tube for a plasma glucose level determination.

SIGNIFICANCE OF TEST RESULTS

A 2-hour postprandial glucose determination greater than 126 mg/dL is consistent with the diagnosis of diabetes mellitus. Diagnosis is not made with a 2-hour postprandial glucose test; an elevation indicates a need for a fasting plasma sugar or oral glucose tolerance test.

INTERFERING FACTORS

- Noncompliance with dietary requirements
- Cushing's disease or Cushing syndrome
- Infection
- Malabsorption syndrome
- Malnutrition
- Severe stress
- Medications such as arginine, beta-adrenergic blockers, epinephrine, glucocorticoids, glucose administered intravenously, hypoglycemic agents, insulin, lithium, phenothiazines, and phenytoin.

NURSING CARE

Nursing actions are similar to those used in other venipuncture procedures (see Chapter 2), with the following additional measures.

Pretest

- Instruct the patient to eat normally before the test.

During the Test

- The patient ingests a meal containing at least 100 g of carbohydrate.
- Instruct the patient not to eat or drink for 2 hours after the meal is ingested.
- Venipuncture is performed to obtain a blood glucose level 2 hours after the meal.

Posttest

- The patient resumes a normal diet.

Glucose-6-Phosphate Dehydrogenase Screen

gloo-kohs-siks-fos-fayt dee-hai-droj-uh-nays skreen

Also called: G-6-PD Screen

SPECIMEN OR TYPE OF TEST: Blood

PURPOSE OF THE TEST

This test is used to detect a G-6-PD enzyme defect in erythrocytes and determine this cause of hemolytic anemia.

BASICS THE NURSE NEEDS TO KNOW

Genetic defects in erythrocyte metabolism are responsible for many forms of hemolytic anemia. The deficiency of the glucose-6-phosphate dehydrogenase (G-6-PD) enzyme in the erythrocyte is the most common cause of sudden hemolysis and is commonly associated with chronic hemolytic anemia. With deficient or diminished enzyme activity, the erythrocytes have a shorter lifespan. The deficiency of this enzyme is hereditary and linked to the X chromosome. This type of hemolytic anemia is seen most frequently in African Americans and is usually a mild condition. A more severe, but rare, form of the disorder affects individuals from Asia and the countries of the Mediterranean.

In individuals with G-6-PD deficiency, a sudden, acute episode of severe hemolytic anemia usually is triggered by the administration of particular drugs, an infection, or an illness. The medications include sulfonamides, antimalarial drugs, aspirin, and a variety of other medications. The ingestion of fava beans may also cause an episode of hemolysis. The illnesses that can trigger hemolytic episodes are usually acute bacterial or viral infections or metabolic disorders, including acidosis. In severe infection, the anemia can be life threatening. Other individuals have a mild or moderate condition, but it can become chronic, particularly if the triggering factor is not eliminated. Finally, some people have the condition, but never experience hemolytic anemia.

NORMAL VALUES G-6-PD enzyme activity is present

HOW THE TEST IS DONE

A lavender-topped tube is used to collect 7 mL of venous blood.

SIGNIFICANCE OF TEST RESULTS

Decreased Values

G-6-PD anemia, mild to moderate
G-6-PD anemia, severe

INTERFERING FACTORS

- Sudden, severe hemolysis

NURSING CARE

Nursing actions are similar to those used in other venipuncture procedures (see Chapter 2), with the following additional measures.

Posttest

- If the patient is diagnosed with G-6-PD deficiency, he or she needs to understand which triggering factors can cause an episode of anemia, and eliminate the causative food (fava beans) or medication (as sulfa drugs). The patient should also be instructed to avoid aspirin or nonprescription medications that contain aspirin.
- During a period of additional stress, as with surgery or infection, an episode of severe hemolysis can occur. If the patient has an episode of severe hemolysis, the nurse should assess for severe pallor and possible abdominal pain. Later, jaundice will occur. The indirect bilirubin level rises. The patient's sclera and skin develop a yellow tinge, and the urine turns darker in color as bilirubin is excreted. Severe episodes last about 7 to 12 days, and then the condition recedes. For mild or severe episodes, the nurse encourages the patient to rest because fatigue accompanies anemia. If the hemolysis is severe enough, the physician may prescribe a transfusion of red blood cells. In addition, extra fluid intake will help promote renal function and urinary output. A nutritious diet will help in the recovery process as the patient begins to manufacture new erythrocytes.

G

Glucose Tolerance Test

gloo-kohs to-luhr-uhns test

Also called: (GTT); (OGGT); Oral Glucose Tolerance Test; (IVGGT), Intravenous Glucose Tolerance Test

SPECIMEN OR TYPE OF TEST: Plasma

PURPOSE OF THE TEST

The glucose tolerance test is performed to confirm the diagnosis of diabetes mellitus.

BASICS THE NURSE NEEDS TO KNOW

Fasting plasma glucose level determinations, if repeated, are usually adequate to diagnose diabetes mellitus if the plasma glucose level is greater than 126 mg/dL. However, if the fasting blood glucose levels are questionable, and clinical indications make diabetes mellitus likely, an oral glucose tolerance test (OGTT) or an intravenous glucose tolerance test (IVGTT) may be performed. Other indications include delivery of an infant weighing more than 9 lb (4.1 kg), frequent vaginal yeast infections, and impotence in males.

The *IVGTT* is similar to the OGTT. It is usually ordered when the patient has a problem with gastrointestinal absorption. It is not preferable to the OGTT because it bypasses normal glucose absorption and, therefore, normal changes in gastrointestinal hormones.

Patient preparation for the IVGTT is the same as that for the OGTT, except that the glucose load (0.5 g/kg of ideal body weight) is given intravenously over 2 to 3 minutes. The fasting blood glucose levels after the IVGTT are similar to those after an OGTT, except that the 30-minute ingestion fasting blood glucose level tends to be higher.

The OGTT confirms the diagnosis of diabetes mellitus if the 2-hour blood glucose level is greater than 200 mg/dL and at least one other blood glucose determination is greater than 200 mg/dL. Blood glucose levels between the diagnostic criteria and normal values are called *impaired glucose tolerance*.

NORMAL VALUES

Baseline fasting blood glucose level: 70–105 mg/dL *or*
SI: 3.9–5.8 mmol/L
30-minute blood glucose level: 110–170 mg/dL *or*
SI: 6.1–9.4 mmol/L
60-minute blood glucose level: 120–170 mg/dL *or*
SI: 6.7–9.4 mmol/L
90-minute blood glucose level: 100–140 mg/dL *or*
SI: 5.6–7.8 mmol/L
120-minute blood glucose level: 70–120 mg/dL *or*
SI: 3.9–6.7 mmol/L

HOW THE TEST IS DONE

After the ingestion of a glucose load, venous blood samplings for plasma glucose are obtained at the time of ingestion and then at 30, 60, 90, and 120 minutes after the glucose load is given.

SIGNIFICANCE OF TEST RESULTS

Diabetes mellitus
Impaired glucose tolerance

INTERFERING FACTORS

- Noncompliance with dietary and fasting requirements
- Alcohol ingestion
- Being bedridden
- Cushing syndrome or Cushing's disease
- Infection
- Malabsorption syndrome
- Malnutrition
- Pregnancy
- Severe stress
- Smoking
- Medications such as amphetamines, arginine, beta-adrenergic blockers, diuretics, epinephrine, glucocorticoids, glucose administered intravenously, insulin, lithium, oral contraceptives, oral hypoglycemic agents, phenothiazines, phenytoin, and salicylates

NURSING CARE

Nursing actions are similar to those used in other venipuncture procedures (see Chapter 2), with the following additional measures.

Pretest

- The nurse takes a medication history to determine if any interfering drugs are being taken. Check with the physician to determine if medications should be withheld. Oral hypoglycemic agents are withheld for 2 weeks before an OGTT is performed. The nurse also questions the patient regarding any recent acute illnesses. The OGTT should be delayed for at least 2 weeks after an acute illness.
- ***Patient Teaching.*** Instruct the patient to take in at least 150 to 250 g of carbohydrates per day for 3 days before the test to optimize insulin secretion.
- ***Patient Teaching.*** Instruct the patient not to drink or eat for 8 hours before the test begins. The patient is also instructed to avoid stimulants and not to smoke or perform any unusual activity for 8 hours before the test.

During the Test

- A fasting blood glucose determination is performed (usually in the early morning between 7 AM and 9 AM).
- Within 5 minutes of obtaining the baseline fasting blood glucose level, the patient drinks 75 g of glucose in 300 mL of water. Children are given 1.5 g of glucose per kilogram of ideal body weight. The glucose solution should be ingested within 5 minutes.
- Venipunctures are performed to obtain blood glucose readings at 30, 60, 90, and 120 minutes after the glucose solution is ingested. If a hypoglycemic reaction is suspected, a 3-hour blood specimen is obtained.
- The nurse observes the patient for a hyper- or hypoglycemic reaction.
- The patient may drink water during the collection period.

Posttest

- The patient resumes taking medications that were withheld.
- A normal diet and activity level are resumed.
- ***Health Promotion.*** The American Diabetes Association recommends that pregnant women at the 24th to 28th week of gestation have an OGTT done using 50 g of glucose. If any abnormality results, a repeat OGTT is done with 100 g of glucose. Many recommend that any pregnant woman at risk for gestational diabetes have the OGTT done in the 16th to 18th week of pregnancy and repeat the test at the 24th to 28th week.

Glucose, Urinary

gloo-kohs, yur-i-ner-ee

Also called: (SMUG); Self-Monitoring of Urine Glucose; Urinary Sugar

SPECIMEN OR TYPE OF TEST: Urine

PURPOSE OF THE TEST

When capillary glucose monitoring is not possible, urinary glucose is measured to determine insulin and dietary requirements of patients with diabetes mellitus. Urinary glucose levels only provide a rough estimate of current blood glucose levels.

BASICS THE NURSE NEEDS TO KNOW

As serum glucose levels rise, the renal threshold for glucose will be reached and glucose will "spill out" into the urine. The presence of glycosuria (glucose in the urine) once played a major role in regulating the diet and insulin therapy of patients with diabetes mellitus. The urine was checked four times a day—before each meal and at bedtime—and insulin coverage given depending on how much glucose was spilled.

Today, patients with insulin-dependent diabetes mellitus (IDDM) and many patients with non-insulin-dependent diabetes mellitus (NIDDM) are regulated by self-capillary blood glucose monitoring. Capillary glucose monitoring is superior to urinary glucose testing because it reflects the patient's current glucose status, whereas urine reflects the blood glucose level at the time the urine was formed.

If the patient is planning to use self-monitoring of urinary glucose (SMUG) to manage his or her diabetes, the renal glucose threshold must be determined; otherwise, the patient may be overtreated or undertreated.

NORMAL VALUES Negative

HOW THE TEST IS DONE

Two methods are commonly used to check for urinary glucose—copper reduction tests (using Clinitest tablets) or the reagent strip method. The latter is more frequently used at home.

SIGNIFICANCE OF TEST RESULTS

Glucosuria may be a result of the following:

Diabetes mellitus
Chronic renal failure
Cushing syndrome
Thyroid disorders
Fanconi syndrome
Hyperalimentation
Pregnancy

INTERFERING FACTORS

- Failure to use fresh urine
- Urine heavily contaminated with bacteria
- Clinitest tablet or dipstick exposed to air, light, heat, or moisture
- Medications such as acetylsalicylic acid, chloral hydrate, glucocorticoids, isoniazid, levodopa, lithium, methyldopa, penicillin G, probenecid, salicylates, streptomycin, tetramycin, and thiazide diuretics

NURSING CARE

Because this test is used for self-monitoring, patient education is an essential part of the nursing role.

Pretest

- ***Patient Teaching.*** Instruct the patient to collect the specimen in a clean container.
- With the Clinitest tablets, heat is created by the chemical action. Warn the patient not to hold the test tube in the hand after dropping the tablet into it.

During the Test

Clinitest Tablet

- Add 5 drops of urine and 10 drops of water to a clean, dry test tube and then drop a Clinitest tablet into the test tube.
- Compare the color change of the urine with the color chart that comes with the tablets.
- Record results.

Dipstick Method (Clinistix, Diastix, TesTape)

- The dipstick is dipped in urine. The waiting time is indicated by the manufacturer.
- Compare the color change with the chart provided and record the results.

Posttest

- Clean the equipment with soap and water and rinse thoroughly.
- Store the tablets and dipstick in a dry, cool place in their original containers.
- Document the results on a flow sheet.
- Adjust insulin dosage as ordered based on the results.
- ***Patient Teaching.*** The nurse consults with the physician and the patient regarding the method of SMUG that will be used at home. Most patients choose to collect their urine in a disposable paper cup. Instruct the patient according to the chosen method (see Nursing Care section above). Provide the patient with the opportunity to practice SMUG.
- The community health nurse assesses the patient's ability to apply hospital learning to the home and reinforces the learning. Periodically, the community health nurse needs to observe the patient's technique to ensure that test results are accurate. Periodic evaluation of the patient's visual acuity is necessary, because the patient must use a color chart to determine glucose level. Instruct the patient to document results and any insulin taken based on the results and to bring the record to the physician, nurse practitioner, or diabetes clinic at each visit.

Glycosylated Hemoglobin Assay

glai-koh-si-lay-ted hee-moh-gloh-bin a-say

Also called: Glycohemoglobin (GHb); Hemoglobin A_{1c}; Hb A

SPECIMEN OR TYPE OF TEST: Blood

PURPOSE OF THE TEST

A glycosylated hemoglobin determination is performed to measure a patient's diabetic control over a period of weeks or months. The maximum period for evaluation of control is the lifespan of the red blood cells (120 days).

BASICS THE NURSE NEEDS TO KNOW

Glycosylated hemoglobin refers to hemoglobin that has hooked up with glucose. The major glycosylated hemoglobin is hemoglobin A_{1c}, which is approximately 4% of the total hemoglobin. The other glycosylated hemoglobins are phosphoxylated glucose (A_{1a}) and phosphoxylated fructose (A_{1b}).

The reaction between glucose and hemoglobin is based on the blood glucose concentration. The higher the glucose concentration, the higher the percentage of glycosylated hemoglobin. Because the reaction is not reversible, once the glucose adheres to the hemoglobin it remains glycosylated. Since the lifespan of a red blood cell is normally 120 days, measuring the glycosylated hemoglobin can assist in diabetic control assessment. It is not affected by recent changes in diet or medication, as fasting blood glucose levels are, so the physician can determine diabetic control over a period of weeks or months. The guidelines of the American Diabetes Association published in 2002 recommend that the A_{1c} test be done routinely in the management of patients with type 1 diabetes and that the patient's goal should be <7%.

The reliability of the test is based on normal hemoglobin levels. If a person has an abnormal hemoglobin value, the accuracy of the HbA_{1c} is suspect. An example of this is the sickle cell trait. Also, any condition that shortens or lengthens the life of the red blood cells will make the results questionable.

NORMAL VALUES (may vary with assay technique used)	
	Normal, healthy person: 5.5%–8.8% of total hemoglobin *or* SI: 0.05–0.08 (fraction of total hemoglobin)
	Diabetic under control: 7% of total hemoglobin
	Hemoglobin A_{1a}: 1.8% of total hemoglobin
	Hemoglobin A_{1b}: 0.8% of total hemoglobin
	Hemoglobin A_{1c}: 3%–6% of total hemoglobin

HOW THE TEST IS DONE

Venipuncture is performed to obtain 5 mL of blood in a lavender- or green-topped tube.

SIGNIFICANCE OF TEST RESULTS

Elevated Values

Poorly controlled diabetes mellitus
Hyperglycemia

INTERFERING FACTORS

- Acetylsalicylic acid (chronic ingestion)
- Anemia

- Chronic renal failure
- Clotting of specimen
- Fetal-maternal transfusion
- Hemodialysis
- Hemorrhage
- Hemolytic disease
- Phlebotomies
- Thalassemias
- Vitamin C and E

G

NURSING CARE

Nursing actions are similar to those used in other venipuncture procedures (see Chapter 2), with the following additional measures.

- ***Health Promotion.*** Patients who have diabetes need to be aware of the need to keep close glycemic control of their condition to prevent complications. The nurse encourages the patient to follow up on prescribed glycosylated testing. The nurse teaches the patient about lowering the A_{1c} to 7% or less to reduce the risk of microvascular and neuropathological complications.

Growth Hormone

grohth hohr-mohn

Also called: (GH); Somatotropin; (STH); hGH

SPECIMEN OR TYPE OF TEST: Serum

PURPOSE OF THE TEST

Growth hormone levels are evaluated to diagnose growth disorders and possible pituitary tumors. Abnormal linear growth may be a result of several factors: genetics, chronic disease, malnutrition, and so forth. Growth hormone levels will assist in determining the cause of the growth disorder and thereby influence therapy and prognosis.

BASICS THE NURSE NEEDS TO KNOW

Growth hormone is synthesized and secreted by the anterior pituitary gland under the direction of the hypothalamus. The hypothalamus controls growth hormone secretion via somatostatin (growth hormone release-inhibiting hormone) and growth hormone releasing hormone. The primary function of growth hormone is the promotion of linear growth, which it does by stimulating the production of somatomedin, which is produced by a variety of organs.

During linear growth and afterward, growth hormone influences protein, carbohydrate, and fat metabolism. It increases protein synthesis, decreases protein catabolism, and activates lipolysis. Excessive growth hormone will decrease carbohydrate use and glucose uptake by the cells.

NORMAL VALUES

Adult male: Undetectable–5 ng/mL *or* SI: 0–5 mcg/L
Adult female: Undetectable–10 ng/mL *or* SI: 0–10 mcg/L
Child: Undetectable–16 ng/mL *or* SI: 0–16 mcg/L
Infants: 2–10 ng/L *or* SI: 2–10 mcg/L
Newborns: 5–53 ng/mL *or* SI: 5–53 mcg/L
Cord blood: 8–41 ng/mL *or* SI: 8–41 mcg/L

HOW THE TEST IS DONE

Five milliliters of venous blood is drawn into a red-topped tube and sent to the lab.

SIGNIFICANCE OF TEST RESULTS

Elevated Values

Pituitary tumor
Hypothalamic tumor
Acromegaly
Gigantism

Decreased Values

Dwarfism
Metastatic or anoxic pituitary destruction

INTERFERING FACTORS

- Failure to fast for 8 to 12 hours before the test
- Administration of radioactive scan within 7 days
- Medications such as amphetamines, arginine, beta blockers, chlorpromazine, corticosteroids, dopamine, glucagon, insulin, levodopa, and oral contraceptives

G

NURSING CARE

Nursing actions are similar to those used in other venipuncture procedures (see Chapter 2), with the following additional measures.

Pretest

- Obtain a drug history to determine if any interfering medication is being taken.
- The nurse inquires if the patient has undergone any recent radioactive scans.
- ***Patient Teaching.*** The nurse instructs the patient to limit activity and not eat or drink for 8 to 12 hours before the specimen is collected.

During the Test

- The nurse takes actions similar to those for other venipuncture procedures.

Posttest

- The patient can resume diet and the medications that were withheld.
- Send the specimen to the lab on ice.
- The nurse informs the patient that normal activity may be resumed.

Growth Hormone Stimulation Test

grohth hohr-mohn sti-myoo-lay-shun test

Also called: Arginine Test; (ITT); Insulin Tolerance Test

SPECIMEN OR TYPE OF TEST: Serum

PURPOSE OF THE TEST

The growth hormone stimulation test is usually performed to evaluate children and infants with retarded growth. It is also used to support the diagnosis of pituitary tumor. A variety of stimulants can be used to stimulate the secretion of the growth hormone, including arginine, glucagon, propranolol, insulin, levodopa, exercise, and corticotropin-releasing hormone (CRH). Arginine and insulin are the most frequently used stimulants.

The *insulin tolerance test* is also used to distinguish primary versus secondary adrenocorticoid insufficiency by measuring adrenocorticotropic hormone (ACTH) levels instead of growth hormone levels.

BASICS THE NURSE NEEDS TO KNOW

Review the preceding section on growth hormone.

NORMAL VALUES

With arginine: >7 ng/mL *or* SI: >7 mcg/L
With insulin (with serum glucose of <40 mg/dL): >20 ng/mL *or* SI: >20 mcg/L
With propranolol and glucagon: >10 ng/mL *or* SI: >10 mcg/L

HOW THE TEST IS DONE

Depending on the substance used, slight variations exist in the method. With arginine, a baseline sample of 5 mL of venous blood is obtained in a red-topped tube. A venous infusion of arginine is then administered. After the arginine infusion is completed (in approximately 30 minutes), 30 minutes are allowed to pass. Three venous samples are then obtained at 30-minute intervals. Ion exchange chromatography is used to analyze the blood samples.

If insulin is used, a baseline venous sample is taken, after which 100 U of regular insulin are given intravenously over 2 to 3 minutes. Venous samples are taken at 15, 30, 45, 60, 90, and 120 minutes after the administration of insulin. Blood glucose levels must fall to below 40 mg/dL within 1 hour after the insulin is given for an accurate evaluation.

SIGNIFICANCE OF TEST RESULTS

Elevated Values

No growth hormone deficiency

Decreased Values

Pituitary dwarfism
Pituitary tumors

INTERFERING FACTORS

- Failure to comply with fasting or activity restrictions
- Alcohol
- Medications such as amphetamines, beta blockers, calcium gluconate, estrogen, spironolactone, and steroids

NURSING CARE

Nursing actions are similar to those used in other venipuncture procedures (see Chapter 2), with the following additional measures.

Pretest

- Assess patients at risk if a growth hormone stimulation test with insulin is planned. This includes patients with cardiovascular disease, epilepsy, a history of a cerebrovascular accident, or adrenal insufficiency.
- The nurse obtains a medication history to determine if any interfering drug is being taken. The nurse also checks with the physician about withholding any interfering medication.
- ***Patient Teaching.*** The nurse instructs the patient to limit physical activity and not to eat or drink for 12 hours before the test.
- ***Patient Teaching.*** Instruct the patient not to drink alcohol for 24 hours before the blood is drawn.
- The nurse reassures the patient and instructs him or her to lie down quietly for 90 minutes before the blood is drawn.

During the Test

- An intravenous catheter (saline lock) is inserted to prevent multiple venous punctures.
- A baseline venous sample is taken.
- If arginine is used, an infusion is given over 30 minutes in the arm opposite the saline lock used for blood sampling. Thirty minutes after the arginine infusion is completed, three additional blood specimens are obtained at 30-minute intervals.
- If insulin is used, regular insulin is given over 2 to 3 minutes. Blood specimens are drawn at 15, 30, 45, 60, 90, and 120 minutes.
- The nurse observes the patient carefully. Stop the test if serious signs of hypoglycemia occur (e.g., vertigo, chest pain).

Posttest

- The patient can resume medication schedule, diet, and physical activities.
- Ensure that the patient who received insulin as a stimulant has adequate food intake.

Growth Hormone Suppression Test

grohth hohr-mohn suh-pre-shun test

Also called: Glucose Loading Test

SPECIMEN OR TYPE OF TEST: Serum

PURPOSE OF THE TEST

This test usually is performed to assess an increase in growth hormone levels and to confirm the diagnoses of gigantism in children and acromegaly in adults.

BASICS THE NURSE NEEDS TO KNOW

The growth hormone suppression test is performed after high levels of growth hormone are found. Normally, the ingestion of glucose causes a decrease in the secretion of growth hormone. In patients with hypersecretion of growth hormone, however, a significant decrease does not occur.

NORMAL VALUES Growth hormone levels decrease to undetectable to <3 ng/mL *or* SI: <3 mcg/L in 30–120 minutes

HOW THE TEST IS DONE

A baseline venous blood sample, 5 mL, is drawn into a red-topped tube. The patient ingests a glucose solution. After 1 to 2 hours, another blood sample is drawn.

SIGNIFICANCE OF TEST RESULTS

If high growth hormone levels are maintained:
Acromegaly
Gigantism

INTERFERING FACTORS

- Noncompliance with activity restrictions and fasting
- Radioactive scans within the previous week
- Medications such as amphetamines, arginine, beta blockers, chlorpromazine, dopamine, glucagon, histamine, insulin, levodopa, nicotinic acid, and steroids

NURSING CARE

Nursing actions are similar to those used in other venipuncture procedures (see Chapter 2), with the following additional measures.

Pretest

- The nurse obtains a medication history to ensure that any interfering drug has not been taken.
- Question the patient or check the patient's chart for any recent radioactive scans.
- ***Patient Teaching.*** The nurse instructs the patient about the need to avoid physical activity for 10 to 12 hours before the test and to lie quietly for 30 minutes before the blood is drawn.
- ***Patient Teaching.*** Instruct the patient not to eat or drink for 12 hours before the sample is taken.

During the Test

- Explain the purpose of the two venipunctures.

NURSING CARE—*cont'd*

- After the first specimen is obtained in the early morning, the nurse instructs the patient to drink the glucose solution *slowly* to minimize nausea.
- Ensure that the second specimen is obtained 1 to 2 hours after the ingestion of glucose.

Posttest

- The patient resumes normal diet and activity.

Guthrie Screening Test

See Phenylalanine, Blood on p. 515.

Haptoglobin

hap-tuh-gloh-bin

Also called: Hp

SPECIMEN OR TYPE OF TEST: Serum

PURPOSE OF THE TEST

Haptoglobin measurement is useful in the work-up for hemolytic conditions. It also is used for monitoring of acute-phase reactions that involve hemolysis of erythrocytes.

BASICS THE NURSE NEEDS TO KNOW

When erythrocytes undergo hemolysis by normal or abnormal processes, circulating haptoglobin binds to the free hemoglobin. These newly formed complexes cannot be filtered through the renal glomeruli so hemoglobin is protected from excretion in the urine. As the complexes are broken down, iron is conserved and stored for use in the manufacture of new erythrocytes. Increases in serum haptoglobin may occur in conditions of inflammation, infection or tissue destruction. A decreased value is more useful as a lab test. Decreased values occur with conditions of abnormal hemolysis of red blood cells. The decrease may be gradual, chronic, or sudden and severe in occurrence. As the red blood cells are destroyed, available haptoglobin is rapidly consumed as it binds to hemoglobin. When the haptoglobin value is suddenly and severely decreased, it is an indicator of acute hemolysis.

NORMAL VALUES

Adult: 30–200 mg/dL *or* SI: 0.03–2.0 g/L
Child: 22–164 mg/dL *or* SI: 0.22–1.64 g/L

HOW THE TEST IS DONE

A red-topped tube is used to collect 10 mL of venous blood.

SIGNIFICANCE OF TEST RESULTS

Elevated Values

Collagen diseases
Corticosteroid therapy
Acute rheumatoid arthritis
Nephrotic syndrome
Infection
Advanced malignancy

Decreased Values

Hemolytic transfusion reaction
Sickle cell anemia
Thalassemia
Folate deficiency
G-6-PD deficiency
Hereditary spherocytosis
Oral contraceptives (estrogen)
Acute thermal injury
Hematoma formation
Malaria
Liver disease

INTERFERING FACTORS

- Hemolysis from a traumatic venipuncture

NURSING CARE

Nursing actions are similar to those used in other venipuncture procedures (see Chapter 2), with the following additional measures.

Pretest

- This test may be used to monitor for a blood transfusion reaction. If prescribed, ensure that the haptoglobin specimen is drawn before starting the transfusion.

Posttest

- The nurse compares the current results with the patient's baseline value to monitor for the level and direction of change. A sudden or severe decrease in the value is an indication of hemolysis of the erythrocytes. The physician must be notified immediately. The cause of an abnormal lab result will determine the interventions that are needed.
- The nurse should assess any fresh sample of urine for change in color. If the haptoglobin level is decreased, free hemoglobin will be filtered out of the blood into the urine. Hemoglobin changes the color of the urine to dark red or brown.

Helicobacter pylori Tests

he-lai-ko-bac-ter pai-lohr-ee tests

SPECIMEN OR TYPE OF TEST: Blood, breath, feces, gastric biopsy

PURPOSE OF THE TEST

This test establishes the presence of *Helicobacter pylori* infection that can cause chronic, active gastritis and peptic ulcers.

BASICS THE NURSE NEEDS TO KNOW

Helicobacter pylori is a gram-negative bacillus that resides under the mucosal layer and in the gastric epithelium of the stomach, causing chronic infection and inflammation. The infection is usually acquired in childhood, particularly in people who are poor or who reside in developing countries where poor sanitary conditions and a lack of running water prevail. If the infection has not been eradicated in childhood, it remains as a life-long infection, with or without symptoms. When it progresses, the infection causes chronic atrophic gastritis, gastric ulcers, and some cases of duodenal ulcer. Less frequently, it causes gastric cancer and gastric lymphoma. There is much that still is not understood about this infection, including how it is transmitted. There are several different tests to confirm the *H. pylori* infection and to document its eradication.

Serology Test

This test identifies the elevated level of immunoglobulin G (IgG) and antibody to the *H. pylori* antigen in the blood of the infected patient. The positive test result is considered a marker for active infection.

Urea Breath Test

Radiolabeled carbon urea is administered to the patient orally. If *H. pylori* is present, the organism produces a unique enzyme, urease. The urease converts the carbon urea to ammonia and radiolabeled carbon dioxide (CO_2) gas. The radiolabeled CO_2 enters the blood and one option is that it can be measured by blood sample. The radiolabeled CO_2 is then exhaled by the lungs and can be measured in the exhaled air. The presence of radiolabeled carbon dioxide is proof that the patient has infection with *H. pylori.* When the urea breath test is done 7 days or more after completing the prescribed course of antibiotics, a negative result is proof that the infection has been eradicated.

H. pylori Antigen Test

This is the newest lab method to detect *H. pylori*. The antigen of *H. pylori* can be detected in the fecal matter of the infected patient. A positive lab analysis confirms the diagnosis of infection with *H. pylori.* After the infection has been treated, the same antigen test can be repeated. A negative result confirms that the infection has been eradicated.

Tissue Biopsy

During an endoscopy procedure, the gastric and duodenal mucosa are examined, and suspicious lesions and areas of inflammation or ulceration are biopsied. If antibiotic therapy has been tried before the tissue biopsy is done, the antibiotics can cause a false-negative result.

Histology

Biopsy tissue slides are prepared and stained for microscopic examination. When present, the characteristic *H. pylori* bacteria are seen and identified.

Rapid Urease Test

H. pylori produces a unique enzyme called *urease*. The urease can be detected by chemical analysis of the tissue sample. The presence of urease presumes the presence of *H. pylori*.

PCR-DNA

From the tissue specimen, polymerase chain reaction (PCR) technique amplifies the DNA sequence of *H. pylori* bacillus. The microbe is identified by its DNA blueprint.

Tissue Culture

After the tissue specimen is cultured, the culture plates are read at intervals of 1, 3, and 5 days to identify the presence of colonies of *H. pylori* bacilli.

NORMAL VALUES

Serology, IgG antibody: Negative
Urea breath test: Negative
Stool antigen: Negative
Tissue biopsy
  Histology: Negative
  Rapid urease test: Negative for *H. pylori*
  PCR-DNA: Negative
  Tissue culture: No *H. pylori* growth

HOW THE TEST IS DONE

Serology

A venipuncture is performed to collect 10 mL of venous blood in a red-topped tube. Some laboratories use a lavender-topped (EDTA) tube or a green-topped (heparin) tube.

Urea Breath Test

The patient ingests a capsule of radiolabeled carbon urea (C^{13} or C^{14}). Exhalation breath samples are collected in a special collection container, every 5 minutes for 30 minutes. The measurement of the radiolabeled CO_2 is done by scintillation scanner.

H. pylori Antigen Test

A stool sample is collected.

Tissue Biopsy

During an esophagogastroduodenoscopy (EGD) procedure, biopsy specimens are obtained.

SIGNIFICANCE OF TEST RESULTS

Positive Values

H. pylori infection
Chronic gastritis
Peptic ulcer disease
Gastric cancer
Gastric lymphoma

INTERFERING FACTORS

- Recent antimicrobial therapy

NURSING CARE

Pretest

- *Serology test.* Nursing actions are similar to those used in other venipuncture procedures (see Chapter 2), with the following additional measures.
- *Breath test.* Inform the client that a small amount of low-dose radiation will be in the capsule, but it will be exhaled. The body will clear out the radiation source within hours and the brief exposure will not harm the patient.
- H. pylori *antigen test.* Instruct the patient to collect a random stool sample to be brought to the lab. Further discussion of the stool collection procedure is presented in Chapter 2.
- *Tissue biopsy.* The reader is referred to the nursing discussion for the procedures of Esophagogastroduodenoscopy (see p. 317) and Gastrointestinal Cytology studies (see p. 339).

Hematocrit

he-mah-toh-crit

Also called: (Hct); Microhematocrit

SPECIMEN OR TYPE OF TEST: Blood

PURPOSE OF THE TEST

The hematocrit is useful in the evaluation of blood loss, anemia, hemolytic anemia, polycythemia, and dehydration.

BASICS THE NURSE NEEDS TO KNOW

The hematocrit is a measurement of the proportion of whole blood volume occupied by erythrocytes. The value is expressed as a percentage or fraction of cells to whole blood. For example, a hematocrit value of 40% means that there are 40 mL of erythrocytes in 1 dL of blood.

Variations of Normal Values

The normal values vary with the gender and age of the individual, and in a few other special circumstances. The normal value for males is slightly higher than that for females. The pregnant female has a slightly lower normal value than that of the nonpregnant female because of the greater blood volume during pregnancy. In men older than age 65, the normal value is slightly lower than that for younger males. For all individuals, the normal value can be 5% to 6% lower when blood is drawn with the patient in a recumbent as opposed to an upright position.

Elevated Values

The hematocrit rises if the number or size of the erythrocytes increases or when the plasma fluid volume is reduced. When the fluid volume is decreased, the red blood cells become concentrated in the smaller fluid volume. The blood is thicker or has increased viscosity.

Decreased Values

The hematocrit falls to less than normal when an excessive loss of erythrocytes occurs, as in hemolytic anemia or after excessive bleeding. It also can occur because fewer red blood cells are made or the erythrocytes are microcytic (smaller). The hematocrit also can decrease because of excessive intravenous fluids or fluid retention that creates greater plasma volume. The fluids exert a dilution effect, meaning that normal numbers of red blood cells are in a larger amount of fluid.

In bleeding or hemorrhage, the hematocrit drops several hours after the bleeding episode. The severity of the drop in value correlates directly with the amount of red blood cells that are lost.

NORMAL VALUES	Male: 41.5%–50.4% *or* SI: 0.415–0.504 (volume fraction) Female: 35.9%–44.6% *or* SI: 0.359–0.446 (volume fraction)
▼ Critical Values	>54% (SI: >0.54 [volume fraction]) *or* <18% (SI: <0.18 [volume fraction])

HOW THE TEST IS DONE

A purple-topped tube with EDTA is used to collect 7 mL of venous blood. As an alternative, two purple-tipped capillary tubes can be used to collect blood from a heelstick, earlobe, or finger puncture. After the blood is collected, the tube is inverted gently five to ten times to mix the anticoagulant and prevent clotting.

SIGNIFICANCE OF TEST RESULTS

Elevated Values

Polycythemia vera
Secondary polycythemia
Addison's disease
Acute thermal injury
Extreme physical exertion
Hemoconcentration
Dehydration
Chronic obstructive lung disease

Decreased Values

Recent hemorrhage
Anemia
Fluid overload
Fluid retention
Cirrhosis
Hemolytic anemia
Hemodilution
Leukemia
Lymphoma

INTERFERING FACTORS

- Hemolysis
- Coagulation of the specimen
- Hemodilution

NURSING CARE

Pretest

- Nursing actions are similar to those used in other venipuncture or fingerstick procedures (see Chapter 2), with the following additional measures.
- The nurse informs the patient that blood will be drawn at intervals to monitor his or her condition.

During the Test

- Ensure that the blood sample is not taken from a vein in the hand or arm with an intravenous line. Hemodilution with intravenous fluids or plasma will lower the hematocrit value falsely.

Posttest

Elevated Hematocrit

- When the patient's condition is due to dehydration and the hematocrit is elevated, fluid and electrolyte replacement is usually administered intravenously, as prescribed. Dehydration can occur quickly in infants and elderly people, often due to infection or diarrhea. Fluid losses also can occur rapidly in conditions such as

Continued

NURSING CARE—*cont'd*

extensive burns. The nurse ensures that the correct solution and the correct amount of solution are given in the prescribed period. If the patient's medical condition allows, the nurse encourages the patient to take extra fluids orally. As the patient is rehydrated, the hematocrit value will fall toward the normal value.

Decreased Hematocrit

- When the patient is hemorrhaging or has just had a severe bleeding episode, both hemoglobin and hematocrit values will decline. These tests are used to help evaluate the patient's hemodynamic status at regular intervals. The nurse monitors the lab results because the decreased hemoglobin and hematocrit values indicate the severity of the blood loss. Likewise, after transfusion replacement of packed cells or whole blood, the nurse monitors the hematocrit and hemoglobin results for rising values that indicate effectiveness of treatment. The nurse ensures that the lab tests are performed at the indicated times.
- Because the loss of blood or fluids often results in hemodynamic instability, the nurse measures and records vital signs at regular and frequent intervals. Abnormal findings would include hypotension (a low blood pressure), tachycardia (a rapid pulse), and dyspnea (labored breathing).
- When the patient has excess fluid volume, often with edema, the underlying conditions that cause fluid retention and fluid overload must be diagnosed and treated medically. In cases such as cirrhosis, congestive heart failure, and renal failure, the hematocrit falls because the normal number of red blood cells is diluted in excess plasma. The nurse carries out the medical treatment protocol that often includes medications, fluid restrictions, and salt restrictions. As excess fluid is excreted, the hematocrit rises toward a more normal value.

▼ Nursing Response to Critical Values

When the hematocrit rises to a critical value or higher, the patient is at great risk of developing a myocardial infarction or a stroke. Those who are most vulnerable are patients with preexisting cardiovascular disease. When the hematocrit decreases to a critical value or lower, the patient may go into shock, particularly when there is associated blood loss or hemorrhage. The nurse must notify the physician immediately of any hematocrit result that is in the critical value range.

The nurse also starts frequent and regular monitoring of vital signs and assessment of the patient's overall condition. The patient may complain of intense chest pain or exhibit signs of neurologic abnormality, including loss of consciousness, aphasia (impairment or loss of speech), hemiparesis (weakness in one side of the body), and hemiplegia (paralysis on one side of the body).

Hemoglobin

hee-moh-gloh-bin

Also called: (Hgb); (Hb)

SPECIMEN OR TYPE OF TEST: Blood

PURPOSE OF THE TEST

The hemoglobin is used to measure the severity of anemia or polycythemia, and it monitors the response to treatment of anemia. It is also used to calculate the mean corpuscular hemoglobin (MCH) and mean corpuscular hemoglobin concentration (MCHC) values.

BASICS THE NURSE NEEDS TO KNOW

Hemoglobin is the oxygen-carrying compound contained in each erythrocyte. The large amount of hemoglobin and the broad surface area of each erythrocyte enable the red blood cells to have a large oxygen-carrying capacity and to function with great efficiency.

Variation in Normal Values

The normal value of hemoglobin varies among individuals of different ages, genders, races, and geographic locations. The normal hemoglobin value is higher in males than in females. After age 10, the hemoglobin value is slightly lower in African Americans than in whites. Men older than age 65 have a slightly lower value than do younger men. The normal value is slightly higher in individuals who live in high-altitude areas. The value is 5% to 6% lower in patients who have their blood drawn when in a recumbent position as opposed to an upright position.

Elevated Values

An elevated hemoglobin value may be a result of either excess production of erythrocytes by the bone marrow or dehydration. In excess production of erythrocytes, the hemoglobin rises because it is present in additional cells. In dehydration, the red blood cell counts and hemoglobin are relatively high because of a normal number and quality of cells that are concentrated in a smaller amount of fluid.

Decreased Values

An individual generally is considered anemic when the hemoglobin value for the male is less than 13 g/dL (SI: <130 g/L) and for the female, less than 11 g/dL (SI: <110 g/L). The low hemoglobin value can be caused by a low red blood cell count, by a lack of hemoglobin in each erythrocyte, or by fluid retention. The low red cell count may be a lack of production by the bone marrow, a loss of red blood cells in bleeding, or a loss of red blood cells from hemolysis (rapid destruction of the erythrocytes). The lack of hemoglobin in the erythrocytes is often due to a lack of iron, an essential mineral used to make heme, the iron-containing molecule in hemoglobin. In fluid retention, red blood cell counts and hemoglobin values are normal, but the cells are diluted in a greater amount of fluid.

NORMAL VALUES

Male: 14.0–17.5 g/dL *or* SI: 140–175 g/L
Female: 12.3–15.3 g/dL *or* SI: 123–153 g/L
Child (5 years): 11.7–13.7 g/dL *or* SI: 117–137 g/L
Infant (5–7 months): 10.8–12.2 g/dL *or* SI: 108–122 g/L
Newborn (1 day): 17.3–21.5 g/dL *or* SI: 173–215 g/L

HOW THE TEST IS DONE

A purple-topped tube with EDTA is used to collect 7 mL of venous blood. As an alternative, two purple-tipped capillary tubes can be used to collect blood from a heelstick, earlobe, or finger puncture. After the blood is collected, the tube is inverted gently five to ten times to mix the anticoagulant and prevent clotting.

SIGNIFICANCE OF TEST RESULTS

Elevated Values

Polycythemia vera
Secondary polycythemia
Acute thermal injury
Dehydration
Hemoconcentration
Chronic obstructive pulmonary disease

Decreased Values

Recent bleeding
Fluid retention
Hemolysis of red blood cells
Pregnancy
Hemorrhage
Anemia
Cirrhosis of the liver
Hyperthyroidism

INTERFERING FACTORS

- Hemolysis
- Coagulation of the specimen
- Lipemia
- White blood cell count greater than 50×10^3 μL (SI: >50×10^9/L)

NURSING CARE

Nursing actions are similar to those used in other venipuncture or capillary puncture procedures (see Chapter 2), with the following additional measures.

Pretest

- The nurse informs the patient of the need for additional lab testing to monitor his or her condition. When the patient is hemorrhaging or has just had a severe bleeding episode, both hemoglobin and hematocrit measurements are taken at regular intervals. The decreased results indicate the severity of the blood loss. Likewise, after transfusion replacement of packed cells or whole blood, the same tests are used to evaluate the effectiveness of treatment. Ensure that the tests are performed at the indicated times.

NURSING CARE—*cont'd*

During the Test

- Ensure that the blood sample is not taken from the hand or arm that has an intravenous line in the vein because of the dilution effect on red blood cell concentration.

Posttest

- The nurse arranges for prompt transport of the specimen to the lab. If a delay is anticipated, refrigerate the specimen to prevent deterioration of the cells.
- When the hemoglobin level is decreased, the nurse can assess abnormal physical responses that include dizziness, pallor, and fatigue associated with physical activity. When the decline in hemoglobin occurs slowly over time, the patient may not experience symptoms of anemia, particularly when resting. With physical activity, however, the patient may report breathlessness or palpitations. The decrease in hemoglobin means that less oxygen can be transported. With exertion, the lungs and heart must work harder to get as much oxygen to cells as possible. As a result, both the pulse and respiratory rate will increase.
- When acute blood loss occurs, both the hemoglobin and hematocrit values will fall. The declines, however, do not occur for several hours after the bleeding occurs. Conversely, if blood transfusion is administered, the new supply of red blood cells will cause the hemoglobin and hematocrit to rise. The nurse monitors the hemoglobin and hematocrit values for anticipated beneficial responses.
- There are numerous causes for an abnormal hemoglobin value. Lab testing will be needed to determine the specific cause and appropriate medical therapy. Additional specific nursing interventions will be implemented when the medical diagnosis is made.

Hemoglobin Electrophoresis

hee-moh-gloh-bin e-lek-tro-fuh-ree-sis

SPECIMEN OR TYPE OF TEST: Blood

PURPOSE OF THE TEST

Hemoglobin electrophoresis is used to detect hemoglobinopathy (genetic disorder of hemoglobin) and identify the type of anemia that results from the abnormal hemoglobin. It is also the test that definitively identifies sickle cell hemoglobin and differentiates between sickle cell disease and sickle cell trait.

BASICS THE NURSE NEEDS TO KNOW

In the normal adult, the three types of hemoglobin found in erythrocytes are HbA, HbA_2, and HbF. Using the electrophoresis method, the test separates the normal from the abnormal hemoglobin types and measures the percentage amounts of each type.

There are more than 400 variants (abnormal or altered types) of hemoglobin, identified by letters other than A, A_2, and F. Of all the abnormal variants, HbS, or sickle cell hemoglobin, is the most predominant. Other relatively common hemoglobin variants are HbC and HbE. *Hemoglobinopathy* is the general term used to describe altered hemoglobin and some forms of hemolytic anemia. Some conditions are asymptomatic or mild, because the genetic defect of hemoglobin is a heterozygous (mixed) type, or trait condition. In the trait condition, the mutant gene is inherited from one, but not both parents. Other conditions are of the homozygous (pure) state that produces the disease. In the disease condition, the individual inherits the mutant gene from both parents.

Hemoglobin A_2

Although this is normal hemoglobin, it is only a small proportion of the total hemoglobin. Hemoglobin electrophoresis evaluates the amount of HbA_2 in the investigation of beta-thalassemia trait and differentiates beta-thalassemia diseases from iron deficiency anemia. The beta-thalassemia diseases are a group of disorders that produce a range of conditions varying from no clinical change to severe hypochromic, microcytic anemia. The amount of HbA_2 is increased in the beta-thalassemia trait. Abnormal elevations of HbA_2 may include up to 7% of the total hemoglobin content.

Hemoglobin F

HbF is the hemoglobin present in fetal life. During infancy, it is gradually replaced by HbA and HbA_2. Adults can have abnormal quantities of HbF in hereditary persistence of fetal hemoglobin. The homozygous state produces mildly microcytic, hypochromic erythrocytes without anemia. The hemoglobin electrophoresis test reveals 100% HbF. The heterozygous state does not cause anemia, but hemoglobin electrophoresis reveals 30% to 40% HbF.

Hemoglobin S

In the homozygous (pure) state, HbS produces the disease of sickle cell anemia, a type of severe hemolytic anemia. Hemoglobin electrophoresis demonstrates a large percentage of HbS, and the affected individual will have many health problems throughout life. In the heterozygous form, or sickle cell trait, hemoglobin electrophoresis demonstrates 30% to 35% HbS. Sickle cell trait produces no disease or hematologic abnormality unless the person experiences hypoxia, acidosis, or thrombosis (a blood clot).

Hemoglobin C

In the homozygous state of HbC disease, a mild hemolytic anemia often exists, but it is usually asymptomatic. On electrophoresis, no HbA is present. Most of the hemoglobin is HbC, with smaller quantities of other forms of hemoglobin. In the heterozygous state 30% to 40% of the hemoglobin is type HbC.

NORMAL VALUES

HbA: 95%–98%
HbA_2: 1.5%–3.5%
HbF: 0%–2%
HbC: Absent
HbS: Absent

HOW THE TEST IS DONE

A lavender-topped tube is used to collect 7 mL of venous blood.

A fingerstick or earlobe puncture may be used to obtain two lavender-tipped capillary tubes of blood.

SIGNIFICANCE OF TEST RESULTS

Elevated Values

Beta-thalassemia minor or major
Hereditary persistence of fetal hemoglobin
Sickle cell disease
Sickle cell trait
HbC disease
HbC trait
Megaloblastic anemia

Decreased Values

Deficiency of HbA$_2$

Sideroblastic anemia
Untreated iron deficiency anemia
Hereditary persistence of fetal hemoglobin

INTERFERING FACTORS

- Blood transfusion in the preceding 4 months
- Hemolysis of the erythrocytes
- Coagulation of the specimen

NURSING CARE

Nursing actions are similar to those used in other venipuncture or fingerstick procedures (see Chapter 2), with the following additional measures.

Pretest

- Ask the patient about any transfusion of blood received within the preceding 4 months. A recent transfusion would make the findings of the test inconsistent.

Posttest

- ***Health Promotion.*** In almost all states of the U.S., newborns are screened for sickle cell disorders. When screening is mandated, it is a universal requirement for all newborns regardless of ethnicity. The sickle cell genetic mutation is more common in black Americans, and the trait condition affects about 9% of this population group. Sickle cell disease primarily affects people of African ancestry, but it is also common in people of Mediterranean countries, India, Spanish-speaking people in the U.S., as well as individuals from Central and South America and the Caribbean Islands. The early identification of sickle cell disease in the newborn means that health care interventions can be started early in the infant's life and a comprehensive treatment plan instituted.

Continued

NURSING CARE—*cont'd*

- The nurse provides support to the parents who have an infant who tested positive for sickle cell trait or disease. The parent often has feelings of concern, guilt, fear, and worry about the well-being of the infant. Encourage the parents or the adult patient to return to the primary physician for the test results and guidance that includes genetic counseling and education about specific health care needs.
- The nurse teaches and reinforces the benefits of treatment, including the maintenance of prophylactic penicillin medication and receiving additional vaccinations along with the regular vaccination protocol. The interventions are very effective in prevention of infections, particularly of the respiratory tract, and thereby lessen the incidences of sickle cell crises. The child will also need balanced nutrition and regular health care visits to monitor growth and development. The nurse encourages the parents of a child with sickle cell disease to maintain the treatment plan and to follow-up with the care that is needed throughout the life of the individual.
- When one child of the family tests positive for the trait or disease, the nurse encourages all members of the family to be tested. If the individual knows his or her genetic status regarding this mutation, he or she can make informed decisions regarding health and reproduction.

Hemosiderin, Urinary

hee-moh-said-uh-rin, yur-i-ner-ee

SPECIMEN OR TYPE OF TEST: Urine

PURPOSE OF THE TEST

Urinary hemosiderin is used to identify hemolytic anemia that is associated with intravascular hemolysis.

BASICS THE NURSE NEEDS TO KNOW

Hemosiderin granules are indicators of hemoglobin in the urine resulting from significant acute or chronic intravascular hemolysis. With the lysis of many erythrocytes, hemoglobin is released into the blood, and the excess hemoglobin is filtered out by the kidneys. In the kidneys, the hemoglobin is converted to ferritin and hemosiderin. The hemosiderin granules are present in the cells or casts in urinary sediment. They appear in the urine on the second or third day after the hemolytic episode. The source of the urinary hemosiderin may also be excretion of excess iron, as from hematochromatosis.

The presence of hemoglobin in the urine may not be detected by a urine reagent strip. When the urinary sediment is stained with Prussian blue stain, however, the iron in urinary hemosiderin appears as blue-stained granules. The results are seen by microscopic examination of the slides that contain urinary cells and casts.

NORMAL VALUES Negative

HOW THE TEST IS DONE

A random sample of 30 to 60 mL of urine is collected in a clean glass container.

SIGNIFICANCE OF TEST RESULTS

Positive Values

Blood transfusion reaction
Chronic hemolytic anemia
Mechanical trauma to erythrocytes
Exposure to oxidant drugs or chemicals
G-6-PD deficiency
Thalassemia major
Severe megaloblastic anemia
Sickle cell anemia
Hematochromatosis
Severe infectious organisms (malaria, *Clostridium perfringens*)

INTERFERING FACTORS

- None

NURSING CARE

There are no special patient care measures needed.

Hepatitis A Antibody

he-puh-tai-tis ay an-tib-od-ee

Also called: HAV, ab; HAVab; Anti-HAV

SPECIMEN OR TYPE OF TEST: Serum

PURPOSE OF THE TEST

The hepatitis A antibodies identify the hepatitis A virus as the cause of the infection. The specific antibody type distinguishes between current infection and past infection with immunity against a repeat infection.

BASICS THE NURSE NEEDS TO KNOW

The hepatitis A virus is transmitted by the fecal-oral route, primarily after ingestion of virus-contaminated water, food, milk, or shellfish. Although the virus is found in the feces of an infected individual for about 3 weeks, the diagnosis is based on identification of the hepatitis A antibodies in the blood.

Two types of hepatitis A antibodies are measured: the immunoglobin M (IgM) type and the immunoglobin G (IgG) type. The IGM type, also called anti-HAV IgM appears early in the course of illness. It is present in the blood within 1 week after the patient develops symptoms. It peaks within 3 months, and during convalescence it subsides, usually in 4 to 6 months. The IgG type, also called anti-HAV total, begins to rise after 4 weeks of infection and persists for life.

NORMAL VALUES	Hepatitis A antibody: Negative IgM type: Negative IgG type: Negative

HOW THE TEST IS DONE

A venipuncture is performed to collect 10 mL of venous blood in a red-topped tube.

SIGNIFICANCE OF TEST RESULTS

Elevated Values

Hepatitis A antibody: Hepatitis A infection
IgM: Current hepatitis A infection, acute or convalescent stage
IgG type: Old hepatitis A infection with immunity to reinfection with the hepatitis A virus

H

INTERFERING FACTORS

- Recent administration of radioisotopes

NURSING CARE

Nursing measures are similar to those used in other venipuncture procedures (see Chapter 2), with the following additional measures.

Pretest

- To alert the laboratory personnel, write on the requisition slip that hepatitis is suspected. When hepatitis is suspected, extra attention to technique should help prevent needlestick injury or contact with blood from splashes.
- Until the specific diagnosis is made, apply standard precautions. Hepatitis A infection is contagious and the virus is present in the feces before the patient feels any symptoms.

Hepatitis B Core Antibody

he-puh-tai-tis bee kohr an-tib-od-ee

Also called: Anti-HB_c

SPECIMEN OR TYPE OF TEST: Serum

PURPOSE OF THE TEST

The hepatitis B core antibody test is used to assess the stage of the hepatitis B infection.

BASICS THE NURSE NEEDS TO KNOW

The hepatitis B core antibody (anti-HB_c) is a marker of hepatitis B infection in the acute or chronic phase of illness or is a marker of past illness. This hepatitis B core antibody appears after 1 to 2 weeks of infection, before symptoms appear. It rises in the acute stage of illness, with a peak and plateau during convalescence several months later. It remains elevated for years and is considered a lifetime marker of past illness. When the subtype antibodies are tested, a positive IgM result indicates an acute infection. A positive IgG type indicates a chronic or carrier state.

NORMAL VALUES

Hepatitis B core antibody: Negative
Type IgM: Negative
Type IgG: Negative

HOW THE TEST IS DONE

A venipuncture is performed to collect 10 mL of venous blood in a red-topped tube.

H

SIGNIFICANCE OF TEST RESULTS

Hepatitis B core antibody: Hepatitis B infection
IgM: Acute or convalescent stage
IgG: Chronic stage or past infection

INTERFERING FACTORS

- Recent administration of radioisotopes

NURSING CARE

Nursing measures are similar to those used in other venipuncture procedures (see Chapter 2), with the following additional measures.

Pretest

- To alert the laboratory personnel, write on the requisition slip that hepatitis is suspected.
- Venipuncture is always performed with gloves, and used needles must be discarded carefuly, according to agency protocol. When hepatitis is suspected, extra attention to technique should help prevent needlestick injury or contact with blood from splashes.
- In giving care and in handling blood and body fluids, use standard precautions. Hepatitis B infection is contagious and the virus is present in the blood and body fluids at about the same time that the patient begins to experience symptoms of hepatitis.

Hepatitis B_e Antibody

he-puh-tai-tis bee-ee an-tib-od-ee

Also called: Anti-HB_e; HB_e Ab

SPECIMEN OR TYPE OF TEST: Serum

PURPOSE OF THE TEST

The hepatitis B_e antibody (anti-HB_e) test helps stage the course of illness and is a prognostic indicator about the status of the hepatitis infection.

BASICS THE NURSE NEEDS TO KNOW

Hepatitis B is transmitted via infected body fluids, particularly blood, but also is transmitted during sexual intercourse, intravenous drug use, and by the infected mother to her baby during delivery.

The hepatitis B_e antibody usually appears in the blood after the hepatitis B_e antigen has disappeared, or about 3 months after the onset of infection. When anti-HB_e does appear, it is an indication that the patient has a decline in infectivity and a lower potential to transmit the infection to other people. The patient is probably starting the convalescent phase of the infection. Conversely, when the hepatitis B_e antigen remains present and the hepatitis B_e antibody does not appear, it is an indication that the patient continues to have an active infection.

NORMAL VALUES

Anti-HB_e: Negative

HOW THE TEST IS DONE

A venipuncture is performed to collect 10 mL of venous blood in a red-topped tube.

SIGNIFICANCE OF TEST RESULTS

Positive Values

Reduced infectivity in convalescence
Reduced infectivity in a carrier state
Reduced infectivity in chronic infection

INTERFERING FACTORS

- Recent administration of radioisotopes

NURSING CARE

Nursing measures are similar to those used in other venipuncture procedures (see Chapter 2), with the following additional measures.

Pretest

- To alert the laboratory personnel, write on the requisition slip that hepatitis is suspected. When hepatitis is suspected, extra attention to technique should help prevent needlestick injury or contact with blood from splashes.
- While giving care, drawing blood, or handling body fluid, use standard precautions. Hepatitis B infection is contagious while the virus is present in the blood and body fluids.

Hepatitis B_e Antigen

he-puh-<u>tai</u>-tis bee-ee <u>an</u>-tuh-jen

Also called: HB_eAg

SPECIMEN OR TYPE OF TEST: Serum

PURPOSE OF THE TEST

The hepatitis B_e antigen determination is used to diagnose the hepatitis B infection and help determine the prognosis for recovery.

BASICS THE NURSE NEEDS TO KNOW

Hepatitis B is transmitted via infected body fluids, particularly blood, but also is transmitted during heterosexual and homosexual intercourse, intravenous drug use, and by the infected mother to her baby at the time of delivery. Nurses and other healthcare workers who are not immunized against hepatitis B infection are vulnerable because of the potential for contact with infected blood, body fluids, and instruments, such as needles, that are contaminated with infected blood.

The hepatitis B_e antigen is one of the antigens produced by the hepatitis B virus. The antigen is produced by particles of the genes (DNA) of the hepatitis B virus. When this antigen is present in the blood, it indicates the acute stage of illness when the patient is most infectious. This antigen usually appears in the blood at about the time the patient has symptoms of illness and it remains in the blood for about 3 to 6 weeks.

When this antigen disappears from the blood and there is an accompanying rise in the HB_e antibodies, the patient is thought to be at the start of the recovery phase. Alternatively, the persistence of the hepatitis antigen in the blood indicates that the patient continues to be infective in a carrier state and may develop chronic liver disease.

NORMAL VALUES Hepatitis B_e antigen: Negative

HOW THE TEST IS DONE

A venipuncture is performed to collect 10 mL of venous blood in a red-topped tube.

SIGNIFICANCE OF TEST RESULTS

Positive Values

Increased infectivity in the acute stage
Increased infectivity and chronic carrier of hepatitis B
Chronic liver disease

INTERFERING FACTORS

- Radioactive scan in the preceding week

NURSING CARE

Nursing measures are similar to those used in other venipuncture procedures (see Chapter 2), with the following additional measures.

Pretest

- To alert the laboratory personnel, write on the requisition slip that hepatitis is suspected. When hepatitis is suspected, extra attention to technique should help prevent needlestick injury or contact with blood from splashes.
- Apply standard precautions until the specific diagnosis is made and continue these precautions when the lab test is positive. Hepatitis B infection is contagious. The virus is present in the blood and body fluids before or at the time the patient feels symptoms of the illness.

Hepatitis B Surface Antibody

he-puh-tai-tis bee sur-fuhs an-tib-od-ee

Also called: HB_sAb; Anti-HB_s

SPECIMEN OR TYPE OF TEST: Serum

PURPOSE OF THE TEST

This test is used to evaluate immunity or the need for vaccination in individuals at high risk to acquire hepatitis B infection. It is also used to evaluate the need for immune globulin after a needlestick injury. For the infected patient, it is used to help determine the antibody response that indicates recovery from hepatitis B infection.

BASICS THE NURSE NEEDS TO KNOW

The hepatitis B surface antibody appears several weeks to several months after the hepatitis B surface antigen has disappeared. The antibody remains in the patient's blood during convalescence and may or may not disappear after recovery. The presence of this antibody usually indicates that recovery is complete and that immunity now exists to any recurrent hepatitis B exposure. If the hepatitis B surface antibody and the hepatitis B core antibody are present simultaneously, immunity to recurrent hepatitis B infection is definite.

NORMAL VALUES

Hepatitis B surface antibody: Negative

HOW THE TEST IS DONE

A venipuncture is performed to collect 10 mL of venous blood in a red-topped tube.

SIGNIFICANCE OF TEST RESULTS

Positive Values

Convalescent stage of the hepatitis B infection
Clinical recovery from hepatitis B infection
Effective response to hepatitis B immunization

INTERFERING FACTORS

- Recent administration of radioisotopes

NURSING CARE

Nursing measures are similar to those used in other venipuncture procedures (see Chapter 2), with the following additional measures.

Pretest

- To alert the laboratory personnel, write on the requisition slip that hepatitis infection is suspected. When hepatitis is suspected, extra attention to technique should help prevent needlestick injury or contact with blood from splashes.
- Until the specific recovery from hepatitis B infection has been proven, continue to apply standard precautions. Hepatitis B infection is contagious and the virus is present in the blood and body fluids.

Hepatitis B Surface Antigen

he-puh-tai-tis bee sur-fuhs an-tuh-jen

Also called: HB_sAg

SPECIMEN OR TYPE OF TEST: Serum

PURPOSE OF THE TEST

The hepatitis B surface antigen is used to identify the specific type of hepatitis and to diagnose the infection in its acute or chronic stage. It is used to screen the blood of potential donors, with rejection of those with positive results. It is also used to evaluate risk in needlestick incidents involving health care personnel.

BASICS THE NURSE NEEDS TO KNOW

Hepatitis B is transmitted via infected body fluids, particularly blood, but also is transmitted during heterosexual and homosexual intercourse, intravenous drug use, and by the infected mother to her baby at the time of delivery. Nurses and other healthcare workers who are not immunized against hepatitis B infection are vulnerable because of the potential for contact with infected blood, body fluids and instruments such as needles that are contaminated with infected blood.

The hepatitis B surface antigen is one of the antigens produced by the hepatitis B virus. The antigen is produced by particles of the genes (DNA) of the hepatitis B virus. When this antigen is present in the blood, it indicates the acute stage of illness when the patient is most infectious. This antigen usually appears in the blood 2 to 4 weeks before the liver enzyme levels become elevated and up to 5 weeks before the patient has symptoms of illness. Hepatitis B surface antigen is the first antigen test to turn positive when hepatitis infection exists.

In a typical pattern of illness, the amount of the hepatitis B surface antigen rises and peaks in the acute stage. The hepatitis B surface antigen level then declines steadily over a period of 12 weeks in the convalescent stage. In a different pattern, if the hepatitis B surface antigen rises to a plateau and remains elevated for 4 to 6 months or more, the patient is probably a carrier of hepatitis B virus or has chronic hepatitis B infection.

NORMAL VALUES Hepatitis B surface antigen: Negative

HOW THE TEST IS DONE

A venipuncture is performed to collect 10 mL of venous blood in a red-topped tube.

SIGNIFICANCE OF TEST RESULTS

Positive Values

Acute, active hepatitis B infection
Active, chronic hepatitis B infection
Chronic carrier of hepatitis B surface antigen

INTERFERING FACTORS

- Recent administration of radioisotopes

NURSING CARE

Nursing measures are similar to those used in other venipuncture procedures (see Chapter 2), with the following additional measures.

Pretest

- To alert the laboratory personnel, write on the requisition slip that hepatitis is suspected. When hepatitis is suspected, extra attention to technique should help prevent needlestick injury or contact with blood from splashes.
- Apply standard precautions until the specific diagnosis is made and continue these precautions when the lab test is positive. Hepatitis B infection is contagious. The virus is present in the blood and body fluids before or at the time the patient feels symptoms of the illness.

Hepatitis B Virus DNA Assay

he-puh-tai-tis bee vai-ruhs dee-en-ay a-say

Also called: HBV DNA Detection

SPECIMEN OR TYPE OF TEST: Serum; liver tissue

PURPOSE OF THE TEST

This test helps diagnose the chronic carrier state of hepatitis B in those cases of mild to severe chronic liver disease. This test is used when the antigen and antibody responses are negative in the patient who is suspected to have hepatitis infection.

BASICS THE NURSE NEEDS TO KNOW

Hepatitis B can be identified by genetic testing of the virus to identify the DNA sequence. If present, the virus will be in the blood and also in liver tissue that is removed by liver biopsy. In addition to identification of the hepatitis B virus, the DNA assay test can calculate the viral load (the measure of how much virus is present).

NORMAL VALUES

Hepatitis B virus: Negative

HOW THE TEST IS DONE

Serum: A venipuncture is performed to collect 10 mL of venous blood in a red-topped tube or 7 mL of blood in a lavender-topped tube.
Tissue: A sample of liver tissue is placed in a sterile container. The container is sealed in a plastic bag.

SIGNIFICANCE OF TEST RESULTS

Positive Values

Hepatitis B infection

INTERFERING FACTORS

- Recent radioisotope scan

NURSING CARE

Nursing measures are similar to those used in other venipuncture procedures (see Chapter 2), with the following additional measures.

Pretest

- To alert the laboratory personnel, write on the requisition slip that hepatitis is suspected. When hepatitis is suspected, extra attention to technique should help prevent needlestick injury or contact with blood from splashes.
- Apply standard precautions until the specific diagnosis is made and continue these precautions when the lab test is positive. Hepatitis B infection is contagious. The virus is present in the blood and body fluids before or at the time the patient feels symptoms of the illness. It may also continue to be present after both antigen and antibody tests have converted to negative results.

Hepatitis C Antibody

he-puh-tai-tis see an-tib-od-ee

Also called: Anti-HCV; HCV Antibody

SPECIMEN OR TYPE OF TEST: Serum

PURPOSE OF THE TEST

This test is used to diagnose hepatitis and the specific virus involved. It is also used to screen the blood of potential donors, with rejection of those with positive results.

BASICS THE NURSE NEEDS TO KNOW

The HCV infection is transmitted in infected blood and body fluids. The most common occurrence is in intravenous drug users who shared contaminated needles. In this high-risk population, the HCV infection is highly likely to become a chronic infection. Chronic HCV infection is the cause of a significant number of cases of cirrhosis of the liver.

The hepatitis C antibody test (anti-HCV) is an important test to detect the presence of antibodies that appear in response to the HCV antigen and infection. Depending on the method of analysis used, the antibodies will be detected in the blood from 6 to 12 weeks after the patient is infected. The HCV antibody test is very highly accurate when testing a patient in the high-risk category. The positive test result indicates active infection, chronic infection, or recovery from a past infection. A follow-up hepatitis C RNA assay test is used to detect the presence of the hepatitis C virus of active or chronic infection.

NORMAL VALUES

Hepatitis C antibody: Negative

HOW THE TEST IS DONE

A venipuncture is performed to collect 10 mL of venous blood in a red-topped tube.

SIGNIFICANCE OF TEST RESULTS

Positive Values

Hepatitis C infection, acute or chronic

INTERFERING FACTORS

- Recent administration of radioisotopes

NURSING CARE

Nursing measures are similar to those used in other venipuncture procedures (see Chapter 2), with the following additional measures.

Pretest

- To alert the laboratory personnel, write on the requisition slip that hepatitis is suspected. When hepatitis is suspected, extra attention to technique should help prevent needlestick injury or contact with blood from splashes.
- Apply standard precautions until the specific diagnosis is made and continue these precautions when the lab test is positive. Hepatitis C infection is contagious and the virus is likely to be present in the blood and body fluids.

Hepatitis C RNA Assay

he-puh-<u>tai</u>-tis see <u>ar</u>-en-ay a-say

Also called: HCV_cDNA

SPECIMEN OR TYPE OF TEST: Serum; liver tissue

PURPOSE OF THE TEST

The test is used to confirm the diagnosis of hepatitis C virus infection and monitor the response to treatment.

BASICS THE NURSE NEEDS TO KNOW

The hepatitis C virus is transmitted by infected blood and body fluids. Today, the most common incidence is in intravenous drug users who shared infected needles. The virus can infect healthcare workers and patients who receive hemodialysis treatments because of the transmission of the virus in serum.

This test uses genetic testing to detect particles of the nuclear material of the hepatitis C virus that are in the blood or liver tissue. The viral RNA material can be detected within 2 weeks of the onset of infection. Many cases of hepatitis C infection become chronic infections with eventual liver damage, cirrhosis, and liver failure. When present in the blood or liver tissue, this test can remain positive for many years or throughout life after the infection has begun.

This hepatitis C-RNA assay test is the most specific test to confirm hepatitis C in acute or chronic infection. The test also may be used to measure the viral load, meaning that the number of viruses may be counted or measured. This is very helpful in detecting decreases in viral load in response to specific medications that treat hepatitis C infection.

NORMAL VALUES

Negative; no hepatitis C viral RNA is detected

HOW THE TEST IS DONE

Serum: A venipuncture is performed to collect 10 mL of venous blood in a red-topped tube.

Tissue: A sample of liver biopsy tissue is placed in a sterile container. The container is sealed in a plastic bag.

SIGNIFICANCE OF TEST RESULTS

Positive Values

Hepatitis C infection, acute, convalescent, or chronic

INTERFERING FACTORS

- Recent administration of radioisotopes

NURSING CARE

Nursing measures are similar to those used in other venipuncture procedures (see Chapter 2), with the following additional measures.

Pretest

- To alert the laboratory personnel, write on the requisition slip that hepatitis is suspected. When hepatitis is suspected, extra attention to technique should help prevent needlestick injury or contact with blood from splashes.
- Apply standard precautions until the specific diagnosis is made and continue these precautions when the lab test is positive. Hepatitis C infection is contagious and the virus is likely to be present in the blood and body fluids.

High-Density Lipoproteins

See Lipid Profile on p. 431.

Histamine Challenge Test

See Pulmonary Function Studies on p. 557.

Histoplasmosis, Antigen and Antibody Tests

his-toh-plas-moh-sis, an-tuh-jen and an-tib-od-ee test

H

SPECIMEN OR TYPE OF TEST: Serum, urine, cerebrospinal fluid

PURPOSE OF THE TEST

These tests are used to help diagnose severe disease caused by histoplasmosis infection and to monitor the patient's response to treatment.

BASICS THE NURSE NEEDS TO KNOW

Histoplasmosis is a fungal disease caused by the *Histoplasma capsulatum* organism. The histoplasmosis infection results from the inhalation of spore-laden dust in the infected excreta of birds, bats, chickens, or turkeys. In the acute form, the spores usually cause pulmonary infection. The infection can also become chronic in the lungs and chest or disseminated in any organ of the body. In acute or disseminated infection, the antigen appears in the blood, urine, and cerebrospinal fluid (CSF), and the laboratory value is positive. The histoplasmosis antibodies are found in the blood. Patients who are immunocompromised (the elderly and those infected with HIV) are vulnerable to develop the disseminated form of the disease.

NORMAL VALUES	Antigen test, blood <1.0 Urine and cerebrospinal fluid: Negative Antibody test: serum: <1:4, Negative

HOW THE TEST IS DONE

Serum (antigen and antibody tests): A venipuncture is performed to collect 10 mL of venous blood in a red-topped tube.

Urine (antigen test): A random sample of urine is placed in a plastic urine container.

CSF (antigen test): During a lumbar puncture, a sample of CSF is collected in a sterile CSF tube.

SIGNIFICANCE OF TEST RESULTS

Positive/Elevated Value

Histoplasmosis

INTERFERING FACTORS

- Positive value for rheumatoid factor
- Other fungal infections
- Histoplasmin skin test

NURSING CARE

Nursing measures are similar to those used in other venipuncture procedures (see Chapter 2), with the following additional measures.

Pretest

- When histoplasmosis is suspected, ask the patient if he or she has had any recent exposure to the feces of birds. Cleaning out the chicken coop is a common source of infection. By geographic region, this infection is endemic in the Ohio and Mississippi River valleys. Also ask the patient if he or she has had a histoplasmosis skin test performed recently. A recent skin test can cause a positive antibody result.

Posttest

- These tests provide some documentation of the cause of this infectious disease, but additional laboratory tests, including a fungal culture will be needed to confirm the medical diagnosis.
- The nurse monitors the patient's vital signs, including temperature. When the client is symptomatic, he or she develops a fever and flu-like manifestations of infection. The illness can infect the lungs and pericardium, causing chest pain and pleuritic pain.
- Schedule a histoplasmosis antibody test in 2 to 3 weeks to evaluate the convalescent phase of the infection.

Holter Monitoring

hohl-ter mon-i-tuhr-ing

Also called: Ambulatory Monitoring

SPECIMEN OR TYPE OF TEST: Electrophysiology

PURPOSE OF THE TEST

The primary purpose of Holter monitoring is dysrhythmia detection. This procedure is helpful in identifying conduction defects and responses to therapeutic measures.

BASICS THE NURSE NEEDS TO KNOW

Holter monitoring permits the recording of cardiac electric activity over time (usually 24 hours) on a cassette tape recorder. It allows the patient to perform normal daily activities so that cardiac responses to these activities can be determined.

NORMAL VALUES Normal rate and rhythm; no ectopy, reentry phenomenon, or changes in segments of the ECG with exercise or medication, or both

HOW THE TEST IS DONE

With Holter monitoring, electrodes are applied to the patient's chest (placement varies with desired leads) and attached to a battery-operated cassette tape recorder. Most recorders permit simultaneous recording of two channels (frequently leads II and V_5 are chosen). Recorders are equipped with an event marker, which alerts the scanning technician that the patient experienced some symptom. A diary is kept by the patient, who records daily activities and the times at which they were performed, when and what medications were taken, and the presence and time at which symptoms occurred. The recordings are analyzed at 60 to 120 times real time by a microcomputer program. Any abnormalities are then recorded on the usual electrocardiograph paper.

SIGNIFICANCE OF TEST RESULTS

Abnormal Values

Conduction disturbances
Dysrhythmias

INTERFERING FACTORS

- Failure of patient to keep records of events and medications taken

NURSING CARE

Pretest

- The nurse checks the Holter monitor's indicator light to determine if the battery is functioning.
- ***Patient Teaching.*** The nurse informs the patient regarding the purpose of the Holter monitoring and the vital role he or she plays in obtaining the needed information.
- ***Patient Teaching.*** The patient is instructed by the nurse to keep a diary of activities and is taught how to trigger the event marker.

During the Test

- Apply electrodes to the chest. Shave the site if the chest is hairy.
- Have the patient demonstrate triggering the event marker. The patient will push the marker whenever pain or other symptoms occur.
- Give the patient a writing pad to record activities during the test time.

Posttest

- Remove electrodes and cleanse the site of gel.
- The nurse checks the skin for signs of irritation.

Homocysteine

hoh-moh-sis-teen

Also called: Total Homocysteine

SPECIMEN OR TYPE OF TEST: Plasma

PURPOSE OF THE TEST

Homocysteine levels may be done to identify people at risk for myocardial infarction or stroke.

BASICS THE NURSE NEEDS TO KNOW

Homocysteine is an intermediate amino acid, which increases with vascular disease. It has been associated with increased risk for coronary artery disease, myocardial infarction, peripheral vascular disease, and stroke.

H

NORMAL VALUES

5–15 µmol/L

HOW THE TEST IS DONE

A fasting venous sample is obtained in a red-topped tube. Send specimen to the lab immediately.

SIGNIFICANCE OF TEST RESULTS

Increased Values

Atherosclerosis
Deficiency in B_6, B_{12}, folic acid, and riboflavin
Hypothyroidism
Inborn errors of cobalamin and folate metabolism
Renal insufficiency

INTERFERING FACTORS

- Ingestion of regular and decaffeinated coffee
- Medications: Corticosteroids, cyclosporine, phenytoin

NURSING CARE

Nursing measures are similar to those used in other venipuncture procedures (see Chapter 2), with the following additional measures.

Pretest

- ***Patient Teaching.*** Instruct patient to fast for 8 to 10 hours before the blood is drawn.
- ***Patient Teaching.*** Instruct patient to avoid drinking coffee.

Homovanillic Acid

See Catecholamines, Urinary on p. 185.

Human Immunodeficiency Virus Tests

hyoo-min im-yuh-noh-de-fi-shun-see vai-ruhs tests

Also called: HIV Tests; Acquired Immune Deficiency Syndrome (AIDS) Tests

SPECIMEN OR TYPE OF TEST: Blood

PURPOSE OF THE TEST

H

The HIV tests are used to diagnose the infection and to monitor progression of the disease. They also are used to screen blood donated for transfusion purposes.

BASICS THE NURSE NEEDS TO KNOW

The human immunodeficiency virus (HIV) is from the retrovirus family of RNA viruses. The two types of HIV are HIV-1 and HIV-2. HIV-1 is the more prevalent type in the United States. HIV infection is transmitted by contaminated blood; by contaminated needles, as in intravenous drug use; by intimate sexual contact with an infected person; and from an infected pregnant woman to her fetus.

HIV Antibody Tests

Several tests are available that detect antibodies to HIV antigen in the patient's serum. About 23 days after the virus enters the patient, the antibody test will convert to a positive value. When HIV antibodies are identified in the blood, it is inferred that HIV antigen and the virus are present. Positive results are verified by a repeat enzyme-linked immunosorbent assay (ELISA) test and an additional antibody test using the Western blot or immunofluorescent assay (IFA) method of analysis.

There are two recently approved methods of detection of the HIV-1 antibodies. The OraQuick rapid HIV-1 antibody test uses point-of-care methodology to produce test results in 20 minutes. The testing can be done in community settings, including physicians' offices, HIV counseling centers, drug treatment centers, and prisons. The ability to perform the test while the patient is at the health care setting and the rapid analysis of the blood will help identify the large group of individuals who are infected with HIV and do not know it. The OraSure HIV-1 Oral Specimen Collection Device is a test method used to detect the HIV-1 antibodies from the cells of the buccal mucosa and the gingival tissue in the mouth. This procedure provides for specimen collection without the use of needles or blood. For both tests, confirmation of a positive value is done by a Western Blot test.

HIV Antigen Test

The p24 core antigen is present in every HIV virion. The antigen will be detected in the patient's blood, 14 days after exposure. The antigen test is used for diagnosis in the early stage of HIV infection. It also reemerges in the blood when the HIV infection progresses to the clinical disease of AIDS. The p24 antigen test is one of the screening tests performed on donated blood.

HIV-DNA Amplification

This test detects proviral DNA molecules of the HIV virus that are in infected lymphocytes. It is used to test neonates born to mothers who have HIV infection.

$CD4^+$

$CD4^+$ lymphocytes (T lymphocytes) are the immune system cells that are killed by the HIV virus. The $CD4^+$ measurement is used as a way to monitor the patient's immune status. If the $CD4^+$ level is 200 cells/mm^3 or less, the low value indicates severe immunosuppression, and the person is at risk to develop opportunistic infections. If the chronically infected HIV patient has this low value, he or she has AIDS and treatment with antiretroviral drugs is recommended. This test is also used in serial monitoring of the immune system's response to the medications.

HIV Viral Load Assay

This test measures the amount of HIV-RNA, the genetic material of HIV in the patient's blood. The test is used to measure the amount of virus copies in the blood at the start of medication treatment and in serial monitoring of the patient's response to the medication. The change in the virus count is a very important measurement. A rising count indicates worsening infection and need for revision of the medication therapy, and a falling level indicates improvement. The changes are used to predict risk for clinical progression and to guide the medical treatment of HIV infection.

NORMAL VALUES

HIV antibody: Negative
p24 Antigen test: Negative
DNA-PCR amplification: No HIV viral DNA detected
$CD4^+$ (T4) lymphocytes: 800–1100 cells/mm^3
Viral load: No HIV viral RNA copies detected

HOW THE TEST IS DONE

p24 Antigen: A red-topped tube is used to collect 10 mL of venous blood.

Antibody test: A red-topped tube is used to collect 10 mL of venous blood.

OraQuick rapid HIV-1 antibody test: A special loop device is used to wipe the drop of blood from a fingerstick puncture or it is dipped into the whole blood specimen from a venipuncture.

OraSure HIV-1 Oral Specimen Collection Device: A special swab is used to obtain cells from the oral mucosa and gingival tissue.

$CD4^+$: A green-topped tube is used to collect 10 mL of venous blood.

HIV-DNA test: Two yellow-topped and two lavender-topped tubes are used collect 10 to 20 mL of venous blood.

Viral load: A lavender-topped tube is used to collect 7 mL of blood.

Note: For the HIV-DNA test and the viral load assay test, the laboratory should specify the type of tube and the volume of blood that is required.

SIGNIFICANCE OF TEST RESULTS

Positive Values

HIV infection
AIDS

Decreased Values

$CD4^+$: AIDS

INTERFERING FACTORS

- Hemolysis
- Insufficient volume of blood

NURSING CARE

Nursing measures are similar to those used in other venipuncture procedures (see Chapter 2), with the following additional measures.

Pretest

- If the nurse draws the blood, standard precautions are used. This means the nurse wears gloves when in contact with blood or body fluids. Needles are disposed of in the puncture-proof container. Proper hand-washing is done after the gloves are removed.
- ***Patient Teaching.*** If the OraSure HIV-1 Oral Specimen Collection Device is to be used, the nurse instructs the patient to discontinue food and fluid intake for 2 hours before the test. The patient should also avoid brushing the teeth, using mouthwash, rinsing the mouth with water, and chewing gum during the 2-hour period. These activities could alter the cellular surface of the tissues and interfere with the accuracy of the test result.

Posttest

- For the patient with confirmed HIV infection, inform the patient that he or she cannot donate blood. If appropriate, instruct that intravenous needles must not be shared.
- ***Patient Teaching.*** The nurse explains that safe sex practices or abstaining from sexual intercourse will help prevent transmission of the infection to others.
- ***Patient Teaching.*** The patient should be taught and encouraged to continue with regular periodic examinations and follow-up laboratory testing. In addition, the obstetrician of the pregnant female patient should be informed of the positive test results.
- ***Patient Teaching.*** The nurse teaches the patient to seek healthcare assistance for symptoms of AIDS, including recurrent respiratory or skin infections, fatigue, diarrhea, weight loss, fever, lymphadenopathy, or a combination of these conditions. The nurse also can assist the patient with education, supportive counseling, and by encouraging referral for prompt medical assistance.

Human Leukocyte Antigen

hyoo-min loo-koh-sait an-tuh-jen

Also called: HLA Typing; Tissue Typing, Crossmatch; Transplant Tissue Typing

SPECIMEN OR TYPE OF TEST: Blood

PURPOSE OF THE TEST

In organ transplantation, human leukocyte antigens (HLA) tissue typing is used to determine tissue compatibility between the donor and the recipient. HLA testing also may be performed to exclude paternity, and it may be used as a source of data in genetic counseling.

BASICS THE NURSE NEEDS TO KNOW

HLAs are genetic products that are major determinants of histocompatibility. These antigens exist in an exact sequence or pattern that is specific and different for each individual. The unique protein sequence is found on every cell of the body, including on leukocytes. The only exception is in identical twins, which have identical HLA antigens.

Circulating leukocytes are in contact with other cells. During the moment of contact, the leukocytes compare the HLA sequence on the cell surface with their own HLA sequence. When the HLA sequence is the same, the leukocyte does not react. When the HLA sequence is different, the leukocyte recognizes the cell as a foreign substance and initiates an inflammatory reaction to inactivate and destroy the cell with a different HLA sequence.

In organ transplantation, HLA matching of the organ donor and transplant recipient is essential. Tissue matching improves the chance of acceptance of the tissue graft and increases the long-term survival of the transplanted tissue. When HLA matching is less than optimal, the recipient's immune system is activated with the recognition of a foreign HLA antigen. Mismatching results in graft-versus-host disease, graft failure, and possible increased sensitization of the recipient when retransplantation is needed.

NORMAL VALUES No destruction of lymphocytes; identification of specific leukocyte antigens or class I and class II alleles

HOW THE TEST IS DONE

Donor Specimen

Two green-topped tubes are each filled with 10 mL of venous blood.

Recipient's Specimen

A red-topped tube is used to obtain 10 mL of venous blood.

HLA Typing

A green-topped, heparinized tube is filled with 7 mL to 10 mL of venous blood.

SIGNIFICANCE OF TEST RESULTS

Abnormal Values

Incompatibility of donor and recipient tissues

INTERFERING FACTORS

- Recent blood transfusion
- Inadequate lymphocytes in the specimen
- Hemolysis of blood sample

NURSING CARE

Nursing measures are similar to those used in other venipuncture procedures (see Chapter 2), with the following additional measures.

Pretest

- Schedule this test before or 72 hours after a blood transfusion.

Posttest

- The patient who is tested to be an organ donor or the person who is in need of an organ transplant has hopes and possible concerns. Either individual may need to talk about the situation. Although nothing will be known until compatibility testing is completed, the nurse can help by listening with an empathetic approach.

H

Hydrocortisone, Serum

See Cortisol, Total on p. 238.

17-Hydroxycorticosteroids

sev-un-teen hai-drok-see-kawhr-tik-oh ster-oyds

Also called: (17-OHCS)

SPECIMEN OR TYPE OF TEST: Urine

PURPOSE OF THE TEST

17-OHCS levels are obtained to assess adrenal function.

BASICS THE NURSE NEEDS TO KNOW

17-Hydroxycorticosteroids (17-OHCS) are urinary steroids (cortisol and cortisone metabolites) used to assess adrenal function. An increase in 17-OHCS in the urine reflects an increase in plasma cortisol. With the direct measurement of plasma cortisol and free cortisol, the frequency of 17-OHCS determinations has significantly decreased.

When assessing 17-OHCS values, it is necessary to consider the patient's body type. Obese or muscular individuals will have higher 17-OHCS levels than those with normal body types because of an increase in cortisol metabolism. To adjust to body type, some clinicians correlate the 17-OHCS to the creatinine clearance.

NORMAL VALUES

Adult male: 4.5–12 mg/24 hr *or* SI: 12.4–33.1 μmol/24 hr
Adult female: 2.5–10 mg/24 hr *or* SI: 6.9–27.6 μmol/24 hr
Children: 8–12 years: <4.5 mg/24 hr *or* SI: <12.4 μmol/24 hr
<8 years: <1.5 mg/24 hr *or* SI: <4.14 μmol/24 hr

HOW THE TEST IS DONE

A 24-hour urine specimen is obtained. The urine is assessed by colorimetric reaction.

SIGNIFICANCE OF TEST RESULTS

Elevated Values

Adrenal cancer
Cushing syndrome
Extreme stress
Hyperthyroidism
Pituitary tumor
Obesity
Severe hypertension
Acromegaly

Decreased Values

Addison's disease
Hypothyroidism
Starvation
Liver failure
Renal failure
Pregnancy
Congenital adrenal hyperplasia
Hypotension

INTERFERING FACTORS

- Failure to collect all the urine during the 24-hour collection period
- Failure to keep specimen on ice or refrigerated
- Medications such as chloral hydrate, chlorpromazine, colchicine, erythromycin, estrogens, oral contraceptives, paraldehyde, quinidine, quinine, reserpine, and spironolactone

H

NURSING CARE

Nursing measures are similar to those used in other timed urine collections (see Chapter 2), with the following additional measures.

Pretest

- Take the patient's medication history to assess for interfering medications.
- ***Patient Teaching.*** The nurse explains the collection procedure to the patient, especially the need to collect *all* the urine for 24 hours.

Continued

NURSING CARE—*cont'd*

Pretest—*cont'd*

- ***Patient Teaching.*** Instruct the patient to avoid excessive physical activity during the testing period.

During the Test

- At the start of the test, the nurse instructs the patient to void at 8 AM and discard this urine. The collection period begins at this time, and all the urine is collected for 24 hours, including the 8 AM specimen of the following morning. The nurse needs to remind the patient during the collection period to save all the urine.
- Keep the urine and collection container refrigerated or on ice during the collection period.

Posttest

- On the requisition slip and specimen label, write the patient's name and the time and date of the start and finish of the test period.
- Arrange for prompt transport of the cooled specimen to the laboratory.

Hysterosalpingography

his-ter-oh-sal-ping-og-ruh-fee

Also called: (HSG); Hysterosalpingogram

SPECIMEN OR TYPE OF TEST: Radiography

PURPOSE OF THE TEST

Hysterosalpingography is used to assess the patency of the fallopian tubes as part of infertility studies of the female. It also can identify abnormal development of the uterus and the presence of a uterine fistula.

BASICS THE NURSE NEEDS TO KNOW

As part of the infertility work-up in the female, the hysterosalpingogram is performed to identify anatomic abnormality of the uterus or occlusion of the fallopian tubes. The lumen of each of these structures is visualized. The tubes can be blocked because of external compression from an abdominal or pelvic abnormality, or internal blockage from scarring can exist. The uterus may have an anatomic abnormality, such as that caused by incomplete development of the uterus, or a congenital abnormality resulting from intrauterine exposure to diethylstilbestrol.

In normal anatomy, the radiopaque dye is instilled into the uterine cavity. Then, the effects of gravity and positional changes promote the flow of dye through the uterus and fallopian tubes and then into the abdominal cavity. If the contrast material does not enter the abdominal cavity, one or both tubes are blocked. The test requires 30 to 45 minutes to complete.

NORMAL VALUES Normal flow of dye through the uterus and fallopian tubes

HOW THE TEST IS DONE

Radiopaque contrast medium is instilled through a catheter into the uterus. The patient's positional changes and a tilting of the table promote gravity flow of the contrast material. Fluoroscopic and x-ray films provide visualization of the interior surfaces of the uterus and fallopian tubes.

SIGNIFICANCE OF TEST RESULTS

Abnormal Values

Partial or complete obstruction of the fallopian tubes
Fibroid tumor of the uterus
Adhesions
Uterine fistula
Foreign body (e.g., intrauterine device)
Uterine malformation

INTERFERING FACTORS

- Menstruation
- Pregnancy
- Active uterine bleeding
- Pelvic inflammatory disease
- Allergy to the contrast medium

NURSING CARE

Pretest

- The nurse schedules this test during the early part of the menstrual cycle, before ovulation occurs. This prevents interference with ovulation, irradiation of the oocytes, or the possibility of an early phase of pregnancy. Ensure that the patient has no current vaginal bleeding or gynecologic infection. When these conditions exist, the contrast material could be absorbed into the vasculature, or its flow could introduce microorganisms into the fallopian tubes.
- The nurse identifies any patient with a history of allergy to iodine or shellfish or a reaction to a previous x-ray study that used iodinated contrast medium. If a positive allergic history exists, the allergy is documented in the patient's record and reported to the physician. Plans are made to premedicate the patient with prescribed steroids or an antihistamine, or both.
- Once the patient is informed of the procedure, obtain written consent and place it in the patient's record.
- ***Patient Teaching.*** In the pretest preparation, instruct the patient to take the prescribed laxative on the night before the test. On the morning of the procedure, cleansing enemas are done until the returns are clear.
- The nurse assists the patient in removing all clothes and putting on a hospital gown.

Continued

NURSING CARE—*cont'd*

Pretest—*cont'd*

- ***Patient Teaching.*** The patient is instructed to void to empty the bladder. This prevents displacement of the uterus and fallopian tubes by an enlarged bladder. The nurse takes the patient's vital signs and records the results.

During the Test

- The nurse places the patient in the lithotomy position.
- The nurse provides reassurance as the physician inserts the vaginal speculum, cleanses the cervix with povidone-iodine, and inserts the cannula. As the contrast material is instilled, the patient may experience temporary sensations of nausea, dizziness, bradycardia, or uterine cramping.
- Between radiographic images, the nurse helps the patient change position so that the contrast medium flows through the fallopian tubes.

Posttest

- The nurse monitors and records the patient's vital signs. On discharge, the patient is instructed to gradually return to pretest activity levels.

◇ Nursing Response to Complications

An allergic reaction to the contrast medium can occur. The response is usually mild.

Mild allergic reaction. The nurse assesses for hives and urticaria. The patient would develop redness and some swelling in the skin. The patient complains of itching. The blood pressure value can be low, with hypotension. In cases of mild allergic reaction, the nurse reports the findings to the physician and prepares to administer diphenhydramine hydrochloride (Benadryl), as prescribed.

Immunoreactive PTH

See Parathyroid Hormone on p. 500.

Impedance Cardiography

See Catheterization, Cardiac on p. 187.

Infectious Mononucleosis Tests

in-fek-shuhs mo-noh-noo-klee-oh-sis tests

Also called: Monotest; Heterophil Antibody Test

SPECIMEN OR TYPE OF TEST: Blood

PURPOSE OF THE TEST

These serologic tests help to diagnose infectious mononucleosis.

BASICS THE NURSE NEEDS TO KNOW

The Epstein-Barr virus is responsible for most cases of infectious mononucleosis. In this viral infection, the patient's immune response produces heterophil antibodies of the IgM class and Epstein-Barr antibodies. Six to 10 days after the symptoms appear, the heterophil antibodies can be detected or measured. The antibody level peaks in 2 to 3 weeks and usually persists for 1 to 2 months.

The monotest is a rapid, simple, and effective test that identifies the presence or absence of infectious mononucleosis antibodies in the patient's serum. When the infectious mononucleosis antibodies are present, the test result is positive. The heterophil antibody test is used when the titer is to be measured. A heterophil titer of 1:128 or higher means that the test result is positive.

NORMAL VALUES

Monotest: Negative
Heterophil titer: <1:56

HOW THE TEST IS DONE

A red-topped tube is used to collect 10 mL of venous blood.

SIGNIFICANCE OF TEST RESULTS

Elevated/Positive Values
Infectious mononucleosis

INTERFERING FACTORS

- Hemolysis

NURSING CARE

Nursing measures are similar to those used in other venipuncture procedures (see Chapter 2), with the following additional measures.

Pretest

- Schedule this test a few days after the onset of illness. Until the antibodies have time to develop, the test results will remain negative. On the requisition slip, include the date of the onset of illness.

Posttest

- The nurse assesses the patient for manifestations of the infection. In infectious mononucleosis, there is an elevated temperature and the patient complains of a sore throat. Nursing assessment of the head and neck reveals an inflamed oropharynx and tonsils. The soft palate may have petechiae. On palpation of the abdomen, enlargement of the liver and spleen may be present.

Insulin

in-suh-lin

Also called: Immunoreactive Insulin

SPECIMEN OR TYPE OF TEST: Serum, plasma

PURPOSE OF THE TEST

Insulin levels are determined to assess for insulin-producing tumors, to confirm suspected insulin-resistant states, and as part of the evaluation of glucocorticoid insufficiency. It is not recommended for routine testing of patients with diabetes mellitus.

BASICS THE NURSE NEEDS TO KNOW

Insulin is a protein hormone produced and secreted by the pancreas. It has a short half-life (3 to 5 minutes) and is broken down by the liver and kidneys. Insulin is secreted in response to food intake. It increases in concentration within 10 minutes of eating, peaks in 30 to 45 minutes, and returns to baseline levels within 90 to 120 minutes. Normally, insulin levels increase as blood glucose levels increase.

Without insulin, carbohydrate, protein, and fat metabolism are affected, resulting in hyperglycemia and metabolic acidosis.

NORMAL VALUES

Fasting: Adult: 5–25 μU/mL *or* SI: 34–172 pmol/L
Newborn: 3–20 μU/mL *or* SI: 21–138 pmol/L
1 hour after eating: 50–130 μU/mL *or* SI: 347.3–902.8 pmol/L
2 hours after eating: <30 μU/mL *or* SI: <208.4 pmol/L

HOW THE TEST IS DONE

Insulin levels may be assessed by random venous sampling or during a glucose tolerance test. A specimen is obtained by venipuncture and collected in either an anticoagulated or red-topped tube, depending on the laboratory.

SIGNIFICANCE OF TEST RESULTS

Elevated Values

Acromegaly
Cushing syndrome
Hyperinsulinism
Insulinoma
Liver disease
Pancreatic lesions
Vagal stimulation

Decreased Values

Type 1 diabetes mellitus
Hypopituitarism

INTERFERING FACTORS

- Noncompliance with test protocol
- Insulin antibodies
- Medications such as ACTH, catecholamines, colchicine, diazoxide, oral contraceptives, phenytoin, steroids, sulfonylureas, thyroid hormones, vinblastine, and radioisotopes

NURSING CARE

Nursing measures are similar to those used in other venipuncture procedures (see Chapter 2), with the following additional measures.

Nursing care varies according to whether a fasting sample is used or the insulin level is being obtained as part of the OGTT (see p. 356 for discussion of this test).

Pretest

- The nurse takes a medication history to determine if any interfering drugs are being taken. Check to determine if these drugs are to be withheld. If the patient is receiving insulin therapy, the insulin is withheld until the test is performed.
- Assess the patient's stress level, which may increase endogenous glucocorticoid secretion.
- ***Patient Teaching.*** If a fasting insulin sample is to be drawn, the nurse instructs the patient not to eat or drink for 7 hours before the blood is drawn.

During the Test

- Observe the patient for hyperglycemia if insulin is withheld and for hypoglycemia because of the fasting state.
- If performed with an OGTT, a blood sample for insulin is obtained each time a glucose level specimen is drawn.

Posttest

- Send the specimen to the laboratory immediately, because it must be centrifuged within 30 minutes and frozen until the assay can be performed.
- The patient resumes normal medication schedule and diet therapies.

Insulin Tolerance Test

See Growth Hormone Stimulation Test on p. 364.

Insulin-Induced Hypoglycemia Test

See Metyrapone Stimulation Test on p. 462.

International Normalized Ratio (INR)

See Prothrombin Time on p. 555.

Intravenous Glucose Tolerance Test

See Glucose Tolerance Test on p. 356.

Intravenous Pyelogram

in-truh-vee-nus pai-loh-gram

Also called: (IVP); Excretory Urogram (EUG); Intravenous Urography (IVU), (IUG)

SPECIMEN OR TYPE OF TEST: Radiography

PURPOSE OF THE TEST

The intravenous pyelogram (IVP) is used to evaluate the structure and function of the kidneys, ureters, and bladder. It assesses the cause of nontraumatic hematuria, locates the precise site of obstruction, and determines the cause of flank pain or renal colic.

BASICS THE NURSE NEEDS TO KNOW

I

An IVP is a basic urologic procedure that uses contrast medium and radiography to visualize the anatomy and function of the urinary tract. The intravenous contrast material is filtered from the blood by the kidneys. The x-ray films record the contrast medium entering the renal pelvis of each kidney and then flowing through the ureters and into the bladder.

When a time delay occurs before the injected contrast medium reaches the renal pelvis, the delay is indicative of poor renal perfusion or poor renal function. The x-ray films also demonstrate abnormalities of position, shape, size, or structure of the organs of the urinary tract. Clear detail and precise location of a stricture, dilation, calculus, obstruction, tumor, or filling defect can be seen.

CT, ultrasound, and digital subtraction angiography are replacing IVP, because the contrast medium used in an IVP can be toxic to the kidneys or can cause a severe allergic reaction.

NORMAL VALUES No anatomic or physiologic abnormalities are noted in the kidneys, ureters, or bladder

HOW THE TEST IS DONE

An initial x-ray film is taken to provide baseline information. After an intravenous injection of contrast material, timed radiographs are taken of the urinary tract. Films at 1 minute visualize the kidneys; at 3 to 5 minutes, the renal collecting system is visualized; at 10 minutes, the ureters are seen; and at 20 to 30 minutes, filling of the bladder is seen. A post-voiding film demonstrates the ability of the bladder to empty. The test requires 1 to 1½ hours to complete.

SIGNIFICANCE OF TEST RESULTS

Abnormal Values

Hydronephrosis
Renal or ureteral calculi
Hydroureter
Polycystic kidney disease

Tumor
Pyelonephritis
Renal tuberculosis
Absent kidney
Congenital anomalies
Nonfunctioning kidney

INTERFERING FACTORS

- Renal failure
- Feces, gas, or barium in the colon
- Recent gall bladder series
- Failure to maintain nothing-by-mouth status

NURSING CARE

Nursing measures are similar to those used in other venipuncture procedures (see Chapter 2), with the following additional measures.

Pretest

- The nurse asks the patient about any history of allergy to shellfish or iodine or of a previous reaction to an x-ray study that used contrast medium. Any allergy is documented on the patient chart, according to hospital policy, and reported to the physician in the radiology department.
- Schedule the IVP before any barium test or gallbladder series that also uses iodinated contrast material.
- Ensure that a signed informed consent form has been obtained from the patient or the person legally designated to make healthcare decisions for the patient.
- ***Patient Teaching.*** The nurse instructs the patient regarding the pretest bowel cleansing procedure that removes gas and fecal matter. This includes taking the prescribed laxative or cathartic the night before the test and an enema or suppository on the morning of the test.
- ***Patient Teaching.*** Instruct the patient to discontinue food intake for 8 hours before the test. Fluids are permitted.
- Since patients who are dehydrated are at high risk for the development of renal failure as a result of the toxic effect of the contrast medium on the kidney tissues, the nurse assesses and reports indications of fluid deficit.
- The nurse ensures that recent BUN and creatinine test results are posted in the chart. These tests help identify patients who are at risk and help determine a safe dose of contrast medium.
- Record baseline vital signs.

During the Test

- Assist the patient as the contrast medium is administered. The nurse informs the patient that it is common to experience a brief burning sensation or a metallic taste in the mouth, or both.

Continued

NURSING CARE—*cont'd*

During the Test—*cont'd*

- Have an emesis basin within reach, because nausea and vomiting may occur.

Posttest

- Take the vital signs and record the results.
- Continue the intravenous fluid replacement as ordered and encourage the patient to take oral fluids.

◆ Nursing Response to Complications

Vasovagal response. During the test, a small number of patients have a vasovagal response to the contrast material. Atropine is kept on hand to overcome this side effect.

Allergic response. An allergic or anaphylactic response can occur immediately or hours after test dye is given. This response varies from a rash and hives to acute respiratory distress. A mild reaction is treated with antihistamines or steroids. A severe reaction is treated with intravenous epinephrine and oxygen, with additional measures taken as needed. An emergency cart is maintained in the radiology suite at all times.

Nephrotoxicity. Patients with diabetes and preexisting renal disease may develop impaired renal function, which can occur from 1 to 4 days after the study is completed. Usually it is a temporary problem and the kidneys return to their baseline level of function.

Intrinsic Factor Antibody

in-trin-sik fak-tuhr an-tib-od-ee

Also called: IF Antibody

SPECIMEN OR TYPE OF TEST: Serum

PURPOSE OF THE TEST

This test is performed to differentiate pernicious anemia from other causes of megaloblastic anemia. It also helps determine the cause of a decreased cobalamin (vitamin B_{12}) level.

BASICS THE NURSE NEEDS TO KNOW

Intrinsic factor is a glycoprotein manufactured by the parietal cells of the gastric mucosa. The function of intrinsic factor is to bond with ingested cobalamin and then facilitate absorption of cobalamin in the ilium. Cobalamin is needed by the bone marrow in the manufacture of new red blood cells. Without cobalamin, the patient develops pernicious anemia, a megaloblastic anemia.

Interference with the function of intrinsic factor is caused by intrinsic factor antibodies. These antibodies are autoimmune complexes that are present in many cases of pernicious anemia. Two types of intrinsic factor antibody exist. Type 1, the "blocking" antibody, interferes with the bonding of intrinsic factor to cobalamin. Type 2, the "binding" antibody, interferes with the attachment of the intrinsic factor-cobalamin complex to the ileal receptor sites.

NORMAL VALUES Negative: No intrinsic factor antibodies are present

HOW THE TEST IS DONE

A red-topped tube is used to obtain 10 mL of venous blood.

SIGNIFICANCE OF TEST RESULTS

Positive Value

Pernicious anemia
Hyperthyroidism (Graves' disease)
Diabetes mellitus (insulin dependent)

INTERFERING FACTORS

- Recent radioisotope scan
- Recent vitamin B_{12} injection

NURSING CARE

Nursing measures are similar to those used in other venipuncture procedures (see Chapter 2), with the following additional measures.

Pretest

- Schedule this test before any radioisotope scan. The radioisotopes of the nuclear scan would interfere with the radioimmunoassay method of analysis used in this test.
- Instruct the patient to withhold any injection of vitamin B_{12} for 48 hours before the test. Recent injection of this vitamin could cause a false-positive result.

Iron Studies

ai-uhrn stu-deez

Also called: Serum iron (Fe); Transferrin (Tf); Siderophilin; Total Iron-Binding Capacity (TIBC); Transferrin Saturation; Iron Saturation

SPECIMEN OR TYPE OF TEST: Serum

PURPOSE OF THE TEST

These tests provide an estimate of total iron storage and information regarding the nutritional status of the individual. They help distinguish between iron deficiency anemia and the anemia of chronic disease. They also confirm the presence of iron overload and hematochromatosis.

BASICS THE NURSE NEEDS TO KNOW

Iron is an inorganic ion that is essential to many vital body processes, including erythropoiesis (the manufacture of red blood cells) and as a component of hemoglobin, needed for the transport of oxygen to tissues. In normal physiology, the total iron content remains relatively constant throughout life. The source of iron intake is from food or mineral supplement. The body has an efficient method to conserve the iron from senescent erythrocytes and reuse it in erythropoiesis and hemoglobin synthesis (Figure 53).

I

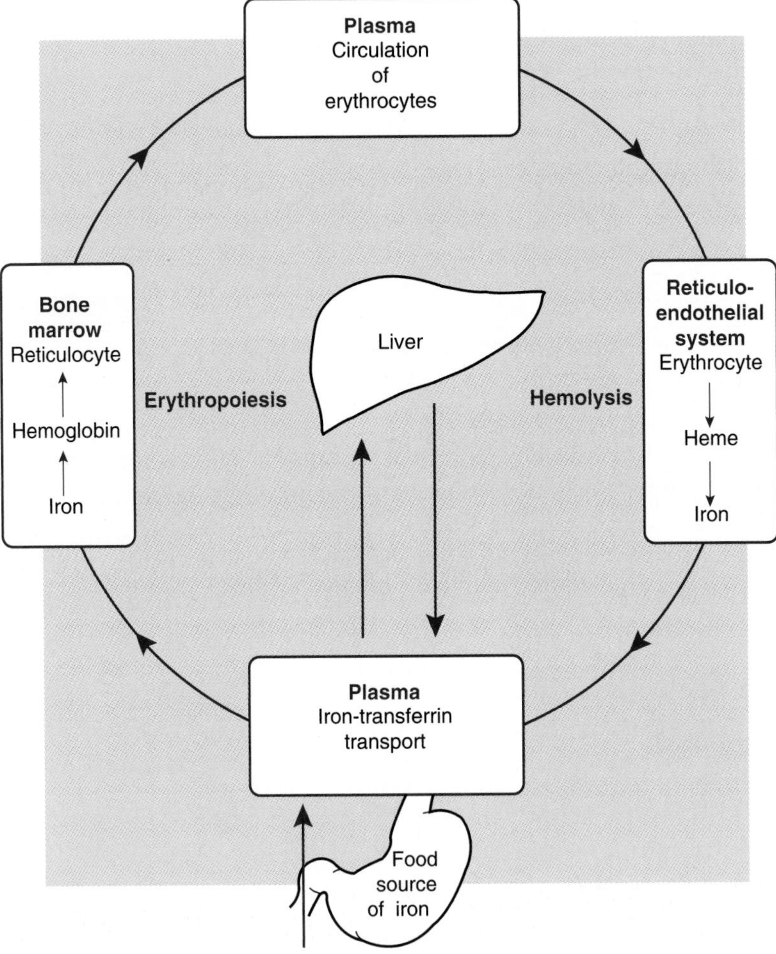

Figure 53. The use and conservation of iron. Some iron is readily available in the plasma and bone marrow for the synthesis of hemoglobin and erythropoiesis. After the hemolysis of old or damaged erythrocytes, the body is very efficient in the conservation and storage of iron in the liver and bone marrow. Whenever the immediate supply of iron is low, the liver releases the stored iron for erythropoiesis.

Iron overload occurs in some types of anemia, in liver disease, in excessive iron replacement therapy, and after multiple transfusions. Iron deficiency occurs when the supply of iron is insufficient to meet the body's demand and the iron reserves are also depleted. The source of the problem can be insufficient intake, impaired absorption, blood loss, or increased demand because of pregnancy or lactation (Table 9).

Laboratory Testing

No single test fully measures iron deficiency, iron overload, and iron storage. A battery of several tests, including the complete blood count, is used to provide a complete assessment. The laboratory assessment of iron stores includes serum iron, transferrin, total iron-binding capacity, transferrin saturation, and ferritin.

Serum Iron

As a single laboratory test, a serum iron determination is used to evaluate iron toxicity. The elevated value can rise to the level of a critical value, indicating serious iron toxicity. The value is decreased in iron deficiency anemia and in the anemia associated with chronic disease.

Transferrin

This is the major protein that binds serum iron and transports it in the blood. In normal physiology, about one third of the transferrin is bound with iron, and the remainder is available in reserve. Transferrin is elevated in iron deficiency anemia and is decreased with iron overload. It is a useful index of nutritional status because it is elevated in uncomplicated iron deficiency but is in the normal to low-normal range in other types of anemia.

Total Iron-Binding Capacity

This is the maximum iron-binding capacity of transferrin and other iron-binding globulins. The serum value also provides data regarding the nutritional status of the individual. The total iron-binding capacity rises in iron deficiency anemia and decreases in the presence of iron overload.

Transferrin Saturation

This is a calculation of the iron storage, expressed as the percentage of transferrin that is saturated with iron. The value is decreased in iron deficiency, but a value of less than 15% indicates iron deficiency erythropoiesis.

TABLE 9 Factors that Contribute to Iron Deficiency

Insufficient Intake	Impaired Absorption	Blood Loss	Increased Demand
Fad diets	Gastric surgery	Gastrointestinal bleeding	Pregnancy
Pica	Celiac disease	Excessive menstruation	Lactation
Poverty	Achlorhydria		

Ferritin

This is a reliable indicator of total iron storage. The level is decreased in iron deficiency anemia and elevated in iron overload. When a ferritin determination is combined with other iron studies, the results differentiate among the different types of microcytic, hypochromic anemias. Iron deficiency anemia is indicated by a serum ferritin value of less than 10 ng/mL (SI: <10 mcg/L).

NORMAL VALUES

Serum Iron
Adult male: 60–150 mcg/dL *or* SI: 10.7–26.9 µmol/L
Child: 50–120 mcg/dL *or* SI: 9–21.5 µmol/L
Infant: 40–100 mcg/dL *or* SI: 7.2–17.9 µmol/L
Newborn: 100–250 mcg/dL *or* SI: 17.9–44.8 µmol/L

Transferrin
Adult (>60 years): 190–375 mg/dL *or* SI: 1.9–3.75 g/L
Adult (16–60 years): Male: 215–365 mg/dL *or* SI: 2.15–3.65 g/L; Female: 250–380 mg/dL *or* SI: 2.50–3.80 g/L
Child (3 months–16 years): 203–360 mg/dL *or* SI: 2.03–3.6 g/L
Newborn: 130–275 mg/dL *or* SI: 1.3–2.75 g/L

Total Iron-Binding Capacity
250–400 mcg/dL *or* SI: 44.8–71.6 µmol/L

Transferrin Saturation
20%–55% *or* SI: 0.20–0.55 fraction saturation

Ferritin
Adult male: 15–200 ng/mL *or* SI: 15–200 mcg/L
Adult female: 2–150 ng/mL *or* SI: 12–150 mcg/L
Child (6 months–15 years): 7–140 ng/mL *or* SI: 7–140 mcg/L
Infant (2–5 months): 50–200 ng/mL *or* SI: 50–200 mcg/L
Newborn: 25–200 ng/mL *or* SI: 25–200 mcg/L

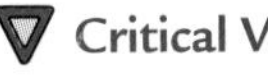

Critical Values: Serum iron: 500 mcg/dL *or* SI: 89.5 µmol/L

HOW THE TEST IS DONE

A red-topped tube is used to collect 10 mL of venous blood.

SIGNIFICANCE OF TEST RESULTS

Elevated Values

SERUM IRON

Anemias (pernicious, aplastic, hemolytic)
Hematochromatosis

Thalassemia
Excess iron replacement
Multiple transfusions
Iron poisoning
Lead poisoning
Vitamin B_6 deficiency
Acute leukemia

Transferrin

Iron deficiency anemia
Elevated estrogen levels
Pregnancy

Total Iron-Binding Capacity

Hypochromic anemias
Iron deficiency anemia
Acute hepatitis
Pregnancy

Ferritin

Thalassemia
Iron toxicity
Hemochromatosis
Viral hepatitis
Nephrosis

Transferrin Saturation

Hemochromatosis
Liver disease
Iron overload
Acute leukemias
Inflammatory diseases
Infectious diseases

Decreased Values

Serum Iron

Iron deficiency anemia
Nephrosis
Hypothyroidism
Acute or chronic infection
Malignancy
Starvation

Transferrin

Inflammation or necrosis
Malignancy
Malnutrition
Multiple myeloma
Hepatocellular diseases
Nephrotic syndrome

Transferrin Saturation
Iron deficiency anemia
Anemia of chronic infection
Malignancy
Total Iron-Binding Capacity
Anemias (non–iron-deficient)
Hemochromatosis
Malignancy
Renal disease
Thalassemia
Ferritin
Iron deficiency anemia

INTERFERING FACTORS

- Recent administration of radioisotopes (ferritin)
- Hemolysis (serum iron, iron saturation)
- Lipemia (transferrin)
- Recent blood transfusion (serum iron)
- Oral iron medication therapy

NURSING CARE

Nursing measures are similar to those used in other venipuncture procedures (see Chapter 2), with the following additional measures.

Pretest

- To obtain the most accurate results, these lab tests should be scheduled before or a few days after a blood transfusion. The blood tests should be done before any nuclear scans, because the radioactive isotopes of the scan interfere with the radioimmunoassay method for testing of ferritin. They also should be performed in the morning. Serum iron has a diurnal rhythm, with the highest value in the early morning. The serum iron values fluctuate widely between day and night and also different days.
- If the patient takes an iron supplement, the nurse includes this information on the requisition slip.
- ***Patient Teaching.*** The nurse instructs the patient to fast from food and fluids for 8 hours before the test for transferrin levels. Lipemia interferes with the transferrin values.

Posttest

Elevated value of iron. The patient who has chronic renal failure and is treated by hemodialysis therapy is vulnerable to development of a chronically elevated serum iron level. The nurse monitors the test results for signs of iron overload. When the patient manufactures too few erythrocytes, there will be an increased blood level and storage of excess iron.

NURSING CARE—*cont'd*

In addition, patients who received multiple transfusions or who have hemochromatosis can develop toxicity from iron overload. The elevated value also may be the result of excessive intake of iron replacement medication.

- The nurse notifies the physician of a serum iron value that is elevated, particularly when there is a blood level of 350 mcg/dL (SI: 63 µmol/L) or higher. Laboratory values in this range or above indicate mild iron toxicity. After the physician establishes the diagnosis and the cause of the iron overload, prescribed measures to lower the iron level can include administration of the antidote, deferoxamine mesylate (Desferal). The medication is given by subcutaneous or intramuscular route. For hemodialysis patients, other measures to lower the chronically elevated iron level include administration of erythropoietin and phlebotomy.

▼ Nursing Response to Critical Values

The lab value of 500 mcg/dL (SI: 89.5 µmol/L) or above is considered to be a critical value indicating a severe iron toxicity. The nurse notifies the physician immediately and assesses the patient for vomiting and severe abdominal pain. The patient will develop metabolic acidosis and an increased anion gap. In severe iron poisoning, other lab values include elevated serum glucose, bilirubin, liver enzymes, and WBC.

With an extreme critical value of 1000 mcg/dL (SI: 179 µmol/L), the problem is usually acute iron toxicity. Unless the problem is reversed, the patient is likely to develop shock and cardiovascular collapse, leading to death. In this extreme situation, the nurse prepares to administer the antidote, deferoxamine mesylate (Desferal), by the intravenous route, as prescribed by the physician. The medication is mixed in an intravenous solution and administered by a slow and controlled infusion rate. If the medication is administered too rapidly, it will cause hypotension and shock, worsening the problem.

Decreased value of iron. In iron deficiency anemia, the nurse assesses for changes in the patient, including pallor, fatigue, and elevated pulse and respirations. A nutritional assessment provides information about the patient's food intake, particularly related to sources of iron.

- *Patient Teaching.* The nurse can teach the patient to increase the intake of dietary sources of iron, including red meat, egg yolk, whole grain bread, fortified cereals, and dried fruits such as raisins. If an oral iron supplement is prescribed, the patient is taught to take the iron tablet or liquid after meals or with a snack. This helps avoid gastric irritation. Replacement iron therapy will cause some constipation and black color of the feces.

Ketone Bodies, Blood

kee-tohn bo-deez, blud

Also called: Ketones

SPECIMEN OR TYPE OF TEST: Serum, Plasma, Whole Blood

PURPOSE OF THE TEST

Serum ketone levels are measured to determine the insulin requirements of patients with diabetes mellitus, who are hyperglycemic.

BASICS THE NURSE NEEDS TO KNOW

Serum ketone levels are measured to distinguish between diabetic ketoacidosis and hyperosmolar coma. With diabetic ketoacidosis, incomplete fatty acid metabolism leads to increasing ketones in the blood. Patients with hyperosmolar coma and extremely high levels of serum glucose produce minimal to no ketones. The mechanism of maintaining nearly normal ketone levels in hyperosmolar coma is not known. It is theorized that these patients have sufficient insulin to break down fatty acids or are glucagon resistant. Without adequate insulin, three major ketone bodies accumulate in the blood: acetone, acetoacetate acid, and beta-hydroxybutyric acid.

K

NORMAL VALUES Negative: <2 mg/dL *or* SI: <0.5 mmol/L

HOW THE TEST IS DONE

Venipuncture is performed to obtain 2 mL of blood in a red-topped or green-topped tube.

SIGNIFICANCE OF TEST RESULTS

Elevated Values

Alcoholic ketoacidosis
Decreased caloric intake (dieting)
Eclampsia
Isopropanol poisoning
Propranolol poisoning
Starvation
Uncontrolled diabetes mellitus
Gierke's disease

INTERFERING FACTORS

- Hemolysis of specimen

NURSING CARE

The nurse's duties are similar to those performed in other venipuncture procedures, as presented in Chapter 2.

Ketones, Urinary

kee-tohnz, yur-i-ner-ee

Also called: Acetoacetate; Acetones

SPECIMEN OR TYPE OF TEST: Urine

PURPOSE OF THE TEST

Urine is tested for ketone bodies to evaluate the patient with diabetes mellitus and to diagnose carbohydrate deprivation. The concentration of urine ketones can be used to adjust insulin requirements in diabetic patients, assist in the diagnosis of diabetic ketoacidosis, and to monitor patients on low-carbohydrate diets.

BASICS THE NURSE NEEDS TO KNOW

Without adequate insulin, three major ketone bodies accumulate in the blood and are excreted in the urine. These ketone bodies are acetone, acetoacetic acid, and beta-hydroxybutyric acid. Ketones form as fats, and fatty acids are broken down.

A variety of commercial products are available to test for ketones in the urine. The most popular products are Acetest tablets, Ketostix, and Keto-Diastix. These products measure acetone and acetoacetate acid levels but not beta-hydroxybutyric acid, which may be the dominant ketone in patients with poorly controlled diabetes mellitus.

Urinary ketone testing is usually performed in conjunction with capillary or urinary glucose testing. It may be carried out randomly to evaluate a suspected diagnosis of uncontrolled diabetes mellitus or periodically during the day to regulate insulin coverage. Ketones should be checked in diabetic patients during acute illness, severe stress, and pregnancy.

NORMAL VALUES Negative

HOW THE TEST IS DONE

With the Acetest tablet, one drop of urine is placed on a tablet. With the Ketostix or Keto-Diastix, the reagent strip is dipped in the urine. The color change of the tablet or on the strip is compared to the chart provided by the manufacturer to determine the presence and concentration of ketones.

SIGNIFICANCE OF TEST RESULTS

Elevated Values

Alcoholic ketoacidosis
Fever
High-fat diet
Hypermetabolic states
Starvation
Uncontrolled diabetes mellitus

INTERFERING FACTORS

- Using products that have been exposed to light or are outdated
- Bacteria in the urine
- Highly acidic urine
- Medications: Ascorbic acid, levodopa

NURSING CARE

- *Health Promotion.* The nurse educates the patient with diabetes mellitus to check his or her urinary ketones whenever the glucose level is over 300 mg/dL (SI: 16.7 mmol/L) or he or she is experiencing an acute illness. Instruct the patient to be aware of possible indications of ketoacidosis; such as nausea, vomiting, or abdominal pain, and to check urinary ketones if these symptoms occur.
- If a diabetic patient is pregnant, the nurse instructs her to inform the manager of her diabetes. During pregnancy, urinary ketones will be assessed periodically.

During the Test

- Instruct the patient to void into a clean, dry container.
- Check voided urine within 60 minutes.
- The method of checking for ketones varies with the product. Follow the manufacturer's guidelines.

Posttest

- Document the results, usually on a flow chart.
- Adjust insulin dosage as ordered based on the results.

L

Lactate Dehydrogenase (LDH)

See Cardiac Markers on p. 178.

Lactate Dehydrogenase, Isoenzymes

See Cardiac Markers on p. 178.

Lactic Acid

lak-tik a-sid

Also called: Lactate; l-Lactate; Blood Lactate

SPECIMEN OR TYPE OF TEST: Venous, plasma, whole blood

PURPOSE OF THE TEST

Lactate levels are used to support the diagnosis of cellular hypoxia. Lactate levels can also predict survival.

BASICS THE NURSE NEEDS TO KNOW

Lactic acid levels may be used to assess cellular oxygenation. If the cells do not receive adequate oxygen, anaerobic metabolism will occur. Lactic acid is the by-product of anaerobic metabolism. Rising lactate levels indicate a need to examine O_2 transport and consumption parameters.

NORMAL VALUES	8.1–15.3 mEq/L *or* SI: 0.9–1.7 mmol/L
▽ Critical Values	>4 mmol/L

HOW THE TEST IS DONE

A venipuncture is performed to obtain 7 mL of blood, which is placed in a gray-topped tube.

SIGNIFICANCE OF TEST RESULTS

Elevated Values

Alcoholism
Diabetic ketoacidosis
Hyperthermia
Liver failure
Malignancies
Peritonitis
Shock states

Decreased Values

Hypothermia

INTERFERING FACTORS

- Noncompliance with dietary and activity restrictions
- The drugs acetaminophen (large dose), ethanol (large dose), epinephrine, fructose, morphine, and sorbitol

NURSING CARE

Nursing measures are similar to those used in other venipuncture procedures (see Chapter 2), with the following additional measures.

Pretest

- ***Patient Teaching.*** The nurse instructs the patient not to eat or drink for 12 hours before the test and to ingest no alcohol for 24 hours before the blood is drawn.
- Instruct the patient to lie quietly for 2 hours before the blood is drawn.

During the Test

- No tourniquet should be applied, and the patient should not clench the fist.

Continued

L

NURSING CARE—*cont'd*

Posttest

- Send the specimen to the laboratory immediately.
- Advise the patient to resume a normal diet and activity level.

▼ Nursing Response to Critical Values

High lactate levels (>4 mmol/L) indicate higher mortality rates. Report elevated values to the physician.

Lactose Tolerance Test

<u>lak</u>-tohs <u>tol</u>-er-uhns test

SPECIMEN OR TYPE OF TEST: Blood, urine, breath

PURPOSE OF THE TEST

L

This test identifies lactose intolerance-lactate deficiency. It is used in the workup for abdominal distension, chronic diarrhea, and abdominal cramps associated with the ingestion of milk. It is also used to investigate the cause of malabsorption.

BASICS THE NURSE NEEDS TO KNOW

Lactose is a sugar present in milk and milk products. For the intestinal absorption of lactose, the person must have lactase enzyme to break down the lactose into simpler sugars. These sugars are then absorbed through the villi of the small intestine and enter the blood circulation. This process results in a normal rise of the plasma glucose level to >30 mg/dL (SI: >1.7 mmol/L) over the normal fasting value of glucose.

When the lactase enzyme is deficient, the client is lactose intolerant. Varying amounts of lactose cannot be absorbed and the sugar remains in the lumen of the intestine. Sugar attracts water into the lumen by osmosis, causing diarrhea. Bacterial fermentation of the sugar causes gas formation, bloating, abdominal cramps, and distension. The lactose intolerance may range from mild to severe, and often worsens with aging.

Abnormal Findings

Glucose Measurements

With lactase deficiency, only some of the simple sugar is absorbed and reaches the blood. There is a small increase in the plasma glucose, but it does not reach the normal value of this test. In the lactose tolerance test, the findings are described as a flat glucose curve or a decreased plasma glucose value of <20 mg/dL (SI: <1.1 mmol/L) over the fasting glucose level.

Lactose Measurements

If urine is collected in this test, lactose intolerance causes higher than normal levels of lactose to be excreted in urine.

Hydrogen Breath Test

As an alternative test, the hydrogen breath test may be done. When lactose is ingested and not absorbed, the lactose passes on in the intestine to reach the colon. There, the bacteria metabolize the lactose and cause hydrogen gas to form. The gas is absorbed into the blood and is exhaled by the lungs. The pulmonary excretion of H_2 gas is increased in the hydrogen breath test. When the hydrogen ion concentration rises to >50 ppm (SI: >2.25 µmol/L) over the normal level, the result is considered abnormal or positive.

These abnormal test results may not indicate lactose intolerance, but can be the result of other causes of intestinal malabsorption.

NORMAL VALUES

Adult

Plasma glucose: >30 mg/dL *or* SI: >1.7 mmol/L (increase over the fasting value)
Urine lactose (24 hour): 12–40 mg/dL *or* SI: 0.7–2.2 mmol/L
Hydrogen breath test: <10 ppm H_2 gas/L of air *or* SI: <0.45 µmol H_2 gas/L of air

Child

Urine lactose (24 hour): <1.5 mg/dL *or* SI: <0.088 mmol/L

L

HOW THE TEST IS DONE

The fasting patient takes an oral dose of lactose with 200 to 300 mL of water.

Plasma glucose: Gray-topped (fluoride) tubes or capillary tubes are used to take serial blood samples at timed intervals for up to 4 hours.

Urine: All urine is collected in a glass container for 24 hours.

Hydrogen breath test: The patient exhales into a special container. The peak respiratory expiration of the hydrogen ions is 3 to 6 hours after the lactose is ingested.

SIGNIFICANCE OF TEST RESULTS

Lactose intolerance
Crohn's disease
Ulcerative colitis
Small bowel resection
Sprue
Viral or bacterial bowel infection
Giardiasis

INTERFERING FACTORS

- Failure to maintain dietary restrictions
- Delayed emptying of the stomach
- Vomiting
- Diabetes mellitus

NURSING CARE

Nursing measures are similar to those used in other venipuncture or capillary puncture procedures (see Chapter 2), with the following additional measures.

Pretest

- ***Patient Teaching.*** Instruct the patient to discontinue food intake for 8 hours before the test. In addition, there can be no eating during the test since food would alter the baseline glucose value. There can be no smoking or gum chewing before or during the test as these activities would alter the gastric motility and gastric emptying; both would alter the test results.

During the Test

- Assess the patient for any signs of watery diarrhea, abdominal cramps, or nausea, because the dosage of lactose can exacerbate symptoms.

Posttest

- The patient can resume eating in 2 hours, after all the blood test samples are obtained.
- For the patient who is medically diagnosed with lactose intolerance, there is a need for nutritional teaching to modify the diet. The goals are to alleviate the abdominal symptoms and, at the same time, maintain calcium intake.
- ***Patient Teaching.*** If the patient is diagnosed with lactose intolerance, the nurse can teach the patient to restrict the intake of milk (lactose). Milk and foods that contain milk or milk products cause varying degrees of abdominal discomfort among people. Lactase enzyme supplement may be helpful, but does not substitute for lactose restriction in the diet. The patient should also be taught that many nondairy foods contain lactose, including bread, baked goods, biscuit and pancake mixes, among others. The nurse also teaches the patient to read the ingredient labels to avoid hidden sources of lactose.
- Most adults can tolerate 8 to12 ounces (1 glass) of milk daily and should be encouraged to continue ingesting the amount that can be tolerated. This will provide some calcium and other needed vitamins and minerals (A, D, riboflavin, and phosphorus). Soy and rice milk are tolerated well. Calcium supplementation in tablet form can be done so that the patient receives 1200 to 1500 mg of calcium per day.

Laparoscopy, Pelvic

lap-uh-ros-kuh-pee, pel-vik

Also called: Peritoneoscopy

SPECIMEN OR TYPE OF TEST: Endoscopy

PURPOSE OF THE TEST

Laparoscopy is used to investigate the cause of pelvic pain, to detect endometriosis or an ectopic pregnancy, to identify a pelvic mass, or to determine if cancer is present.

BASICS THE NURSE NEEDS TO KNOW

The laparoscope is a fiberoptic endoscope used to visualize the size and shape of the ovaries, uterus, and fallopian tubes. The peritoneal cavity and peritoneum are observed for signs of infection, abscess, or adhesions. Biopsy of abnormal tissue may be performed.

NORMAL VALUES

No abnormalities of the ovaries, fallopian tubes, uterus, or peritoneal cavity are noted.

HOW THE TEST IS DONE

Under general or local anesthesia, the surgeon inflates the peritoneal cavity with 2 to 3 L of carbon dioxide. The gas distends the abdominal wall and provides space for the instrument. The laparoscope is inserted through the small incision just below the umbilicus, and the organs are visualized. If a biopsy or other surgical procedure is done, a second incision is made in the lower abdomen for insertion of the additional instruments.

SIGNIFICANCE OF TEST RESULTS

Abnormal Values

Ovarian cyst
Endometriosis
Ectopic pregnancy
Uterine fibroid tumors
Pelvic abscess
Pelvic inflammatory disease
Adhesions
Abnormality of the fallopian tubes
Malignancy

INTERFERING FACTORS

- Failure to maintain a nothing-by-mouth status
- Obesity
- Adhesions

NURSING CARE

Pretest

- After the patient has been informed about the procedure by the physician, the nurse obtains written consent from the patient and places the form in the patient's record. Ensure that all preoperative laboratory work is completed and that the results are posted in the record.
- ***Patient Teaching.*** The nurse instructs the patient to discontinue all food and fluids for 8 hours before the procedure is performed.

Continued

NURSING CARE—*cont'd*

Pretest—*cont'd*

- ***Patient Teaching.*** At the time of the surgery, the nurse assists the patient in removing all clothes and putting on a hospital gown. The nurse also assesses and records the vital signs, including temperature, blood pressure, pulse, and respirations.

During the Test

- The nurse places the patient in the lithotomy position, with the legs supported in stirrups.
- An indwelling catheter is inserted into the bladder and connected to the urinary collection system. This keeps the bladder deflated and protects it from trauma or injury.
- The nurse provides reassurance to the patient until the anesthesia is administered.
- If a biopsy specimen is obtained, place the tissue in a glass container with preservative. Identify the tissue source on the requisition slip.

Posttest

- The nurse assesses the patient by monitoring the vital signs every 30 minutes for 4 hours or until they are stable. The small dressing(s) should remain dry and intact. Once the urinary catheter is removed, the nurse monitors the patient for resumption of voiding and urinary output.
- Once the patient is alert, the nurse encourages ambulation and the oral intake of fluids. Carbonated beverages are avoided for 24 to 36 hours. With the excess carbon dioxide in the abdomen, the intake of carbonated beverage can cause vomiting.
- The nurse provides pain medication as needed. The nurse reassures the patient that some pain in the abdomen and shoulder is to be expected for 24 to 36 hours. The cause is the carbon dioxide gas, which will gradually be absorbed and exhaled from the lungs.
- ***Patient Teaching.*** The nurse instructs the patient to restrict physical activity for a few days until the incisions are healed. The patient is taught to notify the physician of increasing abdominal pain, fever, or abnormal drainage.

Lead, Blood

led, blud

Also called: Pb, blood

SPECIMEN OR TYPE OF TEST: Blood

PURPOSE OF THE TEST

This test is used to detect and measure the level of lead in the blood. It is also used as a screening test for people who are at risk for elevated lead levels.

BASICS THE NURSE NEEDS TO KNOW

Lead is a heavy metal in the environment that can enter the human body orally through respiration of dust that contains lead, and by absorption through the skin. *Plumbism*, or lead toxicity, can occur as an acute condition because of recent exposure, or as a chronic accumulation of lead, over time. An elevated lead level in the body is highly toxic, causing damage to the bone marrow, neurologic system, and kidneys. The blood test is able to measure recent exposure to lead but cannot evaluate the amount of lead already deposited in tissues from past exposure.

In children, the primary source of elevated lead levels is exposure to lead-based paint. The risk is highest for children of low socioeconomic status and with a history of inadequate nutrition including a lack of iron, calcium, and zinc. When a child is screened for a blood lead level, a value of >30 mcg/dL (SI: >1.5 µmol/L) indicates substantial exposure. If the value is >60 mcg/dL (SI: >3.0 µmol/L), the child requires chelation therapy, a medication regimen that will help remove the lead from the body.

Adults are vulnerable to lead exposure because of occupational or recreational exposure, including work with batteries, pottery, welding, printing, smelting, and restoration or demolition of old houses. Based on OSHA requirements, the adult with an occupational exposure and a blood lead level of >40 mcg/dL (SI: >2.0 µmol/L) should be removed from work and undergo chelation therapy.

NORMAL VALUES	Child: <10 mcg/dL *or* SI: <0.5 µmol/L Adult: <50 mcg/dL *or* SI: <2.41 µmol/L
▼ Critical Values	Adult and child: >70 mcg/dL *or* SI: >3.34 µmol/L

L

HOW THE TEST IS DONE

A special, lead-free tube with heparin is used to collect a sample of venous blood.

SIGNIFICANCE OF TEST RESULTS

Exposure to lead
Lead toxicity, acute

INTERFERING FACTORS

- Use of an improper (glass) collection tube

NURSING CARE

Nursing measures are similar to those used in other venipuncture or capillary puncture procedures (see Chapter 2), with the following additional measures.

Pretest

- ***Health Promotion.*** For routine screening, all children should have a blood test at age 1 to determine the lead level. The nurse can teach parents the importance of the test and the need to detect lead content in the child's body at an early stage. In addition, when the test results are elevated for a child or adult, the nurse can teach the patient or parent/guardian about the sources of lead that may be in the patient's environment and the importance of removing the contaminants. The nurse can also advise the family to seek the assistance of the local health department regarding detection of the sources of lead exposure and advice on how to correct the problem.

Continued

NURSING CARE—*cont'd*

Pretest—*cont'd*

- To determine the need for an additional screening test for lead, the CDC recommends that the parent or guardian of the child be asked the following questions:
  1. Does the child reside in or regularly visit a house that was built before 1950?
  2. Does the child live in or regularly visit a home that was built before 1978 and has undergone extensive renovation in the past 6 months?
  3. Do you know any friend of the child who has tested positive for lead?

If the parent answers yes or "I don't know" to any of the questions, the lead screening test is recommended to determine if there has been exposure.

Posttest

- When the lead level is elevated, the nurse should assess the patient for signs of toxicity. At low to moderate levels of lead in the blood, children will develop developmental lags, loss of some mental acuity, hearing loss, and growth delay. At moderate elevations, the child develops anemia, abdominal colic, and neuropathy. A nutritional assessment may also be indicated. In the adult, moderate elevations cause an elevation of the systolic blood pressure, a loss of hearing, infertility, and neuropathy.

L

Nursing Response to Critical Values

At a blood lead level of >70 mcg/dL (SI: >3.34 μmol/L), the patient is at serious risk for developing severe anemia and encephalopathy (brain damage). The patient must be admitted to the hospital and undergo immediate chelation therapy for acute lead poisoning. The nurse notifies the physician of this elevated result.

The nurse would assess for neurologic function, including mental orientation, auditory ability, intact reflexes, and motor function, such as coordination, ambulation ability, and muscle strength. The child should be assessed for signs of developmental delays.

Leukocyte Alkaline Phosphatase

loo-koh-sait al-kuh-lain fos-fuh-tays

Also called: (LAP)

SPECIMEN OR TYPE OF TEST: Peripheral blood

PURPOSE OF THE TEST

This test helps differentiate chronic myelogenous leukemia from leukemoid reaction and other myeloproliferative diseases. It is also useful in the evaluation of Hodgkin's disease and its response to therapy.

BASICS THE NURSE NEEDS TO KNOW

Chronic myeloproliferative diseases are hematologic malignancies that produce rapid, excessive cloning of a multipotential cell of the bone marrow. The cloning produces excessive neutrophils, erythrocytes, platelets, or other related cells.

The leukocyte alkaline phosphatase test produces a characteristic chemical reaction that helps to differentiate among the myeloproliferative disorders. Leukocyte alkaline phosphatase is an enzyme located in neutrophils. In the test method, 100 stained neutrophils are given a rating score of 0 to 4, based on the intensity of the color of the reaction. The scoring is somewhat subject to color interpretation, and the reference range varies among laboratories.

NORMAL VALUES

Rating score of 15–130

HOW THE TEST IS DONE

Fingerstick puncture is used to make six slides with smears of the peripheral blood. Alternatively, a green-topped tube with heparin or oxalate anticoagulant is used to collect 10 mL of venous blood.

SIGNIFICANCE OF TEST RESULTS

Elevated Values

Polycythemia vera
Hairy cell leukemia
Myelofibrosis
Down syndrome
Leukemoid reactions
Hodgkin's disease
Acute lymphoblastic leukemia
Neutrophilia secondary to infection

Decreased Values

Chronic myelogenous leukemia
Acute myeloid leukemia
Thrombocytopenic purpura
Acute monocytic leukemia
Hereditary hypophosphatemia

INTERFERING FACTORS

- Pregnancy
- Acute stress
- Neutropenia
- Delay in the final preparation of slides

NURSING CARE

Nursing measures are similar to those used in other venipuncture or capillary puncture procedures (see Chapter 2), with the following additional measures.

Pretest

- To ensure a valid test, verify that the recent peripheral blood neutrophil count is greater than $1000/mm^3$.

Posttest

- Arrange for immediate transport of the slides or blood specimen to the laboratory. To avoid rejection of the specimen, the slides must be fixed in preservative within 30 minutes.

L

Lipase

li-pays

SPECIMEN OR TYPE OF TEST: Serum

PURPOSE OF THE TEST

Lipase is a test to diagnose acute pancreatitis and can identify other sources of pancreatic disease.

BASICS THE NURSE NEEDS TO KNOW

Lipase is a pancreatic enzyme needed to help digest fatty acids. In pancreatic inflammation, this pancreatic enzyme cannot flow into the intestine because of inflammation or blockage in the pancreas, pancreatic duct, common bile duct, or intestine. Once there is obstruction of the flow, the lipase is secreted into the blood and the serum level rises. In pancreatic disorders, both serum lipase and serum amylase values are elevated on the first day of acute pancreatitis, but the lipase remains elevated in the blood for a few days longer than amylase.

NORMAL VALUES Adult: <200 units/L *or* SI: <3.4 μkat/L

HOW THE TEST IS DONE

A venipuncture is performed to collect 10 mL of venous blood in a red-topped tube.

SIGNIFICANCE OF TEST RESULTS

Elevated Values

Acute pancreatitis
Pancreatic cyst or pseudocyst
Pancreatic duct obstruction
Peritonitis
Strangulated or perforated bowel
Colic from gallstone
Primary biliary cirrhosis

INTERFERING FACTORS

- Heparin
- Narcotics
- Failure to maintain an nothing-by-mouth status

NURSING CARE

Nursing measures are similar to those used in other venipuncture procedures (see Chapter 2), with the following additional measures.

Pretest

- ***Patient Teaching.*** Instruct the patient to discontinue all food and fluid for 12 hours before the test.

NURSING CARE—*cont'd*

- For dialysis patients, draw the lipase blood sample before the dialysis treatment begins, because the heparin used in dialysis would falsely elevate the test result.

Posttest

- If the patient has elevated lab results, assess for signs of pancreatitis. Abdominal pain can range from mild to severe intensity. Nausea, vomiting, and jaundice may occur. Additional nursing assessments depend on the cause and severity of the problem.

Lipid Profile

lip-id proh-fail

Also called: Lipid Panel; Lipoprotein-Cholesterol Fractionation; Serum Lipids

SPECIMEN OR TYPE OF TEST: Serum

PURPOSE OF THE TEST

Lipid levels are used to identify individuals at risk for coronary artery disease (CAD) and as an evaluation tool to determine the effectiveness of "heart healthy" changes in lifestyle.

BASICS THE NURSE NEEDS TO KNOW

Most lipids are bound to protein in the blood and are called lipoproteins. Lipoproteins are usually measured to identify persons at risk for CAD. In the lab, lipoproteins are separated by electrophoresis. Fractionation of the lipoproteins is then performed according to their density. The following groups have been identified:

Very low-density lipoproteins (VLDL), which are made up of 70% triglycerides (triglycerides)

Low-density lipoproteins (LDL), which are made up of 45% cholesterol (low-density cholesterol)

High-density lipoproteins (HDL) (high-density cholesterol)

A high correlation exists between elevated VLDL and LDL levels and CAD. Research has shown that HDL may protect from CAD, because it seems to inhibit the uptake of LDL.

NORMAL VALUES (Vary with reference group)

Lipids, total: 400–800 mg/dL *or* SI: 4.0–8.0 g/L
Cholesterol, total: 120–200 mg/dL *or* SI: 3.11–5.18 mmol/L
LDL: <130 mg/dL *or* SI: <3.37 mmol/L
HDL:
  Male: 44–45 mg/dL *or* SI: 1.24–1.27 mmol/L
  Female: >55 mg/dL *or* SI: 1.425 mmol/L
LDL:HDL ratio: <3
Triglycerides:
  Male:
    <40 years: 46–316 mg/dL *or* SI: 0.52–3.57 mmol/L
    >50 years: 75–313 mg/dL *or* SI: 0.85–3.5 mmol/L
  Female:
    <40 years 37–174 mg/dL *or* SI: 0.42–1.97 mmol/L
    >50 years 52–200 mg/dL *or* SI: 0.59–2.26 mmol/L

HOW THE TEST IS DONE

A venipuncture is necessary for a lipid profile. Two red-topped tubes of 7 mL capacity are required. If a low-density cholesterol level determination is performed as a screening test, a drop or two of blood is obtained from a fingerstick using a sterile lancet, and the blood is collected in a capillary pipette.

SIGNIFICANCE OF TEST RESULTS

Cholesterol

Elevated Values

Alcoholism
Arteriosclerosis
Diabetes mellitus
Hepatitis (early stage)
High-fat diet
Myxedema
Obstructed bile duct
Pancreatitis
Genetic factors

Decreased Values

Hyperalimentation
Hyperthyroidism
Liver disease
Malabsorption
Malnutrition

HDL

Elevated Values

Alcoholism
Diabetes mellitus
Exercise
Myxedema
Nephrotic syndrome
Pancreatitis

Decreased Values

Arteriosclerosis
Hyperalimentation
Hypothyroidism
Malabsorption
Malnutrition

LDL

Elevated Values

Alcoholism
Diabetes mellitus
Nephrotic syndrome
Pancreatitis

Decreased Values
Arteriosclerosis
Hyperalimentation
Malabsorption
Malnutrition

Triglycerides
Elevated Values
Alcoholism
Arteriosclerosis
Diabetes mellitus
Myxedema
Nephrotic syndrome
Pancreatitis
Decreased Values
Hyperalimentation
Malabsorption
Malnutrition

INTERFERING FACTORS

- Diet affects the results of a lipid profile and fractionation outcome. Has the patient been dieting to lose weight? If the patient has had a recent traumatic event or infarction, results will also be affected. Smoking may affect results.
- Medications such as estrogen, steroids, birth control pills, and hypolipid agents cause an inaccurate lipid picture.
- Alcohol intake
- High triglycerides (over 400 mg/dL) will affect low-density cholesterol levels.
- Recent myocardial infarction
- For cholesterol screening, eating a diet high in saturated fats will affect the results.

NURSING CARE

- ***Health Promotion.*** The nurse encourages people between the ages of 45 and 65 to have their cholesterol level checked every 5 years. This is to identify those at risk for atherosclerosis and CAD. A strong family history of CAD may indicate earlier need for evaluation.
- Nursing measures are similar to those used in other venipuncture or capillary procedures (see Chapter 2), with the following additional measures.

Pretest

- ***Patient Teaching.*** The nurse instructs the patient to fast for 10 to 12 hours before the blood sample is taken. If only a low-density cholesterol screening is planned, instruct the patient to refrain from eating a high-fat diet for 12 hours before the blood is drawn.
- Inquire if the patient has been on his or her normal diet for the last 2 to 3 weeks.

Continued

NURSING CARE—*cont'd*

Posttest

- Review results with the patient. The nurse needs to assess patients with elevated low-density cholesterol or high triglycerides for other modifiable risk factors for CAD, such as smoking, obesity, high blood pressure, sedentary lifestyle and hypertension. Goal values for people at risk for coronary artery disease are:
  LDLC: <100 mg/dL
  HDLC: >45 mg/dL in men and >55 mg/dL in females
  Triglycerides: <200 mg/dL
- To reach lipid goals, diet and exercise education may be necessary. If significantly elevated, medication with diet and exercise is usually ordered.
- Home cholesterol screening is now possible. The reported accuracy for the home cholesterol test kits is 98%, which is consistent with tests done in physicians' offices. The accuracy of the home cholesterol test depends on the ability of the user to follow the manufacturer's guidelines. A major problem with home testing is the ability of the patient to understand and interpret the results.
- Before home cholesterol testing is taught, assess the person's medical history. The test is not recommended for anyone with a bleeding disorder or who is receiving anticoagulation therapy. Instruct the person to avoid vitamin A, acetaminophen, and mesalamine for at least 4 hours before the test. Warn the patient to check the packing of the kit for breaks and not to use the test if the foil package is not intact or if sterility of the lancet is questionable.
- Home cholesterol testing requires capillary blood. Instruct the person to wash the hands before testing in warm soap and water. Warn the person not to use alcohol or hydrogen peroxide to clean the skin. Instruct the patient to obtain the blood sample from the side of a fingertip, which has fewer pain sensors and a better blood supply than the center. Instruct the patient to follow the manufacturer's guidelines. Multiple steps are required, with different timings at different steps. Inform the person that cholesterol levels will be affected by diet. One test result is not adequate. Repeating the test is recommended. Instruct the person to notify his or her physician or nurse practitioner if results are greater than 200 mg/dL.

Lipoproteins

See Lipid Profile on p. 431.

Long-Acting Thyroid Stimulator

long–ak-ting thai-royd sti-myuh-lay-tuhr

Also called: (LATS); Thyrotropin Receptor Antibody; Thyroid Stimulation Autoantibody; Thyroid Stimulation Immunoglobulins; TSH Receptor Antibodies

SPECIMEN OR TYPE OF TEST: Serum

PURPOSE OF THE TEST

The determination of long-acting thyroid stimulator levels is performed to support the diagnosis of Graves' disease.

BASICS THE NURSE NEEDS TO KNOW

Long-acting thyroid stimulator is a globulin that binds to thyroid receptor sites and stimulates thyroid activity. It helps to differentiate between Graves' disease and nodular toxic goiter or other disorders.

NORMAL VALUES

Negative

HOW THE TEST IS DONE

Venipuncture is performed and 7 to 10 mL of blood is collected in a red-topped tube.

SIGNIFICANCE OF TEST RESULTS

Elevated Values

Graves' disease
Nodular toxic goiter (rare)

INTERFERING FACTORS

- Radioactive iodine

NURSING CARE

Nursing measures are similar to those in other venipuncture procedures, as presented in Chapter 2.

Pretest

- Schedule any test requiring radioactive iodine for after blood for long-acting thyroid stimulator level is drawn.

Low-Density Lipoproteins

See Lipid Profile on p. 431.

Lumbar Puncture and Cerebrospinal Fluid Analysis

lum-bar punk-chur and suh-ree-broh-spai-nuhl floo-id uh-nal-uh-sis

Also called: (LP); CSF Analysis; Spinal Tap

SPECIMEN OR TYPE OF TEST: Cerebrospinal fluid

L

PURPOSE OF THE TEST

Lumbar Puncture

This procedure is performed to measure the pressure of the cerebrospinal fluid, to detect obstruction in the circulation of this fluid, and to obtain a sample of the cerebrospinal fluid for cellular, chemical, and microbiologic analysis.

Cerebrospinal Fluid Analysis

These laboratory tests are performed to confirm the diagnosis of infection in the central nervous system or to identify a tumor or hemorrhage in the brain, spinal cord, or surrounding lining of the tissues. It may be performed to confirm a chronic central nervous system infection such as neurosyphilis or an inflammatory or autoimmune disorder affecting the central nervous system, such as multiple sclerosis.

BASICS THE NURSE NEEDS TO KNOW

Lumbar Puncture

This procedure is used to obtain the sample of cerebrospinal fluid for analysis. It involves the insertion of a sterile spinal needle between the lumbar vertebrae into the subarachnoid space. Because the spinal cord ends at L1 or L2 in adults, the spinal tap is performed below that level. The level of the tap is usually in the third or fourth lumbar interspace for adults and in the fourth or fifth interspace for children.

Cerebrospinal Pressure

Once the needle is in the subarachnoid space, the pressure of the fluid is measured. A pressure reading greater than 250 mm H_2O is abnormal. If the pressure is in the normal range of <200 mm H_2O, a specimen of up to 20 mL can be removed. Because children have less total fluid in proportion to age and body size, the specimen sample must be considerably smaller. If the child's opening pressure is higher or lower than normal, the specimen is limited to 1 to 2 mL.

Analysis of the Cerebrospinal Fluid

Appearance

The normal cerebrospinal fluid is clear and colorless, with a viscosity similar to that of water. Cloudy fluid is caused by an increased number of cells in the fluid. The cloudiness is sometimes measured on a scale of 0 to 4+ (from clear to cloudy). Discoloration of the fluid indicates that abnormal components are present in the fluid. Gross blood may be present and is caused by a traumatic tap, a subarachnoid hemorrhage, or an intracerebral hemorrhage.

Microscopic Examination

The normal total cell count is low in adults and children of all ages. When a high elevation of leukocytes exists, the cause is often bacterial meningitis. A cloudy specimen is associated with a white blood cell count of more than 200 cells/μL, and a very high count may be greater than 50,000 cells/μL.

The cerebrospinal fluid may be cultured to identify the infectious agent. Immunologic examination also may be performed to detect the specific microbial antigen present in bacterial or fungal meningitis. Immunologic testing may include the testing performed to confirm neurosyphilis. Cytologic examination may be performed to identify the cells of the primary or metastatic tumor. The cells are shed from a malignant tumor that has extended into the ventricles or subarachnoid space.

Differential Cell Count

Normally, lymphocytes and monocytes are the predominant cells in cerebrospinal fluid. In bacterial meningitis, the neutrophil count is greatly elevated. In other causes of meningitis, an increased lymphocyte count exists. The presence of plasma cells can be a result of acute viral infection, a chronic inflammatory condition, or multiple sclerosis. A large increase in eosinophils is indicative of a parasitic or fungal infection. Malignant cells indicate a primary or metastatic tumor. Metastases are commonly from melanoma, leukemia, lymphoma, or cancer of the breast, lung, or gastrointestinal tract.

Chemical Analysis

Glucose

The glucose concentration is proportionate to the level of blood glucose. Within a period of 2 hours before the spinal tap, the glucose level in the cerebrospinal fluid is normally 60% to 70% of the blood level. To interpret the glucose level of the cerebrospinal fluid correctly, a blood specimen must be drawn 30 to 60 minutes before the spinal tap is performed. Higher-than-normal values of glucose in the cerebrospinal fluid reflect hyperglycemia. Lower-than-normal values (<40 mg/dL) of glucose in the cerebrospinal fluid occur with many forms of meningitis, neoplasm, inflammatory disorder, and other conditions.

Protein

Some protein is normally present in the cerebrospinal fluid, but an excessive increase or decrease is indicative of a problem. The increased level may be the result of increased permeability of the blood-brain barrier, allowing protein to pass into the cerebrospinal fluid. It may also be the result of poor resorption of the protein or of an increase in immunoglobulin synthesis. Decreased protein values occur when an increase in water resorption occurs, such as with increased intracranial pressure or with leakage of the cerebrospinal fluid as the result of head trauma. Because a measurement of cerebrospinal fluid protein does not indicate the cause of abnormality, there are numerous additional protein tests that can be performed to help with specificity.

Oligoclonal Bands

If present, oligoclonal bands are detected by protein electrophoresis performed on the cerebrospinal fluid. The presence of these bands is abnormal and supports the diagnosis of inflammatory or autoimmune disorder that affects the central nervous system. A positive test result is very common in patients with multiple sclerosis.

β-Amyloid$_{(1\text{-}42)}$ and T-Tau

These two proteins are potential biochemical markers to identify early stage Alzheimer's disease. If Alzheimer's disease is present, the β-amyloid$_{(1\text{-}42)}$ is decreased or is significantly lower than the normal value. It is not fully understood why the level of this protein declines, but one possible reason is that it forms deposits of senile plaques that are toxic to neurons. If bound in plaque, the protein is not circulating in the cerebrospinal fluid, and the level of the protein declines. At the same time, the T-tau protein

L

level rises significantly in Alzheimer's disease. It is proposed that this happens because of degeneration of axons within the brain, releasing this peptide into the cerebrospinal fluid in quantities that are much greater than normal. When both tests are used in combination, the abnormal results are highly accurate in detecting Alzheimer's disease. These tests, however, are not specific enough to distinguish Alzheimer's disease from some other forms of dementia. Medical research continues to explore the role of these two proteins as clinical markers of Alzheimer's disease.

NORMAL VALUES

Cerebrospinal Fluid Analysis
Pressure: <200 mm H_2O (lateral recumbent position)
Appearance: Clear, colorless

Leukocyte Count
Adult: 0–5 cells/μL *or* SI: 0–5 $\times 10^6$/L
Child (5–18 years): 0–10 cells/μL *or* SI: 0–10 $\times 10^6$/L
Neonate–1 year: 0–30 cells/μL *or* SI: 0–30 $\times 10^6$/L

Differential Count
Adult
Lymphocytes: 40%–80% *or* SI: 0.40–0.80 number fraction
Monocytes: 15%–45% *or* SI: 0.15–0.45 number fraction
Neutrophils: 0%–6% *or* SI: 0.00–0.06 number fraction

Neonate
Lymphocytes: 5%–35% *or* SI: 0.05–0.35 number fraction
Monocytes: 50%–90% *or* SI: 0.50–0.90 number fraction
Neutrophils: 0%–8% *or* SI: 0.00–0.08 number fraction

Glucose
40–80 mg/dL *or* SI: 2.8–4.4 mmol/L

Total Protein
12–60 mg/dL *or* SI: 120–600 mg/L

Oligoclonal Bands
Negative

β-Amyloid$_{(1\text{-}42)}$
>444 pg/mL

T-tau
<195 pg/mL

 Critical Values

Cerebrospinal fluid pressure: >300 mm H_2O

HOW THE TEST IS DONE

Lumbar Puncture

Under sterile conditions and using local anesthesia, the physician inserts a spinal needle between the lower lumbar vertebrae and into the subarachnoid space (Figure 54). After pressure measurements are determined by manometer readings, spinal fluid is collected in three or more sterile tubes.

SIGNIFICANCE OF TEST RESULTS

Elevated Values

Intracranial Pressure

Brain tumor
Intracranial hemorrhage
Hydrocephalus

Leukocytes

Bacterial meningitis

Neutrophils

Bacterial meningitis
Encephalomyelitis

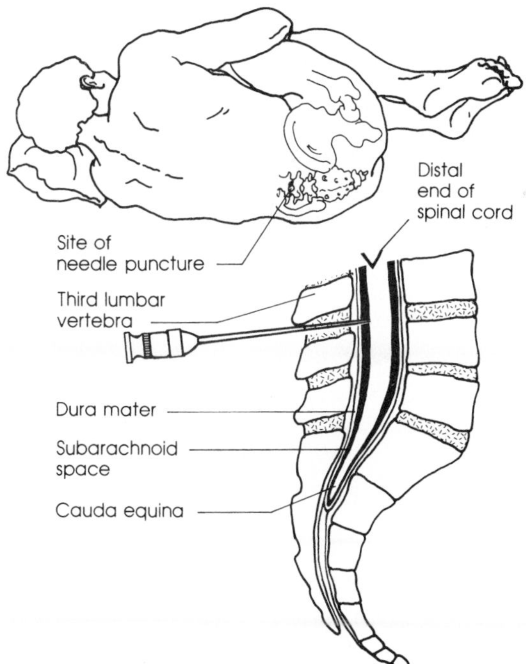

Figure 54. Patient position for lumbar puncture. The flexion of the lumbar spine widens the intervertebral spaces so that the needle can be inserted into the subarachnoid space more easily. (*Reproduced with permission from Dewit, S. C. [1992].* Keane's essentials of medical surgical nursing *[3rd ed., p. 330]. Philadelphia: W. B. Saunders.*)

Cerebral abscess
Cerebral hemorrhage
Cerebral infarction
Metastatic tumor

Lymphocytes

Meningitis
Multiple sclerosis
Parasitic infection

Glucose

Hyperglycemia

Total Protein

Meningitis
Stroke
Extradural abscess
Endocrine disorder
Trauma
Tumor
Herniated disc
Multiple sclerosis
Neurosyphilis

Oligoclonal Bands

Multiple sclerosis
Systemic lupus erythematosus
Neurosyphilis
Jakob-Creutzfeldt disease

T-tau

Alzheimer's disease
Frontotemporal dementia

Decreased Values

Glucose

Acute or chronic meningitis
Meningoencephalitis
Systemic hypoglycemia
Subarachnoid hemorrhage
Neurosyphilis
Sarcoidosis (meningeal)

Total Protein

Trauma
Dural tear
Increased intracranial pressure

β-Amyloid$_{(1-42)}$

Alzheimer's disease
Frontotemporal dementia
Vascular dementia

Jakob-Creutzfeldt disease
Amyotrophic lateral sclerosis

INTERFERING FACTORS

- Infection of skin or epidural abscess at the site of the proposed spinal tap
- Increased intracranial pressure
- Spinal block (incomplete or complete)
- Bleeding disorder

NURSING CARE

Pretest

- After the physician explains the test to the patient, obtain written consent from the patient and enter it into the patient's record. Ask the patient about any history of hemophilia, thrombocytopenia, other bleeding disorder, or anticoagulation therapy. Because these problems will result in prolonged bleeding into the tissues or cerebrospinal fluid, they are a relative contraindication to lumbar puncture.
- Assist the patient in removing all clothing and putting on a hospital gown. Baseline vital signs are taken and recorded in the patient's record.
- Place the patient in a lateral recumbent position with his or her back at the edge of the bed or examining table. Flex the patient's neck and knees toward the chest. As an alternative, the physician may want the patient to sit up and lean over a bedside table. With either position, the flexion of the spine widens the intervertebral spaces.

During the Test

- The nurse assists with the preparation of the equipment and sterile field, the antiseptic cleansing of the skin, and the preparation of the local anesthetic. Usually, 1 to 2 mL of lidocaine is administered subcutaneously by the physician.
- Instruct the patient to remain absolutely still during the insertion of each needle. Hold the patient in position to help prevent movement. Provide reassurance to the patient as the needles are inserted. The administration of the anesthetic causes a stinging sensation. Brief pain also occurs as the spinal needle penetrates the dura and enters the subarachnoid space.
- Assist the patient in placing the legs in extension for the pressure reading. The nurse also assists with the collection of the cerebrospinal fluid. The tubes are marked "1," "2," "3," and so on, in the order in which they are collected. The first tube is used for chemical and immunologic analysis, because blood or tissue fluid will not alter these test results. The second tube is used for microbial analysis, and the third tube for microscopic examination of cells. If only a small amount of fluid is drawn, it is placed in a single tube, and the physician prioritizes the tests.
- Arrange for immediate delivery of the specimen to the laboratory. With delay, lysis of the white blood cells results in a false decrease in the cell count and microbial organisms will be destroyed.

Continued

NURSING CARE—*cont'd*

Posttest

- For nursing assessment, monitor vital signs every 30 minutes until they are stable. At the same time, assess the patient's level of consciousness and responsiveness. Assess the puncture site for swelling, redness, bleeding, hematoma formation, or leakage of cerebrospinal fluid. At regular intervals, assess the patient's motor ability in the lower legs. If spinal blockage or severe compression of the cord occurs after the procedure, paresis can turn into paralysis. In addition, massive hematoma can occur within the subarachnoid space. This would compress the cauda equina and result in paralysis.
- Spinal headache (post-lumbar puncture syndrome) sometimes occurs 24 to 48 hours after the procedure, although the incidence is much lower when a thinner or "atraumatic" needle is used for the lumbar puncture. A spinal headache usually causes pain in the back of the head, neck, and upper back, along with dizziness, orthostatic hypotension, as well as nausea, vomiting, and increased sweating. The symptoms are worsened when the patient stands erect and disappear when the patient is lying flat.
- Bed rest and increased fluid intake do not prevent spinal headache but may be part of the post-procedure protocol. If these measures are used, the nurse instructs the patient to lie flat for about 3 hours. If headache occurs, bed rest is extended for 12 hours. Extra fluid intake is encouraged in the belief that the fluids help replace the volume of fluid removed from the subarachnoidal space.

L

▼ Nursing Response to Critical Values

An opening intracranial pressure reading of 300 mm H_2O or higher is considered a critical value. With a pressure reading at this very elevated level, the patient is in danger of a cerebellar herniation of the brain, with possible fatal consequences. The physician can only remove a very small fluid sample. The pressure also may rise in the posttest period.

The nurse assesses the patient for signs of increased intracranial pressure in the posttest period. Abnormal findings include deteriorating levels of consciousness, including stupor or coma. Additionally, the patient may develop bradycardia, elevated blood pressure, slow or irregular respirations, and papillary changes. These findings are ominous and are reported to the physician immediately. The nurse can prepare to assist with treatment. Intravenous urea or mannitol may be prescribed. After medical treatment, another cerebrospinal fluid pressure reading may be needed to verify that the pressure has declined.

◆ Nursing Response to Complications

The most frequent complication of lumbar puncture is headache. Infection also may occur. Although it is an infrequent complication, increased intracranial pressure may occur. The increase in the intracranial pressure may be caused by meningitis or brain tumor.

Headache. The nurse assesses for the patient's complaints of severe head pain. The patient may also have nausea, vomiting, and dizziness. The nurse instructs the patient to lie flat because that position usually provides relief. Prescribed pain medication, antiemetic medication, and additional oral or intravenous fluids are administered, as needed. The headache often lasts for several days and will disappear spontaneously.

NURSING CARE—*cont'd*

Infection. Meningitis may be a complication of the spinal tap, but it can be the condition that caused the patient to become so ill. The nurse assesses for high fever and the patient's complaints of pain in muscles (myalgia), headache, back pain, and photophobia (sensitivity to light). The nurse also assesses the patient's level of consciousness and any signs of meningeal irritation including a positive Kernig's or Brudzinski's sign. Seizures may occur. Abnormal assessment findings must be reported to the physician, immediately.

Lung Scans

lung skans

Also called: Ventilation Scan; Perfusion Scan; Ventilation-Perfusion Scan; V/Q Scan; Ventilation-Perfusion Scintiphotography

SPECIMEN OR TYPE OF TEST: Radiography

PURPOSE OF THE TEST

Ventilation studies may be performed to evaluate patients with decreased pulmonary function. V/Q scans are usually carried out to diagnose pulmonary emboli.

BASICS THE NURSE NEEDS TO KNOW

For adequate oxygenation, the lungs must receive adequate alveolar ventilation and blood flow to the ventilated alveoli. Thus, two types of lung scans exist: a *ventilation scan* and a *perfusion scan*. Ventilation scans are performed to evaluate the distribution of gas within the lungs. The patient inhales a radioactive gas, and a scanner records the distribution of the gas as it enters and leaves the lungs. Perfusion scans evaluate arterial pulmonary blood flow. A radioactive dye is given intravenously, and a scintillation camera records the distribution of the dye as it passes through the right side of the heart to the pulmonary arterial bed.

Ventilation and perfusion scans (V/Q scans) may be performed together so that they can be compared to identify mismatching of ventilation and perfusion. V/Q scans are most often ordered to confirm the diagnosis of pulmonary emboli. The diagnosis of pulmonary emboli is difficult to confirm. Clinically, pulmonary emboli may be suspected because of chest pain, dyspnea, and hemoptysis, but pulmonary emboli are associated with other pulmonary and cardiac disorders, which makes the diagnosis difficult to confirm. Although pulmonary angiography is the most specific diagnostic tool for pulmonary emboli, it is invasive. A V/Q scan is less invasive and therefore less dangerous. It permits an evaluation of V/Q mismatching. Figure 55 demonstrates how alveolar-capillary blood flow must interface for adequate oxygenation.

When the radioactively tagged albumin is given intravenously, it circulates through the pulmonary vasculature. If a pulmonary artery is occluded, the part of the lung served by that vessel does not "take up" the radioisotope, and the scan is positive.

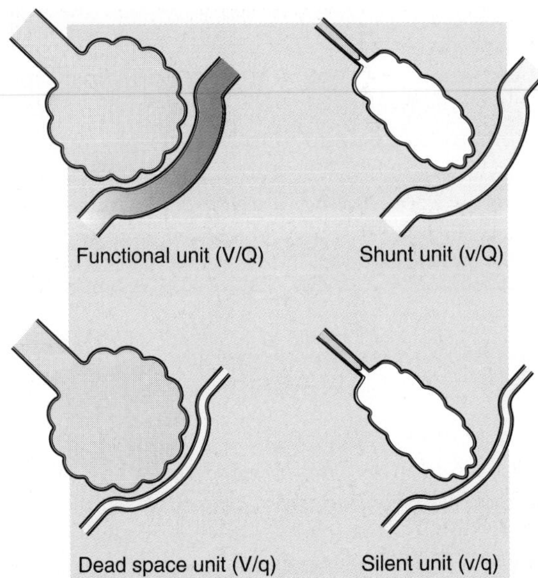

Figure 55. Alveolar-capillary interface. V = ventilated unit; Q = perfused unit; v = unventilated unit; q = unperfused unit.

The scan can verify a pulmonary occlusion. It cannot verify that the tissue is necrotic (pulmonary infarction). With the ventilation scan, decreased areas of ventilation are lighter, indicating poorly ventilated lung tissue. Additional information about Nuclear Scans is presented on p. 473.

NORMAL VALUES Normal ventilation and perfusion
Ventilation-perfusion ratio of 0.85 or greater

HOW THE TEST IS DONE

With a ventilation scan, xenon-133, xenon-127, or krypton-81m is given via inhalation. Multiple scans are taken during (1) washin, as the radioactive gas builds up in the lung; (2) equilibrium, as the gas reaches its plateau within the lung; and (3) washout, as the radioactive gas is exhaled (Figure 56).

For a perfusion scan, serum albumin is tagged with a radioisotope and given intravenously. As the tagged albumin passes through the right side of the heart into the pulmonary artery, a radiation detector scan of the lungs shows the diffusion of the radioactive albumin throughout the pulmonary vessels (Figure 57).

SIGNIFICANCE OF TEST RESULTS

Abnormal Values

Pulmonary Vascular Occlusion Resulting from the Following:

Thrombus
Cysts

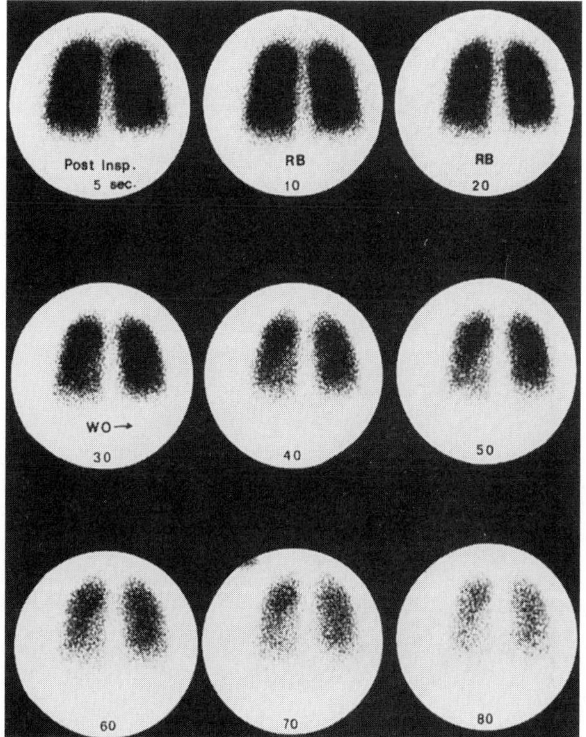

Figure 56. Normal ventilation lung scan. These are images of the lungs made from the patient's back. The patient inhales radioactive gas and rebreathes it for several seconds (RB), then additional images are made as the radioactive gas is allowed to wash out (WO) of the lungs for 30 to 80 seconds. *(Reproduced with permission from Mettler, F. A., Jr. [1996].* Essentials of radiology *[p. 137]. Philadelphia: W. B. Saunders.)*

Abscesses
Carcinomas
Necrotizing pneumonia

Inadequate Ventilation Resulting from the Following:

Atelectasis
Chronic obstructive pulmonary disease
Adult respiratory distress syndrome
Retained secretions
Pleural effusion
Pneumonia
Pneumothorax

INTERFERING FACTOR

- Uncooperative patient

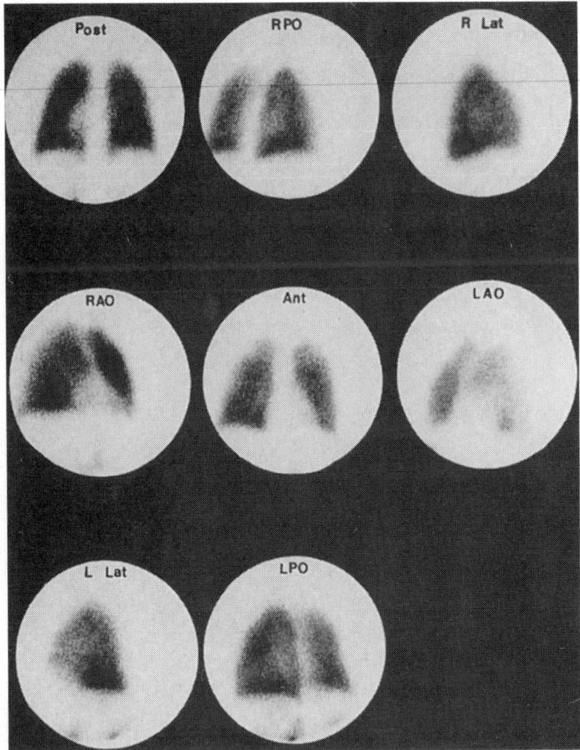

Figure 57. Normal perfusion lung scan. This nuclear medicine study is performed by intravenously injecting numerous very tiny particles that lodge in the pulmonary capillary bed, then obtaining perfusion images of the lungs in various projections. *(Reproduced with permission from Mettler, F. A., Jr. [1996].* Essentials of radiology *[p. 138]. Philadelphia: W. B. Saunders.)*

NURSING CARE

Pretest

- Schedule other radionuclide tests for 24 to 48 hours after the perfusion scan.
- ***Patient Teaching.*** Inform the patient about the procedure and ensure his or her cooperation.
- ***Patient Teaching.*** The nurse explains to the patient that the ventilation scan must be performed in the nuclear medicine department. Some hospitals have portable perfusion scanners.
- ***Patient Teaching.*** Advise the patient that with the ventilation scan, the inhaled gas should be held in the lungs for 20 seconds when the patient is instructed to do so.

During the Test

- Maintain the patient in an upright position for the ventilation scan. This position is maintained for at least 15 minutes.

NURSING CARE—*cont'd*

- If the patient is unable to maintain the upright position, a supine position may be used with the gamma camera underneath the patient.
- After the radioactive gas is inhaled, encourage the patient to hold the breath for 20 seconds.
- Radiolabeled albumin is given to the patient intravenously.
- Six different views of the chest are obtained: anterior, posterior, right and left lateral, and right and left oblique.

Posttest

- The nurse evaluates the patient's response to the test. Most patients need to rest.

Lyme Disease Tests

laim duh-zeez tests

Also called: Tests for *Borrelia burgdorferi*

SPECIMEN OR TYPE OF TEST: Serum; cerebrospinal fluid; synovial fluid, tissue

PURPOSE OF THE TEST

These tests are used to help diagnose the infection of Lyme disease.

BASICS THE NURSE NEEDS TO KNOW

Lyme disease is an infection caused by the spirochete *B. burgdorferi*. The infection is transmitted to the person by a bite from an infected tick of the *Ixodes* species. The infection progresses in two stages. In the early stage, most patients develop a characteristic rash and flu-like symptoms. In the late stage, the spirochete infects different tissues of the body including the heart, joints, and brain. The infection is difficult to diagnose because the symptoms vary among individuals.

Antibodies

In response to the infection, the immune system develops specific antibodies that can be detected by serologic testing of the blood. Unfortunately, antibodies to the spirochete do not appear in the blood until weeks after the tick bite, so antibody test results may not be positive until the late stage of the disease. If the patient has Lyme disease with meningitis, the cerebrospinal fluid may demonstrate the antibodies to *B. burgdorferi*.

DNA Identification

Using polymerase chain reaction (PCR) amplification technology, fragments of the DNA of the *B. burgdorferi* spirochete can be detected and identified from the patient's serum, cerebrospinal fluid, synovial fluid, tissue, or urine. This method is very specific and accurate in the identification of the spirochete at an early stage of infection.

NORMAL VALUES Negative for *B. burgdorferi*

HOW THE TEST IS DONE

A red-topped tube is used to collect 10 mL of venous blood.

SIGNIFICANCE OF TEST RESULTS

Positive Value

B. burgdorferi infection

INTERFERING FACTORS

- Treatment with antibiotics before the testing is done.

NURSING CARE

Nursing measures are similar to those used in other venipuncture procedures (see Chapter 2), with the following additional measures.

Pretest

- Testing should be done before antibiotic therapy is initiated.
- In obtaining a nursing history, the patient may or may not remember a tick bite. After becoming infected, the skin rash often appears within a month. There may be travel or work history that would expose the individual to ticks, particularly by walking through high grass in a field or at the edge of a forest. Lyme disease is more common in the late spring and summer.

Posttest

- ***Health Promotion.*** All people who undertake outdoor activity in tall grass or near the edge of a forest should take personal protective measures to avoid tick bites. These include the use of insect repellant with DEET, and wearing long pants and boots that protect the ankles and overlap the pant legs. Long sleeve shirts and gloves protect the arms and hands when the individual is working in infested areas. The individual should inspect his or her skin for ticks, daily.

Magnesium, Serum

mag-nee-zee-uhm, see-ruhm

Also called: Mg

SPECIMEN OR TYPE OF TEST: Blood

PURPOSE OF THE TEST

The measurement of serum magnesium helps to evaluate electrolyte disorders, hypocalcemia, hypokalemia, and acid-base imbalance. It also is used to monitor patients who have a cardiac disorder, because low magnesium levels are dangerous to these individuals. The test is also performed to monitor the pregnant patient with severe toxemia during the intravenous administration of magnesium sulfate.

BASICS THE NURSE NEEDS TO KNOW

Magnesium is one of the major intracellular cations of the body. Almost all magnesium is stored in soft tissue, muscle, and bone, with only 1% of the total magnesium present in the serum and extracellular fluid. Magnesium is obtained from food. The serum level is maintained in homeostatic balance by the functions of gastrointestinal absorption and excretion and renal resorption and excretion, and excess magnesium is removed from the body in feces and urine.

Elevated Values

An elevation of the serum value of magnesium in the blood is called *hypermagnesemia*.

Most cases of hypermagnesemia are caused by advanced renal failure, with a decreased glomerular filtration rate and a resultant rise in the serum value of magnesium.

Decreased Values

A low level of magnesium in the blood is called *hypomagnesemia*. The deficiency of magnesium is usually associated with deficiencies of calcium and potassium.

Hypomagnesemia often occurs with inadequate food intake, because of impaired intestinal absorption, or as a result of hemodialysis treatment. It may also occur during long-term hyperalimentation or intravenous fluid replacement. Hypomagnesemia together with hypokalemia is associated with a high rate of ventricular dysrhythmias. Patients with a cardiac disorder or an acute myocardial infarction are particularly vulnerable to a depleted magnesium level, and ventricular dysrhythmia or sudden death can occur. Hypomagnesemia is considered more serious than hypermagnesemia.

M

NORMAL VALUES	Adult: 1.5–2.3 mg/dL *or* SI: 0.62–0.95 mmol/L
▼ Critical Values	<1.2 mg/dL (SI: <0.5 mmol/L) *or* >4.9 mg/dL (SI: >2.0 mmpol/L)

HOW THE TEST IS DONE

A red-topped tube is used to obtain 10 mL of venous blood.

SIGNIFICANCE OF TEST RESULTS

Elevated Values

Advanced renal failure
Addison's disease
Administration of multiple magnesium sulfate enemas
Excessive ingestion of magnesium-containing antacids
Magnesium sulfate infusion therapy

Decreased Values

Early renal disease
Chronic glomerulonephritis
Chronic alcoholism

Hypercalcemia
Pancreatitis
Hemodialysis therapy
Prolonged hyperalimentation
Diabetic ketoacidosis (during treatment)
Inadequate dietary intake
Prolonged intravenous therapy
Malabsorption
Prolonged nasogastric drainage
Severe burns
Hypoparathyroidism
Hyperaldosteronism

INTERFERING FACTORS

- Venous stasis
- Hemolysis

NURSING CARE

Nursing measures are similar to those used in other venipuncture procedures (see Chapter 2), with the following additional measures.

Pretest

- ***Patient Teaching.*** The nurse instructs the patient to discontinue all food and fluid for 8 hours before the test.

During the Test

- The blood specimen is obtained without a tourniquet, to avoid false positive results.

Posttest

- The nurse monitors the lab test results for early warnings that the patient is developing difficulty related to the magnesium level. When the patient has a low level of magnesium, the serum potassium and serum calcium levels may also be low.
- With altered levels of magnesium, the nurse assesses the patient for manifestations. With hypermagnesemia, the patient may become sleepy and difficult to arouse (somnolence and neurologic reflexes are decreased). The pulse can become very slow. In hypomagnesemia, there is a hyperactive neuromuscular effect. The patient may experience muscle spasms, weakness, or tremors. Cardiac arrhythmia may occur, particularly if the serum level of potassium is also decreased. Cardiac monitoring or the taking of vital signs at regular and frequent intervals is needed. The nurse performs frequent neurologic assessments, particularly of reflexes and mental alertness.

▼ Nursing Response to Critical Values

When the serum value of magnesium falls to or rises to the critical value, the nurse must notify the physician immediately.

NURSING CARE—*cont'd*

With severe hypermagnesemia, both cardiac and respiratory systems are slowed markedly. In addition to heart block with a pulse of less than 60, the respiratory rate and effort are diminished. The patient may experience respiratory failure, unresponsiveness or coma, a loss of deep tendon reflexes, a heart attack or cardiac arrest. To support breathing and oxygenation, the nurse can institute oxygen therapy at a low flow rate. If the patient is still somewhat responsive, place the patient in semi-Fowler's position. The nurse also prepares for cardiac monitoring of the patient. Additional specific nursing interventions will depend on the medical cause of the problem and the physician's decisions about treatment.

Severe hypomagnesemia causes severe neuromuscular changes, as evidenced by tetany, convulsions, and cardiac arrhythmia. The nurse assesses for tetany, the hyperexcitability of nerves, and spasms of muscles. Reflexes are often described as 3+ or 4+, brisk or hyperactive. Because of the risk of convulsions, the nurse institutes seizure precautions. Vital signs are taken, noting any irregularity of the pulse or heartbeat. The nurse prepares for cardiac monitoring. Cardiac arrest can occur.

Magnetic Resonance Imaging

mag-ne-tik re-zuh-nuhns i-muh-jing

Also called: (MRI)

SPECIMEN OR TYPE OF TEST: Magnetic field scan

PURPOSE OF THE TEST

Magnetic resonance imaging (MRI) is used to assess anatomic structures, organs, and soft tissue, including visualization of any pathologic condition that is present. It can differentiate between benign and malignant growth and may be used to stage cancer or evaluate the response to treatment of a malignancy.

BASICS THE NURSE NEEDS TO KNOW

MRI is a noninvasive imaging technique that uses large, powerful magnets and a radiofrequency coil to obtain cross-sectional images of body tissues. The images of axial planes are similar to those produced by computed tomography (CT), but MRI has a greater ability to produce images of any plane (Figure 58). This is particularly useful in imaging the head, neck, brain, and spinal cord. The MRI is also an important diagnostic procedure used to image vascular abnormality and the soft tissues involved in musculoskeletal function.

MRI is based on the biochemical differences among cells. The nuclei of cells contain many atoms that have electric fields. For example, each hydrogen atom has one proton with a positive charge. When in the presence of the strong magnetic field produced by the MRI magnets, the protons spin and move to realign in a new formation. The radio waves stimulate and detect the magnetized protons as they realign and then return to

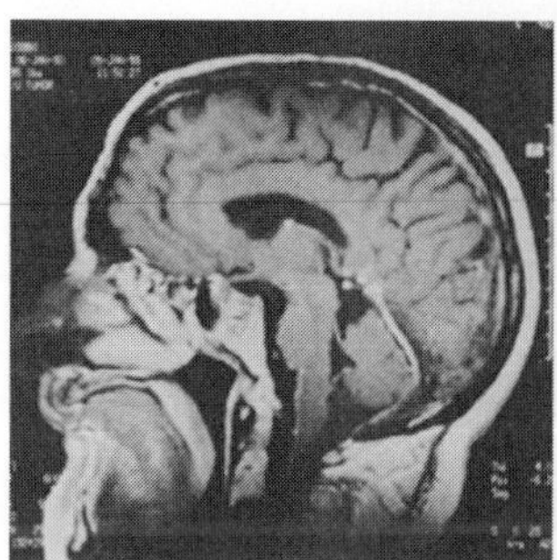
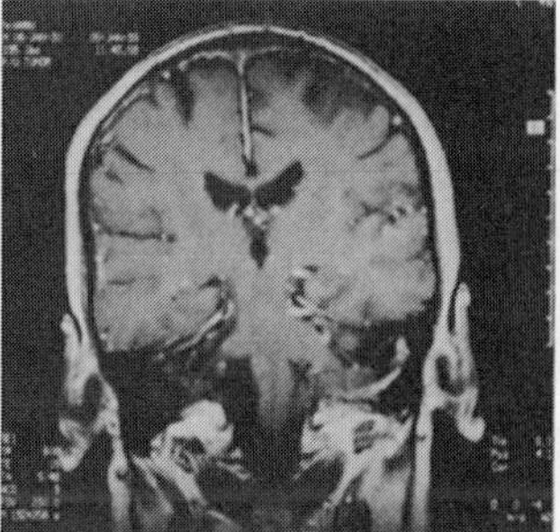
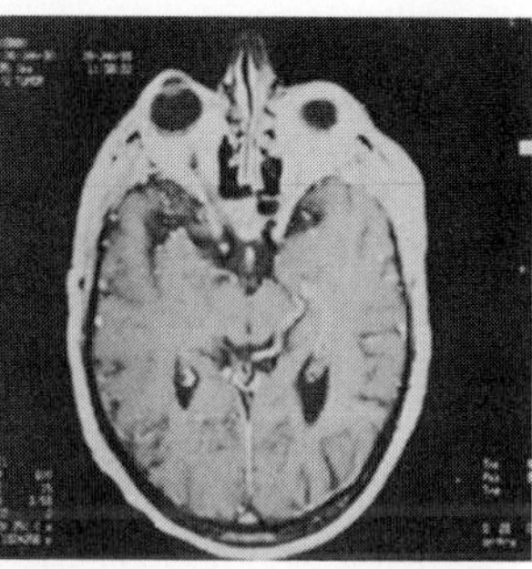

Figure 58. Magnetic resonance imaging (MRI) of the head. MRI can produce images in almost any body plane: *Left*, sagittal; *middle*, coronal; *right*, transverse. *(Reproduced with permission from Thompson, M. A., Hall, J. D., Hattaway, M. P., & Dowd, S. B. [1994].* Principles of imaging science and protection *[Vol. 2, Slide 393]. Philadelphia: W.B. Saunders.)*

their original position. The different tissues have distinct qualities and patterns of movement. These differences are identified by the radiofrequency coil, and the messages are transmitted to the computer for number coding and translation into images of the tissue.

MRI can detect anatomic differences among tissues, including the difference between cystic and solid tissues or the differences among muscle, ligament, and tendon. It can also detect pathologic changes, including fluid-filled growths, edema, inflammation, hematoma, and neoplasm.

Types of Magnetic Resonance Imaging Systems

The conventional MRI uses a *circumferential whole body* scanner. The entire body must be placed into a narrow chamber that is open at both ends. With an *open configuration* scanner, the patient is not completely enclosed in the cylindrical chamber, but the images may not be as clear as with the conventional scanner and the procedure takes longer. The third type of MRI is the *dedicated extremity MRI* (E-MRI). This system uses a special scanner to image the affected extremity only. The imaging is for the middle and lower joints of the arm or leg.

Safety Concerns

Definite risks exist for the patient with a ferromagnetic metal implant. The magnetic forces of MRI are so great that they will twist, damage, or move the metallic object and cause injury. The metallic items that are contraindications for this test are shrapnel, BBs, bullets, or other metal fragments that are imbedded in the body, particularly those located near the eyes or neurologic system. Implants that are contraindications for the test include aneurysmal vascular clips, vascular stents, pacemakers, cochlear implants, joint implants, intrauterine devices, surgical screws, clips, staples, and other implanted, therapeutic devices. Metallic items worn by the patient, including jewelry, body piercing items, a nicotine patch, and dental appliances, must be removed.

A strong ambient magnetic force exists around the outside of the scanner. The examination room must be kept clear of all extraneous metal objects such as oxygen tanks, wheelchairs, canes, crutches, and vacuum cleaners. No person can enter the examination room with coins, keys, stethoscopes, pens, credit cards, scissors, or hairpins. If these items are present, they become missiles that will be pulled into the scanner with force. The patient can be seriously injured by these objects.

Vascular Imaging

Magnetic resonance angiography (MRA) is a noninvasive procedure used to study blood flow and the structure and location of the major blood vessels. Some studies require no contrast medium. When noniodinated contrast is used, there is minimal complication and the contrast is not toxic to the kidneys. In the head and neck, this procedure is used for imaging of the circle of Willis and the carotid arteries. In the evaluation of major arteries of the torso, aneurysm, dissection, and coarctation, vascular imaging of the aorta and the renal, mesenteric, and iliac arteries are done by this method. The MRA is also used to visualize impaired blood flow in cases of peripheral vascular disease. In vascular applications, the procedure often is done prior to medical or surgical intervention. The data help to determine whether the problem can be corrected by endovascular stenting, angioplasty, or surgical repair with bypass or graft replacement of the blood vessel.

Brain and Spinal Cord Imaging

MRI is particularly valuable for assessment of the soft tissue of the brain and spinal cord. Although it cannot image the bones of the skull and vertebrae, it provides clear imaging of the organs and tissue contained within these bones. Because no contrast material is used, the procedure is noninvasive. In the study of the brain, MRI provides images of tumors, cerebral edema, ischemia, multiple sclerosis, and other demyelinating diseases. In the study of the spinal cord, MRI provides images of disc degeneration, spinal cord tumor, epidural fat, and postoperative scar tissue that impinge on the cord or its nerve roots.

Musculoskeletal Imaging

The soft tissue structures of the knee, hip, and shoulder joints are most often examined. MRI provides clear images of tears in the menisci, ligaments, tendons, and muscles that provide the structure for the knee or shoulder joint. The procedure can distinguish between an inflammatory problem that will heal with conservative therapy and a tear that will require surgical repair.

NORMAL VALUES

No anatomic abnormalities are noted

HOW THE TEST IS DONE

While lying on the MRI table, the patient enters the tube of the MRI machine, which contains circular magnets and a radiofrequency coil. In the presence of the magnetic field and radio wave stimulation, changes in and movement of tissue protons occur. These movements are converted by computer to precise images of the tissue in any plane selected.

SIGNIFICANCE OF TEST RESULTS

Abnormal Values

Tumor
Stricture
Stenosis
Thrombus
Embolus
Malformation
Abscess
Inflammation
Edema
Fluid collection
Bleeding or hemorrhage
Organ atrophy
Ligament tear

INTERFERING FACTORS

- Jewelry or other metal in the magnetic field
- Metallic implant in the body
- Uncooperative behavior

NURSING CARE

Pretest

- Although explanations about the test are given by the physician and final instructions are given by the MRI technologist, the nurse can be very helpful by answering the patient's follow-up questions and providing reassurance when the patient is apprehensive. An effective pretest orientation helps the patient be more aware and comfortable with the procedure. A signed consent is required and is placed in the patient's record.
- ***Patient Teaching.*** The nurse teaches the patient that he or she will be on a flat surface and the table will move into the chamber of the MRI machine. The space is small, with only 3 to 10 inches of extra space around the patient. The chamber is usually lighted and has a fan to help cool the air. When the machine's magnets are working, the patient hears loud tapping, chirping, and knocking noises. In some settings, earplugs help lower the level of noise. More recently, headphones are used to block the noise and provide calming music for the patient. The technologist and the patient can also communicate during the procedure. The nurse should also tell the patient that the procedure is painless, although the patient will feel warmth as the machine heats the air within the chamber. The patient will feel vibration in the fillings of the teeth, but the vibrations will do no damage. The imaging time lasts 30 minutes to 1 hour and the patient must remain still throughout that time so that the imaging will be clear.
- ***Patient Teaching.*** Some patients become very anxious and claustrophobic in the narrow, noisy chamber. If the person shows some anxiety, the nurse responds with a calm

NURSING CARE—*cont'd*

demeanor. The patient may be able to maintain a calm feeling by using relaxation techniques, guided imagery, or listening to the music. The elderly patient can become disoriented in the confusing environment. A friend or family member may be allowed to remain in the room during the procedure. If the patient is a child under the age of 3, or who is apprehensive and unable to remain still, a sedative can be given to help the patient with relaxation.

- ***Patient Teaching.*** Prior to the MRI, there must be a specific review of the medical and surgical history with the patient, to eliminate anyone who has contraindications of metal within the body. These are discussed in the section on Safety Concerns. Dental braces and a permanent dental bridge are acceptable. Although they are visible in the MRI images, they are not likely to interfere with the findings.
- ***Patient Teaching.*** At the time of the test, the MRI technologist uses a final checklist to ensure that the patient removes all external sources of metal from the body. Usually, the patient removes all clothing and dons a hospital gown for the procedure. The patient must remove jewelry, including rings, hair ornaments, hair pins, and body piercing items. These objects interfere with the imaging and would become missiles within the machine. They can also heat up and burn the skin.
- ***Patient Teaching.*** If the patient has used eye shadow with metallic fragments or wears glitter in the hair, it must be removed. Patients with tattoos or permanent skin coloring of eyeliner or lip liner will have these areas covered with cool compresses. These tattoos can become red and swollen during the MRI. Some tattoos interfere with the imaging.
- ***Patient Teaching.*** If the patient wears an externally wired device such as a pulse oximeter or EKG leads, they must be detached and removed prior to the test. If left on, the wires would heat up and burn the patient's skin severely during the imaging process.

During the Test

- The technologist reviews with the patient how to communicate during the time in the chamber. The patient is also instructed to remain motionless on the narrow table during the test. If contrast medium is to be administered, it can cause a mild reaction on rare occasions. If an adverse reaction occurs, it is usually limited to nausea, vomiting, or hives that occur about 15 minutes after the intravenous injection.

Posttest

- If sedatives were administered, the nurse monitors the vital signs on a regular basis until the patient is responsive and awake. If no medication was administered, the patient can be discharged from the radiology unit as soon as the imaging is completed. The nurse explains that if intravenous contrast was used, it will be automatically eliminated in the urine within 24 to 48 hours. No special care measures are needed.

Magnetic Resonance Imaging, Pituitary Gland

mag-ne-tik re-zuh-nuns i-muh-jing, pi-too-i-tar-ee gland

Also called: Pituitary MRI

SPECIMEN OR TYPE OF TEST: Imaging

M

PURPOSE OF THE TEST

Magnetic resonance imaging (MRI) of the pituitary gland is performed to identify suspected hypothalamic-pituitary tumors and vascular abnormalities, including aneurysms, infarctions, and malformations.

BASICS THE NURSE NEEDS TO KNOW

MRI has significantly affected endocrine diagnoses because of its ability to identify small lesions of the pituitary gland. In most cases, it has eliminated the need for angiography in patients with suspected aneurysms or vascular malformations. With MRI, the pituitary stalk and gland, as well as the optic chiasm and the intercavernous portion of the carotid artery, are visualized.

NORMAL VALUES

Normal pituitary size and configuration

HOW THE TEST IS DONE

MRI of the pituitary gland is usually performed once without contrast dye and then again with a contrast agent. Usually, gadolinium diethylenetriaminepentaacetic acid is given intravenously as the contrast medium.

SIGNIFICANCE OF TEST RESULTS

Abnormal Values

Adenomas
Aneurysm
Arachnoid cysts
Craniopharyngiomas
Hemochromatosis
Germinomas
Gliomas
Vascular malformations

INTERFERING FACTORS

- Patient has claustrophobia

NURSING CARE

See p. 454 for the nursing care associated with an MRI.

Mammography

ma-mog-ruh-fee

Also called: Mammogram

SPECIMEN OR TYPE OF TEST: Radiography

PURPOSE OF THE TEST

Mammography is used to screen for asymptomatic breast cancer and investigate a symptomatic change in the breast tissue.

BASICS THE NURSE NEEDS TO KNOW

Mammography is used as a screening tool for breast cancer in asymptomatic women because it can identify tumors less than 5 mm in diameter. Because this small size is not palpable on physical examination, mammography can detect cancer at a very early stage of growth.

On the mammography film, malignancy of the breast appears as a dense mass with irregular margins. The malignancy also may appear as numerous tiny clusters of calcification. Additional abnormalities that may indicate malignancy include a newly developed area of density and asymmetry of the breast. Benign growths also are visible and appear more rounded and have well-defined margins.

NORMAL VALUES

The breast tissue is within normal limits

HOW THE TEST IS DONE

X-ray films of each breast are taken from different angles (Figure 59).

SIGNIFICANCE OF TEST RESULTS

Abnormal Values

Benign cyst
Microcalcifications
Fibroadenoma
Malignancy of the breast

INTERFERING FACTORS

- Jewelry and clothing
- Scar tissue from previous surgery
- Body powders, creams, and deodorants
- Silicone breast implants

NURSING CARE

Pretest

- ***Patient Teaching.*** The nurse instructs the patient to omit the use of body creams, powders, and deodorants on the day of the test. The metallic elements in these products interfere with visualization of the tissues.
- ***Patient Teaching.*** At the imaging center, instruct the patient to remove all jewelry and clothing above the waist. The hospital gown is put on with the opening to the front.

During the Test

- Although the nurse does not perform the mammogram, he or she may be asked to describe the procedure.

Continued

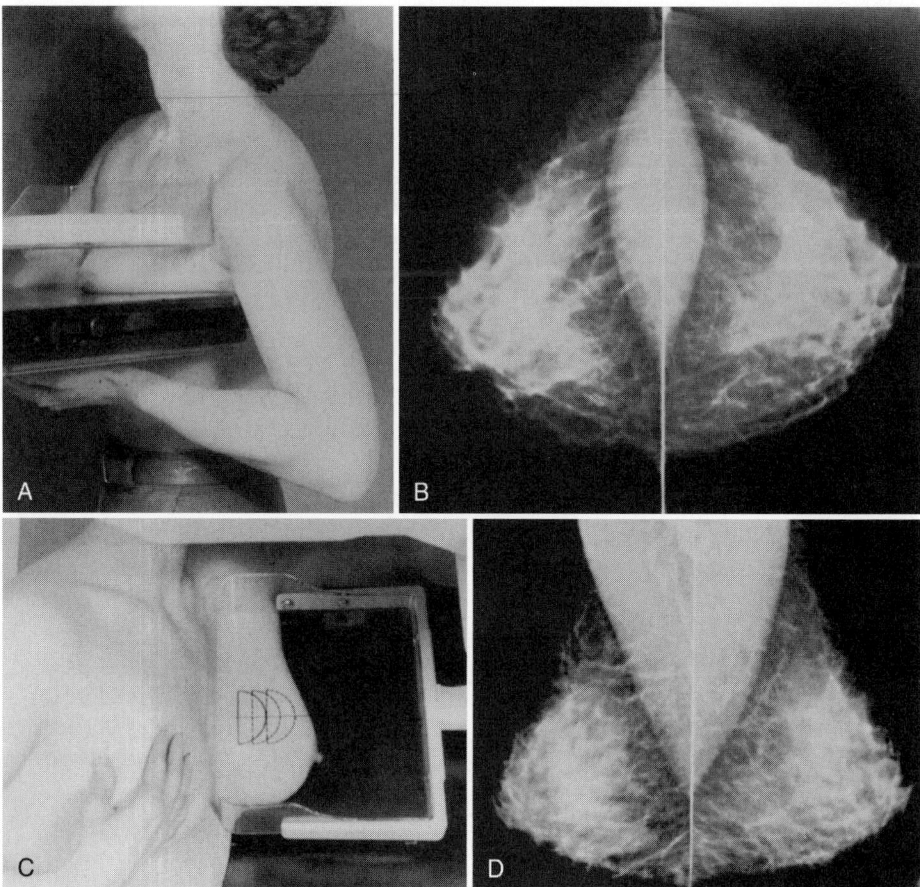

Figure 59. Mammography positioning and corresponding radiographic views. *A,* Positioning for craniocaudal view. *B,* Radiographs depicting properly positioned craniocaudal views. *C,* Positioning for mediolateral oblique view. *D,* Radiographs depicting properly positioned mediolateral oblique views. *(Reproduced with permission from Prue, L. K. [1994].* Atlas of mammographic positioning *[pp. 16, 17, 23, 24]. Philadelphia: W. B. Saunders.)*

M

NURSING CARE—*cont'd*

- The patient is positioned by seating her in front of the machine, with the breast placed on the platform over the x-ray cassette. The compressor is applied to the top of the tissue. The breast is squeezed between the two surfaces to hold the tissue firmly in place. The sensation is one of compression. Each breast is imaged separately.

Posttest

- Explain how the patient will learn of the results. Usually the report is sent to her personal physician.

NURSING CARE—*cont'd*

- ***Health Promotion.*** American Cancer Society recommendations are that all women age 40 and older receive an annual mammogram. Breast self-examination has not been found to contribute to breast cancer survival rates and is no longer recommended. If a woman has a risk for breast cancer because of a positive family history, she may want to begin mammography screening at age 30. In health teaching efforts, the nurse can communicate and encourage women age 40 and older to have a mammography done annually.

Measles Antibody

mee-suhls an-tib-od-ee

Also called: Rubeola Antibody

SPECIMEN OR TYPE OF TEST: Blood

PURPOSE OF THE TEST

The test of the serum is sometimes used to diagnose the cause of a viral rash, particularly in the pregnant female. The immunoglobulin G (IgG) value is used to document measles immunization.

The test of the cerebrospinal fluid is used to diagnose the neurologic complications of measles.

BASICS THE NURSE NEEDS TO KNOW

Measles (rubeola) is a viral infection transmitted by droplet and respiratory secretions from an infected person. At the time that the rash appears in acute measles infection, the levels of IgM and IgG measles antibodies rise. These values peak in about 10 days. Three months after the infection, the IgM antibodies disappear. The IgG antibodies decline somewhat, but the value remains positive for life.

The absence of the IgM and IgG antibodies indicates susceptibility to infection. Measles can be prevented by administration of the vaccine. Four weeks after vaccination, the antibodies appear in the blood.

NORMAL VALUES

Antibody IgM: <1:10; negative
Antibody IgG: <1:5; negative

HOW THE TEST IS DONE

Collect 10 mL of venous blood in a red-topped tube.

M

SIGNIFICANCE OF TEST RESULTS

Elevated Values

Measles Antibody IgM

Measles infection (acute stage)
Multiple sclerosis

Measles Antibody IgG

Past or present measles infection
Immunity to future measles reinfection
Past vaccination with immunity

INTERFERING FACTORS

- None

NURSING CARE

Nursing actions are similar to those used in other venipuncture procedures (see Chapter 2), with the following additional measures.

Pretest

- Teach the patient that the elevated or positive value of the IgG antibody indicates immunity to future measles infection. This occurs as a result of immunization or past infection.

Posttest

- ***Patient Teaching.*** If vaccination has not been done, teach the parents to have their children vaccinated. The vaccine is a combined measles, mumps, and rubella (MMR) vaccine, given at 15 months and again at 4 to 6 years or 11 to 12 years. Despite vaccination programs, outbreaks of measles infection can occur in population groups that have not been vaccinated, including people who have recently immigrated to this country.
- If the antibody titer is negative after vaccination, encourage the person to be revaccinated.

Mediastinoscopy

mee-dee-as-tin-os-kuh-pee

SPECIMEN OR TYPE OF TEST: Endoscopy

PURPOSE OF THE TEST

Mediastinoscopy is performed to determine invasion by lung cancer into the mediastinum; this determination can be used to "stage" lung cancer. Staging assists in determining appropriate treatment modalities. Mediastinoscopy also may be performed for diagnosing suspected granulomatous infections and other intrathoracic diseases, including sarcoidosis.

BASICS THE NURSE NEEDS TO KNOW

Mediastinoscopy is a surgical invasive procedure in which the mediastinum is entered to determine whether cancer has invaded the mediastinum or its lymph nodes. The procedure involves the insertion of an endoscope into the mediastinum, permitting visualization of the lymph nodes and biopsy of mediastinal nodes and tissue.

NORMAL VALUES

No pathologic cells

HOW THE TEST IS DONE

With the patient under general anesthesia, a small incision is made over the suprasternal fossa and a mediastinoscope is gently inserted. The mediastinum, with its lymph nodes, is visualized; it may be photographed and tissue samples removed.

SIGNIFICANCE OF TEST RESULTS

Bronchogenic carcinoma
Esophageal cancer
Granulomatous infections
Lymphomas
Sarcoidosis

INTERFERING FACTORS

- Noncompliance with dietary restrictions
- Phenytoin hypersensitivity (may cause false-positive cytologic findings)

NURSING CARE

The nurse takes actions similar to those for thoracic surgery.

Pretest

- Ensure that an informed consent form has been obtained.
- The nurse supports the patient, who is usually fearful of the outcome.
- ***Patient Teaching.*** Explain the procedure to the patient.
- ***Patient Teaching.*** Instruct the patient not to eat or drink after midnight.
- The nurse performs preoperative care according to hospital protocol.

Posttest

- Take vital signs every 15 minutes until they are stable and then every 4 hours for 24 hours.
- The nurse checks the dressing to observe for bleeding or drainage.
- Reassure the patient that chest discomfort is temporary.
- Advise the patient to resume normal activities and diet when he or she has fully recovered from the anesthesia.

◆ Nursing Response to Complications

Complications are rare but include accidental puncture of the esophagus, the trachea, or a blood vessel. These complications are evident during the procedure. The nurse should anticipate that the physician may require sutures and a suture set.

Methacholine Challenge Test

See Pulmonary Function Studies on p. 557.

Metyrapone Stimulation Test

me-tai-ruh-pohn sti-myoo-lay-shun

Also called: Metyrapone Test

SPECIMEN OR TYPE OF TEST: Serum

PURPOSE OF THE TEST

Metyrapone testing is performed to diagnose secondary adrenal insufficiency and to assess pituitary-adrenal reserves.

BASICS THE NURSE NEEDS TO KNOW

Review the section on Adrenocorticotrophic Hormone (ACTH), Plasma (p. 46). Metyrapone is given to block cortisol synthesis. A decrease in cortisol will normally stimulate ACTH secretion, which, in turn, will increase the secretion of 11-deoxycortisol. If an increase occurs after the metyrapone is given, ACTH and adrenal function are normal. If an abnormal result occurs, that is, no increase in 11-deoxycortisol occurs, the diagnosis of adrenal insufficiency is established; however, it is unknown whether it is primary or secondary adrenal failure.

Insulin may be used as a stimulant, like metyrapone. The *insulin-induced hypoglycemia test* is similar to the metyrapone test. The hypoglycemia causes a stress response normally resulting in the secretion of corticotropin-releasing hormone (CRH), which causes an increase in ACTH secretion. This test allows the assessment of the hypothalamic-pituitary axis.

NORMAL VALUES

11-deoxycortisol level: >7 mcg/dL *or* SI: >202 nmol/L
Serum ACTH: >75 pg/mL *or* SI: >17pmol/L

HOW THE TEST IS DONE

Metyrapone is given orally at midnight, with milk or a snack. The dose is based on the patient's weight. At 8 AM, a venipuncture is performed to obtain 7 to 10 mL of blood in a red-topped tube.

SIGNIFICANCE OF TEST RESULTS

Abnormal response (no change in value)
Adrenal hyperplasia
Adrenal tumor
Ectopic ACTH syndrome

INTERFERING FACTORS

- Recent radioisotope therapy or testing
- Medication such as chlorpromazine, phenobarbital, corticosteroids

NURSING CARE

Nursing actions are similar to those used in other venipuncture procedures (see Chapter 2), with the following additional measures.

Pretest

- The nurse obtains a medication history and asks the physician if any interfering drugs should be withheld. The medications that are listed as interfering factors all enhance steroid metabolism and would alter the test results.
- ***Patient Teaching.*** The nurse explains to the patient the need to take the oral medication on the night before the test and that the specimen of blood will be drawn promptly at 8 AM the next morning. Instruct the patient to ingest nothing by mouth for 12 hours before the test.

◆ Nursing Response to Complications

For a patient with adrenocorticoid insufficiency, the administration of metyrapone, which inhibits cortisol production, may precipitate an addisonian crisis.

Addisonian crisis. The nurse should observe for hypotension, muscle weakness, shock, hyponatremia and hyperkalemia. Report the abnormal assessment findings to the physician immediately. Anticipate need for intravenous access and steroid therapy administration.

Mixed Venous Blood Gases

mikst vee-nus blud ga-ses

SPECIMEN OR TYPE OF TEST: Venous blood

PURPOSE OF THE TEST

Mixed venous blood gases are obtained to assess the O_2 supply and tissue O_2 consumption. Changes in SvO_2 (venous oxygen saturation) indicate a need to determine which factor in O_2 supply and delivery is abnormal: cardiac output, hemoglobin level, tissue O_2 consumption, or SaO_2 (arterial oxygen saturation).

BASICS THE NURSE NEEDS TO KNOW

Mixed venous blood gases provide a method for evaluating the dynamic balance between O_2 supply and O_2 consumption of the body. Since the organs of the body use various amounts of O_2, mixed venous blood gases measure the blood in the pulmonary artery, which contains the venous return from all the body systems. Arterial blood gases

(ABGs) reflect what is available for body use (supply), whereas venous blood gases tell how well the body uses this supply.

With ABGs, the nurse can assess the oxygen supply available to the body tissues and determine oxygen delivery (see Arterial Blood Gases, p. 99). With mixed venous oxygen saturation (SvO_2), the nurse can assess oxygen consumption and whether the person has adequate venous reserves of oxygen.

Venous reserve is that amount of oxygen in the blood that returns to the right side of the heart after systemic circulation. If oxygen demand is greater than oxygen supply, the amount of oxygen in the returning blood decreases. This is assessed by a low SvO_2.

Mixed venous blood gases may be obtained periodically, or the mixed venous oxygen saturation (SvO_2) may be monitored continuously.

SvO_2 monitoring has been made possible by the development of fiberoptic pulmonary catheters. It is measured by light emitted from the catheter and reflected onto red blood cells within the pulmonary artery. The wavelength of reflected light is interpreted by the SvO_2 computer and continuous readings of the SvO_2 in the blood *after* systemic circulation is provided. Because the hemoglobin normally unloads about 25% of its O_2 during systemic circulation, the normal SvO_2 is 75%, with a range of 60% to 80%.

Continuous SvO_2 monitoring is used to evaluate the response to nursing care. For an unstable patient, changes in position, bathing, suctioning, and so forth can increase O_2 consumption, resulting in a corresponding lowering of the SvO_2.

M

NORMAL VALUES

pH: 7.33–7.43 *or* SI: 7.33–7.43
pCO_2: 41–51 mm Hg *or* SI: 5.3–6.0 kPa
HCO_3^-: 24–28 mm Hg *or* SI: 24–28 mmol/L
pvO_2: 35–49 mm Hg
SvO_2: 60%–80%

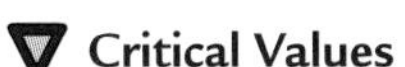

Critical Values

No specific value for SvO_2 is correlated with anaerobic metabolism. A pvO_2 of 28 mm Hg does correlate with lactic acidosis, however, and this pvO_2 corresponds to a SvO_2 of 53%, which seems to be a critical value.

HOW THE TEST IS DONE

A mixed venous sample may be obtained in a heparinized syringe from the distal port of the pulmonary artery catheter, or continuous SvO_2 may be assessed from a fiberoptic pulmonary artery catheter attached to an oximeter.

SIGNIFICANCE OF TEST RESULTS

Elevated Values (SvO_2 greater than 80%)

Anesthesia
Cyanide toxicity
High fractional concentration of oxygen in inspired gas (FiO_2)
Hypothermia

Left-to-right shunt
Neuromuscular blockade
Relaxation
Sepsis, early stages
Sleep
Vasodilation

Decreased Values (SvO_2 less than 60%)
Anemia
Anxiety
Bleeding
Cardiogenic shock
Congestive heart failure
Fever
Hyperthermia
Hypovolemia
Inadequate FiO_2
Large burns
Pain
Pulmonary disease
Multiple trauma
Position changes
Seizures
Severe pain
Shivering
Stress
Strenuous exercise
Suctioning

INTERFERING FACTORS

- Inadequate perfusion
- Poorly positioned pulmonary artery catheter

NURSING CARE

Care is based on the technique used. With a random mixed venous blood gas determination, use the procedures that follow:

Pretest
- Explain the procedure to the patient.
- Check the hemodynamic monitoring system. Ensure proper position of the catheter.
- Gather the following equipment: a 3-mL syringe, two 10-mL syringes, a syringe cap, heparin, and ice.

Continued

NURSING CARE—*cont'd*

During the Test

- Wear gloves.
- Draw up 1 mL of heparin into the 3-mL syringe and draw back to coat the barrel. Expel heparin, leaving heparin in the needle.
- Attach an empty 10-mL syringe to the sampling stopcock at the distal port of the pulmonary artery catheter.
- Turn the stopcock off to the infusion solution.
- Aspirate 5 mL into the syringe to clear the distal line of solution. Close the stopcock to the infusion and syringe.
- Remove the syringe and discard. In special situations, such as in neonates, the blood is saved and returned to the patient after the sample is drawn. Check hospital protocol.
- Attach the 3-mL heparinized syringe to the stopcock.
- Open the stopcock to the syringe and aspirate the blood slowly.
- Close the stopcock, remove the 3-mL syringe, and expel any air bubbles. Cap the syringe.
- Gently roll the syringe in your hand. Place on ice.
- Attach a 10-mL syringe to the stopcock. Open the stopcock to the solution and flush to clear the stopcock of blood.
- Turn solution off to the stopcock port used to obtain the sample and cap the sampling port.
- Flush the line and ensure the patency of the distal port. Check the monitor for pulmonary artery waveform.
- Obtain and send an ABG sample, if ordered.

Posttest

- Send blood to the laboratory immediately; clearly indicate on the slip that the blood is a mixed venous sample.
- Compare ABG and mixed venous blood gas samples.

▼ Nursing Response to Critical Values

If the SvO_2 falls to less than 60% or varies by 10% from the patient's baseline for longer than 3 minutes (10 minutes after suctioning), a full assessment of the patient is needed, including a cardiac output determination.

Mumps Antibody

mumps <u>an</u>-tib-od-ee

Also called: Mumps Serology

SPECIMEN OR TYPE OF TEST: Blood

PURPOSE OF THE TEST

The immunoglobulin M (IgM) antibody test may be used to diagnose mumps infection. The IgG antibody test is used to document immunity.

BASICS THE NURSE NEEDS TO KNOW

Mumps, or parotitis, is a viral infection, transmitted by droplets from an infected individual to the respiratory tract, gastrointestinal tract, or conjunctiva of a susceptible person. The infection produces classic inflammation of lymph glands, salivary glands, and one or both parotid glands. Immunization with the measles, mumps, rubella (MMR) vaccine usually produces immunity to future infection.

The IgM antibodies become elevated to a titer of 1:10 or higher, indicating the early, acute phase of illness. The rise of the IgG antibodies to a titer of 1:5 or higher indicates immunity, obtained by past infection or vaccination.

NORMAL VALUES

Mumps antibody IgM: <1–10; negative
Mumps antibody IgG: <1–5; negative

HOW THE TEST IS DONE

A red-topped tube is used to collect 10 mL of venous blood.

Two specimens are drawn, 10 to 14 days apart, to diagnose the acute (IgM) and convalescent (IgG) phases.

SIGNIFICANCE OF TEST RESULTS

Elevated Values

Mumps Antibody IgM

Acute mumps infection

Mumps Antibody IgG

Past mumps infection, with current and future immunity
Mumps vaccination, with current and future immunity

INTERFERING FACTORS

- None

NURSING CARE

Nursing actions are similar to those used in other venipuncture procedures (see Chapter 2), with the following additional measures.

Pretest

- ***Patient Teaching.*** Teach the patient that the positive value of the IgG antibody titer indicates immunity to future mumps infection.

Posttest

- If vaccination has not been done, teach the parents to have their children immunized for MMR at 15 months and again at 4 to 6 years or 11 to 12 years. Despite immunization programs, outbreaks of mumps still occur in vaccinated and unvaccinated people.
- With a negative IgG titer, the person has no immunity and is susceptible to mumps infection. The nurse encourages the person to be vaccinated or revaccinated to provide immunity.

Myelography

mai-log-ruh-fee

Also called: Myelogram

SPECIMEN OR TYPE OF TEST: Radiography

PURPOSE OF THE TEST

Myelography is performed to identify an obstruction or abnormality that impinges on the spinal cord or its nerve roots.

BASICS THE NURSE NEEDS TO KNOW

As a single procedure, myelography is a radiographic study that uses plain x-ray film with contrast medium to evaluate spinal disorders. Currently, the myelogram is usually performed with *computed tomography (CT myelography)* in the detection of pathologic conditions of the spine. The combination procedure is particularly useful when the CT examination alone has not resulted in a clear diagnosis.

Although CT and MRI have replaced myelography in most instances, myelography is still useful in the evaluation of the postoperative spinal surgery patient, the obese patient, and the patient who has a mobile herniated disc that is demonstrated only in a weight-bearing or flexion-extension position.

In myelography, the radiopaque water-based contrast material is instilled in the subarachnoid space. Once the contrast medium is in place, x-ray films or CT is used to image the spinal cord, spinal nerve roots, and thecal sac (Figure 60). The specific area of the spinal imaging is identified as *cervical*, *lumbothoracic*, or *lumbar*.

NORMAL VALUES No obstruction or structural abnormalities of the spinal canal, discs, cord, or nerve roots are noted

HOW THE TEST IS DONE

Using local anesthesia, the physician uses a lumbar puncture needle to instill iodinated contrast material into the lumbar subarachnoid space. The instillation is guided by fluoroscopic imaging. Once the contrast medium has filled the subarachnoid space or the whole spinal column, the images are taken at the appropriate level. The procedure takes about 45 minutes.

SIGNIFICANCE OF TEST RESULTS

Abnormal Values

Protrusion of an intervertebral disc
Herniated intervertebral disc
Spinal nerve root injury
Syringomyelia
Cervical spondylosis
Tumor of the spinal cord
Lumbar stenosis

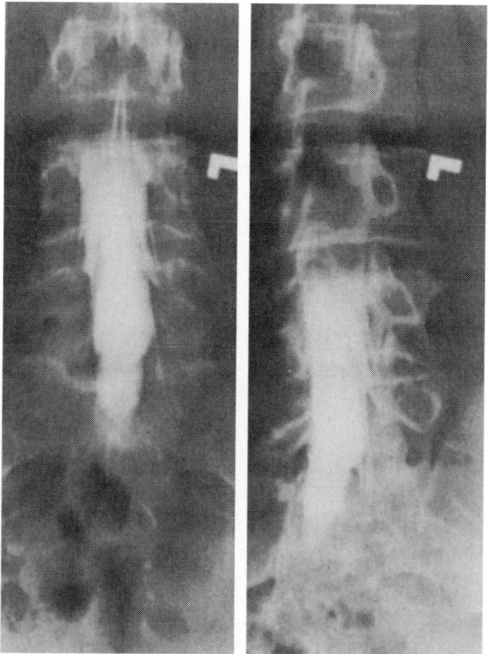

Figure 60. Lumbar myelogram. Posteroanterior (PA) and oblique views of the spinal column. The contrast material is in the subarachnoid space. *(Reproduced with permission from Adler, A. M., Carlton, R. R. [1994].* Introduction to radiography and patient care *[Vol. 1, Slide 206]. Philadelphia: W. B. Saunders.)*

Arachnoiditis
Epidural mass or tumor

INTERFERING FACTORS

- Allergy to iodine
- Incorrect placement of the needle
- Failure to fast from food and fluids

NURSING CARE

Pretest

- After the procedure is explained by the physician, obtain a written consent from the patient and place the signed document in the patient's record.
- Ask the patient about a history of allergy to iodine or shellfish or a reaction to contrast material during a previous x-ray study.

Continued

NURSING CARE—*cont'd*

Pretest—*cont'd*

- ***Patient Teaching.*** The nurse can help the patient by explaining what he or she will feel during and after the procedure. The patient will feel a needle stick as the local anesthetic is injected and a sharp stick as the spinal needle is inserted. The instillation of the contrast feels like a sharp tingling or a burning sensation. The patient receives reassurance that these feelings are expected and of short duration. Once the contrast medium has been instilled, the radiologist will tilt the examining table to allow the contrast medium to flow by gravity through the affected area.
- ***Patient Teaching.*** The nurse instructs the patient about pretest modifications of food and fluid intake. For 8 hours before the test, most institutions require a fast from food. When this procedure is performed in an outpatient setting, instruct the patient to have a responsible adult present to provide transportation home at the end of the procedure. Help the patient to undress completely and put on a hospital gown. Also, assist the patient in moving into the desired positions on the examining table. Most of these patients have problems with back pain and limited mobility because of their spinal injury or disease.
- Monitor baseline vital signs and document the results.
- If the patient is extremely anxious or has muscle spasms, administer 5 mg of diazepam (Valium) by mouth or intravenously, as prescribed. Most patients do not require pretest medication.

During the Test

- Position the patient according to the requirements of the radiologist or the anesthesiologist who administers the local anesthetic and performs the lumbar puncture. Alternative positions include (1) seated at the edge of the table with the legs dangling and the back somewhat flexed, (2) in a lateral position with the head and knees flexed toward the chest, and (3) prone, with a small pillow under the abdomen.
- If hair is present on the lower back, the skin is shaved before it is cleansed. Assist the physician with the skin preparation, draping, and preparation of the local anesthetic. The skin preparation feels wet and cold to the patient.
- Prepare the sterile lumbar puncture tray for the intrathecal administration of contrast medium. Reassure the patient during the injection of the local anesthetic. Help the patient remain still as the lumbar puncture needle is inserted. After the contrast medium has been instilled, place the patient in a prone position, with a shoulder harness and footrest in place. These are used to help the patient maintain position as the table is tilted.

Posttest

- The nurse places the patient in a semi-Fowler's position to ease the lumbar pain and prevent the contrast from rising to a high level in the spinal column. If allowed to flow to a high level, one of the contrast materials will irritate the meninges and could precipitate seizures.
- Monitor vital signs every 15 minutes for 1 hour or until the results are stable in a normal range.

NURSING CARE—*cont'd*

- ***Patient Teaching.*** The nurse instructs the patient to remain on bedrest at home for 24 hours. Two pillows are used to elevate the upper torso and head. The pillows prevent the contrast medium from rising up to the head and causing headache. Encourage the patient to drink extra fluids for the next day or two. The contrast medium will diffuse out of the subarachnoid space and be excreted in the urine. Alcohol and caffeine intake are not permitted for 24 hours because they promote rapid urinary elimination.
- ***Patient Teaching.*** Instruct the patient to notify the physician if inability to urinate occurs. The patient should also report a fever, drowsiness, stiff neck, paralysis, or seizure.

Myoglobin, Serum

See Cardiac Markers on p. 178.

Myoglobin, Urine

mai-oh-gloh-bin, yur-in

SPECIMEN OR TYPE OF TEST: Urine

PURPOSE OF THE TEST

This test is used to identify the presence of myoglobinuria and investigate the cause of damaged muscle tissue.

BASICS THE NURSE NEEDS TO KNOW

Rhabdomyolysis is the breakdown of striated muscle tissue with a release of myoglobin in the urine. With severe injury or ischemia, skeletal or cardiac muscle tissue releases myoglobin into the blood. The kidneys filter the blood rapidly, and the myoglobin is excreted in the urine.

Myoglobinuria (myoglobin in the urine) in large quantities causes the urine to become a shade of red, to dark red, to a darker brown color similar in appearance to a cola beverage. It is difficult to distinguish by appearance between hemoglobin and myoglobin in the urine because the color change is similar. In addition, myoglobin will cause a false-positive value for hemoglobin or for occult blood when tested by dipstick. Myoglobin is nephrotoxic. Large quantities of this protein can occlude the renal tubules and result in acute tubular necrosis and acute renal failure.

Myoglobinuria has many possible causes. In skeletal muscle damage, the underlying cause may be muscle trauma, such as after a "crush injury," severe exercise, or seizure; or immobility, such as from muscle compression during a coma or prolonged unconsciousness. It may also result from toxic exposure, such as carbon monoxide inhalation, or alcohol or cocaine ingestion.

NORMAL VALUES Qualitative method: Negative
Quantitative method: <0.5 mg/dL *or* SI: <5 mg/L

HOW THE TEST IS DONE

A random sample of urine is collected in a plastic container.

SIGNIFICANCE OF TEST RESULTS

Elevated Values

Severe muscle trauma
Arterial insufficiency to a large muscle mass
Severe exercise
Surgical muscle trauma
Myocardial infarction
Prolonged immobility
Drug toxicity (alcohol, cocaine, barbiturates, amphetamine)
Carbon monoxide poisoning
Muscular dystrophy

DERMATOMYOSITIS INTERFERING FACTORS

- Ascorbic acid
- Renal failure

NURSING CARE

Pretest

- The nurse assesses the urine for change in color. If present, myoglobin will cause the urine to be dark red or dark brown.
- If the patient is conscious, request a urine specimen, collected in a plastic container.
- If the patient is unresponsive or cannot assist, obtain the specimen from the port in the urinary catheter drainage system.

Posttest

- Send the specimen to the laboratory without delay. If the result is very elevated, treatment, including rehydration and restoration of electrolyte balance, must be done quickly to protect and preserve renal function.
- The nurse continues to assess the color of the urine. As the muscle tissue heals, there will be less myoglobin in the urine and the urine color lightens toward the characteristic yellow color. In addition, the volume of urinary output is monitored. Urinary myoglobin can cause acute renal failure, with diminished or no urinary output.

Norepinephrine

See Catecholamines, Plasma on p. 183.

Nuclear Scan

noo-klee-uhr skan

Also called: Isotope Scan; Scintigraphy

SPECIMEN OR TYPE OF TEST: Radionuclide study

PURPOSE OF THE TEST

A nuclear scan is used to assess the physiologic function and assist in the localization of abnormality in a designated organ or tissue.

BASICS THE NURSE NEEDS TO KNOW

In most radiologic procedures, the source of the radiation is in a machine that emits radio waves aimed to pass through the patient from the external source. In the nuclear scan, the process is different, because the radiation source is placed within the patient. Once in the patient's body, the radionuclide is taken up, concentrated, and distributed in the targeted organ or tissue. For a short time, it emits gamma rays in the pattern and concentration that correspond to the physiologic uptake of that tissue. A gamma camera or scintillation scanner detects and records the emission of the gamma rays. The data are converted into a visual image by the computer and its special software.

In a nuclear scan, the source of the radiation is a radionuclide, a radioactive isotope that has a short half-life. This means that the isotope emits gamma rays or photons for a few hours and then loses strength. By the time it is excreted in urine or feces, the radioactivity is greatly reduced or negligible. Technetium (Tc 99m) is one of the most common radionuclides. Others include isotopes of iodine, xenon, gallium, indium and thallium are used for scans of specific organs or locations. In nuclear scanning, the radioisotope that is bound to a specific compound is called a radiopharmaceutical. When administered orally or intravenously to the patient, the radiopharmaceutical is taken up or absorbed by the target tissue or organ. The targeted tissue concentrates the radiopharmaceutical and emits radiation that is detected and imaged by the scanner or camera. Some of these scans, their purposes, and the pertinent patient care information are presented in Table 10.

Abnormal Findings

In a nuclear scan, the pathologic condition that affects the target organ or tissue results in abnormal uptake and distribution of the radionuclide. The abnormality may be a space-occupying lesion or tumor, nonfunctioning tissue such as scar tissue, a loss of structural integrity such as a fracture, or another abnormality. The types of abnormalities include deficiency of uptake, excessive uptake, localization of activity in focal areas of tissue, disseminated activity throughout the organ, and asymmetry when the results should be bilateral and symmetrical.

TABLE 10 Nuclear Scans

Name of Scan	Purpose	Patient Position During Scan	Special Measures
Brain and cerebral flow scan (positron emission testing [PET] scan)	To evaluate brain tissue, internal carotid arteries, and their intracranial branches for the detection of cerebrovascular abnormality such as stroke or atherosclerosis To identify brain tissue abnormality such as tumor, hematoma, cyst, atrophy, or edema	Supine	During imaging, the head must be motionless. Fasting is required for at least 4 hr before the test. Water is permitted. To document the circulation in the arteries and brain, initial views are taken immediately after the radiopharmaceutical is administered. Additional images of the brain tissue tissue are taken after 45 min.
Brain imaging scan (single photon emission computed tomography [SPECT])	To visualize the function of brain tissue, particularly in the evaluation of dementia, cerebrovascular disease, and the location of foci of seizure activity	Supine	In the pretest and test periods, the patient must remain in an unstimulated state. The room is kept dark, quiet, and without traffic.
Cerebrospinal fluid imaging scan (cisternogram)	To investigate the passageway and flow of cerebrospinal fluid in the ventricular system of the brain	Supine and possibly Trendelenburg	If leakage of cerebrospinal fluid from the ears or nose is suspected, packing is placed in these orifices.

N

TABLE 10 Nuclear Scans—*cont'd*

Name of Scan	Purpose	Patient Position During Scan	Special Measures
Cerebrospinal fluid imaging scan (cisternogram)—*cont'd*	To help diagnose hydrocephalus To investigate brain trauma, with leakage of cerebrospinal fluid		A lumbar puncture is performed to instill the radiopharmaceutical intrathecally. For adults, images are taken at 2, 6, 24, and 48 hr. For children, images are taken at 1, 2, 4, 6, 8, and 24 hr.
Thyroid scan with technetium (Tc 99m)	To rapidly assess thyroid function and structure To help diagnose hypothyroidism, thyroid nodule, cancer, and Graves' disease	Supine, with neck in hyperextension	This test is preferred for patients who receive propylthiouracil, because the radiopharmaceutical contains no iodine. The radiopharmaceutical is injected intravenously. The patient should not swallow during the imaging stage.
Thyroid scan with iodine-123	To assess thyroid function and structure To help diagnose hypothyroidism, thyroid tumor or nodule, and Graves' disease	Supine, with neck in hyperextension	Thyroid medications and iodine interfere with iodine uptake in the test; these are discontinued in the pretest period, as per physician's orders and test protocol. Pretest, no solid foods are permitted for 4–6 hr.

Continued

N

TABLE 10 Nuclear Scans—*cont'd*			
Name of Scan	**Purpose**	**Patient Position During Scan**	**Special Measures**
Thyroid scan with iodine-123—*cont'd*			The radiopharmaceutical is given orally, 24 hr before imaging begins.
Liver-spleen scan	To assess the physiologic functions of the liver and spleen To identify focal or diffuse areas of deficit, caused by tumor, fibrosis, circulatory abnormality, or trauma	Supine	The patient should fast for at least 4 hr before the test. The radiopharmaceutical is injected intravenously
Hepatobiliary scan	To assess for patency of the hepatic ducts, biliary ducts, and gallbladder To identify defects, abnormal function, and blockage	Supine	Nothing by mouth for 6–8 hr pretest (some protocols require nothing by mouth for a minimum of 2 hr). Scanning time is 4 hr, with possible additional images for up to 24 hr
Thallium scan with thallium-201, resting or exercise	To determine the blood flow to the myocardium, at rest or after maximal stress or exercise	Upright before and during administration of the radiopharmaceutical Supine and lateral for the imaging	Nothing by mouth for 4–6 hr pretest to reduce radiopharmaceutical uptake in nearby organs. Blood pressure and electrocardiogram are monitored during treadmill exercise and imaging phases.

TABLE 10 Nuclear Scans—*cont'd*

Name of Scan	Purpose	Patient Position During Scan	Special Measures
Thallium scan with thallium-201, resting or exercise—*cont'd*			Exercise is performed to the maximal heart rate, using the treadmill. After injection of the radio-pharmaceutical, imaging is performed immediately and after 3–4 hr.
Myocardial infarction scan	To assess the cardiac tissue for damage caused by acute myocardial infarction, particularly when other tests are inconclusive	Supine	Scan is performed 10–72 hr after a possible myocardial infarction or cardiac insult. Imaging is performed 2–3 hr after the radiophar-maceutical is injected.
Gated blood pool ventricu-lography (ventriculo-gram)	To measure cardiac ventricular performance at rest and during stress or exercise To evaluate coronary artery disease, acute cardiomyopathy, valvular disease, and intracardiac shunting	Supine	The patient's erythrocytes are tagged to form the *blood pool;* the image sequence is *gated* (timed or triggered by the R wave of the electrocardio-gram). Stress or exercise studies may be performed. The patient has nothing by mouth for 4–8 hr before the test.

Continued

TABLE 10 Nuclear Scans—*cont'd*			
Name of Scan	**Purpose**	**Patient Position During Scan**	**Special Measures**
Gated blood pool ventriculography (ventriculogram)—*cont'd*			The imaging is performed immediately after the injection of the radiopharmaceutical.
Pulmonary perfusion scan	To assess the integrity of the pulmonary circulation and to identify obstruction as from pulmonary embolus	Seated or supine	The radiopharmaceutical is given intravenously, and imaging is performed immediately thereafter.
Pulmonary ventilation scan	To assess the ventilatory ability of the lungs, particularly in chronic obstructive pulmonary disease and inflammatory lung disease	Seated or upright	After the rapid imaging begins, the patient exhales deeply and inhales delivered by mask for 15 sec; the patient then rebreathes oxygen for 2–3 min followed by normal air for 2–3 min, to clear the lungs.
Meckel's diverticulum scan	To assess for bleeding in the ilium, the distal part of the small intestine	Supine or left posterior oblique	Nothing by mouth for 3–4 hr before the test. After administration of the intravenous radiopharmaceutical, scanning of the lower abdomen is carried out every 30 min, and then scanning of the right lateral midabdomen is performed for 30 min.

TABLE 10 Nuclear Scans—*cont'd*

Name of Scan	Purpose	Patient Position During Scan	Special Measures
Gastrointestinal scan	To identify and locate the source of lower gastrointestinal bleeding; the causes include diverticulitis, vascular abnormality, neoplasm, and inflammatory bowel disease	Supine	After intravenous injection of the radionuclide, images are obtained at 1–5 min intervals for 30–45 min.
Testicular scan	To differentiate among the causes of a painful, swollen testicle To assess for the vascular integrity of the testicle	Supine	After intravenous administration of the radiopharmaceutical, the imaging is performed immediately and again in 15 min.
Bone marrow scan	To identify malignant tumor or abnormal distribution of bone marrow To locate active sites for biopsy	Supine, prone, or sitting	20 min after intravenous administration of the radiopharmaceutical, imaging begins and lasts for 1 hr. Shield the liver and spleen during imaging.

When the targeted organ or tissue is not visualized, no uptake of the radionuclide has occurred. One possible cause is that vascular or ductal obstruction blocks the radionuclide from reaching the target site. Another possible cause is that the organ is nonfunctional.

An area of decreased activity in the target organ is called a defect or a cold spot. Areas of tissue are nonfunctional because of the pathologic change in the tissue. For instance, an abnormal liver scan can demonstrate a defect because of a cyst or abscess that has formed a space-occupying lesion. Multiple focal defects are often the result of metastatic disease.

An area of increased activity in the target organ is called a focal abnormality or hot lesion in otherwise normally functional tissue. The excess activity may also involve the entire organ. For instance, the thyroid scan of the patient with Graves' disease demonstrates increased activity throughout the gland (Figure 61). All the thyroid tissue is hyperactive and absorbs a maximum amount of the iodine radionuclide.

NORMAL VALUES There is normal uptake, distribution, and excretion of the radionuclide by the targeted organ or tissue.

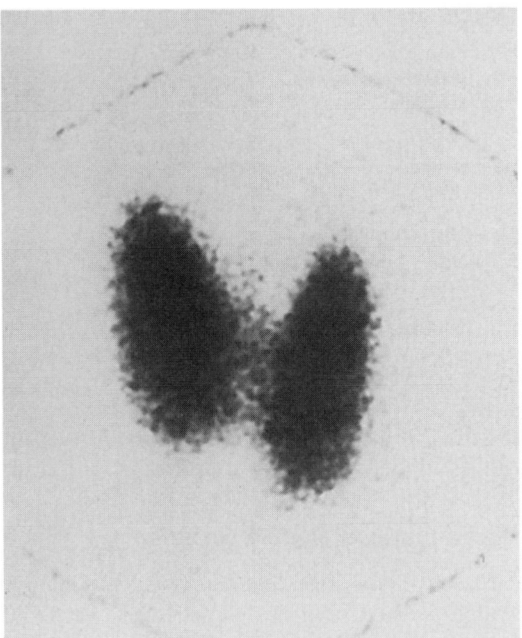

Figure 61. Thyroid scan. Diffusely enlarged thyroid gland in Graves' disease. The scintiscan was made 3 hours after an oral dose of ^{123}I. *(Reproduced with permission from Wagner, H. N., Szabo, Z., & Buchanan, J. W. [1995].* Principles of nuclear medicine *[2nd ed., Fig. 30–91, p. 611]. Philadelphia: W. B. Saunders.)*

HOW THE TEST IS DONE

An oral or intravenous dose of radiopharmaceutical is administered to the patient and a gamma camera or scintillation scanner records the radioactive emissions. These emissions are then converted to images that correspond to the location, distribution, and concentration of the radionuclide in the targeted organ or tissue (Figure 62).

SIGNIFICANCE OF TEST RESULTS

Abnormal Values

Organ atrophy or fibrosis
Congenital defect
Tumor or cyst
Metastatic lesions
Inflammation or abscess
Hyperactivity of organ function
Hematoma
Traumatic disruption of tissue
Vascular obstruction
Obstruction of a duct
Ischemia or necrosis of tissue

INTERFERING FACTORS

- Failure to follow specific pretest dietary or medication restrictions
- Recent intake of iodine
- Pregnancy

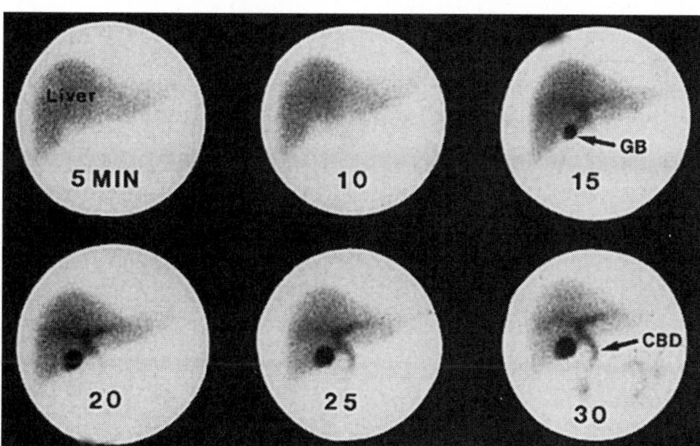

Figure 62. Normal hepatobiliary scan. With normal function of the liver and biliary system, the radionuclide provides visualization of the liver and gall bladder (GB) within 15 minutes and visualization of the common bile duct (CBD) within 30 minutes. *(Reproduced with permission from Mettler, F. A. [1996].* Essentials of radiology. *Philadelphia: W. B. Saunders.)*

NURSING CARE

Pretest

- For the patient who is female and of childbearing age, the nurse asks if she is pregnant, the date of the last menstrual period, or if she is breast-feeding. Pregnancy is a contraindication because of the patient's exposure to radiation. If the patient is breast-feeding, she will have to avoid doing so for a period until the radioisotope clears out of her body. Document the patient's responses and inform the physician of any interfering factors.
- The nurse provides reassurance regarding the scanning process. Other than the venipuncture, the procedure is painless. If the patient is anxious, a family member or friend can be in the room during the scanning procedure. Unlike x-ray imaging, there is no external source of radiation exposure, so that there is no risk to others.
- Sedatives are avoided for the older child or adult. Sedation is sometimes used for the infant or child younger than age 3, particularly when the scan requires an extended period of immobility. A nurse often administers the prescribed sedative and remains readily available to monitor and assist the patient during and after the imaging procedure. The sedative medication is usually chloral hydrate, Nembutal, or phenobarbital.
- ***Patient Teaching.*** The nurse provides the pretest patient instructions, which vary for each scan. Some scans have dietary restrictions to prevent an increase in the circulation to the liver or intestines. Many medications interfere with the absorption of the radio pharmaceutical. Often, after consultation with the patient's physician, medications are withheld and the patient remains under medical supervision during the period of the test. If the scan involves the uptake of radioactive iodine (iodine-123 or iodine-125), the nurse instructs the patient to avoid the intake of iodine from food (shellfish, kelp preparations) and medication sources (some cough medicines, some multivitamin tablets with minerals, Lugol's solution) for 3 to 5 days before the test.

During the Test

- At the time of the test the patient removes all clothing, jewelry, and metal objects. A hospital gown is worn.
- If sedatives are administered to young children, the nurse monitors vital signs regularly. This ensures early detection of any untoward response to the medication.
- The technician instructs the patient to remain still while a bolus dose of radionuclide is administered intravenously. In some studies, the scanning process begins immediately after the injection. In others, there is a waiting period before scanning can begin. The radionuclide requires time to be absorbed and concentrated by the target organ.

Posttest

- For the disposal of any urine or feces, the nurse wears gloves and then performs thorough handwashing. The radionuclide is excreted in urine and feces for several days, although the radioactivity level is minimal after a few hours. The body wastes can be disposed of in the toilet.

NURSING CARE—*cont'd*

- ***Patient Teaching.*** The nurse instructs the patient to wash his or her hands after voiding or a bowel movement. Parents and others should wash their hands after changing the diapers of an infant who has had a nuclear scan. The patient is reassured that the amount of radioactivity is negligible, but that it can remain on the hands unless they are washed.

5′-Nucleotidase

faiv noo-klee-oh-taid-ays

Also called: 5′-NT

SPECIMEN OR TYPE OF TEST: Serum

PURPOSE OF THE TEST

This test may be used to help identify diseases of the hepatobiliary system.

BASICS THE NURSE NEEDS TO KNOW

5′-nucleotidase is a liver enzyme found in the plasma membranes of all cells. Its functions are thought to include help with nutrient absorption by cells and cell reproduction. The test level rises dramatically in conditions of extrahepatic or intrahepatic biliary obstruction and cancer of the liver. The test may rise to four to six times the upper limits of the normal value in cases of hepatobiliary obstruction, but demonstrate a normal value or mild elevation in cases of hepatitis. An elevated value of this test will parallel elevations of gamma-glutamyltransferase (GGT) and alkaline phosphatase (ALP) in the presence of hepatobiliary disease. Unlike ALP, the 5′-nucleotidase will not rise in the presence of bone disease.

NORMAL VALUES Adults: 0–1.6 units *or* SI: 1–1.6 units

HOW THE TEST IS DONE

A venipuncture is performed to collect 10 mL of venous blood in a red-topped tube.

SIGNIFICANCE OF TEST RESULTS

Elevated Values

Hepatic cirrhosis
Intrahepatic cholestasis
Metastatic cancer of the liver
Lymphoma
Common bile duct obstruction
Biliary cirrhosis
Ovarian cancer
Rheumatoid arthritis

INTERFERING FACTORS

- Failure to maintain a nothing-by-mouth status
- Hemolysis of the red cells in the specimen sample

NURSING CARE

Nursing actions are similar to those used in other venipuncture procedures (see Chapter 2), with the following additional measures.

Pretest

- ***Patient Teaching.*** Instruct the patient to fast from food and fluids for 12 hours before the test. This is because lipemia (excess fat in the blood following digestion) will elevate the serum value of this test.

Occult Blood, Feces

uh-kult blud, fee-seez

Also called: Fecal Occult Blood Test, (FOBT)

SPECIMEN OR TYPE OF TEST: Feces

PURPOSE OF THE TEST

O

This test detects small amounts of blood in the gastrointestinal tract. It is used as a screening test for the early diagnosis of bowel cancer.

BASICS THE NURSE NEEDS TO KNOW

Occult blood refers to the blood that is present in feces, but is not visible. In some cases, the blood is not seen because the amount is small. In other cases, the slow, but steady leakage of blood mixes with the feces. Fecal occult blood can originate anywhere from the upper to the lower gastrointestinal tract. This test is used to detect bleeding from adenocarcinoma and premalignant polyps in the colon (Figure 63).

The test, although somewhat helpful, presents difficulties with reliability because of false-positive and false-negative results. Recent dietary intake of meat may cause a false-positive result because the test detects hemoglobin, myoglobin, and erythrocytes in the meat. Ascorbic acid (vitamin C) depresses peroxidase activity. Because the test detects the enzyme activity of peroxidase enzyme, vitamin C intake may cause a false-negative result. Other fruits and vegetables contain peroxidase, and recent intake causes a false-positive result. Some medications are irritating to the intestinal tract and cause bleeding that is unrelated to cancer or precancerous polyps (Box 3). Finally, only 30% of the adenocarcinomas or precancerous polyps of the colon bleed in sufficient amounts to be detected by this test. This means that the fecal occult blood test alone cannot detect 70% of the tumors that are present.

NORMAL VALUES Feces: Negative for occult blood

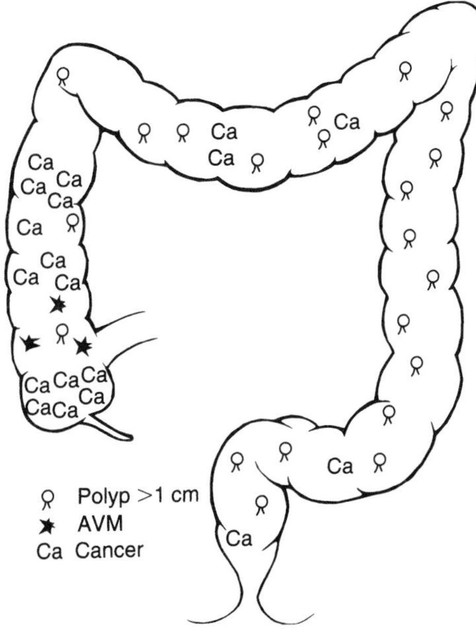

Figure 63. Sites of occult bleeding in the colon. Cancer, benign polyps, and arteriovenous malformations are three causes of occult bleeding. Their location and characteristic pathologic features are identified in follow-up colonoscopy. *(Reproduced with permission from Church, J. M. [1992]. Colonoscopy for the diagnosis and treatment of colorectal bleeding.* Seminars in Colon and Rectal Surgery, 3:*43.)*

HOW THE TEST IS DONE

Specimens of three separate stools are collected in different containers.

In performing the analysis, an applicator stick is used to place a thin smear of feces on filter paper. After 3 to 5 minutes, the specimen has penetrated the paper. The paper is turned over and a few drops of reagent are placed on the area of the specimen. After 30 seconds to 1 minute, the result is read. The appearance of color, usually blue, is considered positive.

SIGNIFICANCE OF TEST RESULTS

Positive Values

Esophageal varices
Hiatal hernia
Mallory Weiss tears in the esophagus
Gastritis
Peptic ulcer
Intussusception
Dysentery
Crohn's disease
Parasitic disease

BOX 3 Food and Medication Restrictions for the Fecal Occult Blood Test
Foods
Horseradish
Turnips
Red meat
Artichokes
Broccoli
Cauliflower
Black grapes
Melon
Bananas
Plums
Pears
Medications
Aspirin
Nonsteroidal anti-inflammatory drugs
Iron replacement
Vitamin C
Steroids
Reserpine

Benign polyps of the colon
Diverticular disease
Arteriovenous formation in the colon
Adenocarcinoma of the colon
Kaposi's sarcoma

INTERFERING FACTORS

- Recent dietary intake of animal protein, vegetable peroxidase, or vitamin C
- Recent intake of alcohol and some medications that cause intestinal irritation
- Failure to refrigerate the specimens
- Presence of toilet bowl cleaner that contains chlorine
- Presence of urine, soap, or toilet paper

NURSING CARE

- ***Health Promotion.*** The nurse can educate and encourage healthy people older than age 50 to have an annual fecal occult blood test. Many people do not have routine health screening performed for various reasons. Health education can correct the perceptions of the public that "I have no symptoms and feel well, so I do not need the test." Cancer of the colon and precancerous polyps can be detected before symptoms occur. Early detection is very important for successful intervention that leads to a cancer-free outcome.

NURSING CARE—*cont'd*

Pretest

- ***Patient Teaching.*** Instruct the patient to avoid the foods presented in Box 3 for 3 days before the test. Vitamin C must be omitted for 5 days before the test. If possible, the medications that cause intestinal irritation should be stopped for 7 days before the test. To avoid intestinal irritation, alcohol should also be omitted.
- ***Patient Teaching.*** The nurse also instructs the patient about how to collect a stool specimen. The reader is referred to Chapter 2 for additional information about collection procedure.

Posttest

- If the fecal occult blood test is positive, further diagnostic testing is essential. A colonoscopy will be ordered to determine the cause of the bleeding in the colon. The nurse provides caring support to the patient and strongly encourages that the patient complete the additional diagnostic testing that is prescribed.

Opiates, Urinary

oh-pee-ayts, yur-i-nar-ee

SPECIMEN OR TYPE OF TEST: Urine

PURPOSE OF THE TEST

The test for urinary opiates is almost always used to identify the presence of drugs of abuse in the opiate classification.

BASICS THE NURSE NEEDS TO KNOW

Urinary opiate testing includes identification of the presence of the drugs morphine, codeine, opium, heroin, hydrocodone (Hycodan), hydromorphone (Dilaudid), oxycodone (Roxicodone, Percocet, Percodan), and oxymorphone (Numorphan). Morphine and codeine are taken for the relief of pain, as prescription medications. However, they also have a high potential for abuse.

The opiate screen is used medically to obtain a rapid laboratory result when treating a patient who is suspected of a drug overdose. A test value of 300 ng/mL is the cutoff value. Above that level, the urine sample is determined to be positive. This cutoff value may be too low because the ingestion of poppy seeds on bread, bagels or Danish pastry could produce the positive result. Recently, the cutoff value for morphine and codeine has been raised to 2000 ng/mL. When this value is used, it eliminates false-positive errors. If the test is positive, confirmatory tests for the specific opiate are performed, particularly when the case is one involving forensics or medico-legal decisions. If the test result will be part of forensic evidence, the established procedure for chain-of-custody must be followed.

NORMAL VALUES Negative; <2000 ng/mL

HOW THE TEST IS DONE

A random sample of 30 to 60 mL of urine is obtained.

SIGNIFICANCE OF TEST RESULTS

Positive Values

Recent use of opiates

INTERFERING FACTORS

- None

NURSING CARE

Pretest

- The nurse assesses the patient for opiate use. The patient or parent of the affected neonate is asked about the use of any drug or medication in the past 24 hours. The patient who has taken a lower amount of the opiate drug may "nod," meaning that he or she alternates between drowsiness and alertness. The patient may also appear restless or experience nausea and vomiting. If the dose of the opiate was large, the patient may be unconscious. The assessment findings also include very constricted pupils and skin that is cold, sweaty, and cyanotic. The patient's rate of breathing is abnormally slow. If the drug effects are not reversed, the patient may die of a drug overdose.

Posttest

- The urine specimen must be sent to the laboratory immediately and refrigerated until the analysis is performed.

Osmolality, Plasma

ahz-muh-lal-i-tee, plaz-muh

SPECIMEN OR TYPE OF TEST: Plasma, serum

PURPOSE OF THE TEST

Plasma osmolality is determined to assess the person's fluid status and identify antidiuretic hormone (ADH) abnormalities.

BASICS THE NURSE NEEDS TO KNOW

Osmolality is a measure of the number of particles dissolved in a solution. In the blood, osmolality is created by sodium, chloride, bicarbonate, proteins, glucose, and urea dissolved in the plasma. Osmolality is affected by an increase or decrease in fluid volume or by an increase or decrease in blood particles.

NORMAL VALUES	Adults: 285–300 mOsm/kg H_2O *or* SI: 280–300 mmol/kg Children: 270–290 mOsm/kg H_2O *or* SI: 270–290 mmol/kg
Critical Values	>320 mOsm/kg *or* SI: >320 mmol/kg <265 mOsm/kg *or* SI: <265 mmol/kg

HOW THE TEST IS DONE

Venipuncture is performed to obtain 1 mL of blood in a red-topped tube.

Osmolality may also be calculated with the following equation:

$$2(Na^+) + BUN/2.8 + Glu/18$$

SIGNIFICANCE OF TEST RESULTS

Increased Values

Alcoholism
Aldosteronism
Dehydration
Diabetes insipidus
High-protein diet
Hypercalcemia
Hyperglycemia
Hypernatremia
Hyperkalemia

Decreased Values

Addison's disease
Fluid overload
Hyponatremia
Liver failure with ascites
Syndrome of inappropriate antidiuretic hormone

INTERFERING FACTORS

- Hemolysis of specimen
- Medications
- Diuretics
- Mineralocorticoids

NURSING CARE

The nursing actions are similar to those of other venipuncture procedures.

Nursing Response to Critical Values

Assess patient fluid and electrolyte status. High osmolality will cause fluid to shift out of the cells causing cellular dehydration, and low osmolality will cause fluid to shift into the cells causing cells to swell. Notify the physician, especially if the patient is increasingly stuporous. Initiate seizure precautions for high osmolality levels.

Osmolality, Urine

ahz-muh-lal-i-tee, yur-in

SPECIMEN OR TYPE OF TEST: Urine

PURPOSE OF THE TEST

Urine osmolality is determined to assess the ability of the kidneys to concentrate or dilute urine and to identify antidiuretic hormone (ADH) abnormalities.

BASICS THE NURSE NEEDS TO KNOW

Osmolality is a measure of the number of particles that are dissolved in a solution. Thus, urine osmolality varies based on the person's fluid status and the metabolic waste products being excreted. If the patient is overhydrated, the urinary osmolality decreases as output increases. If the person is dehydrated, the urine osmolality increases as the output decreases. Urine osmolality is based on the concentration ability of the kidneys and the serum levels of sodium, chloride, bicarbonate, proteins, glucose, and urea.

NORMAL VALUES

24-hour Urine Specimen (with Normal Diet and Fluid Intake)
500–800 mOsm/kg H_2O *or* SI: 500–800 mmol/kg H_2O

Random Urine Specimen
Adults and children: 250–1200 mOsm/kg H_2O *or* SI: 250–1200 mmol/kg H_2O
Neonates: 75–300 mOsm/kg H_2O *or* SI: 75–300 mmol/kg H_2O

HOW THE TEST IS DONE

If a random urine specimen is desired, 10 mL of urine is collected in a sterile container and sent to the laboratory. For a 24-hour specimen, all urine voided in a 24-hour period is collected and sent to the laboratory.

SIGNIFICANCE OF TEST RESULTS

Increased Values

Addison's disease
Azotemia
Cirrhosis of the liver
Dehydration
Diabetes mellitus
Diarrhea
Hyperglycemia
Hypernatremia
Syndrome of inappropriate antidiuretic hormone

Decreased Values

Aldosteronism
Diabetes insipidus

Glomerulonephritis
Hypocalcemia
Hyponatremia
Overhydration
Sickle cell anemia

INTERFERING FACTORS

- Noncompliance with nothing-by-mouth status
- Glucosuria
- Recent scans requiring radiopaque dyes
- Medications
- Antibiotics
- Diuretics
- Volume expanders

NURSING CARE

Nursing care is similar to that for other 24-hour urine collection or random sample specimen procedures as described in Chapter 2. For a random specimen, perform the following.

Pretest

- ***Patient Teaching.*** Instruct the patient not to eat or drink overnight before the urine is collected for a random specimen.

During the Test

- Obtain 10 mL of urine in a sterile container.

Posttest

- Send the specimen to the laboratory immediately.
- The results should be interpreted in relation to the serum osmolality.

Ova and Parasites, Feces

oh-vuh and pa-ruh-saits, fee-seez

Also called: Stool for Ova and Parasites; Stool for O and P

SPECIMEN OR TYPE OF TEST: Feces

PURPOSE OF THE TEST

The microscopic examination of the feces is used to identify the presence of specific parasites in the intestinal tract.

BASICS THE NURSE NEEDS TO KNOW

Numerous parasites can infect individuals and then live in the intestinal tract and other organs during parts of the parasitic life cycle. Many ova, cysts, larvae, or spores from fecal-contaminated soil enter the person via a fecal-oral route (Figure 64). Common methods of transmission are from unwashed hands, eating contaminated raw fruits and vegetables, and drinking from a feces-contaminated water supply. Other parasites invade the body through the skin and then migrate through body tissue to the intestinal lumen or are transmitted by eating undercooked meat, raw fish, or plants that are contaminated by the parasite. As these various parasites reach the intestine, they mature to the adult stage of development and deposit ova that can be recovered in stool samples.

The procedure for stool collection is based on the type of parasite infection that is suspected. Traditionally, the method of fecal sample collection is to obtain three separate specimens on different days. This maximizes the chance of identification of the ova in at least one of the samples. A patient may be infected with more than one type of parasite.

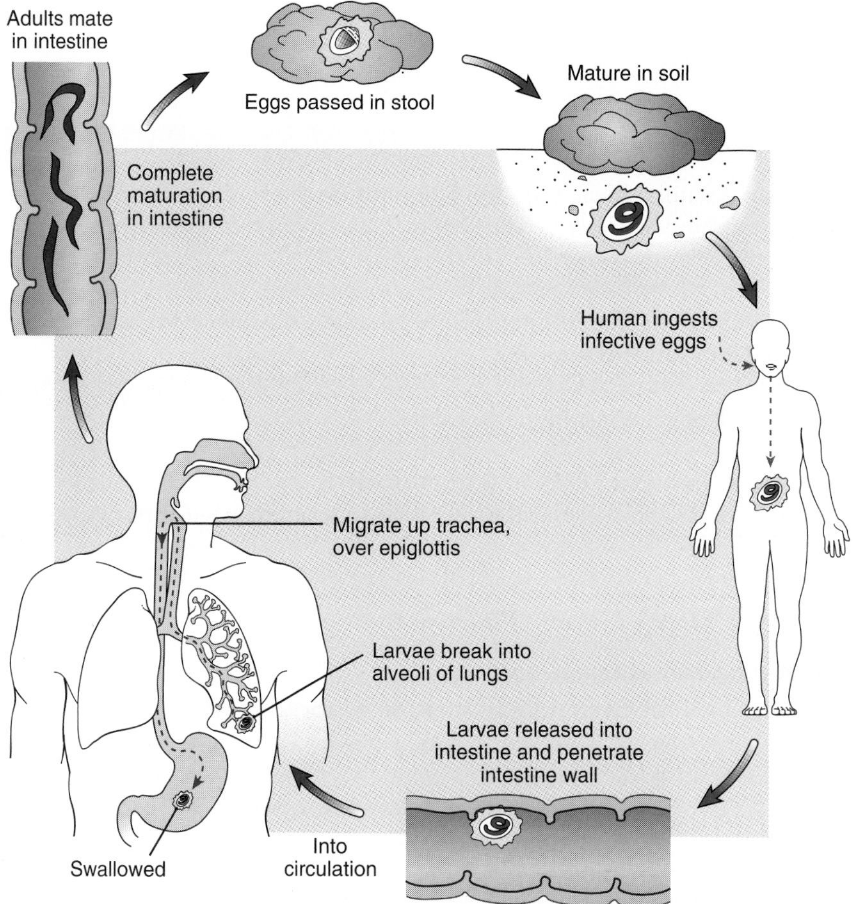

Figure 64. Life cycle of *Ascaris lumbricoides*. The eggs of this roundworm parasite enter the person via fecally contaminated soil, on food, or on unwashed hands. The eggs, larvae, and worms live in and migrate through the body. As the worms mature, new eggs are deposited in the colon and feces. *(Reproduced with permission from Mahon, C., & Manuselis, G. [1995].* Textbook of diagnostic microbiology. *Philadelphia: W. B. Saunders.)*

NORMAL VALUES

Negative; no parasites or ova are present

HOW THE TEST IS DONE

Stool collection: Collect a small sample of feces directly into a clean, wide-mouthed container and close the lid. A common requirement is to collect one specimen each day for 3 days.

Perianal swab (for pinworm): Transparent tape is placed on a tongue depressor, sticky side out. Press the tape firmly on the perianal skin. Remove the tape and place it on a glass slide, sticky side down.

SIGNIFICANCE OF TEST RESULTS

Positive Values

Amebiasis
Cryptosporidiosis
Ascariasis
Pinworm
Giardiasis
Tapeworm
Hookworm

INTERFERING FACTORS

- Antibiotic therapy in the 3- to 4-week pretest period
- Soil, water, or urine contamination of the sample
- Barium sulfate administration in the 2- to 3-week pretest period
- Mineral oil, castor oil, antacids, or antidiarrheal medication in the week before the test

NURSING CARE

Pretest

- Schedule this test before any barium studies, because the barium obscures the microscopic visualization of the ova.
- ***Patient Teaching.*** The nurse instructs the patient regarding correct collection procedure. The fecal matter should be evacuated directly into a clean, dry container or into a clean, dry basin and then transferred into the container. For this test, the feces should not be removed from the toilet bowl. The patient should not use a laxative to assist in evacuation because it would interfere with the microscopic examination of the sample.

Posttest

- If the nurse collects the specimen, he or she wears gloves and, after removing the gloves, washes hands thoroughly. Intestinal parasites are a highly transmissible source of infection via the fecal-oral route or via contact with the skin. The nurse must take precautions to prevent possible self-infection from poor hygiene practices.

Continued

NURSING CARE—*cont'd*

Posttest—*cont'd*

- The nurse includes the time and date of the collection on the laboratory slip and the container. On the laboratory requisition form, pertinent data are included regarding the patient's clinical history, such as immunosuppression or AIDS, or possible sources of infection, such as backpacking in the mountains or travel to another country. In rural areas of Central and South America, and in the Caribbean, parasitic infection is endemic.

Papanicolaou Smear

pah-puh-nee-kuh-lou smeer

Also called: PAP Smear

SPECIMEN OR TYPE OF TEST: Cytology study

PURPOSE OF THE TEST

The Papanicolaou smear is used to detect inflammation, infection, premalignant changes, and malignancy of the cervix.

BASICS THE NURSE NEEDS TO KNOW

The Papanicolaou (Pap) smear is an inexpensive screening test that examines cervical cell scrapings for abnormality. Most commonly, the reported results are classified according to the Bethesda system. When abnormality is present, the changes can be of infectious, inflammatory origin or they can be squamous cell or glandular cell abnormalities. The abnormalities are graded in severity.

The borderline lesion (inconclusive result) is defined as atypical squamous cells of undetermined significance (ASC-US). The squamous intraepithelial lesions (SIL) are graded from low grade to high grade. The low-grade squamous intraepithelial lesion (LSIL) consists of condyloma, mild dysplasia (CIN I)—a precancerous state—or both. A high-grade squamous intraepithelial lesion (HSIL) ranges from moderate dysplasia (CIN II) to severe dysplasia (CIN III)—carcinoma in situ. Invasive carcinoma or adenocarcinoma is also included in the HSIL category.

Populations at Risk

In general, older, urban women with a low-income or poverty status and less education, and those who are of an ethnic minority group are at high risk for poor health and disease. The ethnic groups who are at higher risk for cancer of the cervix are women who are Hispanic, African American, and Native American. These population groups have a lower screening rate, a higher risk for cervical cancer, and a higher risk for a late diagnosis of this disorder. After having an abnormal Pap smear, these women also have a low rate of follow-up diagnostic and treatment measures.

NORMAL VALUES Bethesda system classification: Normal; within normal limits

HOW THE TEST IS DONE

Using a vaginal speculum to enhance visibility, the physician or nurse practitioner collects the patient's secretions and cells from the cervix and vagina. The fluid and tissue scrapings are placed on glass slides and sprayed with or immersed in a fixative. When the liquid-based/thin prep method shows a result of ASC-US, the laboratory then tests the specimen sample for DNA of the human papilloma virus (HPV).

SIGNIFICANCE OF TEST RESULTS

Abnormal Values

Cervical dysplasia or cervical intraepithelial neoplasia
Genital infection (viral, fungal, parasitic)
Cervicovaginal endometriosis
Condyloma
Human papillomavirus
Lymphogranuloma venereum
Carcinoma in situ
Squamous cell carcinoma
Adenocarcinoma

INTERFERING FACTORS

- Menstruation
- Recent douching
- Vaginal infection or medication
- Recent sexual intercourse
- Drying of the specimen
- Inadequate specimen
- Lubricating jelly on the speculum

P

NURSING CARE

Pretest

- Schedule the test for when the patient is not menstruating.
- ***Patient Teaching.*** The nurse instructs the patient to refrain from sexual intercourse, douching, and vaginal medication for 48 hours before the test. Sexual intercourse can cause inflammation of the tissue. Douching can remove surface cells before the test sample is obtained. Medication obscures the microscopic examination of the cells. If vaginal infection is present, it will be treated and the Papanicolaou test postponed for 2 to 4 weeks.

During the Test

- The nurse assists the patient to lie on the table in the lithotomy position with the legs supported by stirrups. The elderly patient may need extra assistance in positioning because of stiffness and arthritic pain.
- After the tissue and fluid samples are obtained, apply the fixative by spraying the samples or immersing them in solution. Identify each slide with the patient's name.

Continued

NURSING CARE—*cont'd*

Posttest

- On the requisition slip, the nurse writes the patient's name, age, date of last menstrual period, and the source of the specimen. The pertinent clinical data are also included, such as history of an abnormal Papanicolaou smear, carcinoma, radiation, chemotherapy, abnormal vaginal bleeding, exposure to diethylstilbestrol, a visible lesion, or recent pregnancy.
- When the woman is informed of abnormal Papanicolaou test results, she often requires additional information about the meaning of the results and the follow-up measures. The nurse recognizes the patient's anxiety or confusion and intervenes appropriately to help with the emotional stress. Additional information and repetition of the instructions may be needed. The nurse can provide information and support, help to clarify misconceptions and encouragement to complete the follow-up testing
- ***Health Promotion.*** The American Cancer Society guidelines on the need and frequency of Pap testing are presented in Box 4. In the roles of health teaching and health promotion, the nurse should encourage women to have the Pap test and to return for results and follow-up appointments, as recommended. The nurse can also work in collaboration with community-based health programs, as they have been effective in providing breast and cervical screening tests to low income and uninsured women. For all women, the goal is to detect cervical tissue changes and premalignant conditions before they become advanced or change into malignant tumors. Early detection and treatment greatly reduce the morbidity and mortality of cancer of the cervix.

BOX 4 Guidelines for Need and Frequency of Pap Testing

- A young woman should begin having Pap tests about 3 years after starting vaginal intercourse, or at age 21. The test should be repeated annually (or every 2 years when the liquid-based/Thin Prep test method is used).
- Beginning at age 30, the woman who has had three consecutive, normal Pap tests can be screened every 2 to 3 years. Women who are at increased risk for cervical cancer (history of cervical cancer, HIV, weakened immune system) should be screened more frequently, as recommended by her physician or health care provider.
- Women age 70 or older, who have three or more consecutive normal Pap tests and no abnormal results in the past 10 years, can choose to stop having Pap tests.
- Women who have had a hysterectomy with removal of the cervix do not need Pap tests (unless the surgery was done for cancer or a precancerous condition). Women who had hysterectomy without removal of the cervix should continue to follow current guidelines for Pap testing.

From News Briefs (2003). American Cancer Society updates guidelines on Pap tests. Clinical Journal of Oncology Nursing, 7(3), 268.

Paracentesis and Peritoneal Fluid Analysis

pa-ruh-sen-tee-sis and per-i-toh-ne-al floo-id uh-nal-uh-sis

Also called: Abdominal Paracentesis; Abdominal Tap

SPECIMEN OR TYPE OF TEST: Peritoneal fluid

PURPOSE OF THE TEST

Abdominal paracentesis is used to obtain a sample of the peritoneal fluid as part of the investigation of ascites, the effect of blunt abdominal trauma, or the cause of an acute abdomen when perforation of the intestine is suspected.

BASICS THE NURSE NEEDS TO KNOW

A healthy person has less than 50 mL of peritoneal fluid and no distension of the peritoneal (abdominal) cavity. The abnormal accumulation of fluid in the peritoneal cavity is called ascites. When the ascites is advanced, the fluid volume can increase to 750 to 1500 mL or more. The peritoneal fluid can be aspirated by a needle that penetrates into the peritoneal cavity (Figure 65). Laboratory analysis of the fluid specimen includes cytologic study, chemistry analysis, and microbiologic examination, as requested.

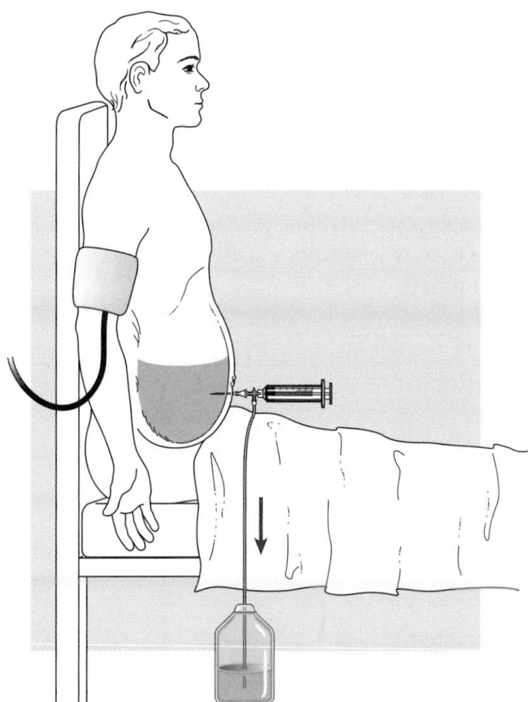

Figure 65. Paracentesis. The three-way stopcock controls the direction of the peritoneal fluid into the syringe or the drainage tubing and collection container.

As the specimen is collected by the physician, the nurse can assess the quality of the fluid visually. Normal peritoneal fluid should be clear and colorless or pale yellow. Abnormal fluid can appear bright red and bloody, indicating bleeding, possibly from organ rupture resulting from blunt trauma to the abdomen. Cloudy fluid is often due to infection, a strangulated bowel, or organ rupture. Greenish fluid can result from perforation of the duodenum or gall bladder, causing bile peritonitis. Milky fluid may result from malignancy, cirrhosis of the liver, adhesions, or infection.

NORMAL VALUES

Peritoneal Fluid Analysis
Appearance: Clear, odorless, colorless or pale yellow, scanty
Ammonia: <50 mcg/dL
Amylase: 138–404 amylase units/L
Bacteria and fungi: None present
Cells: No malignant cells present
Glucose: 70–90 mg/dL *or* SI: 3.89–4.99 mmol/L
Protein: 0.3–4.1 g/dL *or* SI: 3–41 g/L
Red blood cells: None
White blood cells: <300 cells/μL

HOW THE TEST IS DONE

Paracentesis

Under local anesthesia, the physician inserts a long thin needle or trocar through the skin and into the peritoneal cavity. The insertion site is midline, about 2 inches (5 cm) below the umbilicus. Either a syringe or a three-way stopcock with polyethylene tubing is used to draw off the fluid. The procedure takes 30 to 45 minutes to complete.

Peritoneal Fluid

For cell counts, a lavender-topped tube is used to collect 7 mL of fluid. For culture, blood culture bottles are used. For cytology studies, at least 100 mL of fluid is collected in a sterile jar or collection bag.

SIGNIFICANCE OF TEST RESULTS

Malignancy (liver or peritoneum)
Pancreatitis
Hepatic cirrhosis
Peritonitis (bacterial, fungal, parasitic, tuberculosis)
Traumatic organ rupture (bowel, liver, spleen)
Ruptured appendix
Duodenal ulcer, perforated
Intestine, perforated
Bowel, strangulated, infracted
Hypoproteinemia
Congestive heart failure

INTERFERING FACTORS

- Contamination of the fluid by urine, feces, blood, or bile
- Pregnancy
- Coagulation disorder
- Intestinal obstruction
- Abdominal wall infection
- Uncooperative behavior
- History of multiple abdominal surgeries
- Portal hypertension

NURSING CARE

Pretest

- Because of the risk of bleeding, obtain the hematocrit, prothrombin time, partial thromboplastin time, and platelet values within 48 hours of this procedure. The lab values are entered into the patient's record and the nurse notifies the physician of abnormal results. After the physician has informed the patient about the procedure, a signed consent is needed and is placed in the patient's record.
- Prior to the procedure, the nurse records the patient's baseline vital signs, temperature, and measurements of the weight and abdominal girth.
- Just before the procedure, have the patient void to empty the bladder completely. This helps prevent an inadvertent puncture of the organ during the procedure.
- The nurse positions the patient in full Fowler's position. If a removal of a large volume of fluid is anticipated, the physician will establish a central venous pressure (CVP) line to monitor venous pressure. Record the baseline CVP value.

During the Test

- The nurse stands at the patient's shoulder and provides reassurance to alleviate fear. Some pain is felt by the patient as the needle or trocar penetrates the peritoneum. Encourage the patient to remain immobile.
- The nurse assists with the collection of the fluid. In addition, vital signs are taken and documented every 15 minutes. Because hypovolemic shock can occur as the fluid is removed, the nurse assesses the patient for signs of impending shock, including pallor, dizziness, diaphoresis (cold, moist skin, sweating), a rising pulse rate, and a falling blood pressure.
- Once the procedure is completed, the physician removes the needle and applies a small bandage to the puncture site. On removal of a trocar, a suture or two will be used to close the hole and a small bandage covers the wound.

Posttest

- Vital signs and a CVP reading are done and the abdominal girth is measured. The data are recorded in the chart. The nurse also documents that the paracentesis was done, and includes the patient's tolerance of the procedure. The entry includes the amount, color, odor, and characteristics of the fluid that was withdrawn. The amount of peritoneal fluid removed is also entered as output on the record of intake and output. All specimens are labeled appropriately, including the identification of the specimen as peritoneal fluid. The collection bottles and specimens are sent to the laboratory, without delay.

Continued

NURSING CARE—*cont'd*

Posttest—*cont'd*

- The nurse continues to monitor the vital signs frequently and take CVP readings every hour for 6 hours or until the patient is stable. The dressing is checked frequently for excess drainage or bleeding. With the removal of large amounts of fluid from the peritoneal cavity, there may be a rapid shift of fluid, albumin, and potassium from the blood to the peritoneal cavity. The nurse remains alert for hypotension, shock, a rapid pulse, an irregular pulse, and a very low CVP as indicators of a serious shift of fluid and electrolytes.

◆ Nursing Response to Complications

The two complications of a paracentesis are hemorrhage and perforation of the intestine. If one of these complications occurs, the symptoms usually become apparent in the posttest period. The nurse would notify the physician immediately of abnormal assessment findings.

Bleeding or hemorrhage. The patient with a hemorrhage into the peritoneal cavity will demonstrate hypotension, tachycardia, dyspnea, diaphoresis, and pallor. The CVP value will drop soon after the bleeding begins, and the hematocrit will drop after a few hours. The patient may feel abdominal discomfort or acute abdominal pain. Ecchymosis appears on the skin in dependent areas, as toward the back and buttocks.

Peritonitis. The patient is at risk to develop infection in the peritoneal cavity. The nurse should assess for acute abdominal pain, a board-like abdomen, abdominal distension, shock, and a fever.

Parathyroid Hormone

pa-ruh-thai-royd hohr-mohn

Also called: (PTH); Parathormone; Immunoreactive PTH

SPECIMEN OR TYPE OF TEST: Serum, plasma

PURPOSE OF THE TEST

A parathyroid hormone determination is performed to diagnose suspected parathyroid disorders. It may be performed to differentiate among clinical diagnoses that result in calcium and phosphate abnormalities.

BASICS THE NURSE NEEDS TO KNOW

Parathyroid hormone is produced and secreted by the parathyroid glands. Its role in the body is the regulation of calcium. Its secretion is based on a negative feedback mechanism with calcium (Figure 66).

Parathyroid hormone affects calcium levels by stimulating osteoclast activity and inhibiting osteoblast activity in the bone. This causes bone reabsorption, which shifts calcium and phosphate out of the bone into the blood. Parathyroid hormone

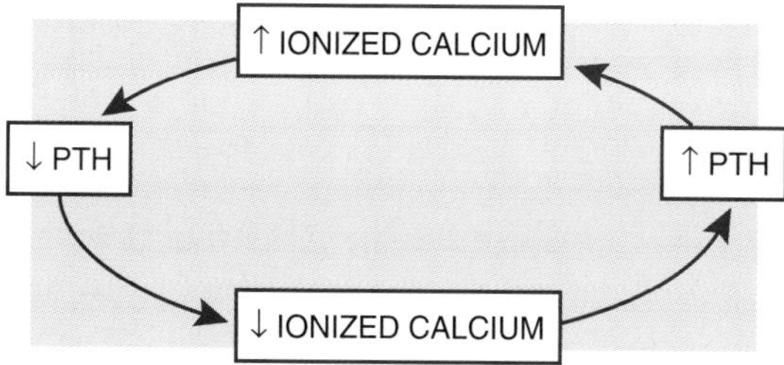

Figure 66. Regulation of parathyroid hormone (PTH) secretion.

also causes increased reabsorption of calcium at the kidney's distal tubules and decreased reabsorption of phosphate at the proximal tubules. The result of parathyroid hormone activity is an increase in calcium in the blood with a decrease in plasma phosphate levels.

NORMAL VALUES

(Interpreted in relation to serum calcium and phosphate levels)
Intact parathyroid hormone: 210–310 pg/mL *or* SI: 210–310 ng/L
N-terminal fraction: 230–630 pg/mL *or* SI: 230–630 ng/L
C-terminal fraction: 410–1760 pg/mL *or* SI: 410–1760 ng/L

HOW THE TEST IS DONE

Parathyroid hormone is measured by radioimmunoassay (RIA), which can measure biologically active intact parathyroid hormone. This fraction represents only a small portion of the total parathyroid hormone. Alternatively, RIA can measure C-terminal or N-terminal portions of the hormone. Two venous samples, 3 mL each in red-topped tubes, are needed. If a plasma sample is requested, a green-topped tube is used.

SIGNIFICANCE OF TEST RESULTS

Elevated Values

Hyperparathyroidism

Decreased Values

Hypoparathyroidism
Lung, kidney, pancreatic, or ovarian cancer

INTERFERING FACTORS

- Noncompliance with fasting requirements
- Elevated lipid levels
- Medications, such as, lithium and thiazide diuretics

P

NURSING CARE

The actions of the nurse are similar to those carried out in other venipuncture procedures (see Chapter 2), with the following additional measures.

Pretest

- Check with the physician if any medications are to be held.
- ***Patient Teaching.*** The nurse instructs the patient not to eat or drink for 12 hours before the test.

Posttest

- The patient may resume a normal diet.
- Send the specimen to the laboratory on ice.

Parietal Cell Antibody

puh-rai-e-tuhl sel an-tib-od-ee

Also called: Antiparietal Cell Antibody

SPECIMEN OR TYPE OF TEST: Serum

PURPOSE OF THE TEST

The parietal cell antibody test is useful in the diagnosis of pernicious anemia and some cases of atrophic gastritis.

BASICS THE NURSE NEEDS TO KNOW

P

The parietal cells of the gastric mucosa manufacture intrinsic factor, the glycoprotein that promotes intestinal absorption of cobalamin (vitamin B_{12}). When the parietal cells are destroyed, cobalamin deficiency and pernicious anemia develop. Parietal cell antibodies can be detected in most cases of pernicious anemia and atrophic gastritis. The two conditions often coexist and are characterized by the absence of parietal and chief cells in the gastric mucosa.

NORMAL VALUES Negative; no parietal cell antibodies are present.

HOW THE TEST IS DONE

A red-topped tube is used to collect 10 mL of venous blood.

SIGNIFICANCE OF TEST RESULTS

Positive Values

Pernicious anemia
Atrophic gastritis
Hashimoto's thyroiditis
Gastric ulcer
Sjögren syndrome

INTERFERING FACTORS

- None

NURSING CARE

Nursing actions are similar to those used in other venipuncture procedures (see Chapter 2). No other special nursing care measures are needed.

Partial Thromboplastin Time

par-shuhl throm-boh-plas-tin taim

Also called: (PTT); Activated Partial Thromboplastin Time (aPTT)

SPECIMEN OR TYPE OF TEST: Blood

PURPOSE OF THE TEST

This test helps identify bleeding or clotting disorders that are hereditary or acquired conditions. It is used to monitor the effect of heparin anticoagulant therapy and to adjust the dosage of the medication based on the test results.

BASICS THE NURSE NEEDS TO KNOW

The partial thromboplastin time (PTT) measures the number of seconds needed for a clot to form. The test results include the patient's value and the control value. The control value of the test is the reference or normal value that is used to evaluate the patient's test result. The PTT test is used to monitor the results of anticoagulation therapy with heparin, hirudin, or argatroban. The goal of anticoagulation therapy is to maintain the PTT in a therapeutic range about 1.5 to 2.5 times the normal value. With a prolonged PTT, the patient takes longer to make a clot, and a thrombus or embolus is less likely to develop.

If the patient has an impairment of the intrinsic coagulation system that causes a prolonged PTT, the medical treatment may be a transfusion of whole blood or plasma so that the clotting factors are increased and the PTT value returns to normal.

The PTT is measured by newer laboratory methodology called activated partial thromboplastin time (APTT). The common name of PTT continues to be used in the clinical area, but refers to this newer methodology. The normal values reported in this text are those of the activated partial thromboplastin time.

NORMAL VALUES	Average value: 25–35 seconds Newborn: <90 seconds Premature infants: <120 seconds
▼ Critical Value	>100 to 150 seconds

P

HOW THE TEST IS DONE

A blue-topped tube with sodium citrate is used to obtain 4.5 mL of venous blood. As an alternative, a heelstick, earlobe, or finger puncture may be used to collect capillary blood in siliconized sodium citrate micropipettes. To mix the anticoagulant with the blood, the specimen tube is tilted gently from side to side five to ten times.

When multiple specimens are drawn, the PTT test specimen is obtained last. When this is the only test specimen taken, a double-tube technique must be used to prevent specimen contamination with tissue thromboplastin. With the double-tube technique, a 1- to 2-mL blood sample is obtained and discarded; the blue-topped tube is then used to collect the test sample.

SIGNIFICANCE OF TEST RESULTS

Elevated Values

Anticoagulant therapy
Deficiency of one or more coagulation factors
Hemophilia
Disseminated intravascular coagulation (DIC)
Circulatory anticoagulants such as lupus anticoagulants
Liver failure
Vitamin K deficiency

Decreased Values

Hypercoagulable states (with thrombus formation)

INTERFERING FACTORS

- Inadequate blood sample

NURSING CARE

Nursing actions are similar to those used in other venipuncture procedures (see Chapter 2), with the following additional measures.

Pretest

- When heparin is given in intermittent doses, the time for PTT monitoring is 6 hours after the anticoagulant is given. This timing provides accurate information and allows the physician to adjust the heparin dose as needed.
- When a continuous intravenous infusion of heparin is started, the PTT is drawn every 6 hours after the initial dose of anticoagulant for the first day and 6 hours after the dosage of medication is changed. Once the therapeutic range of anticoagulation is achieved, the PTT is tested once a day.

Posttest

- For the patient receiving anticoagulants, assess the venipuncture site for signs of bleeding or ecchymosis. To promote clotting at the venipuncture site, the nurse uses sterile gauze to apply pressure to the site or raises the patient's arm above the head while maintaining pressure on the site.

NURSING CARE—*cont'd*

- When the patient receives heparin anticoagulation therapy, the nurse monitors each PTT result for a value in the therapeutic range. If the result is elevated beyond the therapeutic range, the nurse notifies the physician. The physician may lower the dose of the anticoagulant or the intravenous infusion with heparin may be discontinued for a short time. Protamine sulfate, the antidote to heparin is kept available for a severe, excess anticoagulation result. If needed, the nurse injects the protamine sulfate subcutaneously, as prescribed.
- ***Patient Teaching.*** The nurse teaches the anticoagulated patient how to protect from a bleeding episode. The patient should use an electric razor for shaving and a soft toothbrush to avoid scraping of the gingiva (gums) of the oral cavity. Over-the-counter medications of aspirin and remedies that contain aspirin are to be avoided because they interfere with platelet aggregation. The patient is taught to observe for signs of abnormal bleeding in the skin, gingiva, vomitus, stools, and urine.

▼ Nursing Response to Critical Values

If the PTT value is in the critical value range, the physician must be notified. The patient is at risk for spontaneous bleeding or hemorrhage.

The nurse assesses the patient for spontaneous bleeding, oozing of blood, bruising, and petechiae. The nurse observes the skin, mucus membranes, and gingiva of the oral cavity, and the urine and stool for manifestations of bleeding. The vital signs are taken, observing for hypotension and tachycardia. The nurse asks the patient if he or she has a headache because this can be an early sign of an intracranial bleeding episode. Until the physician is contacted, the nurse must withhold the next dose of heparin.

Patch Test, Skin

pach test, skin

SPECIMEN OR TYPE OF TEST: Skin Sensitivity Test

PURPOSE OF THE TEST

This test is used to identify the particular allergen that causes contact dermatitis. It is also used to differentiate contact dermatitis from other causes of eczematous disease.

BASICS THE NURSE NEEDS TO KNOW

Allergic contact dermatitis causes an eczematous skin change. It is an inflammatory skin response to that occurs when the skin is in contact with a particular antigen. The person is sensitized to the antigen over time, without the immediate development of a skin reaction. Eventually, re-exposure to the antigen induces a vigorous cell-mediated immune (allergic) response at the site of contact with the antigen.

Because one part of the treatment of the skin eruption is to remove the patient from further contact with the antigen, the antigen must be identified. In some cases, a patch test is used to identify one or more suspected antigens by evoking a skin reaction to suspected allergens.

The patch test may be carried out by placing the suspected allergen, such as a small piece of clothing, a bit of a cosmetic substance, or a diluted solution of chemical components, on the skin. Industrial substances or laboratory chemicals are never used in testing, because they can produce an irritant dermatitis or a chemical burn. The most common allergens or sources of contact dermatitis are listed in the section of abnormal results.

The physician grades the results of the skin testing according to severity of the reaction. An erythematous (red), macular (flat), or papular (raised) lesion is labeled as an undecided, doubtful, or weak result. An erythematous, edematous, papular, or vesicular (fluid-filled) area of skin where a particular allergen was placed is identified as a strongly positive reaction. A raised, red, edematous area with large vesicles, bullae (fluid-filled blisters), or possible ulceration is identified as an extreme reaction.

NORMAL VALUES

Negative; no abnormal skin reactions are noted.

HOW THE TEST IS DONE

Samples of selected allergens used by the patient or of a number of standard allergens are taped to the patient's skin for 48 hours of contact exposure (Figure 67). The readings of the results are performed after 48 hours and again after 72 hours to 7 days, as prescribed.

SIGNIFICANCE OF TEST RESULTS

Abnormal Values

COMMON CAUSES OF CONTACT DERMATITIS

Nickel (snaps, belt buckles, rings, watchbands, bracelets, earrings)
Formaldehyde (permanent-press clothing, skin and nail products)
Chromates (cement, cutting oil)
Topical medication with neomycin, benzocaine, or ethylenediamine
Epoxy resins (adhesives, glues)
Hair dyes
Lanolin
Chemicals in sunscreen creams
Permanent-wave solutions
Fragrances in perfumes and soaps

INTERFERING FACTORS

- Concurrent dermatitis from another source
- Exposure of the patch site to water or excessive perspiration
- Inaccurate interpretation of the results
- Inaccurate timing for reading of the results

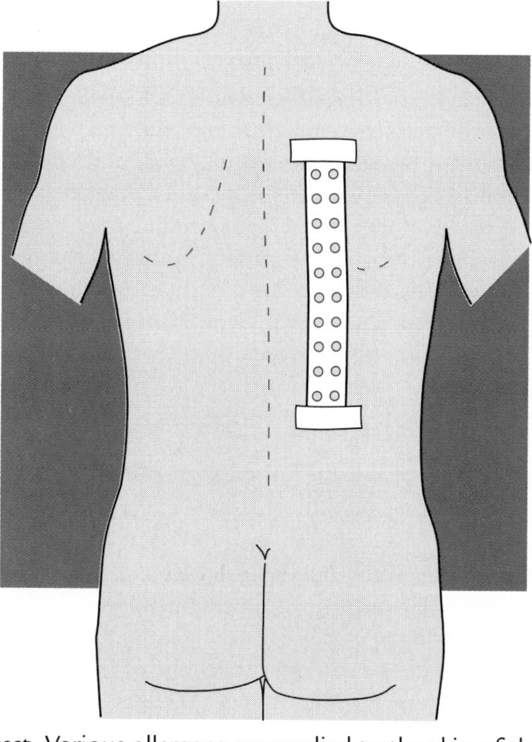

Figure 67. Patch test. Various allergens are applied to the skin of the patient's back. Those allergens that cause an allergic skin response are identified as the sources of contact dermatitis.

NURSING CARE

Pretest

- Schedule this test after an episode of acute dermatitis has subsided and after treatment with corticosteroids has ceased. After the physician has informed the patient about the test, a written consent from the patient is needed.
- If the products the patient uses are to be tested, instruct the patient to bring them in beforehand. The patch test must be prepared, and a detailed list of the ingredients must be written.

During the Test

- The nurse or physician tapes the allergen patch to the patient's upper back between the scapula and the spinal column. A diagram on paper is made to identify the location of each allergen.

Posttest

- ***Patient Teaching.*** The nurse instructs the patient to refrain from showers and physical exercise during the following 48 hours. This is because water and perspiration will loosen the tape of the patch. The patient is also told that if itching, irritation, or pain occurs under one of the discs of allergen, it should be removed immediately.

Continued

NURSING CARE—*cont'd*

Posttest—*cont'd*

- ***Patient Teaching.*** The patient is instructed to return in 48 hours for the first evaluation of the results. The patch is removed at that time. After a 30-minute to 1-hour wait, the skin is assessed for any reaction in the area of the allergens. The nurse instructs the patient to return for the second appointment to reevaluate the skin because a delayed reaction can occur. This second reading is done at 96 hours (4 days) after the patch is applied. The patient is advised that exercise and showers are permitted while waiting for the second evaluation, but that soap must not be used, and that the patient must not scrub, scratch, or rub the skin in the test area.

Percutaneous Umbilical Cord Sampling

per-kyuh-tay-nee-uhs um-bi-li-kuhl kohrd sam-pling

Also called: (PUBS); Cordocentesis

SPECIMEN OR TYPE OF TEST: Blood

PURPOSE OF THE TEST

This procedure primarily is used to obtain a specimen of fetal blood for the assessment of Rh isoimmunization, a fetal anemia. It may also be used to identify chromosomal abnormality, detect fetal infection, measure acid-base balance, and to detect other hematologic abnormalities.

P

BASICS THE NURSE NEEDS TO KNOW

The percutaneous umbilical blood sampling can be performed in the second or third trimester, but for the purpose of genetic studies, the procedure is performed around the 15th to 16th week of gestation. The normal values of fetal cord blood vary based on the gestational age of the fetus.

Fetal Blood Analysis

Red Cell Isoimmunization

This occurs when the fetus has Rh-positive red blood cell antigens and the mother has Rh-negative erythrocytes. The maternal antibodies are transmitted to the fetus and cause fetal hemolysis of erythrocytes. If the erythrocyte incompatibility is not prevented or controlled, the fetus experiences a hemolytic anemia called *erythroblastosis fetalis* or *Rh disease*. The fetal cord blood is tested for blood type, the presence of Rh antigens, the hematocrit level, and the reticulocyte count. The treatment is individualized, but an intrauterine blood transfusion can be given to the fetus.

Prenatal Chromosomal Analysis

The karyotype consists of the characteristics of the chromosomes, their number, form, size, structure, and grouping. Chromosomal abnormality in the fetus is identified.

Congenital Infection

Infection in the pregnant woman can cross the placental barrier and infect the fetus. The fetal blood analysis for infection includes measurement of fetal antibodies, white blood cells, eosinophils, liver enzymes, and platelets. Viral culture of the fetal blood and the amniotic fluid may be performed to identify the infectious organism. Because fetal antibodies do not develop until the 22nd week of gestation, fetal cord blood samples cannot verify the infection before this time.

Thrombocytopenia

This is a low platelet count, which can cause fetal intracranial bleeding during pregnancy, labor, or the neonatal period. In most cases, the mother has immune thrombocytopenia and passively transmits the maternal antiplatelet antibodies to the fetus. If the fetus is affected severely, the fetus can receive an intrauterine platelet transfusion, administered via the umbilical vein.

NORMAL VALUES

Hematologic evaluation: Within normal limits for gestational age
Chromosomal analysis: Normal karyotype
Biochemistry analysis: Within normal limits for gestational age
Immunoglobulin G (IgG) antibodies: Within normal limits
IgM antibodies: Within normal limits

HOW THE TEST IS DONE

Guided by ultrasound imaging, the physician inserts a sterile 20- to 22-gauge spinal needle through the maternal abdomen and uterus. The needle is then advanced into the umbilical cord until it is placed in one of the umbilical veins (Figure 68). Once the needle placement is verified, a syringe is used to aspirate 0.5 to 3 mL of venous blood. The blood is then transferred to microtubes for the specific laboratory analyses.

SIGNIFICANCE OF TEST RESULTS

Hemolytic Anemia

Rh disease
Minor antigen disorders

Chromosome Disorder

Cystic fibrosis
Sickle cell anemia
Muscular dystrophy
Hemophilia A, B
Inborn errors of metabolism
Down syndrome
Retinoblastoma
Wilms' tumor
Thalassemias

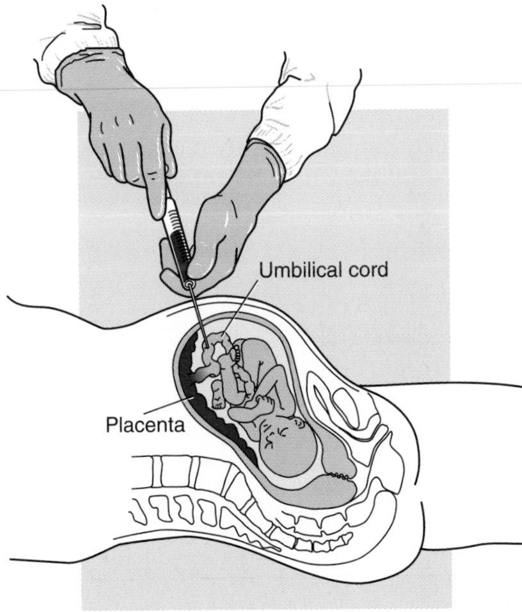

Figure 68. Percutaneous umbilical cord sampling. The needle is advanced through the skin and into the uterus. Once the needle punctures the umbilical cord and one of the uterine veins, cord blood is aspirated by syringe.

Phenylketonuria
Enzyme G-6-PD deficiency

Infection
Toxoplasmosis
Rubella
Varicella
Cytomegalovirus
Human parvovirus B19

Platelet Disorder
Thrombocytopenia

INTERFERING FACTORS

- Maternal obesity
- Uncooperative behavior
- Severe polyhydramnios
- Unfavorable fetal position
- Specimen contamination

NURSING CARE

Pretest

- Once the woman has been informed of the procedure by her physician, obtain her written consent for the procedure and the genetic testing. The signed form is placed in the patient's record.
- Assist the patient in removing all clothes and putting on a hospital gown.
- Place the patient in a lateral position on the examining table.
- Assess and record the mother's vital signs and the fetal heart rate.
- The nurse provides emotional support. The patient's anxiety level is often high because of concern for the safety of the fetus, fear of the procedure, or concern about the potential for abnormal test results.

During the Test

- The nurse cleanses the woman's abdomen with the appropriate povidone-iodine or surgical soap solution, and then places the surgical drape. As the physician administers the local anesthetic, the nurse provides reassurance to the patient. The injection causes a slight stinging sensation in the abdominal area.
- The nurse begins the frequent assessment and recording of the fetal heart rate. The fetal cardiac contractions can be counted during the imaging of the fetus on the ultrasound monitor.
- Prepare any additional medications, as prescribed. If the fetus moves excessively, the mother may receive intravenous sedation to limit fetal movement. As an alternative, the fetus may receive an intravenous sedative or muscle relaxant via the umbilical vein.
- Once the blood is obtained, the nurse assists with depositing it in the microtubes. Ensure that all blood samples and requisition forms are properly labeled. The data include the mother's name and age and the gestation of the pregnancy. Each requisition slip clearly identifies the specimen as fetal blood (cord blood) obtained by percutaneous umbilical cord sampling.

Posttest

- Once the needle is removed, the nurse begins to monitor the fetal heart rate and takes the mother's vital signs. In the recovery area, external fetal monitoring of the fetal heart rate and uterine contractions continues. It is common for the mother to have mild uterine cramping for a short while. The fetal monitoring is discontinued when the fetal heart rate remains stable in a normal range and the uterine contractions cease.
- At regular intervals, the nurse observes the abdomen for signs of bleeding. The small sterile dressing that covers the puncture site should remain dry and intact.
- Prophylactic antibiotics are administered, as prescribed. The nurse also administers prescribed $Rh_0(D)$ immune globulin (RhoGAM) to the Rh-negative mother. This will help prevent Rh disease of the newborn in a future pregnancy.
- ***Patient Teaching.*** In preparation for discharge, the nurse instructs the patient to rest for the remainder of the day. The patient should take her temperature at least two times per day. She should report a fever to her physician without delay. She is instructed to return to the physician for a follow-up evaluation and to learn the test results.

Continued

NURSING CARE—*cont'd*

Posttest—*cont'd*

- ***Patient Teaching.*** When serious or severe chromosomal abnormality exists, the parents experience emotional distress. Genetic counseling is an essential component of care before testing and after the test results are known. This helps the parents make an informed choice about the continuation of the pregnancy. In obstetric management, the alternatives include continuation or termination of the pregnancy. If the pregnancy is continued, plans are made for intensive antepartal monitoring, for possible cesarean section for fetal distress during labor, and for the special postdelivery needs of the newborn.

◆ Nursing Response to Complications

Although the PUBS procedure is a potential risk for the fetus, the overall complication rate is 1% to 2% or less. Bleeding is the most common problem. Many patients have minimal bleeding that ceases a few minutes after the needle is removed, but more severe bleeding can occur. Other complications include fetal bradycardia, maternal or fetal infection, and premature labor. The nurse assesses for complications and notifies the physician of abnormal findings.

Bleeding. Prolonged bleeding from the umbilical cord is identified by continued staining or wetness of amniotic fluid on the mother's abdominal dressing. The drainage is pink. Fetal movements may be hyperactive or lethargic.

Fetal bradycardia. Fetal bradycardia can be observed on the fetal monitor. Bradycardia is identified by a fetal heart rate <120. In addition, the fetus is lethargic, with fewer than normal movements.

Maternal infection. If the mother develops infection, she experiences chills and fever. She also may have uterine cramping. The nurse monitors the temperature and examines the abdomen for signs of redness, swelling, or purulent drainage. If the fetus develops an infection, it is lethargic, with fewer than normal movements.

Premature labor. Premature labor may develop, as characterized by continual uterine contractions recorded on the fetal monitor. The mother may complain of backache, uterine cramping, or rhythmic contractions. There may be leakage of amniotic fluid from the vagina because of premature rupture of the membranes.

Pericardiocentesis

pe-ri-kar-dee-oh-sen-tee-sis

Also called: Pericardial Fluid Analysis

SPECIMEN OR TYPE OF TEST: Pathology

PURPOSE OF THE TEST

Analysis of pericardial fluid is performed to determine the cause of and appropriate therapy for acute pericarditis, subacute effusive-constrictive pericarditis, neoplastic pericardial disease, and pericardial effusion of unknown cause.

BASICS THE NURSE NEEDS TO KNOW

Pericardiocentesis is a diagnostic and therapeutic procedure in which the pericardial space is accessed with a needle or cannula, and fluid is aspirated. For diagnostic purposes, the fluid is then analyzed. For therapeutic purposes, either fluid is drained on a one-time basis or a catheter is inserted and left in place for 1 to 48 hours (rarely, it may be kept in for 72 hours).

Normally, the pericardial space between the visceral and parietal pericardium contains approximately 20 to 50 mL of clear serous fluid. If the pericardium becomes inflamed or diseased or is disrupted, pericardial effusion may occur. As fluid builds up in the pericardial space, cardiac tamponade may result. Cardiac tamponade will eventually lead to a decrease in cardiac output, with an increase in right atrial pressure, pulsus paradoxus, and hypotension. If progressive and untreated, cardiac tamponade will result in death.

NORMAL VALUES Pericardial fluid is sterile, clear, and colorless or straw-colored.

HOW THE TEST IS DONE

Pericardiocentesis for diagnostic purposes is not an emergency situation and can be performed in the controlled environment of an operating room or special procedure room. The procedure begins after skin preparation and infiltration of a local anesthetic, usually 1% lidocaine without epinephrine. A small incision is made in the skin, the site being determined by the desired approach.

The physician inserts a needle and approximately 20 mL of fluid is removed for analysis. If cytologic studies are performed, a heparinized container is necessary. The fluid is usually analyzed for color; hemoglobin concentration; hematocrit value; red blood cell, white blood cell, and differential counts; and protein and glucose determinations. In addition, Gram stains and culture, fungal stains and culture, and cytologic studies are performed. Additional fluid is removed if viral and parasite studies, immunologic and serologic screens, or lipoelectrophoresis are planned.

If therapeutic pericardiocentesis is desired after the specimens are obtained, a catheter is inserted and positioned to allow drainage.

SIGNIFICANCE OF TEST RESULTS

Bacterial, viral, or fungal infection
Malignancy

INTERFERING FACTORS

- Pericardiocentesis requires a patient who is cooperative and who will lie still during the procedure. Uncooperative patients may require sedation.
- Those receiving anticoagulant therapy, with bleeding disorders or thrombocytopenia, are not appropriate candidates.
- If cultures of the fluid are planned, administration of antibiotics will affect the results.

NURSING CARE

Pretest

- Ensure that an informed consent form has been signed.
- Check laboratory work for bleeding problems. Take medication history to check for anticoagulant use.
- Obtain a baseline ECG if ordered.
- The nurse documents baseline vital signs and heart sounds.
- ***Patient Teaching.*** The nurse explains the procedure to the patient.
- ***Patient Teaching.*** The nurse instructs the patient to maintain nothing-by-mouth status for 4 to 6 hours before the test.
- Administer sedation as prescribed.
- Shave site if necessary.

During the Test

- Position the patient. Usually a recumbent position is used, with the torso and head elevated 30 to 45 degrees.
- Ensure that an intravenous infusion is present and patent.
- The nurse maintains telemetric or cardiac monitoring and reports any abnormality immediately. Vital signs are taken frequently. Have a defibrillator and emergency drugs on hand.
- The nurse continuously reassures and supports the patient, who will feel the local anesthetic being infiltrated and may experience a sharp pain when the pericardium is infiltrated.

Posttest

- The patient may return to pretest activities gradually if vital signs are stable.

P

◇ Nursing Response to Complications

Complications from pericardiocentesis include puncture or laceration of the cardiac chamber, laceration of a coronary artery, ventricular fibrillation, pneumothorax, and peritoneal puncture. Puncture or laceration of the cardiac chamber and laceration of the coronary artery will cause cardiac tamponade.

Cardiac tamponade. A feared complication of a pericardiocentesis is cardiac tamponade, which is due to bleeding into the pericardial sac. As blood accumulates into the pericardial sac, the heart is restricted. The nurse will observe a decrease in cardiac output, muffled heart sounds, increase in right atrial pressure, and pulsus paradoxus. Notify the physician immediately. If the size of the pericardial effusion is significant, emergency surgery may be necessary.

Ventricular fibrillation. The mechanical trauma of a pericardiocentesis may cause ventricular fibrillation during the procedure. The nurse observes the cardiac monitor and informs the physician if this lethal dysrhythmia occurs. The nurse anticipates this response to the procedure by having a code cart available with its emergency medications.

Pneumothorax. Anxiety, restlessness, dyspnea, tachypnea, pallor, and decreased breath sounds are indications of pneumothorax. Notify the physician immediately and anticipate an order for chest x-ray to evaluate the size of the pneumothorax.

Persantine Scan

See Stress Test, Cardiac on p. 596.

PET Scan

See Positron Emissions Tomography on p. 532.

Phenylalanine, Blood

fen-uhl-al-uh-neen, blud

Also called: PKU Test; Phenylketonuria Test; Phenylalanine Screening Test; Hyperphenylalaninemia Screen; Guthrie Screening Test

SPECIMEN OR TYPE OF TEST: Serum, plasma, whole blood

PURPOSE OF THE TEST

The blood phenylalanine test is performed to detect phenylketonuria (PKU) and other causes of hyperphenylalaninemia. It is also used to monitor patients who have PKU and are being maintained on a phenylalanine-restricted diet.

BASICS THE NURSE NEEDS TO KNOW

In normal amino acid metabolism, the enzyme phenylhydroxylase is needed to convert phenylalanine to tyrosine. When this enzyme or its cofactor BH_4 is absent, the levels of phenylalanine and phenylpyruvic acid, a phenylalanine metabolite, rise in the blood and urine.

Phenylketonuria (PKU) is an inherited disorder of amino acid metabolism that is characterized by elevated levels of phenylalanine and phenylpyruvic acid. Unless early detection and proper dietary intervention occur, the elevated blood level of phenylalanine will cause central nervous system damage and mental retardation.

The phenylalanine level is not elevated at birth because no dietary intake of protein has occurred. In the infant who has a defect in amino acid metabolism, the serum level begins to rise within 24 hours after starting to feed with milk or formula. The ideal time to screen the blood for phenylalanine is 48 to 72 hours after birth or 2 days after the newborn begins to feed.

State laws require PKU testing of all newborns within a specified period. If the blood phenylalanine test is performed in the first 24 hours of life, the test should be repeated after feeding has begun. The repeat test greatly reduces the chance of a false-negative result.

The blood phenylalanine test is a screening tool that identifies only hyperphenylalaninemia. Further testing is needed to verify the cause of the elevated blood level. If an elevated result occurs, the test is repeated in 24 hours to ensure accuracy.

Premature or low-birth-weight infants have higher serum values than do full-term infants of normal weight. This false-positive serum elevation is caused by immaturity of the liver. Antibiotics also interfere with the Guthrie method of analysis and cause a false-positive result.

NORMAL VALUES	**Guthrie Test** <2 mg/day/L *or* SI: 121 μmol/L **Fluorometry Method** Full-term newborn: 1.2–3.4 mg/dL *or* SI: 73–206 μmol/L Premature newborn: 2–7.5 mg/dL *or* SI: 121–454 μmol/L Adult: 0.8–1.8 mg/dL *or* SI: 48–109 μmol/L
▼ Critical Values	Guthrie test: >4 mg/day/L *or* SI: >242 μmol/L

HOW THE TEST IS DONE

A heelstick puncture is used to obtain two to three drops of blood. The blood sample is collected by capillary tube or PKU card or filter paper.

SIGNIFICANCE OF TEST RESULTS

Elevated Values

Phenylketonuria
Severe burns
Hyperphenylalaninemia
Liver disease
Sepsis
Galactosemia

P

INTERFERING FACTORS

- Over saturating the filter paper with blood
- Little to no ingestion of milk
- Insufficient quantity of blood
- Antibiotics (Guthrie method of analysis)
- Recent exchange transfusion

NURSING CARE

- ***Health Promotion.*** The nurse needs to instruct mothers who are going home with their newborns that, before they have been breast-feeding or taking infant formula for 24 hours, to have their babies tested or retested for PKU within 2 weeks of discharge. All states in the United States and many other countries, worldwide, mandate phenylalanine testing of all newborns within 28 days. The goal is to identify PKU at a very early stage and provide effective dietary treatment so that mental retardation does not occur.

NURSING CARE—*cont'd*

Pretest

- Nursing actions are similar to those used in other capillary puncture procedures (see Chapter 2), with the following additional measures.
- The nurse needs to verify when the baby started on milk or breast-feeding.
- Ensure that the laboratory requisition slip includes the name, date, time of the test, date of birth, and time of the first milk feeding. Note the administration of antibiotics or blood transfusion.

During the Test

- With the filter paper or card, only one side of the paper is blotted to fill the circles. The paper should not be turned over to soak the other side. Cord blood cannot be used for this test.

Posttest

- Arrange for prompt transport of the specimen to the laboratory.

▼ Nursing Response to Critical Values

Nutritional guidance and support are necessary, if the elevated PKU level is verified. Dietary restrictions are necessary. The nurse can provide information about a phenylalanine-restricted diet, as well as provide the parents with emotional support.

Phenylalanine, Urinary

fen-uhl-al-uh-neen, yur-i-nar-ee

Also called: PKU Urine Test

SPECIMEN OR TYPE OF TEST: Urine

PURPOSE OF THE TEST

The urine phenylalanine test is used to assist in the detection of hyperphenylalaninemia, including phenylketonuria (PKU). The test is used to monitor the effect of dietary treatment for patients who have a defect in amino acid metabolism.

BASICS THE NURSE NEEDS TO KNOW

In normal amino acid metabolism, phenylalanine is converted to tyrosine. The enzyme phenylalanine hydroxylase and other cofactors must be present for this conversion to take place. When the enzyme or its cofactors are absent and an intake of protein exists as the source of amino acids, the levels of phenylalanine and phenylpyruvic acid (the phenylalanine metabolite) rise in the blood. The increase of amino acids in the plasma concentration results in an increase in glomerular filtration, but the renal tubules cannot resorb all the excess. Thus, the overflow of phenylalanine and phenylpyruvic acid is excreted in the urine.

In hyperphenylalaninemia, the presence of phenylpyruvic acid is not detectable in the urine for 2 to 6 weeks after birth. Phenylpyruvic acid is not present in the urine at birth, because an intake of protein from breast milk or infant formula must first occur.

Once the serum level of phenylpyruvic acid rises to 10 to 20 mg/dL, the metabolite appears in the urine. Because of this time delay, the phenylalanine urine test is not used as a screening test for PKU.

PKU is one type of aminoaciduria. It is an inherited disorder of amino acid metabolism caused by the absence of phenylalanine hydroxylase. If the condition remains undetected or uncontrolled by dietary therapy, damage to the central nervous system and mental retardation will occur.

NORMAL VALUES

Ferric chloride method: Negative
Phenastix method (urine reagent dip strip): 5–10 mg/100 mL

HOW THE TEST IS DONE

A freshly voided specimen of urine is collected in a plastic urine collection container.

SIGNIFICANCE OF TEST RESULTS

Phenylketonuria
Non-PKU hyperphenylalaninemia

INTERFERING FACTORS

- Improper collection procedure
- Diluted urine

NURSING CARE

- *Patient Teaching.* For testing infants and small children, the nurse teaches the parent to apply a urine collection bag and transfer the urine to a collection container. (See also: Pediatric Urine Collection, Chapter 2, p. 35.) If the patient has PKU, instruct the parent on the use of dipstick method, used to monitor the child's condition.

Phosphorus, Serum

fos-fuh-ruhs, seer-uhm

Also called: HPO_4^-; Phosphate, Blood

SPECIMEN OR TYPE OF TEST: Blood

PURPOSE OF THE TEST

Serum phosphorus helps diagnose kidney disorders and acid-base imbalance. It is also used to detect disorders of calcium, bone, or endocrine origin.

BASICS THE NURSE NEEDS TO KNOW

Phosphorus is a mineral element present in bone cells and extracellular fluid, including serum. Phosphorus from dietary intake provides for necessary replacement of the mineral. The homeostatic balance of the mineral in the extracellular fluid is maintained, and excess phosphorus is excreted in the feces and urine.

An inverse relationship exists between the serum levels of phosphorus and calcium. If the serum level of either mineral falls, the serum level of the other mineral rises. Serum phosphorus concentrations have a diurnal rhythm. The level is highest in the morning and lowest in the evening. The normal values also vary over a lifespan, with the highest serum values occurring in infants and children and the lowest values occurring in elderly individuals.

Elevated Value

An elevated level of serum phosphorus is called *hyperphosphatemia.* In the adult, the lab value is greater than 4.7 mg/dL (SI: >1.5 mmol/L). Severe hyperphosphatemia produces no symptoms but does cause hypocalcemia. With a rapid elevation of serum phosphorus to a level of >6 mg/dL (SI: >1.94 mmol/L), the serum calcium level declines and causes symptoms of hypotension and tetany from calcium depletion. The most common cause of hyperphosphatemia is severe renal insufficiency.

Decreased Value

A decreased value of the serum phosphorus level is called *hypophosphatemia.* In the adult, the laboratory value is less than 2.7 mg/dL (SI: 0.87 mmol/L). Causes include inadequate food intake, impaired intestinal absorption, increased phosphate storage in bones, and increased renal excretion of phosphate. Hypophosphatemia is a serious problem because it can affect neuromuscular, neuropsychiatric, skeletal, gastrointestinal, and cardiopulmonary function.

NORMAL VALUES	Adult: 2.5–4.5 mg/dL *or* SI: 0.81–1.45 mmol/L Child: 4.0–6.0 mg/dL *or* SI: 1.29–1.94 mmol/L Infant: 4.5–7.5 mg/dL *or* SI: 1.45–2.72 mmol/L
▼ Critical Value	<1 mg/dL (SI: <0.32 mmol/L)

P

HOW THE TEST IS DONE

A red-topped tube is used to collect 10 mL of venous blood. For infants and small children, a heelstick puncture and capillary tube are used to collect a blood sample.

SIGNIFICANCE OF TEST RESULTS

Elevated Values

Renal failure
Hypovolemia
Dehydration
Milk-alkali syndrome
Acromegaly
Osteolytic metastatic bone cancer
Postanesthesia hyperthermia
Cirrhosis of the liver
Pulmonary embolism
Diabetic ketoacidosis

Vitamin D toxicity
Respiratory acidosis
Sarcoidosis
Lactic acidosis
Hypoparathyroidism

Decreased Values
Osteomalacia
Osteoblastic bone cancer
Acute gout
Vitamin D deficiency
Renal tubular disease
Hyperparathyroidism
Serum calcium elevation
Vomiting, diarrhea
Sepsis
Acute respiratory infection
Prolonged intravenous glucose therapy
Prolonged nasogastric drainage
Severe malabsorption
Starvation
Respiratory alkalosis

INTERFERING FACTORS

- Hemolysis
- Carbohydrate-rich meals
- Recent phosphate enema

NURSING CARE

Nursing actions are similar to those used in other venipuncture procedures (see Chapter 2), with the following additional measures.

Pretest

- Schedule the test for early morning to avoid diurnal fluctuations.
- Do not administer a phosphate enema just before the test, because some of the phosphate is absorbed by the colonic mucosa and would cause a rapid elevation of the test value.
- ***Patient Teaching.*** The nurse instructs the patient to discontinue all food and fluids for 8 hours before the test. It is best to obtain a fasting specimen, because carbohydrate intake and recent food intake tend to decrease the serum phosphate level.

Posttest

- The nurse monitors the lab results for abnormal values. Severe depletion of phosphate can cause many physical changes in the patient's body. A rising serum calcium level may accompany a low phosphorus level and respiratory alkalosis may cause

NURSING CARE—*cont'd*

hypophosphatemia. The patients who are most commonly affected by hypophosphatemia are the elderly and postoperative patients, as well as patients who undergo long-term hemodialysis treatment.

Nursing Response to Critical Values

The physician must be notified immediately when the phosphorus level is decreased to the critical value level. There may be resultant cardiac, respiratory, musculoskeletal and central nervous system dysfunction. This includes decreased cardiac contractility and cardiac output, respiratory failure, tremor, weakness, convulsions, slurred speech, coma, and myopathy. About 20% of patients with a critical low level of hypophosphatemia will die.

The nurse takes vital signs. The respiratory assessment findings often include dyspnea, adventitious sounds, and weak respiratory effort. The nurse also assesses for neurologic changes, including tremors, slurred speech, ataxia, stupor, or coma. As an initial intervention, the nurse maintains the patient on bedrest with siderails, in semi-Fowler's to full Fowler's position to enhance breathing and cardiac output. The nurse also initiates seizure precautions, and prepares for cardiac monitoring.

Platelet Aggregation

playt-let ag-re-gay-shun

Also called: Aggregometer Test; Platelet Function Studies

SPECIMEN OR TYPE OF TEST: Blood

P

PURPOSE OF THE TEST

The platelet aggregation test is used to evaluate platelet function and to detect a hereditary or acquired platelet bleeding disorder.

BASICS THE NURSE NEEDS TO KNOW

After an injury to a blood vessel, platelets are the first component of clotting to respond. The platelets adhere to the blood vessel wall at the site of injury and form a plug that prevents additional blood loss. The platelets change shape, become sticky and are capable of binding plasma proteins, including fibrinogen. The platelets then adhere to each other in platelet aggregation (Figure 69).

With abnormal platelet function, the patient has deficient clotting ability and a tendency to bleed. There are inherited and acquired causes of platelet dysfunction, but the most common cause is medication that interferes with platelet function. Aspirin or aspirin-containing compounds and numerous other medications can result in decreased or absent platelet function.

NORMAL VALUES More than 60% of platelets aggregate in response to each chemical substance that stimulates platelet aggregation

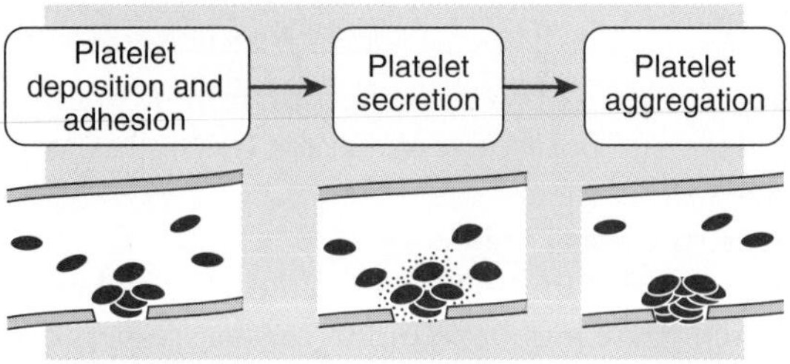

Figure 69. Platelet response to vascular injury.

HOW THE TEST IS DONE

Three blue-topped or plastic tubes with sodium citrate are used to obtain 10 mL of venous blood.

SIGNIFICANCE OF TEST RESULTS

Decreased Values

Aspirin or other medication that interferes with platelet aggregation
Uremia
Liver disease
Bernard-Soulier syndrome
Myeloproliferative disorder
Wiskott-Aldrich syndrome
von Willebrand's disease
Disseminated intravascular coagulation (DIC)

INTERFERING FACTORS

- Lipemia
- Caffeine
- Thrombocytopenia
- Aspirin, antisteroidal medications

NURSING CARE

Nursing actions are similar to those used in other venipuncture procedures (see Chapter 2), with the following additional measures.

Pretest

- The nurse should make a list of all prescribed and over-the-counter medications the patient is taking. Aspirin, antihistamines, nonsteroidal anti-inflammatory agents, penicillin, antimicrobials, and psychotropic drugs and many others interfere with platelet aggregation and can cause a bleeding disorder. Schedule this test for 7 to 10 days after medications that disrupt platelet function have been discontinued.
- ***Patient Teaching.*** The nurse instructs the patient to fast from food or to eat only low-fat foods for 8 hours before the test. Caffeine intake must be avoided on the day of the test. The patient is instructed to discontinue taking aspirin, aspirin-containing medications, and nonsteroidal antiinflammatory medications for 7 days before the test.

NURSING CARE—*cont'd*

Posttest

- Ensure that the venipuncture site has sealed and that the patient is not bleeding. The nurse uses sterile gauze to apply pressure to the puncture site, as needed. Keeping pressure on the site, the patient can also raise his or her arm overhead. The combination of pressure and elevation should help the process of coagulation and stop the bleeding.
- If the platelet aggregation results are abnormal, the nurse should observe for characteristic bleeding in the patient. This can include spontaneous bruising, epistaxis, and bleeding from mucous membranes, particularly the gingiva of the oral cavity, intestine, or bladder. With trauma or surgery, the patient may bleed profusely. General anesthetic medications can also decrease platelet aggregation ability.

Platelet Count

playt-let kount

Also called: Thrombocyte Count

SPECIMEN OR TYPE OF TEST: Blood

PURPOSE OF THE TEST

The platelet count is used to assess the ability of the bone marrow to produce platelets and to identify the destruction or loss of platelets in the circulation. It is also used to evaluate the untoward effects of chemotherapy or radiation treatment.

P

BASICS THE NURSE NEEDS TO KNOW

Platelets function to initiate the process of coagulation. When there is a nick or opening in a blood vessel, platelets quickly aggregate, adhere to the endothelial surface of the blood vessel, and plug the opening. As additional platelets and clotting factors arrive, the clot becomes firm and seals off the opening effectively (Figure 70).

Variation in Normal Values

In laboratory testing, considerable variation exists in the normal platelet count reference range. Newborns have a wider range of normal values than do adults. The normal value is slightly decreased during menstruation and pregnancy. The platelet count is also reduced relative to the excess fluid in the blood. This dilution effect occurs with the administration of fluids, including intravenous fluids and packed red cell transfusions. When the platelets are counted, variation exists between the reference range performed by manual counting and that carried out by an automated counter. The nurse should use the reference value of the laboratory that performs the cell count.

Elevated Values

Thrombocytosis is an excess number of platelets (>400,000 cells/μL *or* SI: >400 × 10^9/L) in the blood. The condition may be reactive, in response to acute inflammatory disease,

Capillary
Anteriole
Break in vessel wall
Blood vessel contracts
Platelet plug forms
Damaged cells and platelets begin reaction, prothrombin activates
Prothrombin converts to thrombin
Fibrinogen converts to fibrin, clot is formed

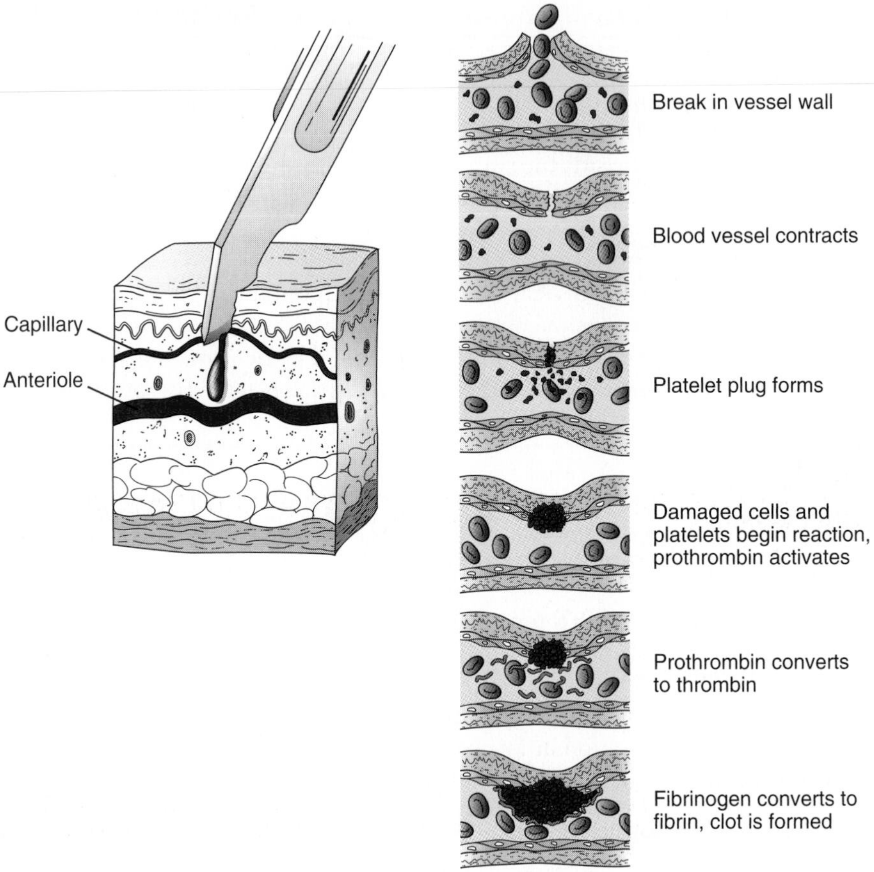

Figure 70. Process of clot formation. The platelets create a plug at the break in the blood vessel, followed by the process of clot formation.(*Reproduced with permission from Stepp, C. A., & Woods, M. A. [1998].* Laboratory procedures for medical office personnel *[p. 111]. Philadelphia: W. B. Saunders.*)

blood loss, or trauma. This condition rarely causes symptoms and is self limiting. The elevated level of platelets returns to a normal value as the underlying condition is corrected. Thrombocytosis also may be a symptom of myeloproliferative disease, such as chronic myelocytic leukemia. When the platelet count rises severely, there is potential for a hemorrhage or thrombosis. Hemorrhage probably results from defects in the platelets and the inability to form a clot. Thrombosis in either veins or arteries can occur as platelets aggregate and trap erythrocytes in the microcirculation. Common sites of vascular occlusion include the splenic, hepatic, and pulmonary veins; the mesenteric and axillary arteries; and the fingers and toes.

Decreased Values

Thrombocytopenia is a decreased number of platelets (<100,000 cells/μL *or* SI: <100 × 10^9/L) in the blood. This condition causes a prolonged bleeding time because the patient's clotting ability is seriously compromised. The decrease in platelets is caused by three possible categories of pathophysiologic change: (1) deficient platelet production, (2) rapid platelet destruction, and (3) abnormal pooling of the platelets (Table 11). The most common cause is the accelerated destruction of platelets. The bone marrow responds with accelerated production of new cells, but when the platelet destruction is rapid and extensive, the response of the marrow is inadequate. With inadequate numbers of platelets, the patient is vulnerable to bleeding, particularly into the skin.

NORMAL VALUES	150,000–400,000 cells/μL *or* SI: 150–400 × 10^9/L
▼ Critical Values	<50,000 cells/μL *or* SI: <50 × 10^9/L >1,000,000 cells/μL *or* SI: >100 × 10^9/L

TABLE 11 Pathophysiologic Causes of Thrombocytopenia

Category	Pathophysiology	Cause
Deficient platelet production	Impairment of bone marrow with reduced numbers of stem cells or megakaryocytes	Drugs, aplastic anemia, radiation chemotherapy, malignancy of the bone marrow
	Ineffective thrombopoiesis	Deficiency of iron, vitamin B_{12}, folic acid
	Defective production or regulation of thrombopoietin	Inherited genetic disorder
Platelet destruction	*Intracorpuscular destruction* Defects in platelet structure with short platelet life span	Inherited genetic disorder
	Extracorpuscular destruction Immunologic destruction of platelets by immunoglobulin G antibodies	Autoimmune processes Infection
	Excess clotting or mechanical damage to platelets	DIC Infection Cardiac valve replacement Microvascular clotting disorder
Abnormal distribution or pooling	Splenic disorder with hypersplenism	Malignancy, infection infiltrates, congestion

P

HOW THE TEST IS DONE

A purple-topped tube with EDTA is used to collect 7 mL of venous blood. As an alternative, two purple-tipped capillary tubes are used to collect blood from a heelstick, earlobe, or finger puncture. After the blood is collected, the tube is gently inverted five to ten times to mix the anticoagulant and prevent clotting.

SIGNIFICANCE OF TEST RESULTS

Elevated Values

Polycythemia vera
Myelofibrosis
Chronic myelocytic leukemia
Thrombocythemia
Posthemorrhage regeneration
Iron deficiency anemia
Multiple myeloma
Postsplenectomy response
Acute or chronic infection
Inflammatory diseases
Hodgkin's disease
Lymphoma
Chronic renal disease
Renal cysts

Decreased Values

Idiopathic thrombocytopenic purpura
Megaloblastic anemia
Liver disease
Infection
Massive blood transfusion
Malignancy of the spleen
Radiation-chemotherapy
Leukemia
Fanconi syndrome
Wiskott-Aldrich syndrome
Uremia
Systemic lupus erythematosus
Aplastic anemia
Severe iron deficiency anemia
Parasitic diseases (malaria, toxoplasmosis, histoplasmosis)
Disseminated intravascular coagulation (DIC)
Thyroid disease
Eclampsia

INTERFERING FACTORS

- Platelet clumping
- Multiple transfusions

NURSING CARE

Nursing actions are similar to those used in other venipuncture procedures (see Chapter 2), with the following additional measures.

Pretest

- The nurse instructs the patient to avoid strenuous exercise before the test, because exertion and stress elevate the test results temporarily.

Posttest

- Assess the venipuncture site for signs of bleeding or ecchymosis. If the patient has a low platelet count, the venipuncture site can leak blood because of a failure to form a clot. To promote clotting, use sterile gauze to apply pressure to the site, or raise the arm above the head while maintaining pressure on the site.
- ***Patient Teaching.*** When the platelet count is decreased, institute measures to protect the patient from trauma, bruising, or cuts. The nurse teaches the patient to avoid bruising or bleeding, Suggested measures include using an electric razor to avoid shaving nicks in the skin, using a soft toothbrush to avoid scratching the gingiva, and walking carefully near tables and other wooden furniture to avoid bumping into a corner or hard surface. The nurse also teaches the patient to avoid the use of aspirin because this medication interferes with the platelets' ability to form a clot. The patient must learn to read the labeled ingredients on over-the-counter medications, to avoid anything containing acetylsalicylic acid. This compound is commonly present in medications to relieve flulike symptoms, colds, and headaches. If the patient us unsure, he or she can ask the pharmacist for assistance.

▼ Nursing Response to Critical Values

If the lab results indicate a critical value in either a lack or an excess of platelets, the nurse should notify the physician immediately. When the platelet count is at or below the critical value on the low side, there is a high risk of spontaneous hemorrhage. The nurse takes baseline vital signs and begins to assess at regular intervals for signs of bleeding. Superficial bleeding in the skin is evidenced by petechiae, purpura, or ecchymosis. Epistaxis (a nosebleed) or bleeding from the gingiva in the mouth may occur. Hematuria (blood in the urine) may occur. If the patient recently delivered a baby, she may exhibit vaginal bleeding or bleeding from the incision of a caesarean section. Hemorrhage into the brain will cause a stroke. If the platelet count is at or above the critical value on the high side, thrombosis can occur. The clot can develop anywhere throughout the body, including the brain, abdominal organs, and heart. The nurse takes baseline vital signs and begins to observe for symptoms of sudden onset, including acute pain, neurologic symptoms, or a change in the level of consciousness.

Plethysmography, Arterial

pleth-iz-mog-ruh-fee, ar-tee-ree-uhl

Also called: Pulse Cuff Recording, (PCR)

SPECIMEN OR TYPE OF TEST: Manometry

PURPOSE OF THE TEST

Plethysmography is a noninvasive test that evaluates the arterial blood flow in the extremities. It detects the presence of peripheral arterial vascular disease.

BASICS THE NURSE NEEDS TO KNOW

Using blood pressure cuffs, plethysmography measures changes in the blood volume of the extremities. Normally, arterial flow is approximately equal to venous flow within an organ or extremity. If the venous blood flow of an extremity is interrupted by use of low pressure in the air cuffs, a subsequent increase occurs in the arterial blood volume of the extremity. This change in arterial volume can be detected by the plethysmograph. The machine records the linear waveform pattern on a strip of graph paper, much like the recording of an ECG.

In normal arterial circulation, the waveform has a pulsatile pattern, with a characteristic rise, sharp peak, dicrotic notch, and down slope in each pulsation (Figure 71). When the artery is stenosed or obstructed, a smaller volume of blood can pass through the arterial lumen. The abnormal waveform pattern is of low amplitude and reduced slope, with the loss of the dicrotic notch.

NORMAL VALUES

No evidence of arterial peripheral vascular disease; normal arterial waveform pattern

HOW THE TEST IS DONE

Plethysmographic cuffs are inflated at different levels on the extremities, and arterial waveforms are recorded. The test takes about 30 minutes to complete.

P

SIGNIFICANCE OF TEST RESULTS

Abnormal Values

Peripheral vascular disease
Arterial occlusive disease
Arterial embolus
Arterial trauma

INTERFERING FACTORS

- Smoking
- Caffeine
- Alcohol
- Cold room temperature
- Anxiety

NURSING CARE

Pretest

- After the physician explains the procedure to the patient, obtain written consent from the patient.
- ***Patient Teaching.*** The nurse instructs the patient to refrain from smoking and ingesting alcohol and caffeine before the test, because stimulants, depressants, and vasoconstrictive substances will alter the results.

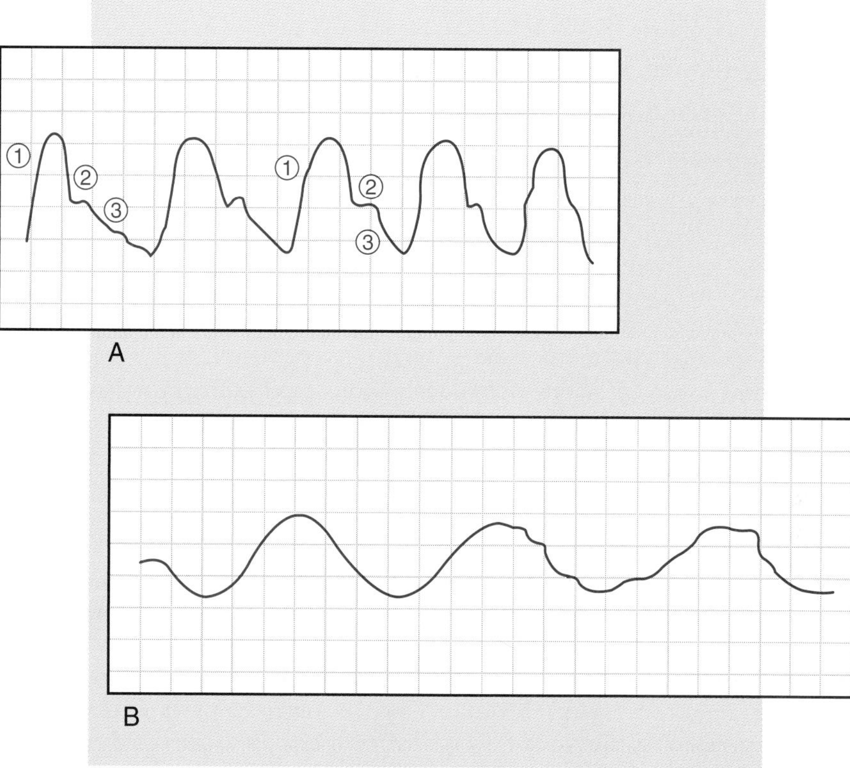

Figure 71. Normal versus abnormal arterial plethysmographic waveforms. *A,* The normal waveforms have characteristic *1,* sharp rise to peak; *2,* dicrotic notch; and *3,* downslope to baseline. *B,* Abnormal waveforms show a loss of the dicrotic notch, lower height, and rounding out of the peaks.

P

NURSING CARE

- The nurse assists the patient in removing all clothing and putting on a hospital gown. Restrictive clothing can alter the circulatory flow to the extremities.
- Place the patient in a supine position with a pillow under the head. Maintain a comfortable room temperature and dim the room lighting. Cool temperatures, anxiety, and muscle tension will alter the results. The nurse also informs the patient to refrain from talking and moving during the test.

During the Test

- The pressure cuffs are applied to both legs at the level of the upper thighs, above and below the knees, and above the ankles.
- At the first cuff site, inflate the cuff to 75 mm Hg for 2 to 3 seconds and then lower the pressure to 65 mm Hg.
- Record four to five waveforms. Label the recording with the correct identification of the cuff level and right or left side. Repeat this procedure at each cuff site.

Posttest

- Deflate and remove the cuffs.

Plethysmography, Venous

ple-thiz-mog-ruh-fee, vee-nus

Also called: Impedance Plethysmography, Venous

SPECIMEN OR TYPE OF TEST: Manometry

PURPOSE OF THE TEST

Venous plethysmography is used to help detect deep vein thrombosis and to screen patients who are at high risk for the development of venous thrombosis.

BASICS THE NURSE NEEDS TO KNOW

Using blood pressure cuffs and electrodes, venous plethysmography measures the change in blood volume of the extremities. The electrodes and the recorder produce a linear waveform pattern that is recorded on a graph-paper strip, as in the recording of an ECG.

In normal venous circulation, the blood moves toward the heart from the distal extremities. If a vein is compressed temporarily by a blood pressure cuff, the venous flow is interrupted. Distal to that compression point, the veins become engorged. On deflation of the cuff and release of the compression, the vein quickly empties of its excess blood and resumes normal venous outflow.

When a deep vein is obstructed by a thrombus, back-up of the venous blood and engorgement of the distal vessel also occur. Once the vein is compressed temporarily by the blood pressure cuff, the blood flow is further interrupted. Increased engorgement of the distal vein cannot occur, because the vein has already filled to capacity. On deflation of the cuff and release of the compression, only minimal venous blood flow resumes, because the thrombus continues to obstruct the lumen.

P

As the compression is applied to a normal vein, the venous plethysmographic waveform pattern shows a gradual rise in height from the baseline. This phase is called venous capacitance and represents the filling of the distal vein to its fullest capacity. On release of the compression, the waveform drops rapidly and returns to baseline (Figure 72). In an obstructed vein, the release of the pressure cuff relieves the venous compression, but limited venous outflow and slow emptying of the engorged vein occur. Correspondingly, the waveform demonstrates a limited, slow return to baseline.

NORMAL VALUES Normal waveform patterns with adequate venous capacity and maximum venous outflow; no evidence of deep vein thrombosis

HOW THE TEST IS DONE

Plethysmographic cuffs and electrodes are applied to the thigh and calf to control and monitor venous blood flow. The cuffs are inflated, and the recorded waveforms demonstrate the filling of the vein to maximal capacity. On rapid release of the cuffs, the waveform demonstrates the venous outflow of the distal vein. The total time required to complete the test is 30 to 45 minutes.

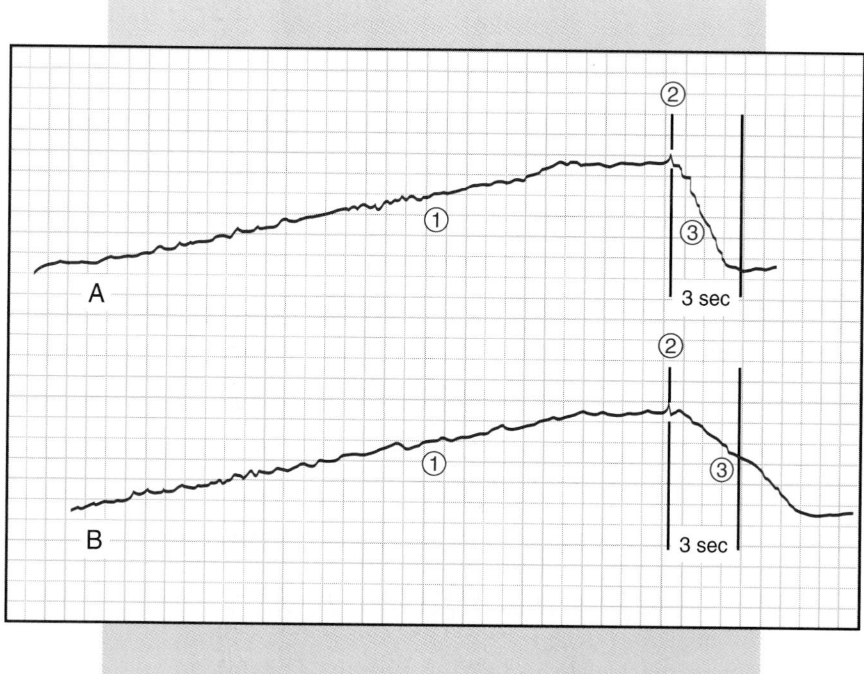

Figure 72. Normal versus abnormal venous plethysmographic waveforms. *A,* The normal waveform demonstrates *1,* venous filling; *2,* release of the thigh cuff; and *3,* rapid venous outflow that completes in 3 seconds. *B,* The abnormal waveform demonstrates *1,* venous filling; *2,* release of the thigh cuff; and *3,* slow venous outflow. It takes longer than the normal 3 seconds for the waveform to return to the baseline level.

SIGNIFICANCE OF TEST RESULTS

Abnormal Values

Venous thrombosis
Thrombophlebitis
Venous obstruction (partial or complete)

INTERFERING FACTORS

- Nicotine, alcohol, and caffeine
- Anxiety and muscle tension
- Uncooperative patient behavior
- Compression of pelvic veins (caused by a tumor or tight bandages)
- Low cardiac output
- Shock
- Arterial occlusive disease

NURSING CARE

Pretest

- After the physician has informed the patient about the procedure, obtain written consent from the patient.
- ***Patient Teaching.*** Instruct the patient to refrain from smoking and ingesting alcohol and caffeine before the test, because stimulants and depressants alter the test results.
- Help the patient remove all clothing and put on a hospital gown. Any compression from restrictive clothing alters the venous circulation from the extremities. Maintain a comfortable room temperature and dim the lights, because anxiety and muscle tension alter the results. Place the patient in the supine position with the legs elevated above the heart and supported by pillows. The affected leg and hip are externally rotated, and the knee is flexed.
- ***Patient Teaching.*** Advise the patient to refrain from movement and talking during the test.

During the Test

- Place blood pressure cuffs on the thigh and calf of the affected leg.
- Apply the conductive gel and electrodes to the skin.
- Inflate the cuff on the calf to 15 mm Hg of pressure. The cuff and electrode monitor the inflow of the venous system.
- Inflate the cuff on the thigh to 50 mm Hg of pressure. This pressure level obstructs the venous outflow but allows the arterial flow to fill and engorge the distal vein segment.
- Start the recorder to trace the waveform. Once the tracing has risen to its maximum level and formed a plateau, the venous filling is completed.
- Quickly release the pressure on the thigh cuff to open the venous outflow of the vein. The waveform pattern will continue and provide the linear recording of the return to the baseline reading.
- Repeat the procedure until three to five waveforms are recorded. Label the paper, correctly identifying the extremity.
- Repeat the entire procedure on the opposite extremity to provide comparison data.

Posttest

- Remove the deflated cuffs and electrodes.
- Wipe the conductive gel off the skin.

Positron Emission Tomography

pos-i-tron i-mi-shun tuh-mog-ruh-fee

Also called: PET Scan

SPECIMEN OR TYPE OF TEST: Nuclear scan

PURPOSE OF THE TEST

The positron emission tomography (PET) scan is used to provide images of the brain and other specific target organs. It detects areas of metabolic change in the tissue at a very early stage of disease. It is also used to guide or manage treatment of disease, monitor the tissue response to drug therapy, and in cancer staging.

BASICS THE NURSE NEEDS TO KNOW

The PET scan is a form of nuclear scan that uses cyclotronproduced isotopes for the radiopharmaceuticals. These radioisotopes produce excellent contrast for specific tissues and measure blood flow, blood volume, glucose, and oxygen metabolism. Glucose provides the energy for the cells to function. The measurement of glucose metabolism or oxygen perfusion and metabolism in a specific area or organ reflects the functional activity of the cells. In abnormal function, the images demonstrate decreased or increased metabolism or perfusion. These changes in metabolism or perfusion are distinctly different responses than those of normal tissue (Figure 73).

In an early stage of Alzheimer's disease, this new technology is able to demonstrate the characteristic hypoperfusion and hypometabolism in the temporoparietal lobes of the brain. It also provides images of the altered brain metabolism of Parkinson's disease. Before cardiac surgery, the PET myocardial perfusion study is used to identify viable myocardial tissue and nonviable tissue that would not benefit from improved coronary artery circulation. In oncology, PET imaging can detect tumor and differentiate a malignant (high metabolic) tumor from a benign (low metabolic) growth. It is also used as a whole body scan to locate and evaluate distant metastases and to monitor the tumor response to treatment.

NORMAL VALUES The imaged organ demonstrates normal perfusion and metabolism

P

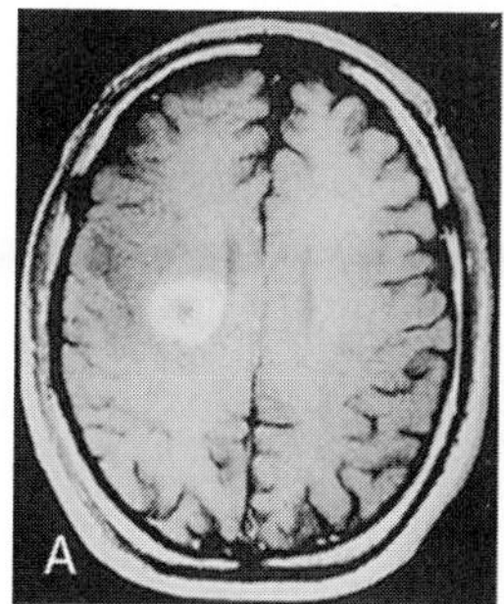

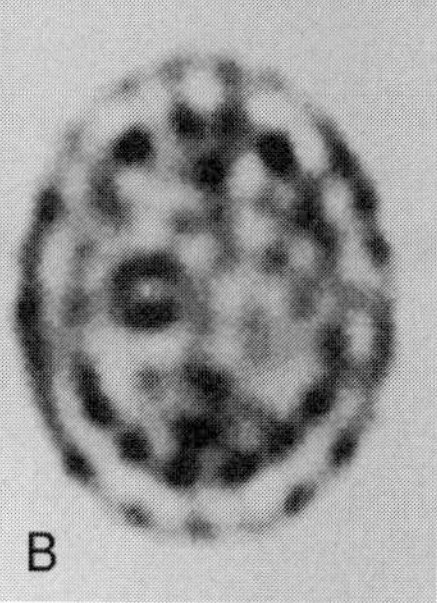

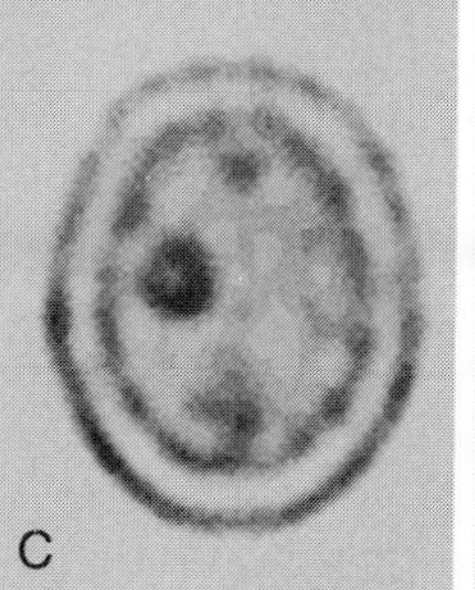

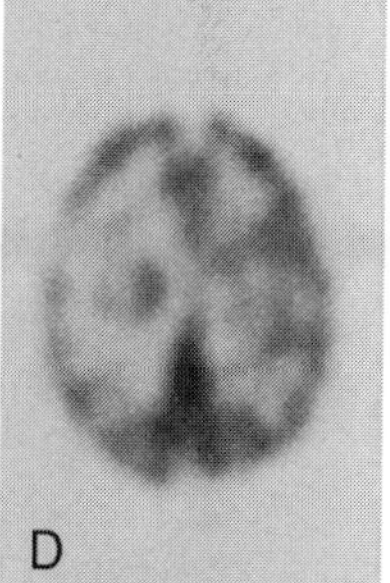

Figure 73. Comparison of brain images from magnetic resonance imaging (MRI) and positron emission tomography (PET) scan. *A*, MRI of a cross-section of the brain. *B–D*, Fluorodeoxyglucose positron emission tomography (FDG-PET) images in a 27-year-old patient with glioblastoma of the brain. In the PET scan, there is significantly increased glucose metabolism in the tumor, shown in three levels of the brain *(B, C, D)*. The PET scan image of (C) corresponds to the MRI image (A) and demonstrates the tumor in both techniques. *(Reproduced with permission from Wagner, H. N., Szabo, Z., & Buchanan, J. W. [1995].* Principles of nuclear medicine *[2nd ed., Fig. 46–1, p. 1047]. Philadelphia: W. B. Saunders.)*

HOW THE TEST IS DONE

A special radiopharmaceutical is injected intravenously or inhaled as a gas. Once the radioactive substance enters the targeted tissue(s) by perfusion and metabolism, the emitted positrons combine with electrons to emit gamma rays. The gamma rays are detected by a special camera that rotates around the body or section of the body (such as the head). The signals captured by the camera are then converted by computer and software to provide images of the body tissue. The patient may be at the imaging center for several hours, but the imaging time lasts about 45 minutes.

SIGNIFICANCE OF TEST RESULTS

Abnormal Findings

Tumor, benign or malignant
Metastatic cancer
Epilepsy
Alzheimer's disease
Dementia
Parkinson's disease
Psychiatric disorder
CNS degenerative disorder
Cardiac or brain ischemia

INTERFERING FACTORS

- Failure to follow the dietary restrictions in the pretest period.
- Caffeine, alcohol, nicotine
- Recent biopsy, surgery, radiation therapy or chemotherapy.

NURSING CARE

Pretest

- If the patient has a history of cancer diagnosis or treatment, schedule this test according to the time-delay protocol of the nuclear medicine institution and in consult with the physician and radiologist. If the scan is done too soon after biopsy or surgery, a false-positive result can occur. If the scan is done too soon after radiation therapy or chemotherapy, a false-negative result can occur.
- ***Patient Teaching.*** The nurse visits the hospitalized patient, or phones the patient who lives at home, to interview the patient and teach about the PET scan procedure and the pretest instructions. The purpose of the nurse's call is also meant to establish personal contact, to answer the patient's questions, and allay anxiety. Patients who know they have cancer or suspect a brain disorder or heart disease are likely to worry about this test and its potential findings. In addition, if the patient is late for the appointment or does not show up, the financial costs of the now unusable radiopharmaceutical and the loss of scheduled scanning time are very high. The nurse works with the patient to promote cooperation and trust.

NURSING CARE—*cont'd*

- ***Patient Teaching.*** The nurse teaches the patient to discontinue food intake for 6 to 8 hours before the test. Intake of water is permitted and the patient should continue with his or her prescribed medication schedule. When glucose metabolism is to be measured by the PET scan, recent food or sugar intake would alter the test results. The patient is also instructed to discontinue the use of alcohol, caffeine, and smoking for 24 hours before the test, as these substances alter the test result. The nurse assesses for claustrophobia and anxiety because the patient will not be allowed to move in the scanner for about 45 minutes. Oral sedation may be needed to overcome these problems and is used routinely for some types of cancer imaging. If sedation is used, the patient will need someone to provide transportation after the test is completed.
- On the morning of the scan, the nurse takes and documents vital signs, height, weight, and blood glucose level. An intravenous line is established so the nuclear technologist can administer the radiopharmaceutical. The patient must change into a hospital gown, remove any metallic objects as jewelry, and void before the test.

During the Test

- The patient is assisted to lie on the scanning table. If the brain is to be scanned, the patient's head will be placed inside the scanner. The patient is reminded to remain still. He or she may be asked to perform certain activities inside the scanner, as speaking, reasoning, or listening to music at particular times during the scanning process.
- If the whole body is to be scanned, the patient lies on the scanning table and the table moves slowly through the ring of the scanner. The patient is given a call light to summon help if needed. Music in the room helps to promote relaxation. The patient is reminded to refrain from movement or speaking during the test.

Posttest

- The patient is assisted to a sitting position and given a glass of juice to drink. The glucose helps to prevent fainting or dizziness. The nurse monitors for orthostatic hypotension as the patient stands up.
- ***Patient Teaching.*** The nurse instructs the patient to drink extra fluids, to help eliminate the radiopharmaceutical in the urine. The level of radioactivity is now minimal because of the short half-life, but the patient should wash his or her hands after each voiding, to rid the skin of any possible contamination.

Potassium, Serum

poh-ta-see-uhm, seer-uhm

Also called: K^+

SPECIMEN OR TYPE OF TEST: Blood

PURPOSE OF THE TEST

Serum potassium is used to evaluate electrolyte balance, acidbase balance, hypertension, renal disease or renal failure, and endocrine disease. It is used to monitor patients receiving treatment for ketoacidosis as well as those receiving hyperalimentation, dialysis, diuretic therapy, or intravenous therapy.

BASICS THE NURSE NEEDS TO KNOW

Potassium is a major electrolyte that is present in all body fluids. Most of the potassium is concentrated in the intracellular fluids, with only a very small amount of the total potassium in the extracellular fluids, including the blood. The renewable source of potassium is the daily food intake. The extracellular potassium level remains within a relatively narrow range. The regulation of the extracellular potassium concentration is performed by the kidneys, with excretion of excess potassium in the urine (Figure 74).

Considerable danger is associated with either depletion or excess of potassium. Abnormal potassium concentration causes disturbances in the membrane potential and altered function of neuromuscular tissue, including the loss of cardiac contractility. With depletion or excess of this cation, the patient is at risk for the development of shock, respiratory failure, or cardiac dysrhythmias (Figure 75), including ventricular fibrillation.

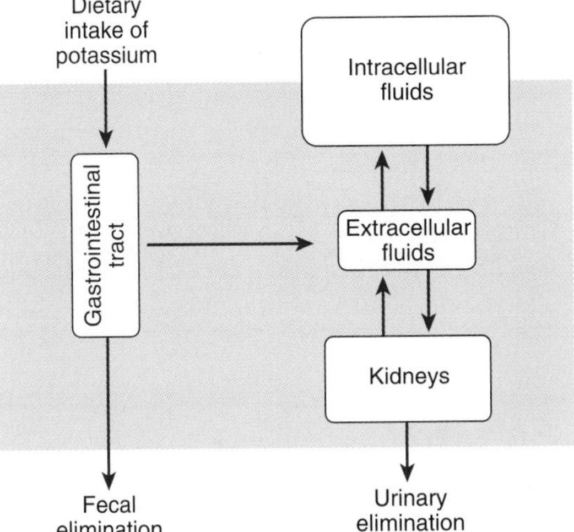

Figure 74. Homeostatic balance of potassium. Once the potassium is absorbed from the small intestine, most of it is stored within cells and a small amount remains in the extracellular fluids, including blood. Excess potassium is excreted from the body in feces and urine. The kidneys are the best regulators of potassium homeostasis.

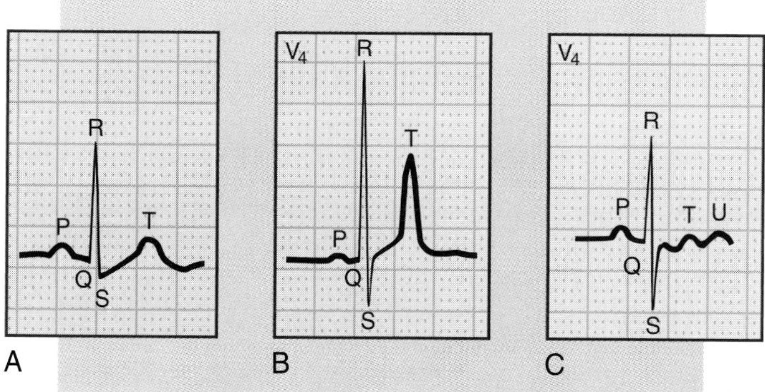

Figure 75. ECG changes in potassium imbalance. *A*, Normal ECG pattern. *B*, Moderate hyperkalemia with tall, peaked T waves. *C*, Moderate hypokalemia with a flattened T wave and elevation of the U wave.

Elevated Value

An elevated level of potassium in the extracellular fluid and blood is called *hyperkalemia*. The most common source of hyperkalemia is renal disease. The potassium value also rises with mineralocorticoid deficiency or metabolic acidosis. Additionally, damage to tissue and cells causes a release of intracellular potassium into the extracellular fluids.

In renal disease, the glomeruli may be unable to filter the blood, causing a rise in the serum value and a decrease in the excretion of potassium in the urine. In acute renal failure, the potassium level begins to rise with the onset of oliguria (scanty urinary output). In chronic renal failure, the potassium level does not begin to rise until there is a 75% reduction in the glomerular filtration rate.

Decreased Value

A decreased amount of potassium in the extracellular fluid is called *hypokalemia*. It can occur with fluid losses from the gastrointestinal tract, skin, or kidneys. The most common cause of urinary potassium loss is from diuretic therapy. Hypokalemia can also result from a decreased dietary intake or from alkalosis. In alkalosis, the potassium has increased entry into the cells, and the intracellular concentration of potassium increases.

NORMAL VALUES	Adult: 3.5–5.1 mEq/L *or* SI: 3.5–5.1 mmol/L
Critical Values	Adult: <2.5 mEq/L (SI: <2.5 mmol/L) *or* >6.5 mEq/L (SI: >6.5 mmol/L)

HOW THE TEST IS DONE

A green- (heparin) or red-topped tube is used to collect 5 or 10 mL of venous or arterial blood.

SIGNIFICANCE OF TEST RESULTS

Elevated Values

Rapid or excessive intravenous potassium replacement
Dehydration
Renal failure
Potassium-sparing diuretics
Massive hemolysis
Acidosis
Diabetic ketoacidosis
Traumatic crush injury
Severe burns
Addison's disease

Decreased Values

Diuretic therapy
Intravenous fluid therapy without potassium replacement
Vomiting or diarrhea
Severe burns
Renal tubular acidosis
Excessive sweating
Fistula drainage
Bartter syndrome
Alkalosis
Aldosteronism

INTERFERING FACTORS

- Hemolysis

NURSING CARE

Nursing actions are similar to those used in other venipuncture or arterial puncture procedures (see Chapter 2), with the following additional measures.

During the Test

- Avoid the use of a tourniquet when drawing the blood, if possible. If the tourniquet is applied loosely, the fist should not be clenched. These measures prevent hemolysis of erythrocytes and a false elevation of the potassium value. The blood sample should be drawn from the arm that does not have an intravenous fluid administration. The fluid and possible electrolyte concentration would alter the test results.

Posttest

- Monitor the test results and notify the physician of any abnormal value. Untreated hyperkalemia or hypokalemia can cause changes in the myocardium and the neuromuscular system, including very serious cardiac arrhythmias (Table 12). For patients

NURSING CARE—*cont'd*

who are at risk for potassium imbalance, vital signs should be monitored routinely. The nurse also monitors the heartbeat to detect any changes in rate or rhythm.

- The nurse monitors and documents intake and output because fluid losses from intestinal drainage, vomiting, diarrhea, fistula drainage, burned skin, and urinary diuresis all can cause loss of potassium. Impaired renal function and diminished urinary output cause a rise in the potassium level.

▼ Nursing Response to Critical Values

Once the values reach a critical level (high or low value), the patient is in a life-threatening situation, with danger of severe cardiac dysrhythmia, cardiac arrest, and death. The nurse immediately notifies the physician of the abnormal test value.

The nurse assesses the patient for manifestations of potassium imbalance. With hyperkalemia, the manifestations include muscle weakness, decreased reflexes, ascending paralysis, respiratory arrest, and a slow or irregular heartbeat. In hypokalemia, the manifestations include weakness, cramps of the legs or body, tetany, anorexia, nausea, tachycardia, bradycardia, premature atrial contractions, and premature ventricular contractions.

The nurse prepares for an electrocardiogram (ECG) or for cardiac monitoring. In addition, the nurse prepares for the administration of prescribed medication or intravenous therapy to correct the potassium imbalance. Specific treatment will depend on the type and severity of the imbalance and its cause.

TABLE 12 ECG* Changes Associated with Critical Values of Serum Potassium

P

Serum Potassium Level	ECG Manifestations
Hyperkalemia	
>6.5 mEq/L (SI: >6.5 mmol/L)	Peaked T waves
7–8 mEq/L (SI: 7–8 mmol/L)	Prolonged P-R interval
	Loss of P waves
	Widening of the QRS complexes
>8–10 mEq/L (SI: >8–10 mmol/L)	Sine wave pattern
	Cardiac standstill; asystole
Hypokalemia	
2–2.5 mEq/L (SI: 2–2.5 mmol/L)	Sagging of the S-T segment
	Flattened or depressed T wave
	Elevation of the U wave
<2 mEq/L (SI: <2 mmol/L)	Smaller T waves
	Increased height (amplitude) of U waves

*ECG, Electrocardiogram.

Progesterone

proh-jes-ter-ohn

SPECIMEN OR TYPE OF TEST: Blood

PURPOSE OF THE TEST

Serum progesterone levels are used to determine ovulation and to assess the function of the corpus luteum, particularly in cases of habitual abortion, first trimester bleeding, and infertility.

BASICS THE NURSE NEEDS TO KNOW

In the menstruating female, progesterone is produced by the ovaries. Progesterone functions to help prepare the endometrium of the uterus for the implantation of the fertilized ovum. In the menstruating female, the corpus luteum of the ovary produces a small but steady supply during the preovulatory or follicular phase of the menstrual cycle. After ovulation, the progesterone level rises over a 4- to 5-day period in the luteal phase of the menstrual cycle. The serum level reaches and maintains its peak for about 1 week and then falls rapidly before the start of menstruation. A normal value in the luteal phase indicates that the patient is ovulating normally. In testing for the cause of infertility in the female, serial blood samples are obtained during the menstrual cycle to determine the day of ovulation.

During pregnancy, progesterone is synthesized in great quantity by the placenta, and the serum level rises progressively throughout the term of the pregnancy. Serial testing may also be done throughout a pregnancy to monitor for abnormal gestational development of the fetus, such as inevitable abortion.

NORMAL VALUES

Menstruating Female

Follicular phase: 15–70 ng/dL *or* SI: 0.5–2.2 nmol/L

Luteal phase: 200–2500 ng/dL *or* SI: 6.4–79.5 nmol/L

Pregnant Female

First trimester: 725–4400 ng/dL *or* SI: 23.0–140.0 nmol/L

Second trimester: 1950–8250 ng/dL *or* SI: 62.0–262.4 nmol/L

Third trimester: 6500–22,900 ng/dL *or* SI: 206.7–728.2 nmol/L

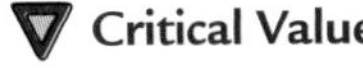 **Critical Value** <150 ng/dL (SI: <4.77 mmol/L)

HOW THE TEST IS DONE

A red-topped tube is used to obtain 10 mL of venous blood.

SIGNIFICANCE OF TEST RESULTS

Elevated Values

Congenital adrenal hyperplasia

Molar pregnancy

Ovarian tumor

Decreased Values
Threatened abortion
Short luteal phase syndrome
Ectopic pregnancy

INTERFERING FACTORS

- Recent radioactive isotope scan

NURSING CARE

Nursing actions are similar to those used in other venipuncture procedures (see Chapter 2), with the following additional measures.

Pretest

- Schedule this test for before or at least 7 days after a nuclear scan. The measurement of progesterone is performed by the radioimmunoassay method of analysis. The radioisotopes of a nuclear scan would interfere with the analysis and results of the progesterone test.
- When a series of blood tests throughout the menstrual cycle is required, make sure that the patient understands the testing plan and schedule of test dates.

Posttest

- On the requisition slip, write the pertinent data, including the patient's sex, the date of the patient's last menstrual period, and the trimester of pregnancy. These data are used to help determine whether the results are within normal limits. If the patient is in her first trimester and is bleeding, a serum progesterone value >250 ng/dL (SI: >7.95 nmol/L) indicates a viable intrauterine pregnancy.

▼ Nursing Response to Critical Values

In the pregnant female who is bleeding in the first trimester, a progesterone level that is at or below the critical value indicates a failing intrauterine pregnancy or an ectopic pregnancy. The nurse alerts the physician of this very low result.

The nurse uses effective listening skills to help support the patient who has a history of miscarriage or who is pregnant and has intrauterine bleeding. The patient may express apprehension or anxiety about a possible loss of this pregnancy.

Prostate-Specific Antigen

pro-stayt–spe-si-fic an-tuh-jen

Also called: PSA

SPECIMEN OR TYPE OF TEST: Serum

PURPOSE OF THE TEST

In combination with the digital rectal examination, prostate specific antigen (PSA) is recommended as a screening tool for all men older than age 50 and for men older than age 40 who have additional risk factors, including African-American men and those with a positive family history of prostate cancer. As a tumor marker for adenocarcinoma of the prostate gland, the test is used to monitor the postsurgical patient who has had a radical prostatectomy. It is used to evaluate for recurrence or residual tumor and helps identify the need for additional treatment.

BASICS THE NURSE NEEDS TO KNOW

The PSA test lacks specificity to distinguish between benign prostatic hypertrophy and an early stage of prostatic malignancy. Elevated value for benign prostatic hypertrophy may be in the same range as the value for stage A of malignant growth.

NORMAL VALUES	**Male** 40–59 years old: <4 ng/mL *or* SI:<4 mcg/L 60–69 years old: <4.5 ng/mL *or* SI: <4.5 mcg/L 70–80 years old: <6.5 ng/mL *or* SI: <6.5 mcg/L
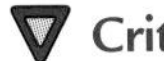 Critical Value	>10 ng/pmL

HOW THE TEST IS DONE

A red-topped tube is used to collect 7 to 10 mL of venous blood.

SIGNIFICANCE OF TEST RESULTS

Elevated Values

Adenocarcinoma of the prostate
Benign prostatic hypertrophy
Prostatitis
Urinary retention
Prostatic infarct

INTERFERING FACTORS

- Prostatic manipulation
- Recent urethral instrumentation

NURSING CARE

- ***Health Promotion.*** Nurses need to advise all men older than age 50 to have a PSA done annually. Men who are at risk (African-American and those with a family history of prostatic cancer) should start annual PSA testing at age 40. The nurse needs to reassure the patient that the test requires a simple venous blood sample; in addition, a digital rectal examination (DRE) should be done annually to improve chances of cancer detection.

Pretest

- Collect the specimen before any prostate manipulation. A digital rectal examination within 48 hours will affect the results.
- Schedule the blood test for at least 2 to 4 weeks after any urethral instrumentation procedure, such as a transurethral resection, prostatic biopsy, or cystoscopy, because these procedures will cause a release of the PSA.
- ***Patient Teaching.*** Because a fasting specimen is preferred, the nurse instructs the patient to cease food intake for 8 hours before the test.

NURSING CARE—*cont'd*

Posttest

- Arrange for prompt transport of the specimen to the laboratory.

Nursing Response to Critical Values

Although elevated values may be suggestive of cancer, the diagnosis can only be confirmed by biopsy of the prostate gland. The nurse listens to the patient's feelings of apprehension and provides support, but urges him to continue with the diagnostic testing to obtain a complete medical diagnosis.

Prostatic Acid Phosphatase

proh-sta-tik a-sid fos-fuh-tays

Also called: (PAP); Acid Phosphatase

SPECIMEN OR TYPE OF TEST: Serum, plasma, vaginal secretions

PURPOSE OF THE TEST

Acid phosphatase is used to assist with the staging of metastatic adenocarcinoma of the prostate gland. After treatment for the malignancy, it assists in the evaluation for recurrence of the disease.

Prostatic acid phosphatase is present in prostatic secretions and, therefore, in semen. In cases of suspected rape, the vaginal secretions are tested for the presence of acid phosphatase.

BASICS THE NURSE NEEDS TO KNOW

Acid phosphatase is an enzyme present in high concentrations in the prostate gland and its secretions. Its value in serum is elevated with metastatic cancer of the prostate, but it may remain in a normal range during the early stage of the disease.

For many years, prostatic acid phosphatase was used as a tumor marker to diagnose and help stage adenocarcinoma of the prostate gland. Today, the prostate-specific antigen test has surpassed the prostatic acid phosphatase test in the diagnosis and evaluation of carcinoma of the prostate gland. The prostatic acid phosphatase test is still used with the prostate-specific antigen test in the evaluation and staging of metastatic prostate cancer.

The tartrate-resistant method of analysis remains an important diagnostic test for hairy cell leukemia.

NORMAL VALUES

Male

4-Nitrophenyl phosphate method at 37° C: 0.13–0.63 unit/L

Tartrate resistance fraction: 0.2–3.5 unit/L *or* SI: 2.2–10.5 units/L

Thymolphthalein monophosphate method at 37° C: <1.9 units/L

Female

Vaginal secretions: <2 units/L

P

HOW THE TEST IS DONE

A red- or purple-topped tube is used to collect 7 mL of venous blood.

SIGNIFICANCE OF TEST RESULTS

Elevated Values

Metastatic cancer of the prostate
Hairy cell leukemia
Gaucher's disease
Hemolytic diseases
Niemann-Pick's disease
Advanced Paget's disease
Benign prostatic hypertrophy
Prostatitis
Metastatic cancer of bone
Prostatic infarct

INTERFERING FACTORS

- Hemolysis
- Warming of the specimen
- Failure to maintain nothing-by-mouth status
- Lipemia
- Manipulation of the prostate

P

NURSING CARE

Nursing actions are similar to those used in other venipuncture procedures (see Chapter 2), with the following additional measures.

Pretest

- To avoid a false-positive elevation, schedule test for several days after any diagnostic test that manipulates the prostate gland (transurethral resection, bladder catheterization, digital rectal examination).
- ***Patient Teaching.*** The nurse instructs the patient to discontinue all food and fluids for 8 hours before the test, because lipemia interferes with the laboratory analysis.

Posttest

- Arrange for prompt transport of the specimen to the laboratory.

Protein Electrophoresis, Serum

proh-teen e-lek-tro-phuh-ree-sis, seer-uhm

SPECIMEN OR TYPE OF TEST: Serum

PURPOSE OF THE TEST

Serum protein electrophoresis is used in the detection of hepatobiliary disease and monoclonal gammopathy, and in the evaluation of nutritional status.

BASICS THE NURSE NEEDS TO KNOW

In the blood, total protein consists of albumin and globulins. The process of electrophoresis uses an electric field to separate these fractional components in greater detail and measure the amount of each component. Different diseases cause alterations in the concentration of the plasma proteins and characteristics of the patterns of protein electrophoresis. One pattern in particular—the tall narrow spike in the M protein of gamma globulin—is an abnormality that is characteristic of multiple myeloma and several other diseases that produce abnormal, elevated amounts of immunoglobin M (Figure 76).

Albumin

This is the largest component and makes up two thirds of the total plasma proteins. The functions of albumin are to (1) maintain the oncotic pressure (the pressure that holds water in the blood vessels), (2) maintain a reserve nitrogen pool for tissue growth and repair, and (3) serve as a carrier protein for numerous substances, such as medications, lipids, bilirubin, hormones, minerals, and fat-soluble vitamins.

Globulins

The three main subgroups of globulins are alpha, beta, and gamma globulins. *Alpha$_1$ globulin* is alpha$_1$-antitrypsin, a protease inhibitor that inactivates trypsin in the blood. *Alpha$_2$ globulin* consist of two important plasma proteins: haptoglobulin and alpha$_2$ globulin. Haptoglobulin binds the hemoglobin that has been released from the lysis of erythrocytes. Alpha$_2$ macroglobulin is a protease inhibitor. Because of its large size relative to other globulins, it cannot pass into glomerular filtrate. In nephrotic syndrome, when other globulins are lost via glomerular filtrate, the concentration of Alpha$_2$ macroglobulin increases dramatically.

Beta$_1$ globulin consists mainly of transferrin, the iron-transporting protein. It carries ferric ions from intracellular storage to the bone marrow. *Beta$_2$ globulin* consists primarily of the low-density lipoprotein that transports cholesterol to the cells. Other beta-globulins are fibrinogen and complement factors.

Gamma globulins consists of the immunoglobulins G, A, D, E, and M. They are usually identified as IgG, IgA, IgD, IgE, and IgM. Each of these plasma proteins is designed to carry out antibody activity by binding with and neutralizing specific antigens.

NORMAL VALUES

Adult

Albumin: 3.2–5.6 g/d/L *or* SI: 32–56 g/L
Alpha$_1$ globulin: 0.1–0.4 g/d/L *or* SI: 1–4 g/L
Alpha$_2$ globulin: 0.4–1.2 g/d/L *or* SI: 4–12g/L
Beta globulins: 0.5–1.1 g/d/L *or* SI: 5–11 g/L
Gamma globulins: 0.5–1.6 g/d/L *or* SI: 5–16 g/L

HOW THE TEST IS DONE

A venipuncture is performed to collect 10 mL of venous blood in a red-topped tube.

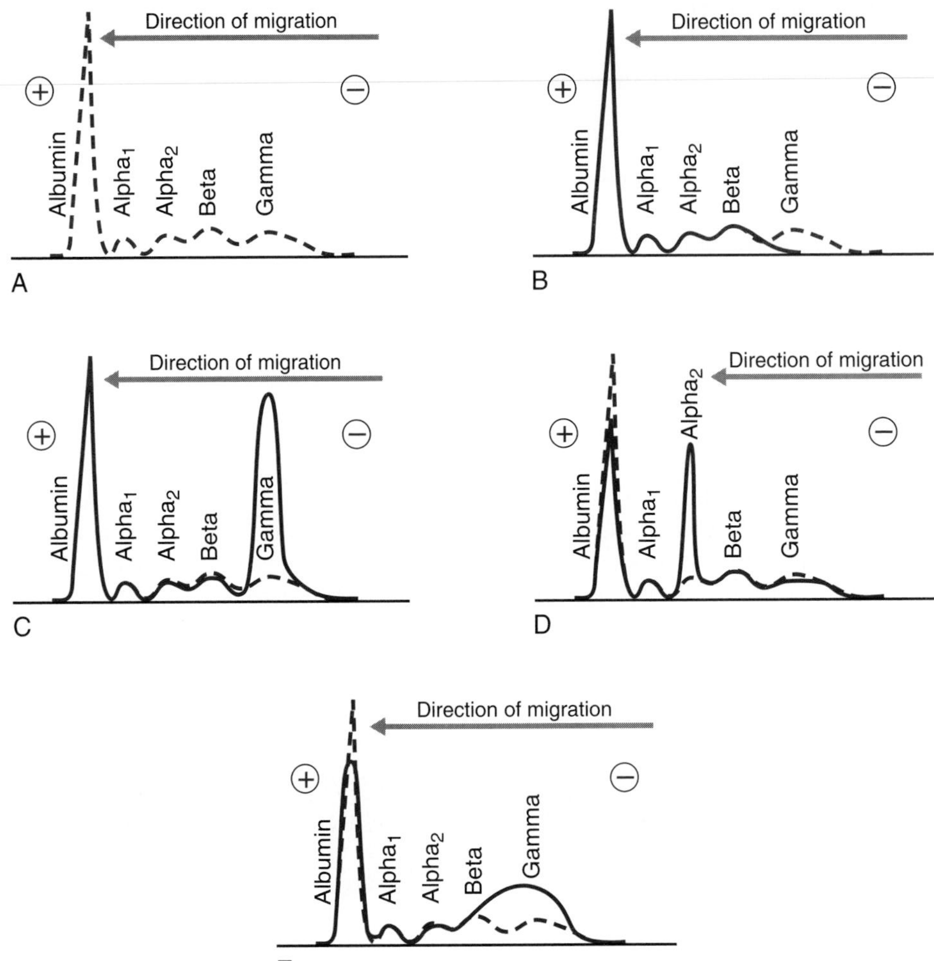

Figure 76. Serum protein electrophoresis: normal versus abnormal patterns. *A*, Normal pattern. *B*, Hypogammaglobulinemia indicated by an almost absent gamma region. *C*, Monoclonal gammopathy, marked by a single spike in the gamma region. *D*, Nephrotic syndrome, indicated by a loss of most serum proteins and a rise in alpha$_2$-macroglobulin. *E*, Active hepatocellular damage (cirrhosis) marked by fusion of the beta and gamma regions and an increase in immunoglobulin A in that region. *(Adapted with permission from Lehmann, C. A. [1998].* Saunders manual of clinical laboratory science. *Philadelphia: W. B. Saunders.)*

P

SIGNIFICANCE OF TEST RESULTS

Elevated Values

Albumin

Dehydration

Alpha$_1$ Globulins

Inflammatory disease
Neoplastic disease (cancer)

Alpha$_2$ Globulins

Nephrotic syndrome
Cancer
Rheumatic fever
Acute infection

Beta Globulins

Hyperlipoproteinemia
Monoclonal gammopathies

Gamma Globulins

Polyclonal gammopathies
- Chronic liver diseases (hepatitis, cirrhosis)
- Collagen diseases (systemic lupus erythematosus, rheumatoid arthritis)
- Infection
- Inflammation (sarcoidosis)
- Cancer

Monoclonal gammopathies
- Multiple myeloma
- Waldenström's macroglobulinemia
- Amyloidosis
- Malignant lymphoma

Decreased Values

Albumin

Metastatic cancer
Heart failure
Malnutrition
Thermal injury
Nephrotic syndrome
Protein-losing enteropathies (Crohn's disease, ulcerative colitis, intestinal fistula)

Alpha$_1$ Globulins

Hereditary alpha$_1$-antitrypsin deficiency

Alpha$_2$ Globulins

Hemolysis
Hepatocellular damage

Beta Globulins

Hypobetalipoproteinemia

Gamma Globulins

Response to cancer chemotherapy or immunosuppressive medications
Lymphocytic leukemia

Lymphosarcoma
Multiple myeloma
Immune deficiency

INTERFERING FACTORS

- None

NURSING CARE

Nursing actions are similar to those used in other venipuncture procedures (see Chapter 2 for additional information). No other patient preparation is necessary.

Protein Electrophoresis, Urinary

proh-teen e-lek-tro-phuh-ree-sis, yur-i-nar-ee

Also called: 24-Hour Urine Protein Electrophoresis

SPECIMEN OR TYPE OF TEST: Urine

PURPOSE OF THE TEST

Protein electrophoresis of the urine is used to identify the different types of protein loss in the urine and to evaluate patients with known or suspected multiple myeloma.

BASICS THE NURSE NEEDS TO KNOW

Normally, a small amount of protein exists in the urine. Less than half the protein in urine is albumin; the remainder consists of plasma proteins, including many small globulins.

When excessive protein appears in the urine, the causes can be broadly categorized as glomerular disorders, tubular disorders, or overflow proteinuria. In the first two categories, the problems are related to renal damage. The third category is characterized by excessive protein produced by nonrenal disease. The proteins are filtered by the glomeruli, but the excessive amount of protein prevents complete resorption by the tubules. Thus, an "overflow" of protein into the urine occurs.

Protein electrophoresis has replaced the *Bence Jones Protein test.* The Bence Jones protein is one of the proteins of overflow proteinuria. Its presence in the urine is associated with multiple myeloma, macroglobulinemia, and malignant lymphoma.

P

NORMAL VALUES

Total protein: 40–150 ng/24 hr *or* SI: 40–150 mg/24 hr
Albumin: <50% of the total protein
Total globulin: 60%–67% of the total protein

HOW THE TEST IS DONE

A 24-hour urine specimen is collected and sent to the lab on ice.

SIGNIFICANCE OF TEST RESULTS

Glomerular-Pattern Proteinuria

Glomerular diseases
Nephrotic syndrome

Overflow-Pattern Proteinuria
Multiple myeloma
Waldenström's macroglobulinemia
Lymphoma
Amyloidosis

Tubular Pattern Proteinuria
Fanconi syndrome
Cystinosis
Wilson's disease
Pyelonephritis
Renal transplant rejection

INTERFERING FACTORS

- Hematuria
- Incomplete collection of all urine for 24 hours

NURSING CARE

Nursing actions are similar to those used in other timed urine collections (see Chapter 2), with the following additional measures.

Pretest

- ***Patient Teaching.*** Instruct the patient to collect a 24-hour urine specimen. Remind the patient that all urine is to be collected in the container. Keep the urine refrigerated or on ice during the collection period.
- ***Patient Teaching.*** Instruct female patients to collect the urine at a time when no menstrual flow occurs.

Posttest

- The nurse ensures that the specimen container and the requisition slip have the complete patient identification and the time and date of the start and finish of the collection period. Send to the lab on ice.

Protein, Total, Serum

proh-teen, toh-tuhl, seer-uhm

Also called: Total Serum Proteins

SPECIMEN OR TYPE OF TEST: Serum

PURPOSE OF THE TEST

Total serum protein testing provides general information about the patient's nutritional status and the severity of diseases of the liver, bone marrow, and kidneys. The test is also used to investigate the cause of edema.

Serum albumin is used to evaluate nutritional status, the oncotic pressure of the blood, and the losses of protein associated with some severe renal, hepatic, skin, and intestinal diseases.

The globulin value identifies the need for additional testing to determine which globulins are elevated or decreased.

The albumin-to-globulin ratio identifies the proportionate amounts of these two proteins in the blood.

BASICS THE NURSE NEEDS TO KNOW

Liver tissue manufactures the serum proteins albumin and fibrinogen, other coagulation factors, and most of the alpha and beta globulins. The various plasma proteins are amino acids that function to (1) maintain oncotic pressure in the blood vessels; (2) provide a reserve source of protein for tissue growth and repair; (3) provide transport for lipids, lipid-soluble substances, iron, copper, magnesium, and calcium; (4) act as immunologic agents; (5) provide factors for coagulation; (6) provide numerous enzymes for a variety of activities.

Total Serum Protein

Total serum protein provides a broad indicator of the quantity and concentration of all plasma proteins except fibrinogen. The total serum protein consists of the amounts of albumin and globulins combined. The test is nonspecific because it does not provide information about specific globulin components or identify the cause of the abnormal value. A low total serum protein value (<4.0 g/dL or SI: <40g/L), together with a low albumin value, causes edema to occur.

Albumin

P

Albumin is the largest component of the plasma proteins and is responsible for most of the colloidal osmotic pressure within the blood. Albumin also serves as a reserve nitrogen source for tissue growth and healing, and it is a transport vehicle for many substances. If water or plasma is lost from the vascular fluid, a high level of albumin will occur. Because of the reduced fluid volume, the albumin shows a relative rise in more concentrated blood.

Decreased albumin can occur from a variety of sources. Liver disease or malnutrition may result in decreased protein synthesis (protein manufacture). Albumin can be lost in renal disease, inflammatory disease of the intestine, or loss of skin as in advanced dermatitis or extensive burns. Lastly, the albumin level may be decreased because of a hypermetabolic disorder that consumes the protein at a very fast rate.

A low serum albumin level causes a low blood pressure. If the liver is unable to respond and manufacture sufficient new albumin, fluid will leak out of the blood vessels and the blood pressure falls because of hypovolemia. Edema will result from a serum albumin level of 2.0 to 2.5 g/dL (SI: 20 to 25 g/L) or less.

Globulin

Globulin measurement refers to the total of all the globulin proteins: alpha, beta, and gamma globulins. Each component globulin has a specific function, but generally, the globulins are either enzymes or immunologic agents (antibodies).

Albumin-to-Globulin Ratio

Albumin-to-globulin ratio is a calculation obtained by dividing the albumin value by the globulins value. In normal conditions, there is substantially more albumin than globulins in the blood. A normal ratio is greater than 1. If there is a severe loss of albumin or a greater amount of globulin synthesis, the ratio drops to less than 1.

NORMAL VALUES	**Adults and Older Children*** Total protein: 6–7.8 g/dL *or* SI: 60–78 g/L Albumin: 3.2–4.5 g/dL *or* SI: 32–45 g/L Globulin: 2.3–3.5 g/dL *or* SI: 23–35 g/L Albumin-to-globulin ratio: >1
▼ Critical Values	Albumin: <1.5 g/dL *or* SI: <15g/L

*Values in babies and very young children are lower than those of adults.

HOW THE TEST IS DONE

A venipuncture is performed to collect 10 mL of venous blood in a red-topped tube or 5 mL of venous blood in a green-topped tube.

For newborns, a capillary tube is used to collect blood from a heelstick puncture.

SIGNIFICANCE OF TEST RESULTS

Elevated Values

Total Protein

Dehydration
Hyperimmunoglobulinemia
Polyclonal or monoclonal gammopathies

Albumin

Dehydration

Globulin

Inflammatory conditions
Waldenström's macroglobulinemia
Multiple myeloma
Collagen diseases
Sarcoidosis
Cirrhosis
Chronic, active hepatitis

Decreased Values

Total Protein

Protein losing enteropathies
 Crohn's disease
 Ulcerative colitis
 Intestinal fistula
Acute burns of the skin
Nephrotic syndrome
Severe protein deficiency

Chronic liver disease
Malabsorption syndrome
Agammaglobulinemia

Albumin

Rapid hydration or overhydration with intravenous fluids
Infection and fever
Malnutrition
Cirrhosis
Chronic alcoholism
Nephrotic syndrome
Cancer
Protein-losing intestinal diseases
  Crohn's disease
  Ulcerative colitis
  Draining fistula
Skin burns
Severe skin disease
Hyperthyroidism

Globulin

Agammaglobulinemia
Hypogammaglobulinemia
Protein-losing intestinal disease
Multiple myeloma

Albumin-to-Globulin Ratio

Cirrhosis and other liver diseases
Chronic glomerulonephritis
Nephrotic syndromes
Waldenström's macroglobulinemia
Sarcoidosis
Collagen diseases
Severe infections
Severe or chronic inflammatory disease
Ulcerative colitis
Cachexia
Multiple myeloma
Severe burns

INTERFERING FACTORS

- Prolonged bedrest
- Massive intravenous transfusion
- Venous stasis
- Peripheral vascular collapse
- Hyperlipidemia
- Hyperbilirubinemia

NURSING CARE

Nursing actions are similar to those used in other venipuncture and capillary puncture procedures (see Chapter 2), with the following additional measures.

Pretest

- The nurse instructs the patient to fast from food and fluid for 8 hours before the test. The fats in food intake would elevate the test results.

During the Test

- The blood sample should be drawn from the arm that does not have an intravenous fluid administration set because intravenous fluids will dilute the blood and lower the test values falsely. The venipuncture procedure should be done efficiently because a prolonged application of the tourniquet will elevate the test results falsely.

▽ Nursing Response to Critical Values

If the albumin level drops to the critical value of <1.5 g/dL (SI: <15 g/L), the patient is so severely depleted of albumin that the blood pressure cannot be maintained. Usually, the decline in albumin and blood pressure is gradual, but at this critical level, the patient is likely to be in hypovolemic shock and could develop vascular collapse, leading to death. The nurse notifies the physician of the laboratory test result and of any abnormal assessment findings.

The nurse takes the vital signs and notifies the physician of the lab results and the assessment results. In shock, the blood pressure is below 120/80 and the pulse is greater than 120. Respirations are usually rapid (>24), and dyspnea is common. The patient's color is pale or cyanotic and the skin feels cold and clammy.

Protein, Urine, 24-Hour

proh-teen, yur-in, twen-tee–fohr-our

Also called: Protein Quantitative

SPECIMEN OR TYPE OF TEST: Urine

PURPOSE OF THE TEST

The urine protein test is used to help confirm the presence of renal disease.

BASICS THE NURSE NEEDS TO KNOW

Protein is minimally present in the urine of individuals with normal renal function. The urinary proteins consist of albumin and many small globulins. In normal renal anatomy and physiology, the albumin molecules are large and most cannot be filtered through the glomerular membrane. The smaller globulins are filtered by the glomeruli, but most are resorbed by the proximal tubules. Additional glycoproteins are secreted by cells in the distal tubules and the ascending Henle's loop. These minimal losses of protein into the urine are considered normal. A value greater than 150 mg/24 hr is called proteinuria.

Urinary protein levels can increase after strenuous exercise, with salt depletion, or during a period of dehydration or febrile illness. These events cause a higher level of proteinuria but are not considered indications of renal or urinary tract disease.

NORMAL VALUES

40–150 mg/24 hr *or* SI: 40–150 mg/24 hr

HOW THE TEST IS DONE

A 24-hour urine specimen is collected in a large, clear, glass or plastic container.

SIGNIFICANCE OF TEST RESULTS

Elevated Values

Glomerulonephritis
Renal transplant rejection
Tubular necrosis
Chronic pyelonephritis
Nephrotic syndrome
Diabetic glomerulosclerosis
Renal failure
Urinary tract infection
Toxemia of pregnancy
Multiple myeloma
Congestive heart failure
Malignant hypertension

INTERFERING FACTORS

- Contamination of the specimen with mucus, vaginal or prostatic secretions, or white blood cells
- Dilute urine from excessive fluid intake
- Failure to collect all urine
- Warming of the specimen

P

NURSING CARE

Nursing actions related to timed urine collection procedures are presented in Chapter 2, with the following additional measures.

Pretest

- ***Patient Teaching.*** Instruct the patient to collect all urine for a 24-hour period. The specimen must be refrigerated or kept on ice throughout the test period. The nurse advises the patient to drink a regular amount of fluids during the test period.

During the Test

- Have the patient void at 8 AM and discard the urine.
- The test period starts at this time, and all urine is collected for 24 hours, including the 8 AM specimen of the following morning.
- Ensure that the patient's name and the time and date of the start and finish of the test are written on the label and requisition slip.

Posttest

- Keep the specimen refrigerated until it is transported to the laboratory.

Prothrombin Time

proh-throm-bin taim

Also called: (PT); Pro Time

SPECIMEN OR TYPE OF TEST: Serum

PURPOSE OF THE TEST

The prothrombin time test is used to evaluate the extrinsic coagulation system; to help screen for coagulation deficiency of Factors I, II, V, VII, and X; and to monitor oral anticoagulant therapy. It also is used to investigate the effects of liver failure and disseminated intravascular coagulation (DIC) and to screen for vitamin K deficiency.

BASICS THE NURSE NEEDS TO KNOW

The prothrombin time test measures the amount of time needed to form a clot. The clot formation is dependent on the functional integrity of coagulation Factors II, V, VII, and X. A deficiency of any of these factors prolongs the prothrombin time. Each test includes the control time in the report of the patient's value. The control time is the normal reference value to be used in the evaluation of the patient's test result.

One use of the prothrombin time test is to monitor the effect of anticoagulant warfarin (Coumadin) therapy. This anticoagulant prolongs the prothrombin time and prevents deep vein thrombosis, pulmonary embolism, myocardial infarction, and other conditions with potential for clot formation. The response to oral anticoagulation varies among individuals and is unpredictable. If an excessive level exists, there is a risk for hemorrhage. If the level is inadequate, there is an ongoing risk is for thrombus formation.

International Normalized Ratio

The Internationalized Normalized Ratio (INR) is a special mathematical calculation of the prothrombin time, used to monitor the effect of an oral anticoagulant. For the patient receiving oral anticoagulant therapy with warfarin (Coumadin), the therapeutic range of the INR is 2.0 to 3.0. For the patient with a mechanical heart valve, the therapeutic range of the INR is 2.5 to 3.5.

Some diseases cause an increased value of the prothrombin time. Severe liver disease and injured liver cells are unable to use fat-soluble vitamin K to manufacture clotting factors.

An elevated prothrombin time value also will occur when fat-soluble vitamin K cannot be absorbed from the intestine because of hepatobiliary or pancreatic obstruction. When vitamin K cannot reach the liver, it is unavailable for the manufacture of clotting factors. DIC is an acute disorder of coagulation that results in formation of microthrombi and bleeding. As part of a DIC panel of tests, the prothrombin time is severely elevated in this disease (see also Disseminated Intravascular Coagulation Screen, p. 274).

NORMAL VALUES	PT: 10–14 seconds INR: 1.00–1.30
▼ Critical Values	PT: >30 seconds INR: 4–5 or higher

HOW THE TEST IS DONE

A blue-topped tube with sodium citrate is used to obtain 4.5 mL of venous blood. As an alternative, a heelstick, earlobe, or finger puncture may be used to collect capillary blood in siliconized sodium citrate micropipettes.

SIGNIFICANCE OF TEST RESULTS

Elevated Values

Excess anticoagulant therapy
DIC
Fibrinogen deficiency
Prothrombin deficiency
Deficiency of vitamin K
Liver disease
Hepatobiliary or pancreatic obstruction

INTERFERING FACTORS

- Lipemia

NURSING CARE

Nursing actions are similar to those used in other venipuncture procedures (see Chapter 2), with the following additional measures.

Pretest

- If the patient receives intermittent doses of heparin, the nurse ensures that the blood is drawn at least 2 hours after the last dose. Recent heparin administration prolongs the prothrombin time excessively.
- ***Patient Teaching.*** The nurse instructs the patient to discontinue intake of alcohol and caffeine for 24 hours before the test. Lipemia from these substances interferes with the accuracy of the test.

During the Test

- If the patient receives intravenous heparin, the blood should be drawn from a vein in the opposite arm from that which has the intravenous infusion or heparin lock device.

Posttest

- Ensure that the venipuncture site has sealed and that the patient is not bleeding. The nurse uses sterile gauze to apply pressure to the puncture site as needed. Keeping pressure on the site, the patient can also raise his or her arm overhead. The combination of pressure and elevation should help promote coagulation.

NURSING CARE—*cont'd*

- As warfarin (Coumadin) therapy is started, the PT and INR measurements are generally done once a day. While the dosage is being increased, the nurse monitors the laboratory results for an excess anticoagulation effect. After the therapeutic range has been reached and is stable, the PT and INR testing is done about once a month.
- ***Patient Teaching.*** The nurse instructs the patient to maintain a routine, prescribed schedule of blood testing to monitor the anticoagulant effect. The nurse also teaches the patient to recognize early signs of bleeding that could indicate excessive anticoagulation. If bleeding occurs, the patient should notify the physician of the problem, immediately.

▼ Nursing Response to Critical Values

The physician should be notified immediately of a severe elevation of the PT or INR result, because a high risk of hemorrhage exists. The nurse assesses the patient for signs of spontaneous bleeding, including petechiae (small red hemorrhagic spots on the skin), ecchymosis (bruising), hematoma, blood in the urine, feces, or gastric secretions, and bleeding in the mucous membranes, particularly the gingiva (gums) in the oral cavity. Vital signs are taken and monitored frequently thereafter, until the risk of bleeding has diminished.

If the patient receives warfarin (Coumadin) anticoagulant medication and the INR value is severely elevated, the nurse should withhold the next dose until the physician responds. The physician may reduce or discontinue the medication temporarily. When the INR is >5 without bleeding, the nurse also prepares to give the antidote of vitamin K, as prescribed. If this is not successful or the patient is bleeding, the physician may prescribe fresh frozen plasma, to be given intravenously. This infusion provides replacement of coagulation factors that will help stop the bleeding.

P

Pulmonary Function Studies

pul-muh-na-ree funk-shun stu-deez

SPECIMEN OR TYPE OF TEST: Spirometry

PURPOSE OF THE TEST

Pulmonary function studies are performed to evaluate the patient's respiratory status, especially those experiencing shortness of breath or other breathing difficulty. These studies may be used to evaluate the therapy for or progression of obstructive and restrictive lung disease. Portions of the test are used as parameters for weaning patients from mechanical ventilation and as part of preoperative evaluations.

A challenge or provocation test is included as part of the pulmonary function studies in patients with suspected hypersensitivity of the airways. *Bronchial provocation tests* or *bronchial challenge tests* are performed for patients who have symptoms suggestive of asthma but who do not show evidence of air flow limitations. They may be used to assess airway function over time and to evaluate various therapeutic interventions.

BASICS THE NURSE NEEDS TO KNOW

Spirometry is a method of measuring the volume of gas that moves into and out of the lungs. The patient breathes through a tube connected to the spirograph, which records on a moving sheet of paper the volume of gas displaced in the spirometer. Two or more volumes form a pulmonary capacity (Figure 77).

The pulmonary volumes consist of the tidal volume (Vt), inspiratory reserve volume (IRV), expiratory reserve volume (ERV), and residual volume (RV).The Vt, the normal volume of air inhaled or exhaled during a single breath in a resting state, is normally 5 to 7 mL/kg body weight. Minute volume (MV) is obtained by multiplying the Vt by the respiratory rate.

The IRV is the amount of air that can be inspired over and above the inspired Vt. The ERV is the air remaining in the lungs, which can be expelled after a normal exhalation. The RV is the amount of air remaining in the lungs that cannot be forcibly expelled.

Pulmonary capacities consist of vital capacity (VC), inspiratory capacity (IC), functional residual capacity (FRC), and total lung capacity (TLC).

The VC is the amount of air that can be expelled from the lungs after a maximum inspiration: VC = Vt + IRV + ERV. A timed VC expresses the volume of air expelled forcibly over a certain amount of time. This forced expiratory volume (FEV) provides an index of pulmonary function. It is the amount of gas exhaled over a given period. It is reported with a subscript to indicate time in seconds. The FEV_1 is the amount of air expelled in the first second of forced exhalation after a maximal inspiration. FEV_2 refers to the amount of air expelled in the first 2 seconds, and FEV_3 is the amount of air expelled in 3 seconds. FEV is reported as a percentage of the forced vital capacity (FVC).

In cases of obstructive and restrictive lung disease, FEV_1 decreases. With obstructive lung disease, this decrease in FEV_1 is the result of increased resistance to outflow. With restrictive lung disease, the decrease in FEV_1 is the result of a decreased ability to inhale an adequate volume of air. Therefore, with restrictive lung disease, an FEV_1 to FVC ratio is a more accurate parameter for evaluating patient status and treatment.

P

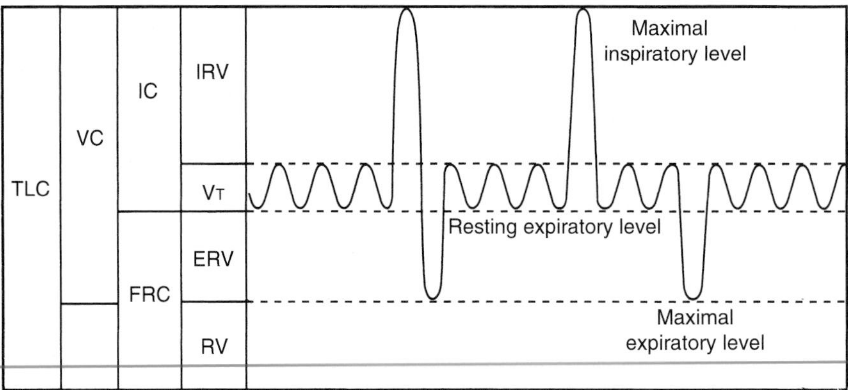

Figure 77. Pulmonary volumes and capacities.

In addition to FEV, the average rate of flow for a specific segment of the FVC may be measured while the FVC is being assessed. The segment measured is usually between 25% and 75% of the FVC. Previously called the maximum midexpiratory flow rate (MMEF), it is now called forced expiratory flow ($FEF_{25\%-75\%}$). The $FEF_{25\%-75\%}$ is the mean rate of expiratory air flow between 25% and 75% of the FVC.

The IC is the maximal amount of air that can be inspired: IC = Vt + IRV. The FRC is the amount of air left in the lungs after a normal resting exhalation: FRC = ERV + RV. The TLC is the amount of air in the lungs after a maximal inspiration: TLC Vt + IRV + ERV + RV.

In addition to the volumes and capacities, maximum voluntary ventilation (MVV) may or may not be determined. The MVV is the total amount of air that is moved into and out of the respiratory tract over 12 seconds with the patient's maximum effort to breathe quickly and deeply. The result is multiplied by 5 and expressed in liters per minute. It is sometimes called maximum breathing capacity.

An estimated volume of pulmonary function is called dead space volume (Vds). The Vds is that portion of inhaled air or gas that does not take part in gas exchange. It is made up of the anatomic dead space (area from the nose and mouth to the terminal bronchioles) and alveolar dead space (areas of the lungs that are not perfused). Physiologic Vd consists of the anatomic Vd and the alveolar Vd. Normally, no measurable alveolar Vd exists. However, anatomic Vd usually is 1 mL of Vd per pound of body weight or 2 mL of Vd per kilogram of ideal body weight. The alveolar Vd increases with pathologic states that decrease blood flow to the lungs.

Pulmonary volumes may also be used to assess alveolar ventilation. *Alveolar ventilation* is estimated by taking the Vt and subtracting the Vds (Vt –Vds).

Varied measurements of the work of breathing can be obtained with pulmonary function studies, including the assessment of respiratory muscle strength. These measurements include the *Pimax test, Pdimax test, sniff test,* and *Pemax test*. The Pimax test involves measuring the intrathoracic pressure while the patient attempts to inspire as forcibly as possible against an occluded airway after a maximal exhalation. The Pdimax test measures transdiaphragmatic pressure (Pdi) while the patient tries to inspire as forcibly as possible against an occluded airway after a maximal exhalation. The sniff test is similar to the Pimax and Pdimax tests, only instead of attempting to inspire, the patient attempts a forceful maximal sniff. The Pemax test is measured while the patient attempts to forcibly exhale against an occluded airway after a maximal inspiration. Maximum cooperation of the patient is required.

A challenge or provocation test is included as part of the pulmonary function studies in patients with suspected hypersensitivities of the airways. *Bronchial provocation tests* or *bronchial challenge tests* are performed as part of the pulmonary function studies for patients who have symptoms suggestive of asthma but who do not show evidence of air flow limitations. They also may be used to assess airway function over time and to evaluate various therapeutic interventions. The provocation tests are contraindicated for anyone whose baseline FEV is less than 1.5 L, who has a history of severe responses to identifiable antigens, or who has had a viral infection of the upper airway within 8 weeks before the test.

Various substances can be used in the provocation test. Inhalation challenges are performed with methacholine or histamine. The *methacholine challenge test* and the *histamine challenge test* use nonspecific agents, which are usually administered with a nebulizer. Specific agents may also be given by inhalation. These specific antigens are given in varying concentrations. When indicated, the patient may be exposed to occupational inhalants.

Instead of inhalational stimulants, oral challenges may be given, but these take several hours or days. Substances ingested are acetylsalicylic acid (aspirin), tartrazine, sodium salicylate, metabisulfite, and monosodium glutamate.

An *exercise challenge* may be used to induce bronchospasms, which are characteristic of hyperresponsive airways when they occur after short-term exercise. Before the test is performed, a baseline FEV_1 is obtained. The exercise challenge is accomplished with either a treadmill or an exercise bike under controlled environmental temperature and humidity. With 5 to 10 minutes of exercise, the heart rate usually reaches at least 80% of the predicted maximum heart rate. The exercise is stopped, and the FEV_1 is measured.

The provocation tests are considered abnormal if there is a 20% or greater fall in FEV_1. At the end of the provocation test, a bronchodilator may be given by inhalation, and postbronchodilator pulmonary function may be evaluated.

NORMAL VALUES

Adults (70-kg man; values are 20% to 25% lower in women)
Tidal volume (Vt): 500 mL
Inspiratory reserve volume (IRV): 3100 mL
Expiratory reserve volume (ERV): 1200 mL
Residual volume (RV): 1200 mL
Vital capacity (VC): 4800 mL
Inspiratory capacity (IC): 3600 mL
Functional residual capacity (FRC): 2400 mL
Total lung capacity (TLC): 6000 mL
FEV_1: 84%
FEV_2: 94%
FEV_3: 97%

P

HOW THE TEST IS DONE

Pulmonary function studies are usually performed in the respiratory therapy department or in a physician's office. To establish a closed system with the spirometer, a nose clip is placed over the patient's nose, and the spirometer's mouthpiece is held in the mouth with the patient's lips maintaining an airtight seal. The patient is then instructed when to breath normally, inhale maximally, and exhale maximally. This procedure is repeated several times.

SIGNIFICANCE OF TEST RESULTS

Elevated Values

FRC

Chronic obstructive pulmonary disease

FEV
Chronic obstructive pulmonary disease

Decreased Values
V_T
Atelectasis
Fatigue
Pneumothorax
Pulmonary congestion
Restrictive lung disease
Tumors
IRV
Asthma
Exercise
Obstructive pulmonary disease
ERV
Ascites
Kyphosis
Obesity
Pleural effusion
Pneumothorax
Pregnancy
Scoliosis
RV
Advanced age
Obstructive pulmonary disease
FEV
Restrictive pulmonary disease
FRC
Adult respiratory distress syndrome
IC
Restrictive pulmonary disease
VC
Diaphragm restriction
Drug overdose with hypoventilation
Neuromuscular diseases
Restrictive or depressed thoracic movement

INTERFERING FACTORS

- Fatigue
- Lack of patient cooperation
- Smoking
- Abdominal distention or pregnancy
- Poor seal around mouthpiece (or tube)
- Medications
- Analgesics, bronchodilators, sedatives

NURSING CARE

Pretest

- Assess the patient's cardiac status. Hold the test and notify the physician if the patient has a history of angina or recent myocardial infarction.
- ***Patient Teaching.*** The nurse can maximize patient cooperation by explaining the procedure and the need for full participation. Demonstrate the nose clip and mouthpiece. The patient should wear dentures if necessary for a proper mouth seal. Instruct the patient not to smoke for 6 hours before the test.
- The nurse checks with the physician about administering bronchodilator and intermittent positive-pressure breathing therapy before the test.
- Ensure that no constricting clothes are worn.
- Ensure that oral intake is light to prevent stomach distention.
- The nurse instructs the patient to void immediately before the test.
- Schedule the test before any other tests or procedures that may fatigue the patient.

During the Test

- If an abnormal response to a specific substance occurs during a provocation test, a placebo substance should be given to ensure that the bronchospasms were not induced by the spirometry.

Posttest

- Advise the patient to resume normal diet and activity. The patient can resume taking medications and therapies as prescribed.

Radioactive Iodine Uptake Study

ray-dee-oh-<u>ak</u>-tiv ai-oh-dain <u>up</u>-tayk <u>stu</u>-dee

Also called: (RAIU)

R

SPECIMEN OR TYPE OF TEST: Nuclear Imaging

PURPOSE OF THE TEST

The radioactive iodine uptake test assesses thyroid function to confirm the diagnosis of hyper- or hypothyroidism.

BASICS THE NURSE NEEDS TO KNOW

Radioactive iodine uptake can be a helpful index of thyroid function, because the thyroid gland takes up from the extracellular fluid only the amount of iodine it needs for the synthesis of the thyroid hormones. The iodide not used is excreted in the urine. The thyroid gland does not distinguish between radioactive and nonradioactive iodine.

Generally, the greater the amount of thyroid hormone produced, the greater the need for iodine and the higher the radioactive iodine uptake. Usually, radioactive iodine uptake increases with hyperthyroidism and decreases with hypothyroidism.

NORMAL VALUES After 24 hours: 10%–30% uptake by the thyroid gland

HOW THE TEST IS DONE

Sodium iodine-123 is given to the patient orally. After 24 hours, a gamma scintillation counter is used to measure the radioactivity of the thyroid gland.

SIGNIFICANCE OF TEST RESULTS

Elevated Values

Hashimoto's thyroiditis
Hyperthyroidism
Hypoalbuminemia
Iodine-deficient goiter
Lithium ingestion

Decreased Values

Excessive iodide intake
Hypothyroidism
Thyrotoxicosis as a result of ectopic thyroid metastasis, subacute thyroiditis, or thyrotoxicosis factitia

INTERFERING FACTORS

- Dietary intake of iodized foods (e.g., salt, bread)
- Iodine-deficient diet
- Previous radiographic studies with iodine-based dye
- Severe diarrhea
- Renal failure
- Noncompliance with dietary restrictions
- Medications such as anticoagulants, antihistamines, antithyroid medications, corticosteroids, lithium, multivitamins, penicillin, phenothiazides, phenylbutazone, salicylates, and thyroid hormones

R

NURSING CARE

Pretest

- The nurse obtains a medication history to determine if any interfering drugs were taken.
- Schedule any x-ray studies requiring dyes for after the radioactive iodine uptake study.
- Ensure that a signed consent form has been obtained.
- ***Patient Teaching.*** Instruct the patient not to eat or drink for 12 hours before the test.
- ***Patient Teaching.*** Describe the scanning equipment to the patient. The probe is placed over the anterior portion of the neck. Emphasize that no discomfort is involved but that the patient must lie absolutely still while the scan is performed. The nurse informs the patient that the oral radioactive iodine must be ingested. It has little or no taste. It comes in capsule or liquid form. Explain to the patient the need for two scans, because the uptake of the radioactive iodine is usually maximized at 24 hours but some thyroid conditions may cause the peak uptake to occur earlier.

Continued

NURSING CARE—*cont'd*

Pretest—*cont'd*

- Transport the patient to the nuclear medicine laboratory when scheduled.

During the Test

- Two hours after ingestion of the radioactive iodine, a light meal may be consumed.

Posttest

- The patient resumes a normal diet.
- The nurse monitors the patient for allergic response to the dye.
- Wear gloves for 24 hours after the test when handling the patient's bedpan or urinal. Wash hands with soap and water after removing gloves.
- ***Patient Teaching.*** Instruct the patient to wash hands with soap and water after voiding for 24 hours. The radionuclide has low dose radioactivity and has a 13-hour half-life. The nuclear material is excreted in the urine. For about 1 day, radioactive material could remain on the hands and can be removed by handwashing.

Radionuclide Thyroid Scanning

ray-dee-oh-noo-klaid thai-royd skan-ing

SPECIMEN OR TYPE OF TEST: Nuclear imaging

PURPOSE OF THE TEST

Radionuclide thyroid scanning is done to support the diagnosis of hyper- or hypothyroidism, thyroid cancer, and cyst.

BASICS THE NURSE NEEDS TO KNOW

R

To produce its hormones, the thyroid gland must extract iodide from the extracellular fluid. Once it has taken up enough iodide to meet its needs, the iodide left in the extracellular fluid is excreted in the urine. The thyroid gland cannot distinguish between dietary iodine and radioactive iodine. Thus, it will take up the radioactive iodide, which can be scanned by a gamma camera. The functioning of the thyroid gland can be evaluated by the amount of radioactive iodide it takes up. In thyrotoxic states, more iodide is needed and the uptake is increased, whereas in hypothyroid states, less than normal amounts of iodide are needed, thus less is taken up by the thyroid gland.

Additional information on nuclear scans is presented on pp. 473 to 483.

NORMAL VALUES Normal anatomic position and size, with homogenous (equally distributed) uptake of the isotopes throughout the glandular tissue

HOW THE TEST IS DONE

Radioactive iodine is given orally or Tc 99m is given intravenously. Scanning is done with a gamma camera.

SIGNIFICANCE OF TEST RESULTS

Increased Uptake

Hyperthyroidism

Decreased Uptake

Hypothyroidism
Cretinism

In addition to an increase or decrease in uptake by the thyroid gland, scanning may also identify "hot" or "cold" spots. Cold nodules are areas of the gland that take up less or no radioactive iodine. Hot nodules are areas that take up more radioactive iodine than does the surrounding tissue. Cold spots may indicate cancer, whereas hot spots are usually not malignant. An echogram (sonogram) may be obtained to distinguish if the cold spot is a solid or semicystic lesion or a pure cyst. Pure cysts are rarely cancerous.

INTERFERING FACTORS

- Ingestion of foods and medications containing iodine
- Recent radiology studies using iodine-based contrast

NURSING CARE

Pretest

- The nurse asks the patient if he or she is allergic to iodine or seafood.
- Ask women if they are pregnant or breast-feeding.
- Ask if any x-ray studies requiring contrast media have been performed within the past 2 months.
- ***Patient Teaching.*** Instruct the patient to avoid iodized salt or iodinated salt substitutes and seafood for a week before the test. The nurse also instructs the patient not to eat or drink for 12 hours before the test. Warn the patient that when the intravenous radioactive iodine is given, he or she may feel warm, flushed, and nauseated. The nurse tells the patient deep breathing may relieve the nausea.
- The nurse checks with the physician to determine if the medications that interfere with the test are to be withheld.
- Make sure that an informed consent form is signed.
- ***Patient Teaching.*** Inform the patient that the procedure takes approximately 20 minutes.
- Transport the patient to the nuclear medicine laboratory.

During the Test

- Iodine-123 is given orally and imaging is done after 24 hours. When Tc 99m is given intravenously, imaging is done 20 minutes later. The different types of contrast media are taken up by the thyroid at different time intervals.

Posttest

- The patient resumes a normal diet.

Continued

NURSING CARE—*cont'd*

Posttest—*cont'd*

- ***Patient Teaching.*** Instruct the patient to wash hands with soap and water after voiding for 24 hours. The radionuclide iodine-123 has low dose radioactivity and has a 13-hour half-life. The nuclear material is excreted in the urine. For about 1 day, radioactive material could remain on the hands and can be removed by handwashing.

Red Blood Cell Count

red blud sel kount

Also called: (RBC); Red Cell Count; Erythrocyte Count

SPECIMEN OR TYPE OF TEST: Blood

PURPOSE OF THE TEST

The red blood cell count may be part of a routine complete blood count, or it may be done separately at regular intervals when the patient's health condition includes an altered number of erythrocytes. The red cell count also is used to evaluate anemia and polycythemia.

BASICS THE NURSE NEEDS TO KNOW

The maintenance of a normal number of erythrocytes in the blood is dependent on the ability of the bone marrow to replace continuously the erythrocytes that are lost or destroyed. Because of the fragility of the cell membrane, the lifespan of the RBC is approximately 120 days. The bone marrow must produce approximately 1 million new erythrocytes per second to maintain adequate replacement.

R

The stimulus for additional production of erythrocytes is cellular oxygen deficiency that triggers the flow of erythropoietin by the kidneys. Erythropoietin stimulates the manufacture of new red blood cells by the bone marrow.

Numerous factors can create an imbalance between erythrocyte production and destruction. With excess production and a normal rate of destruction, the red blood cell count is elevated. With either diminished production or excess destruction of red cells in the blood, their number is decreased.

Variation in Normal Values

The normal red cell count is higher in men than in women, and it is higher in individuals who live at high altitudes. The normal value is lower in men older than age 65 than in younger men. The red cell count is 5% to 6% lower when the blood is drawn from a recumbent patient than from one in an upright position.

Elevated Values

Increases in the red cell count may be a result of hyperactivity of the bone marrow cells or of an increase in erythropoietin from renal disease. Relative polycythemia may also produce an increased red cell count. When this problem is caused by dehydration, there are a normal number of erythrocytes, but they are more concentrated in the diminished fluid volume of the plasma.

Decreased Values

Decreases in the red blood cell count can occur from an excessive loss of cells, as in hemorrhage. It can also occur because of rapid or accelerated hemolysis of the red blood cells. When the bone marrow tissue is damaged, or when a lack of erythropoietin from renal disease exists, too few red cells are produced, and the blood count is low.

NORMAL VALUES Male: $4.5–5.9 \times 10^6/\mu L$ *or* SI: $4.5–5.9 \times 10^{12}/L$
Female: $4.5–5.1 \times 10^6/\mu L$ *or* SI: $4.5–5.1 \times 10^{12}/L$

HOW THE TEST IS DONE

A purple-topped tube with EDTA is used to collect 7 mL of venous blood. As an alternative, two purple-tipped capillary tubes can be used to collect blood from a heelstick, earlobe, or finger puncture. After the blood is collected, the tube is gently inverted five to ten times to mix the anticoagulant and prevent clotting.

SIGNIFICANCE OF TEST RESULTS

Elevated Values

Polycythemia vera
Secondary polycythemia
Hemoconcentration
Dehydration
Renal carcinoma
Cerebral hemangioblastoma
Renal cyst

Decreased Values

Anemia
Hemolytic anemia
Aplastic anemia
Hemodialysis treatment
Immune response with hemolysis
Hemodilution
Excess intravenous fluids
Cirrhosis
Recent hemorrhage or blood loss
Bone marrow failure
Glucose-6-phosphate dehydrogenase deficiency
Sickle cell anemia and other hemoglobinopathies
Leukemia
Hodgkin's disease

INTERFERING FACTORS

- Hemolysis
- Coagulation of the specimen
- Hemodilution

NURSING CARE

Nursing measures include care of the venipuncture or capillary puncture site as described in Chapter 2, with the following additional measures.

Pretest

- Plan to obtain the specimen when the patient is calm and rested. Exercise, exertion, and fear all increase the red blood cell count.

During the Test

- Ensure that the arm or hand that has an intravenous line or saline lock is not used to obtain the specimen. Intravenous fluid dilutes the blood and falsely decreases the cell count.

Posttest

- When value of the red cell count is lower than normal, the patient is anemic. The nurse also monitors the laboratory results of the hemoglobin and hematocrit, as these values will also be lower than normal. In some conditions, such as glucose-6-phosphate dehydrogenase deficiency, sickle cell anemia, or other hemoglobinopathy, the patient must contend with a chronic, life-long anemia problem. In other cases, such as during treatment with chemotherapy or radiation, the effect of bone marrow suppression, or after a hemorrhage, the anemia is a more recent development. Medical intervention depends on the origin of the red blood cell or bone marrow problem.
- The nurse assesses for signs of anemia, including pallor, fatigue, dyspnea on exertion, palpitations, and dizziness. The patient's main problems are activity intolerance and fatigue. The problems occur because there are too few red blood cells to supply sufficient oxygen to the cells, and the heart must work harder to increase the circulation and use the red cells that are available. The nurse can assist the patient to cope with these problems in various ways. Sample nursing interventions include instructing the patient to rest before and after periods of activity, limiting the physical activities, encouraging the patient to perform self-care activities as tolerated, providing assistance when the patient is fatigued and encouraging the patient to move more slowly on arising from a bed or chair. The nurse and the patient can work together to identify when symptoms such as palpitations, dyspnea, or fatigue occur and adjust the plan of care accordingly.

Red Blood Cell Morphology

red blud sel mohr-fo-lo-jee

Also called: Peripheral Blood Smear; Blood Smear Morphology

SPECIMEN OR TYPE OF TEST: Whole blood

PURPOSE OF THE TEST

The cells of the blood are examined to help identify causes of anemia and to evaluate the function of the bone marrow.

BASICS THE NURSE NEEDS TO KNOW

Morphology refers to the shape and structure of cells. Red blood cell morphology is a microscopic or automated analyzer examination of stained red blood cells to identify any altered shapes or structures. In most hematologic diseases, specific characteristic changes can be seen in the blood cells. Changes in the size, structure, and shape of the cells or changes in the number and distribution of the cells may occur, or a combination of these changes may be seen. The microscopic visualization of these changes helps diagnose or confirm the hematologic diagnosis. In addition to red cell morphology, the peripheral smear can be used to examine white blood cell and platelet morphology.

The Shape and Structure of Red Blood Cells

Normal erythrocytes are circular discs of uniform size, color, shape, and appearance. The red cells should be paler in the center than in the periphery. They are described as *normocytic* (normal in size) and *normochromic* (normal in color). The patient can be anemic despite these normal characteristics. A normocytic, normochromic anemia is one that is caused by hemolysis of erythrocytes or blood loss. The cells are normal, but too few of them exist.

Abnormal erythrocytes vary in size, color, hemoglobin content, shape, staining properties, and structure. The altered size is caused by a defect in erythropoiesis. The bone marrow can be adversely affected by genetics, poor nutrition or changes in either bone marrow cells or bone marrow function.

Abnormal color is to the result of an alteration in hemoglobin content. Too little hemoglobin causes a pale color. The problem may be to the result of iron deficiency or abnormal hemoglobin synthesis.

Poikilocytosis refers to abnormally shaped red cells. Abnormal erythrocyte structure includes the presence of a nucleus that identifies these cells as normoblasts, basophilic stippling, Howell-Jolly bodies, or Heinz bodies. The variations of some of the characteristics of erythrocytes, and their relationships to hematologic disease, are presented in Table 13.

NORMAL VALUES

Normal cell shape and structure

HOW THE TEST IS DONE

A purple-topped tube with EDTA is used to collect 7 mL of venous blood. As an alternative, two purple-tipped capillary tubes can be used to collect blood from a heelstick, earlobe, or finger puncture.

For the peripheral blood smear, two slides are prepared immediately using drops of venous or capillary blood.

SIGNIFICANCE OF TEST RESULTS

See Table 13 for abnormal values.

Table 13 Characteristics of Erythrocytes: Relationships to Hematologic Diseases

Characteristics	Interpretation	Pathophysiology	Disorders
Size			
Normocytic	Normal cell size	Adequate response by the bone marrow	None
		Shortened lifespan of the erythrocytes—increased hemolysis	Acute blood loss Hemolytic anemia
		Impaired release of iron from the reticuloendothelial system	Anemia of chronic disease
Macrocytic or megalocytic	Larger than normal cell size	Marrow disorder with defective DNA that affects cell development during erythropoiesis	Deficiency of vitamin B_{12} or folic acid Megaloblastic anemias
		Uptake of cholesterol and bile salts by the erythrocyte membranes	Liver disease and obstructive jaundice
Microcytic	Smaller than normal cell size	Deficiency of heme, a lack of iron, or impaired hemoglobin synthesis	Iron deficiency anemia, thalassemia, sideroblastic anemia, lead poisoning, vitamin B_6 deficiency
Color			
Normochromic	Normal hemoglobin content	Normal iron stores, normal hemoglobin synthesis	Anemia caused by hemorrhage, with loss of erythrocytes
Hyperchromic	Erythrocyte saturated with hemoglobin	A relative increase of hemoglobin within the erythrocyte that has a small diameter and small cell membrane; the cell is spherical	Spherocytosis

Hypochromic	Erythrocyte with diminished hemoglobin	Iron deficiency in proportion to erythropoiesis	Iron deficiency anemia
		Defective hemoglobin synthesis	Thalassemia, lead poisoning, sideroblastic anemia
Shape			
Elliptocyte	Elliptical or oval shape	Cytoplasm and cholesterol in the cell membrane are polarized in areas of convexity; increased hemolysis can occur	Hereditary elliptocytosis, thalassemia, iron deficiency anemia, sickle cell disease, other hemolytic diseases
Spherocyte	Sphere-shaped cell	Genetic disease of the bone marrow; the abnormal cells have a shorter life span	Hereditary spherocytosis, immune disease, and other hemolytic anemias
Target cell	Hemoglobin is distributed on the perimeter and in the center, giving a "target" appearance	Deficient hemoglobin for the normal cell size	Hemoglobin C, D, S diseases, thalassemia, iron deficiency anemia
		Too large a cell membrane and cell size for a normal amount of hemoglobin	Obstructive jaundice, liver disease
Sickle cell	Crescent-shaped cells	In conditions of deoxygenation, the hemoglobin S becomes elongated and rigid; cell membranes also become sickle shaped	Sickle cell trait, sickle cell disease, other sickling hemoglobinopathies
Poikilocytosis	Varied, irregular shapes of cells (teardrop, tennis racket, horned, and helmet shapes)	Irreversible alteration of cell membrane from rapid erythropoiesis or extra-medullary erythropoiesis	Megaloblastic anemia, hemolytic anemia, uremia, liver disease, metastatic cancer, toxicity, idiopathic myelofibrosis

Continued

R

TABLE 13 Characteristics of Erythrocytes: Relationships to Hematologic Diseases—*cont'd*

Characteristics	Interpretation	Pathophysiology	Disorders
Size			
Schistocyte	Red cell fragments	Partial splitting or phagocytosis of the cell, without loss of hemoglobin	Hemolytic anemia, disseminated intravascular coagulation, malignant hypertension, cancer, cardiac valve prosthesis, burns, uremia
Structure			
Nucleated	Normoblasts are immature red cells with nuclei	Normal in fetus or infant, but not in adults; extreme demand on bone marrow to produce cells rapidly	Erythroblastosis fetalis, thalassemia major
		Extramedullary erythropoiesis	Idiopathic myelofibrosis
		With neutrophilia, the bone marrow cells are altered	Leukemia, metastatic cancer of the bone marrow, multiple myeloma, Gaucher's disease
Basophilic stippling	Basophilic granules in cells	Abnormal hemoglobin synthesis and increased erythropoiesis	Lead poisoning, megaloblastic anemia
Howell-Jolly bodies	Remnants of nuclear material in cells	Abnormal erythropoiesis	Postsplenectomy, megaloblastic anemia, hemolytic anemia
Heinz bodies	Irregular patches of hemoglobin in cells	Genetic abnormality of hemoglobin formation; hemoglobin is oxidized and nonfunctional	Cell injury, hemoglobinopathy hemolytic anemia

INTERFERING FACTORS

- Hemolysis
- Coagulated specimen

NURSING CARE

Nursing measures include care of the venipuncture or capillary puncture site as described in Chapter 2. No other special nursing measures are required.

Red Cell Indices

See Complete Blood Count on p. 222.

Renin

re-nin

Also called: Plasma renin activity (PRA)

SPECIMEN OR TYPE OF TEST: Plasma

PURPOSE OF THE TEST

Plasma renin levels are determined as part of hypertension screening and to diagnose primary aldosteronism.

BASICS THE NURSE NEEDS TO KNOW

Renin is a proteolytic enzyme produced and secreted by the juxtaglomerular cells of the kidneys. Renin is secreted whenever a reduction of blood pressure to the kidneys occurs. Renin in the circulation acts on angiotensinogen to form angiotensin I, which is converted to angiotensin II—a powerful vasoconstrictor and stimulant for aldosterone secretion. This action is called the renin-angiotensin-aldosterone system or axis (see Figure 11 on p. 54).

Because renin is a powerful vasoconstrictor, its role in hypertension has been studied. Most patients with hypertension have normal renin levels. Some hypertensive patients with excessive fluid retention have low renin levels, and other hypertensive patients have high renin levels.

It has been difficult to correlate renin levels with clinical states, because renin levels vary between individuals and laboratory techniques vary in the measurement of these levels. In addition, many factors will influence secretion rates of renin, including dietary ingestion of sodium. For this reason, some clinicians correlate renin levels with the sodium content of the patient's diet. The sodium content of the diet is measured by a 24-hour urine sodium level test.

Another method to evaluate renin is to perform a *sodium-depleted renin test*, during which a diuretic (usually furosemide) is given.

NORMAL VALUES (depend on method used and sodium status of the patient)	**Adult**
	With normal sodium:
	Supine position: 0.5–1.6 ng/mL/hr *or* SI: 0.1–0.4 ng/L/sec
	Upright position: 1.9–3.6 ng/mL/hr *or* SI: 0.5–1.0 ng/L/sec
	With low sodium:
	Supine position: 2.2–4.4 ng/mL/hr *or* SI: 0.6–1.2 ng/L/sec
	Upright position: 4.0–8.1 ng/mL/hr *or* SI: 1.1–2.5 ng/L/sec
	After furosemide:
	Upright position: 6.8–15.0 ng/mL/hr *or* SI: 1.9–4.2 ng/L/sec

HOW THE TEST IS DONE

The procedures vary. A random renin test simply requires a venipuncture to obtain 10 mL of blood in a lavender-topped chilled tube. The specimen is placed on ice and immediately sent to the laboratory. If the renin level is to be correlated with sodium intake, a 24-hour urine specimen for sodium and creatinine is required.

If a renin determination from a renal vein is planned, it is carried out under fluoroscopy; a catheter is inserted into the renal vein via the femoral vein access.

SIGNIFICANCE OF TEST RESULTS

Elevated Values

Hypertension
Cirrhosis
Hypovolemia
Hypokalemia
Addison's disease
Chronic renal failure

Decreased Values

Fluid retention with high-sodium diet
Primary aldosteronism
Excessive licorice intake
Hypertension with fluid retention
Cushing syndrome

INTERFERING FACTORS

- Noncompliance with dietary and medication restrictions
- Improper positioning during the test
- Medications such as antihypertensives, clonidine, diuretics, estrogen, minoxidil, nitroprusside, propranolol, reserpine, and vasodilators

NURSING CARE

The actions of the nurse vary depending on the technique used.

Pretest

- Instruct the patient on the technique.
- If a random sampling is ordered, instruct the patient to maintain a prone position or an upright position for 2 hours before the test. The position is based on physician preference.
- If a renal vein level determination is ordered, the nurse explains the need to go to the radiology department for fluoroscopy. Explain equipment, groin preparation, and local anesthesia.
- If a sodium depletion renin test is ordered, assess the patient's cardiovascular status before a diuretic is given.
- ***Patient Teaching.*** Instruct the patient to maintain a low-sodium diet for 3 days before the test.

Posttest

- If the femoral approach to the renal vein is used, assess the site for hematoma and bleeding.

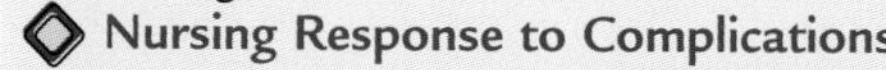

Nursing Response to Complications

The only complications expected with renin evaluation are those associated with femoral vein access. The complications are bleeding and hematoma formation.

Resin Triiodothyronine Uptake

rez-in trai-ai-oh-doh-thai-roh-neen up-tayk

Also called: T_3 resin Uptake Test; RT_3U; T_3 Uptake Ratio; Triiodothyronine Resin Uptake Test; T_3 Uptake

SPECIMEN OR TYPE OF TEST: Serum, plasma

PURPOSE OF THE TEST

The resin triiodothyronine uptake test is performed to diagnose hyper- and hypothyroidism.

BASICS THE NURSE NEEDS TO KNOW

The resin triiodothyronine uptake test is determined to estimate the *free triiodothyronine index* (FT_3I). In many institutions, the assay of free triiodothyronine has replaced the index, because the index is an estimate of the free hormone levels.

The resin triiodothyronine uptake test assesses the capacity of the blood proteins to bind with thyroid hormones. It does not measure the hormones themselves.

NORMAL VALUES

25%–35% *or* SI: 0.25–0.35
Free triiodothyronine index 24–67.

HOW THE TEST IS DONE

Venipuncture is performed to obtain a serum specimen (serum is preferred over plasma) to which radioactive triiodothyronine is added. Radioactive triiodothyronine is used instead of thyroxine because more triiodothyronine is bound to the resin, which has a lower affinity to endogenous protein-binding sites. After the resin is mixed with the radioactive triiodothyronine in serum, it is removed, and the amount of radioactivity absorbed is measured. The tube used may be red, lavender, or green topped, depending on the lab.

The measurement of the free triiodothyronine index is obtained by multiplying the resin uptake and the total thyroid hormone concentration.

SIGNIFICANCE OF TEST RESULTS

Elevated Values

Hyperthyroidism

Decreased Values

Hypothyroidism

INTERFERING FACTORS

- Renal failure
- Recent radioisotope scans
- Malnutrition
- Metastatic disease
- Liver dysfunction
- Critical illness
- Medications such as ACTH, androgens, barbiturates, chlorpromazine, estrogen, furosemide, glucocorticoids, heroin, lithium, methadone, phenylbutazone, propylthiouracil, and thyroid replacement

NURSING CARE

The nurse takes actions similar to those taken in other venipuncture procedures, as discussed in Chapter 2.

Reticulocyte Count

re-tik-yuh-loh-sait kount

Also called: Retic Count

SPECIMEN OR TYPE OF TEST: Blood

PURPOSE OF THE TEST

The reticulocyte count is used to evaluate erythropoiesis, distinguish among different types of anemia, assess the severity of blood loss, and evaluate the bone marrow response to treatment of anemia.

BASICS THE NURSE NEEDS TO KNOW

Reticulocytes are immature erythrocytes. The cells are formed by the bone marrow and 1 to 2 days after they are released into the blood circulation, they mature into erythrocytes (red blood cells) with a full complement of hemoglobin in each cell.

Elevated Values

An increase in reticulocytes indicates the ability of the bone marrow to produce erythrocytes. The elevated value is considered a healthy response to a loss of erythrocytes from hemorrhage or hemolysis. It is also a healthy response to anemia or to a reduced amount of hemoglobin in the red blood cells. The reticulocyte count also may rise after effective treatment of anemia. When the demand for erythrocytes is high, the marrow releases very immature reticulocytes into the blood rather than allow these blood cells to mature for the full time in the marrow. The rise in the reticulocyte is a very positive finding for the patient who has received a bone marrow transplant. After a bone marrow transplant, the rising reticulocyte count means that the transplanted tissue is beginning to function.

Decreased Values

The reduced number of reticulocytes indicates that erythropoiesis is decreased in the bone marrow. The cause may be a lack of stimulation by erythropoietin, a disease that affects the bone marrow cells, or a faulty maturation process in the bone marrow.

NORMAL VALUES

Adult: Percentage of cells: 0.5%–1.5% *or* SI: 0.005–0.015 (number fraction)
Cell count: 25,000–75,000/μL *or* SI: 25–75 × 10^9/L
Newborn: Percentage of cells: 3.0%–7.0% *or* SI: 0.03–0.07 (number fraction)

R

HOW THE TEST IS DONE

A purple-topped tube with EDTA or a green-topped tube with heparin is used to collect 7 mL of venous blood. As an alternative, two purple-tipped capillary tubes can be used to collect blood from a heelstick, earlobe, or finger puncture. After the blood is collected, the tube is inverted five to ten times to mix the anticoagulant and prevent clotting.

SIGNIFICANCE OF TEST RESULTS

Elevated Values

Hemolytic anemia
Hemorrhage
Chronic blood loss

Decreased Values

Aplastic anemia
Iron deficiency anemia
Anemia of chronic disease

Sideroblastic anemia
Red cell aplasia
Renal disease
Endocrine disease
Pernicious anemia
Radiation therapy
Nonfunctioning bone marrow

INTERFERING FACTORS

- Multiple blood transfusions
- Coagulation of the specimen
- Hemolysis

NURSING CARE

Nursing measures include care of the venipuncture or capillary puncture site as described in Chapter 2, with the following additional measures.

Pretest

- If possible, the nurse schedules this test before a blood transfusion is started. Once blood is administered, dilution of the cells occurs, and the reticulocyte count decreases in proportion to the fluid volume. If multiple transfusions were already given, the results of this test are invalid. The reticulocytes are from the transfused blood and do not indicate the current status of the patient's bone marrow function.

During the Test

- The blood sample should not be taken from the arm in which there is intravenous tubing. The fluid administration dilutes the blood and causes a low cell count.

Posttest

- The reticulocyte count gives early, but generalized information about bone marrow function in forming the cells that will become new red blood cells. Additional laboratory tests will be needed to determine the cause of a low reticulocyte count.

Rheumatoid Factor

roo-muh-toid fak-tor

Also called: (RF)

SPECIMEN OR TYPE OF TEST: Serum, synovial fluid

PURPOSE OF THE TEST

The test for rheumatoid factor is used in the diagnosis and prognosis of rheumatoid arthritis.

BASICS THE NURSE NEEDS TO KNOW

Rheumatoid factor is a group of immunoglobulins that are directed against other immunoglobins to form complexes. These immune complexes are found in the blood and synovial fluid. When the immune complexes are at high levels within joints, they may contribute to tissue injury.

At a level of 80 international units/mL or higher, rheumatoid factor is present or positive in the serum of the majority of patients with rheumatoid arthritis and some other rheumatic conditions. A high correlation exists between the presence of rheumatoid factor and rheumatoid arthritis; however, the exact nature of the relationship is unknown. Synovial fluid also can be analyzed for rheumatoid factor, using the patient's joint fluid instead of serum. The test results are comparable.

In rheumatoid arthritis, the highest serum values occur in patients who have severe active disease. The test is not specific to rheumatoid arthritis, however, as patients with Sjögren syndrome also have high serum values of rheumatoid factor. Additionally, positive results at low levels (80 international units/mL or lower) occur in some normal elderly individuals and in those with chronic infection or inflammation from another cause.

NORMAL VALUES Negative: 0–39 international units/mL

HOW THE TEST IS DONE

A red-topped tube is used to collect 10 mL of venous blood.

SIGNIFICANCE OF TEST RESULTS

Positive Values

Rheumatoid arthritis
Sjögren syndrome
Systemic lupus erythematosus
Dermatomyositis
Scleroderma
Polymyositis
Waldenström's disease
Sarcoidosis
Infectious mononucleosis
Subacute bacterial endocarditis
Tuberculosis
Chronic lung disease
Chronic liver disease

INTERFERING FACTORS

- Severe lipemia
- Circulating immune complexes

NURSING CARE

Nursing measures include care of the venipuncture site as described in Chapter 2. No other special nursing measures are required

Rubella Antibody

roo-bel-uh an-tib-od-ee

Also called: German Measles Antibody

SPECIMEN OR TYPE OF TEST: Blood

PURPOSE OF THE TEST

Rubella antibody titer is used to detect the presence of rubella antibodies in the acute or convalescent phase of illness or post vaccination. It also identifies immunity from future infection. The presence of immunoglobulin M (IgM) antibody in the newborn strongly supports the presence of congenital infection.

BASICS THE NURSE NEEDS TO KNOW

Rubella is a viral infection that is transmitted by droplet infection from the nasopharynx of the infected person to the susceptible individual. The virus also can cross the placental barrier of the infected pregnant woman. Rubella infection in the fetus has devastating consequences, particularly if it occurs in the first trimester of pregnancy.

When the rubella IgM and IgG antibodies are negative, the person has not been infected with the rubella virus. It also means that no immunity exists and that the person is susceptible to infection. A positive value of IgM antibody is an indicator of acute infection. In rubella infection, this antibody titer stays positive for 4 to 5 weeks and then disappears. The IgG antibody also rises in infection but then remains elevated for life. The positive value of the IgG antibodies indicates post infection or post vaccination, with immunity to future rubella infection.

If the pregnant woman contracts rubella infection, the fetus could become infected if the virus passes through the placenta. The genetic material (RNA) of the rubella virus can be detected in the amniotic fluid and in the WBCs of fetal blood. If a newborn infant is suspected of congenital rubella, rubella titers are performed. The presence of IgM antibodies in this infant is a strong indicator of the congenital infection.

R

NORMAL VALUES

IgM antibody: Negative
IgG antibody: Negative

HOW THE TEST IS DONE

A red-topped tube is used to collect 10 mL of venous blood.

SIGNIFICANCE OF TEST RESULTS

Positive Values

IgM Antibody

Rubella, acute infection

IgG Antibody

Immunity to future rubella infection

Congenital rubella infection in the fetus or newborn

INTERFERING FACTORS

- None

NURSING CARE

Nursing measures include care of the venipuncture site as described in Chapter 2, with the following additional measures.

Pretest

- ***Patient Teaching.*** The nurse teaches that when IgG antibodies are elevated and positive, the person need not worry about future exposure to rubella infection because he or she has immunity.

Posttest

- If the pregnant woman did not have previous immunity and now tests positive for IgM or IgG antibodies, the fetus has been exposed to rubella infection. The expectant parents will be advised of the risks for the fetus. The nurse provides emotional support to the parents during this stressful time as they learn of the potential harm to the fetus.
- ***Health Promotion.*** If vaccination has not been done, the nurse teaches parents to have their children immunized with the measles, mumps, and rubella (MMR) vaccine at 15 months and again at 4 to 6 or 11 to 12 years of age.
- The nurse also recommends health screening for rubella antibodies to determine susceptibility or immunity. If the young nonpregnant female is negative for rubella IgG antibodies, she should be vaccinated. This will provide her with protection from the infection and will protect the fetus during subsequent pregnancy.

Rubeola Antibody

See Measles Antibody on p. 459.

Severe Acute Respiratory Syndrome Tests

se-veer uh-kyoot res-pir-uh-toh-ree sin-drohm tests

Also called: SARS Tests

SPECIMEN OR TYPE OF TEST: Blood, nasal, and throat secretions; mucus; stool

PURPOSE OF THE TEST

The various specimens are collected to identify the DNA of the SARS virus as the cause of the acute respiratory infection and to distinguish this source of infection from other infectious organisms that cause respiratory illness or pneumonia.

BASICS THE NURSE NEEDS TO KNOW

SARS is a newly discovered corona virus that causes severe and sometimes fatal respiratory illness. The infected person transmits the virus to others via respiratory droplets and person-to-person contact. Possible additional modes of transmission include fomites (as dust particles that are inhaled) or fecal matter. Most cases are transmitted to those who are in close contact with the infected person, such as members of the patient's household, professionals who care for the infected patient, and research laboratory personnel who work with the virus.

NORMAL VALUES

Serology
Immunoglobulin M (IgM) antibodies: Negative
Immunoglobulin G (IgG) antibodies: Negative
Polymerase chain reaction (PCR) testing: Negative for the DNA of the SARS virus

HOW THE TEST IS DONE

All specimens are potentially hazardous and are collected under conditions of strict precautions for airborne droplet and person-to-person contact transmission. The laboratory and epidemiology departments should be contacted before specimen samples are collected. Once the specimens are collected, each is placed in a separate biohazard bag. The bagged specimens are placed in a leak-proof, nonbreakable container with ice for transport to the laboratory.

Samples will be collected from various sources in the body where the virus is known to locate. Other potential infectious organisms may be the cause of the acute respiratory illness.

Blood: A venipuncture is used to collect 5 to 10 mL in a serum separator tube and 5 to 7 mL in a purple-topped EDTA tube.

Nasopharyngeal wash, swab, or aspirate: For the wash or aspirate specimen, 1 to 2 mL of sodium chloride is sprayed into both nasal passages, and the aspirated solution is placed in a sterile container with a leak-proof top. For the swab specimen, a different culture swab is placed in each side of the nose for a few seconds to absorb the secretions. The swabs are then placed in the culture tubes that contain transport media.

Throat (oropharyngeal) culture: With a cultural swab, the posterior pharynx and tonsillar areas are swabbed and the applicator with secretions is placed in the culture tube that contains transport media.

Sputum: The patient rinses the mouth and then performs deep coughing to produce sputum. If the specimen must be obtained by suction, the procedure involves increased risk of transmission from the aerosolization associated with the procedure. The physician collects the specimen during bronchoalveolar lavage, tracheal aspiration, or a bronchoscopy. Any sputum specimens are placed in a sterile cup with a screw-topped, tightly sealed lid.

Feces: Ten to fifty mL of feces is placed in a clean, dry fecal collection container or a urine container. Either one must have a lid.

SIGNIFICANCE OF TEST RESULTS

Abnormal Values

SARS
Influenza

Respiratory syncytial virus (RSV)
Legionella pneumophila
Mycoplasma pneumoniae
Pneumococcal pneumonia

INTERFERING FACTORS

- Inadequate specimen

NURSING CARE

Pretest

- Because of the high risk of nosocomial spread of the virus, the nurse implements Standard (tier 1) precautions for aerosol droplet and person-to-person contact. Guided by the department of epidemiology, the nurse ensures that all personnel follow correct infection control procedures at all times.
- Initially, the patient presents with a fever and complaints of a cough, flu-like symptoms and difficulty breathing. The nurse assesses for additional risk factors that could indicate SARS infection. These include travel within the past 10 days to mainland China, Taiwan, or Hong Kong, working in health care with a patient who had pneumonia from an unknown cause or known SARS infection, and working in a research laboratory with the SARS virus. If the patient has one or more of these risk factors, the nurse places the patient in a private room, instructs the patient to put on a mask, and notifies the physician. Transmission-based (tier 2) precautions for airborne, droplet, and contact transmission will be instituted.

During the Test

- When tracheal suctioning, endotracheal tube insertion or suctioning, or bronchoscopy is used to obtain sputum, the risks of transmission by aerosolization increase. The patient must be placed in a negative pressure room and any health care personnel in the room must wear a respirator (N95 or higher level), goggles or face shield, gloves, and gown.

Posttest

- The specimens are bagged and packed according to infection control procedures and procedures for biohazards. Usually, the hospital laboratory works with the Department of Health and the Center for Disease Control (CDC), regarding analysis of the specimens.

S

Sickle Cell Tests

si-kuhl sel tests

Also called: Dithionite Test; Metabisulfate Test; Sickle Cell Solubility Test; Sickledex

SPECIMEN OR TYPE OF TEST: Blood

PURPOSE OF THE TEST

The sickle cell test is a screening test to detect HbS, the sickling hemoglobin; to evaluate hemolytic anemia; and to help identify the cause of hereditary anemia.

BASICS THE NURSE NEEDS TO KNOW

The normal adult forms of hemoglobin are identified as HbA, HbA_2, and HbF. Sickle cell hemoglobin (HbS) is the most common of the abnormal hemoglobins. The term *sickled* is used because in deoxygenated states, HbS converts the erythrocytes into sickle or crescent shapes (Figure 78).

Sickle cell disease is an autosomal recessive genetic disorder. The homozygous (pure) form of HbS produces the disease of sickle cell anemia. If both parents have the trait mutation, every pregnancy will have a one in four chance of producing a child with sickle cell anemia. The heterozygous (mixed) form of HbS produces sickle cell trait. The infant inherited the sickle cell gene from one parent but not the other. Because all infants are born with 100% hemoglobin F (HbF), sickle cell anemia and sickle cell trait may not be detected by this test method until the baby is age 3 to 6 months. By this time, affected infants have replaced the HbF with HbS, and the test result is positive.

This test has a number of limitations. When the test result is positive, it can only indicate that sickling hemoglobin is present but cannot determine if the positive value is to the result of sickle cell anemia or sickle cell trait. Hemoglobin electrophoresis is the preferred method to confirm the diagnosis and differentiate between sickle cell disease and sickle cell trait. Another limitation is the 3 to 6 month delay in the infant's age before this test can be used. The infant diagnosed with sickle cell disease should begin

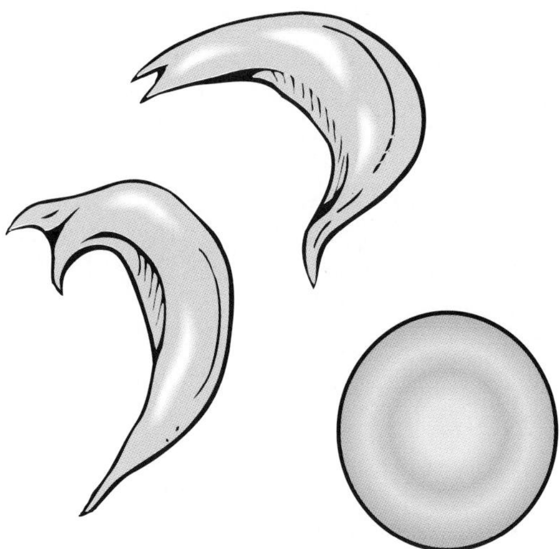

Figure 78. Sickled cells differ significantly from normal cells. *(Reproduced with permission from Stepp, C. A., & Woods, M. A. [1998].* Laboratory procedures for medical office personnel *[Figure 12–24, p. 164]. Philadelphia: W. B. Saunders.)*

comprehensive medical therapy in the first 2 months of life, without the added delay for completion of testing. Today, instead of this test, most states in the United States require hemoglobin electrophoresis as a newborn screening test. Additional discussion of sickle cell anemia and health promotion measures are presented in the test Hemoglobin Electrophoresis (p. 377).

NORMAL VALUES Negative

HOW THE TEST IS DONE

A lavender-topped or green-topped tube is used to collect 7 mL of venous blood. As an alternative method, a fingerstick or earlobe puncture can be performed to obtain a capillary specimen.

SIGNIFICANCE OF TEST RESULTS

Positive Values
Sickle cell anemia
Sickle cell trait

INTERFERING FACTORS

- Hemolysis
- Coagulation of the specimen
- Blood transfusion within the past 3 to 4 months

NURSING CARE

Nursing measures include care of the venipuncture or capillary puncture site as described in Chapter 2, with the following additional measures.

Pretest

- No special nursing intervention is needed.

Posttest

- Provide support to parents who become upset when they learn of the abnormal findings. Additional testing must be performed before any diagnosis is confirmed. With a positive screening test result, assist with the scheduling of a hemoglobin electrophoresis test to determine the exact diagnosis (trait versus disease). Genetic testing may also be used to identify sickle cell trait or disease. Genetic counseling is provided to the parents when the follow-up test confirms the presence of the genetic trait or disease.

S

Sigmoidoscopy and Anoscopy

sig-moid-os-kuh-pee and an-os-kuh-pee

SPECIMEN OR TYPE OF TEST: Endoscopy

PURPOSE OF THE TEST

Sigmoidoscopy is used as a screening test for cancer of the colon. It also is used to investigate the source of unexplained rectal bleeding or infection in the lower colon, to evaluate the postoperative anastomosis of the lower colon, and to diagnose or monitor inflammatory bowel disease. Anoscopy is used to investigate anal symptoms such as bleeding, pain, discomfort, or prolapse.

BASICS THE NURSE NEEDS TO KNOW

Sigmoidoscopy uses a flexible, fiberoptic endoscope (sigmoidoscope) to examine the sigmoid colon and rectum. *Anoscopy* uses a short, blunt anoscope to examine the anus and rectum. Anoscopy is usually performed in conjunction with sigmoidoscopy or colonoscopy.

Sigmoidoscopy is one of the procedures recommended for screening for colorectal cancer. About 50% of colon cancer and polyps of the colon are located in the left colon, between the anus and the splenic flexure. During a sigmoidoscopy procedure, the polyps can be removed and suspicious tissue can be biopsied or cultures taken. Sigmoidoscopy is one method of screening for colorectal cancer. It can be done in the physician's office, without conscious sedation or pain medication. One of the drawbacks of sigmoidoscopy is that 50% of the polyps and cancerous tumors are located between the right colon and transverse colon, beyond the view of the sigmoidoscope. In addition, if polyp or tumor is encountered by sigmoidoscopy, the patient will have to have a follow-up colonoscopy to view the remainder of the colon.

NORMAL VALUES

No tissue abnormalities are seen in the sigmoid colon, rectum, or anus

HOW THE TEST IS DONE

The patient is placed in a lateral or knee-chest (jackknife) position. The well-lubricated instrument is inserted into the anus and advanced to the desired depth. A tissue biopsy or culture specimen may be obtained during the procedure. The time needed for the examination is 5 to 10 minutes.

SIGNIFICANCE OF TEST RESULTS

Abnormal Values

SIGMOIDOSCOPY

Colitis
Polyps
Colorectal cancer
Gay bowel syndrome
Irritable bowel syndrome
Sigmoid volvulus
Crohn's disease
Intestinal ischemia
Parasitic disease

Anoscopy

Hemorrhoids
Fissure
Fistula in ano
Crohn's disease
Pilonidal sinus with abscess
Abscess formation
Polyps
Anal herpes
Colorectal carcinoma
Anal condylomas
Perianal hematoma
Prolapsed rectum

INTERFERING FACTORS

- Uncooperative patient behavior
- Severe bleeding
- Suspected bowel perforation
- Peritonitis
- Acute diverticulitis
- Paralytic ileus

NURSING CARE

- ***Health Promotion.*** In national guidelines and recommendations for routine screening for colorectal cancer, various medical approaches can be used, including colonoscopy, sigmoidoscopy, barium enema, and fecal occult blood test. For sigmoidoscopy, the schedule of the screening test for healthy individuals older than age 50 is to have a sigmoidoscopy at 50, and every 3 to 5 years thereafter, together with an annual fecal occult blood test.
- ***Health Promotion.*** The nurse can help teach people of the importance of colorectal cancer screening. The onset of this disease is usually after age 50 and the risk of developing colorectal cancer increases with each decade thereafter. Screening offers prevention by removal of polyps before they become cancerous and early detection of tumor before symptoms occur. Prevention and early intervention for colorectal cancer has a higher rate of cure.
- ***Health Promotion.*** There is a need for education of the public as to the benefits of regular screening tests. For many years, people were taught to observe for symptoms of disease and then seek medical advice and diagnosis. Today, the emphasis is on screening to detect abnormality before the problem is advanced enough to cause symptoms. The educational focus should include "unlearning" old information as well as learning the new and greatly improved methods of detection.

Continued

NURSING CARE—*cont'd*

Pretest

- Once the physician has explained the test to the patient, the patient signs a consent form. The nurse ensures that the form is placed in the patient's record.
- ***Patient Teaching.*** The nurse explains how the patient will cleanse the bowel before the procedure. Because the protocol for bowel preparation varies, the nurse will teach the protocol that the examining physician uses. The preparation usually consists of administering a combination of laxative and one or two Fleet enemas. The goal is to empty the lower colon of fecal matter.

During the Test

- Assist the patient into a knee chest or side-lying position and drape the patient.
- The nurse provides reassurance and helps promote patient relaxation during the procedure. The patient may be instructed to take a few deep breaths to help relax sphincter muscles as the instrument is inserted. During the passage of the instrument, the patient may feel cramping pain as air is instilled. The nurse can rub the patient's back to help relieve the pain or distract the patient from temporary discomfort.
- The nurse also assists the physician with the collection of tissue or other specimens.

Posttest

- Label any specimen containers with the name of the procedure and the tissue source. Send specimens to the laboratory without delay.
- ***Patient Teaching.*** The nurse instructs the patient that flatulence and mild gas pain may be experienced from the air that was put into the colon during the examination. When a biopsy is performed, it is normal to see a small amount of blood in the stool. These after-effects are temporary. The nurse advises the patient to contact the physician for problems of severe pain, nausea, vomiting, or heavy bleeding.

Single Photon Emission Computed Tomography Scan, Brain

sing-guhl foh-ton e-mi-shun kuhm-pyoo-tuhd tuh-mo-gruh-fee skan, brayn

Also called: SPECT Scan

SPECIMEN OR TYPE OF TEST: Radionuclide scan

PURPOSE OF THE TEST

The cerebral single photon emission computed tomography (SPECT) scan images the brain and is used to investigate cerebrovascular diseases, dementia, epilepsy, and head trauma. It may be used to assess and diagnose a disorder as well as to evaluate the brain's response to treatment.

BASICS THE NURSE NEEDS TO KNOW

The SPECT scan uses a radionuclide that emits gamma rays and a multidetector rotary camera to produce images of the brain. Once it is injected into the vascular system, the radiopharmaceutical perfuses across the blood-brain barrier and into the brain tissue (Figure 79). It is used to evaluate cerebral blood flow and perfusion of the brain tissue and detects cerebral ischemia at an early stage.

In the investigation of cerebrovascular disease, SPECT can be used for detection of acute ischemia, determination of the cause of stroke, and assessment of a transient ischemic attack. In the study of dementia, this method can help identify the cause of dementia and distinguish among Alzheimer's disease, multi-infarct dementia, and frontal lobe dementia. In epilepsy, this test can help identify the seizure focus in conjunction with other neurologic procedures. In cases of head trauma, SPECT can identify mild head injury that is not visible on the CT scan.

NORMAL VALUES No abnormalities of brain tissue and brain function are noted

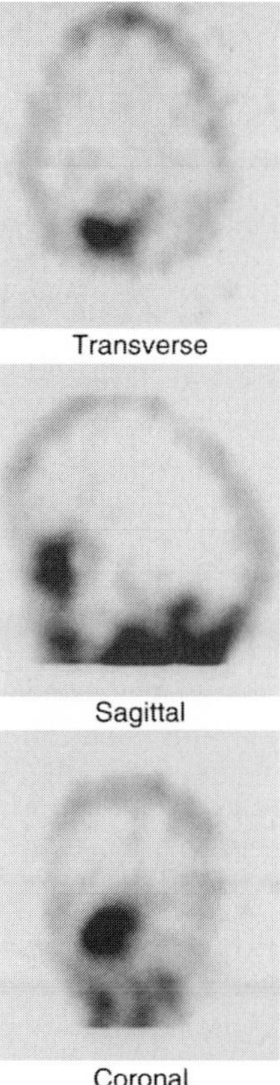

Figure 79. Recurrent brain tumor in the occipital region. The three different views of the SPECT scan demonstrate intense and irregular tracer concentration within the tumor. *(Reproduced with permission from Wagner, H. N., Szabo, Z., & Buchanan, J. W. [1995].* Principles of nuclear medicine *[2nd ed., p. 1138]. Philadelphia: W. B. Saunders.)*

HOW THE TEST IS DONE

After the radiopharmaceutical is injected, a gamma camera records the radioactive emissions. The emissions are then converted to images that correspond to the location, distribution, and concentration of the radionuclide in the brain. The imaging is performed about 1 to 2 hours after the radiopharmaceutical is introduced. The normal imaging time is 20 to 30 minutes.

SIGNIFICANCE OF TEST RESULTS

Abnormal Values

Stroke
Human immunodeficiency virus encephalopathy
Intracranial hemorrhage
Multi-infarct dementia
Transient ischemic attack
Epilepsy
Hypertensive encephalopathy
Intracranial trauma
Alzheimer's disease

INTERFERING FACTORS

- Movement of the head during imaging
- Failure to remove metal objects from the imaging field

NURSING CARE

Pretest

- After the physician explains the procedure, the nurse ensures that written consent is obtained from the patient. The form is then entered in the patient's record.
- The nurse instructs the patient to avoid caffeine intake (e.g., coffee, tea, and cola) for 24 hours before the test.
- The nurse or technician assists the patient in removing all clothes and putting on a hospital gown. All jewelry and metal objects are removed from the head, hair, and neck. The patient is placed in supine position on the scanning table. Minimal restraints are applied, to prevent a fall from a narrow table that has no side rails.
- The person who needs a SPECT scan is usually elderly and suffering from dementia or has residual trauma to the brain. The unfamiliar room and the procedure may be confusing or frightening to this type of patient. Instructions may be difficult to follow. If these conditions exist, the patient will need simple instructions and close guidance. Because no radiation hazard to people in the room exists, a member of the family or a familiar person can assist and help calm the patient during the test.
- Remind the patient to keep the head still during the injection of the radiopharmaceutical and during the imaging procedure. Explain that the room will be kept calm for 10 minutes before and after the radiopharmaceutical is administered. During this quiet time, the patient should keep his or her eyes open. Blinking is allowed. Earplugs are unnecessary.

NURSING CARE—*cont'd*

- The quiet, stimulus-free environment promotes a resting basal state of brain activity. The patient keeps his or her eyes open during administration of the radionuclide so that the occipital lobes are more clearly visible.

During the Test

- The patient's head is positioned in alignment with the body. An intravenous line is established for the administration of the radiopharmaceutical. To maintain a quiet environment, dim the lights in the room, keep noise to a minimum, and prevent traffic in the room. During the scanning process, the patient will hear the quiet sounds of the scanner, but no pain or discomfort is experienced.

Posttest

- The intravenous line is removed and a small bandage is applied to the venipuncture site.
- ***Patient Teaching.*** Because the kidneys will remove the radionuclide from the blood and excrete it in the urine, the nurse instructs the patient to wash his or her hands after voiding. This prevents radioisotopes from remaining on the skin. By 6 hours after the test, the radioactivity level of the isotope is minimal to none.

Sniff Test

See Pulmonary Function Studies on p. 557.

Sodium, Serum

soh-dee-uhm, seer-uhm

Also called: Na^+

SPECIMEN OR TYPE OF TEST: Blood

PURPOSE OF THE TEST

The serum sodium level is used to monitor electrolyte balance, water balance, and acid-base balance. It also is used in the evaluation of disorders of the central nervous system, musculoskeletal disorders, or diseases of the kidneys or adrenal glands.

BASICS THE NURSE NEEDS TO KNOW

Sodium is a major electrolyte found in all body fluids and is responsible for osmolarity and intravascular osmotic pressure.

With the change of sodium concentration in the blood, resultant changes occur in the water content into or out of cells. Thus, the alteration of sodium content is responsible for dehydration or overhydration within cells or in extracellular fluids. The daily intake of sodium is balanced by an equivalent amount of sodium excretion in urine.

Elevated Values

An elevation of serum sodium that is caused by sodium retention or an excessive loss of water is called *hypernatremia.* When a loss of water occurs, the concentration of sodium and the osmolarity of the blood increase. In nonrenal causes of hypernatremia, a loss of body fluid occurs without adequate replacement. This can occur in diuresis, profuse sweating, diarrhea, burns, and respiratory infection. Renal losses of fluid may result from advanced renal failure.

Decreased Values

A low level of serum sodium is called *hyponatremia.* The cause is usually an excessive loss of sodium or excessive water retention. The origin of the problem is frequently due to a renal problem. Metabolic alkalosis, ketonuria, or endocrine deficiency may also cause hyponatremia. In all these conditions, excessive loss of sodium or excessive resorption of water by the kidneys occurs. Nonrenal causes of sodium loss include fluid and electrolyte losses from the gastrointestinal tract, "third space" losses, and severe thermal injury.

NORMAL VALUES	Adult: 136–145 mEq/L *or* SI: 136–145 mmol/L Child (1 year or older): 134–143 mEq/L *or* SI: 134–143 mmol/L Infant (0-7 days): 133–146 mEq/L *or* SI: 133–146 mmol/L
▼ Critical Values	<125 mEq/L (SI: <125 mmol/L) *or* >150 mEq/L (SI: >150 mmol/L)

HOW THE TEST IS DONE

A green- or red-topped tube is used to obtain 5 to 10 mL of venous blood. For infants and small children, a heelstick or finger puncture and a capillary tube are used to obtain capillary blood.

SIGNIFICANCE OF TEST RESULTS

Elevated Values

Dehydration
Cushing syndrome
Aldosteronism
Inadequate thirst
Diabetic acidosis
Azotemia
Excessive saline infusion
Profuse sweating

Decreased Values

Acute or chronic renal failure
Diuretic therapy

Diabetic ketoacidosis
Ketonuria
Vomiting or diarrhea
Burns
Acute water intoxication
Cirrhosis
Congestive heart failure
Nephrotic syndrome
Central nervous system disturbance (trauma, tumor)
Salt-wasting nephritis
Hypothyroidism
Glucocorticoid deficiency
Addison's disease
Hypopituitarism
Bicarbonaturia

INTERFERING FACTORS

- Hemolysis

NURSING CARE

Nursing measures includes care of the venipuncture or capillary puncture site as described in Chapter 2, with the following additional measures.

Pretest

- The blood sample should be collected without use of a tourniquet to avoid clotting or hemolysis. The arm that has an intravenous infusion should not be used, to avoid hemodilution and false results.
- No fasting is required for this test. The test for sodium is usually part of the electrolyte panel of sodium, chloride, potassium, and carbon dioxide.

Posttest

- For the patient with disturbances in sodium values, the nurse should measure daily input and output of fluids. These measurements include recording all oral and intravenous intake and all fluid output as from urine, drainage, vomiting, diarrhea, and fistula drainage. Depending on the cause of the sodium imbalance, the patient may be dehydrated from excessive sodium and water losses or inadequate sodium and fluid replacement. The patient also may be edematous with retention of excess sodium and water in tissue as well as from inadequate kidney function and diminished urinary output.

▼ Nursing Response to Critical Values

Once the values reach either critical level, the patient can have significant dysfunction of the brain and nervous system. The nurse immediately notifies the physician of the abnormal test value. Specific treatment will depend on the type and severity of the imbalance and its cause.

Continued

S

NURSING CARE—*cont'd*

The nurse assesses the patient for manifestations of severe sodium imbalance. With severe hypernatremia, the manifestations include somnolence, confusion, coma, and respiratory paralysis. When the sodium value reaches the elevated critical level in less than 24 hours, the mortality rate is greater than 70%. With moderate hyponatremia, the patient is asymptomatic. Once the sodium value declines to the critical level or lower, the manifestations include lethargy, weakness, somnolence, seizures, and coma. Death can occur from this very severe hyponatremia.

Sodium-Depleted Renin Test

See Renin on p. 573.

Specific Gravity, Urinary

spe-si-fik gra-vi-tee, yur-i-nar-ee

SPECIMEN OR TYPE OF TEST: Urine

PURPOSE OF THE TEST

Specific gravity reflects the ability of the kidneys to concentrate and dilute urine. It assesses renal function and the hormonal regulation of fluid balance—specifically the antidiuretic hormone.

BASICS THE NURSE NEEDS TO KNOW

The specific gravity of urine is the ratio of the weight of a given volume of urine to the weight of the same volume of distilled water at a constant temperature. The urine specific gravity will vary within the individual based on his or her diet and fluid status. Increased fluid intake normally decreases the specific gravity of urine. Decreased fluid intake normally increases the urine specific gravity.

S

NORMAL VALUES 1.003–1.029

HOW THE TEST IS DONE

Urine specific gravity is measured as part of urinalysis (see p. 651), by hydrometer or by a reagent strip.

SIGNIFICANCE OF TEST RESULTS

Elevated Value

Dehydration
Fever
Profuse sweating
Vomiting, diarrhea, or both
Glycosuria
Proteinuria
Congestive heart failure

Adrenal insufficiency
Altered secretion of antidiuretic hormone

Decreased Value
Overhydration
Diuresis
Hypotension
Pyelonephritis
Glomerulonephritis
Renal tubular dysfunction
Severe renal damage
Diabetes insipidus

INTERFERING FACTORS

- Excessive protein in the urine
- Alkaline urine

NURSING CARE

- The actions of the nurse are dependent on the method used to measure the specific gravity. See p. 37 for the Random Specimen Urine Collection procedure.

Hydrometer Method (rarely used in hospitals)

- If a hydrometer (urinometer) is used, perform the following.

Pretest

- Obtain a urinometer calibrated to measure urine specific gravity at room temperature.
- Put on gloves.

During the Test

- Instruct the patient to void into a clean container.
- Allow the urine to reach room temperature.
- Wearing gloves, the nurse pourfresh urine into the urinometer's cylinder until it is three-fourths full.
- Remove any foam with filter paper.
- Gently insert the rod into the urine in the cylinder, using a gentle spinning motion.
- Read the specific gravity at eye level (Figure 80).

Posttest

- Disinfect the urinometer.
- Remove gloves and wash hands.
- Document the specific gravity.

Reagent Strip Method

- Reagent strips are replacing the use of hydrometers in measuring specific gravity. The reagent strip pad will change color according to the concentration of ions in the urine.

Pretest

- Check the vial of reagent strips for product dating. Do not use them after the manufacturer's expiration date. Always store strips in the manufacturer's darkened container. Do not expose the container to direct sunlight or extreme heat.
- Put on gloves.

Continued

NURSING CARE—*cont'd*

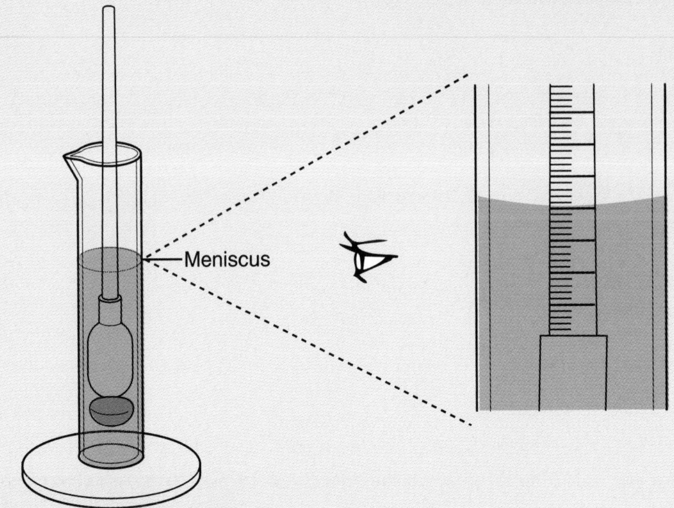

Figure 80. Hydrometer. *(Reproduced with permission from Stepp, C. A., & Woods, M. [1998].* Laboratory procedures for medical office personnel. *Philadelphia: W. B. Saunders.)*

During the Test

- Instruct the patient to void into a clean container.
- Dip the reagent strip into the urine.
- Wait the time specified by the manufacturer.
- Compare the resultant color with the chart provided.

Posttest

- Remove gloves and wash hands.
- Document the specific gravity.

S

Stress Testing, Cardiac

stres tes-ting, kar-dee-ak

Also called: Graded Exercise Testing (GEX); Graded Exercise Stress Testing (GEST); Exercise Stress Testing; Exercise Electrocardiography

SPECIMEN OR TYPE OF TEST: Electrophysiology

PURPOSE OF THE TEST

Stress testing is an invaluable technique for (1) assessing the at-risk population, (2) diagnosing chest pain syndromes and dysrhythmias associated with ischemia,

(3) evaluating the effectiveness of therapy (surgical or pharmacologic), and (4) identifying the initial level of function in cardiac rehabilitation programs and evaluating the results.

BASICS THE NURSE NEEDS TO KNOW

Stress testing is an important noninvasive procedure for evaluating the cardiovascular status of patients who are known to have cardiac disease or are at risk for cardiac disease. The test increases the demand placed on the heart by increasing physical activity. Through electrocardiograph tracings, it can be determined whether the heart is able to meet the increased oxygen demand.

NORMAL VALUES

Increased heart rate
No ST segment changes
No dysrhythmias

HOW THE TEST IS DONE

Stress testing requires the use of a bicycle ergometer or a treadmill with continuous electrocardiac recording. The test is performed in a series of stages in which the patient exercises for 3 minutes. A variety of protocols are used in stress testing. The Bruce protocol involves gradual increase in speed and incline of the treadmill. The Ellestad protocol involves increasing speeds and intervals of shorter duration. At the end of each stage, a 12-lead electrocardiograph (ECG) is recorded. After each stage, the workload or "graded load" is increased. This is accomplished by increasing the speed or resistance of the bicycle or treadmill. The stress testing continues until the patient reaches 85% of the maximum heart rate, becomes symptomatic, or displays electrocardiographic changes consistent with ischemia. The maximum heart rate is usually determined by normograms. A gross estimate of the maximum heart rate is 220 beats per minute minus the patient's age.

If a patient is physically unable to exercise to the point of 85% of the maximum heart rate, a *dipyridamole (Persantine) scan* may be performed. Dipyridamole may be given intravenously or by mouth. It causes coronary artery dilation similar to the response of the coronary arteries to exercise. After peak effect is reached (85% maximum heart rate), a Thallium Scan is performed (see p. 604). A follow-up scan is performed 4 hours later.

The use of adenosine is similar to dipyridamole stress testing. Adenosine also has a vasodilating effect, but has a much shorter half-life then dipyridamole. It may also be used with the thallium scan.

SIGNIFICANCE OF TEST RESULTS

A 1-mm depression of the ST segment is a positive stress test, indicating myocardial ischemia.

INTERFERING FACTORS

- Severe anxiety may interfere with the patient's ability to participate fully in the stress testing.
- False-positive results may be due to bundle branch block, ventricular hypertrophy, or digitalization. False-negative results may be due to the use of beta-blockers.

NURSING CARE

Pretest

- Inform the patient about the purpose and procedure of the test.
- Routine cardiac medications are usually continued.
- Assess for the following contraindications to stress testing: chest pain; hypertension; thrombophlebitis; second- or third-degree heart block; serious dysrhythmias; severe congestive heart failure; and neurologic, musculoskeletal, or vascular problems that would impede mobility on the bicycle or treadmill.
- ***Patient Teaching.*** Instruct the patient not to eat, smoke, or drink alcohol for 3 to 4 hours before the test.
- ***Patient Teaching.*** If the adenosine stress test is being done, the nurse explains to patient the need to avoid theophylline-based drugs, dipyridamole, over-the-counter drugs, and caffeine for 24 hours. The nurse also instructs the patient to wear comfortable clothes and rubber-soled walking shoes. Warn the patient that during the exercise, he or she will feel his or her heart racing. The nurse instructs the patient to report chest pain during the procedure.

During the Test

- Have emergency equipment and drugs available (code cart).
- The patient is attached to electrodes for recording a 12-lead ECG.
- A blood pressure cuff is put in place for quick access. A baseline blood pressure reading is obtained.
- As the graded exercises begin, a multichanneled ECG is recorded. A 12-lead ECG is recorded, and the blood pressure is checked as each workload ends (every 3-minute increment).
- Observe for signs to stop the stress testing, for example, falling blood pressure, three consecutive premature ventricular contractions, chest pain, or exhaustion. The stressing may or may not be discontinued if ST depressions occur, blood pressure does not rise, or frequent or coupled premature ventricular contractions or bundle branch block occurs.
- If dipyridamole or adenosine is used, assess for the following side effects: myocardial infarction, dysrhythmias, bronchospasm, chest pain, nausea, headache, flushing hypotension, and dizziness. Have aminophylline available to treat serious side effects.

Posttest

- Cardiac monitoring is continued for 5 to 10 minutes after the testing to evaluate the patient's physiologic response.
- Blood pressure is checked.
- Remove conduction jelly and assist in dressing the patient if necessary.The nurse evaluates the patient's physical and emotional response to the testing.
- Instruct the patient to rest and not take hot showers or baths for 2 to 4 hours.

◆ **Nursing Response to Complications**

Stress testing is performed in a controlled environment; however, dysrhythmias and myocardial ischemia may occur.

NURSING CARE—*cont'd*

Dysrhythmias. During the stress test the nurse in the stress laboratory will continuously observe the cardiac monitor for dysrhythmias and inform the physician of their presence. The nurse anticipates this complication by having antiarrhythmia medications on hand.

Myocardial ischemia. Myocardial ischemia may be evident by electrocardiographic changes and by patient complaint of chest pain. Stress testing is immediately stopped if chest pain occurs.

Sweat Test

swet test

Also called: Chloride, Sweat; Cystic Fibrosis Sweat Test; Iontophoresis Sweat Test

SPECIMEN OR TYPE OF TEST: Sweat

PURPOSE OF THE TEST

The chloride sweat test is used to diagnose cystic fibrosis in children.

BASICS THE NURSE NEEDS TO KNOW

Cystic fibrosis is an inherited (genetic) disorder that causes abnormal secretion by the exocrine glands of the pancreas and other distinct exocrine glands of the body. In cystic fibrosis, increased sodium and chloride content exists in the sweat gland secretions. Because the chloride ion concentration on the skin can be measured, the chloride sweat test is the preferred method to diagnose cystic fibrosis in infants and children.

In children up to age 20, an elevated sweat chloride value greater than 60 mEq/L (SI: >60 mmol/L) is considered abnormal and consistent with cystic fibrosis. A value of 41 to 60 mEq/L (SI: 41 to 60 mmol/L) is considered borderline and the test must be repeated. Because other disorders can cause elevation of the sweat chloride concentration, the family history and clinical manifestations of cystic fibrosis disease are included in the interpretation of the test results. In most cases of cystic fibrosis, the test becomes positive within 3 to 5 weeks after birth.

Cystic fibrosis DNA detection may be performed by other methodologies. To test the fetus, a sample of amniotic fluid can be analyzed for the abnormal genetic changes, including cystic fibrosis (see Amniocentesis and Amniotic Fluid Analysis, p. 65). To test the child or adult, including the pregnant woman for the abnormal genetic changes of cystic fibrosis, a sample of cells from the mucosal surface of the inner cheek can be analyzed for the abnormal DNA of cystic fibrosis (see Genetic Testing for Cystic Fibrosis, p. 343).

NORMAL VALUES Infants and children: 5–40 mEq/L *or* SI: 5–40 mmol/L

HOW THE TEST IS DONE

A sample of sweat is obtained by stimulating skin sweat production with pilocarpine and low-voltage electric current in a process called *iontophoresis*. The electric current introduces small amounts of pilocarpine into the skin. The pilocarpine drug stimulates a sweat response. On removal of the electrodes, the sweat is collected on filter paper or gauze pads, weighed, and then analyzed for chloride content.

SIGNIFICANCE OF TEST RESULTS

Elevated Values

Cystic fibrosis
Hypothyroidism
Adrenal insufficiency
Malnutrition
Renal insufficiency
Glucose-6-phosphate deficiency

INTERFERING FACTORS

- Dermatitis or skin lesion
- Improper placement of the electrodes
- Inadequate sweat collection
- Salt depletion in the body
- Excessive sweating with fever or exercise prior to the test

NURSING CARE

Pretest

- ***Patient Teaching.*** The nurse explains the test procedure to the parents and the child who is old enough to understand. The electrodes will be applied to the skin on the inner aspect of the forearm or, for the infant, on the back. Reassure them that the electrodes do not cause a shock or pain. The patient will feel a mild, tingling sensation.
- Encourage the parents to accompany the child during the test and to bring a book or favorite toy for the child. These distractions will help to pass the time and ease the child's apprehension.
- This test must not be performed on the child who is receiving oxygen or who is in a mist tent. Danger of explosion exists when electric current mixes with oxygen.

Posttest

- The nurse assesses the skin. It may appear reddened at the site of the electrode placement, but is not considered a serious problem.

Syphilis Serology

si-fi-lis ser-o-loh-jee

Also called: Venereal Disease Research Laboratory Test (VDRL); Rapid Plasma Reagin Test (RPR); Fluorescent Treponemal Antibody Absorption Test (FTA-ABS); Microhemagglutination Assay-*Treponema Pallidum* (MHA-TP)

SPECIMEN OR TYPE OF TEST: Blood, cerebrospinal fluid

PURPOSE OF THE TEST

These blood tests are used to screen for or confirm the diagnosis of syphilis. The VDRL is used to monitor the response to therapy.

BASICS THE NURSE NEEDS TO KNOW

Treponema pallidum is the spirochete that causes syphilis. The spirochete is usually transmitted as the result of sexual contact with an infected partner. In addition, a pregnant woman with primary or secondary stage syphilis can transmit the spirochete to her fetus.

Several laboratory tests can be used to detect syphilis antibodies that are produced in response to the infection. The results are reported as reactive, weakly reactive, or nonreactive. Each blood test has distinct advantages and disadvantages at the various phases of the disease. False-positive results can occur.

The Venereal Disease Research Laboratory (VDRL) test is an effective screening test for syphilis. In most cases, the blood becomes reactive 1 to 3 weeks after a chancre—the first symptom—appears. It is 100% reactive in the secondary phase and remains reactive in most cases of latent syphilis. This is the only test used on cerebrospinal fluid to assess for neurosyphilis. After effective treatment has eradicated the spirochete, the VDRL results become negative or nonreactive.

The rapid plasma reagin test (RPR), and automated reagin test (ART) are used to screen for the disease. A positive test result should be followed up with one of the specific treponemal tests to confirm the diagnosis.

The fluorescent treponemal antibody absorption test (FTA-ABS) identifies the specific antibodies to *T. pallidum* that are present in the serum. This test is the most sensitive for all stages of syphilis. It is used to confirm positive test results with the VDRL, ART, or RPR, but it cannot itself be used as a screening test. This test also cannot be used to monitor treatment, because once the results are reactive, they remain reactive for life.

The microhemagglutination assay-*T. pallidum* (MHA-TP) is specific and sensitive in identification of all phases of syphilis, except the primary stage. The test is used to confirm a positive result of a reagin screening test. It is not used as a screening test itself and cannot monitor the results of treatment, because once the results are reactive, they remain reactive throughout life.

NORMAL VALUES

Negative; nonreactive

HOW THE TEST IS DONE

Serum: A red-topped tube is used to collect 10 mL of venous blood.
Cerebrospinal fluid: A sterile tube is used to collect a sample of cerebrospinal fluid during a lumbar puncture.

SIGNIFICANCE OF TEST RESULTS

Syphilis

INTERFERING FACTORS

- Lipemia
- Alcohol

NURSING CARE

Nursing measures include care of the venipuncture or capillary puncture site as described in Chapter 2, with the following additional measures.

Pretest

- ***Patient Teaching.*** The nurse instructs the patient to avoid alcohol intake for 24 hours before the test. Fasting from food for 8 hours is also recommended, but water is permitted. The alcohol and food restrictions help to reduce the serum lipid content that interferes with test results.

Posttest

- The nurse instructs the patient to abstain from sexual contact until the results are known. When the test results are positive for this sexually transmitted disease, the patient should inform all sexual partners of the test results. Sexual partners are advised to undergo testing. Syphilis, a communicable disease, is reported to the state health department.
- The nurse administers the medication to treat the infection. Penicillin is the antibiotic of choice, given intramuscularly or intravenously, as prescribed. Instruct the patient to refrain from sexual contact for at least 1 month after treatment. Cure of the infection is verified by VDRL testing.
- ***Health Promotion.*** The nurse should educate the patient about how this infection is transmitted, and how to protect from reinfection by using safe sex practices. The patient should understand how to recognize the symptoms and the importance of following through with the prescribed treatment until the infection is cured.

Testosterone, Total, Free

tes-tos-ter-ohn, toh-tuhl, free

Also called: (T)

SPECIMEN OR TYPE OF TEST: Blood

PURPOSE OF THE TEST

The measurement of serum testosterone is used to diagnose precocious sexual development in the boy who is younger than age 10. It helps diagnose deficient activity of the testes or ovaries. It is part of the testing that determines the cause of male infertility or sexual dysfunction. In the female, it helps determine the cause of hirsutism or virilization.

BASICS THE NURSE NEEDS TO KNOW

Total testosterone consists of the measurement of testosterone that is free, loosely bound to albumin, and the part that is strongly bound to sex-hormone–binding globulin. Free testosterone is the amount of the total hormone that is unbound in the serum. Total testosterone is usually the test used when measurement of testosterone is needed.

In the male, almost all the testosterone is synthesized by the testes. In the female, small amounts are synthesized by the ovaries and adrenal glands. Testosterone is the dominant androgen and, in the male, is responsible for spermatogenesis. Androgens affect many other organs and tissues, resulting in increased total body mass and *hirsutism*, the distribution of body hair. When hirsutism is excessive, it is caused by excessive testosterone or its hormonal precursor, androstenedione. In the female, the testosterone level is one of the tests to investigate hirsutism.

NORMAL VALUES

Total Testosterone

Adult male: 280–1100 ng/dL *or* SI: 9.72–38.17 nmol/L
Adult female: 15–70 ng/dL *or* SI: 0.52–2.43 nmol/L
Male child (1–5 years): 0.3–30.0 ng/dL *or* SI: 0.10–1.04 nmol/L
Female child (1–5 years): 2–20 ng/dL *or* SI: 0.07–0.69 nmol/L

Free Testosterone

Adult male: 50–210 pg/mL *or* SI: 174–729 pmol/L
Adult female: 1.0–8.5 pg/mL *or* SI: 3.5–29.5 pmol/L
Male child (6–9 years): 0.1–3.2 pg/mL *or* SI: 0.3–11.1 pmol/L
Female child (6–9 years): 0.1–0.9 pg/mL *or* SI: 0.3–3.1 pmol/L

HOW THE TEST IS DONE

A red-, green-, or lavender-topped tube is used to collect 5 to 10 mL of venous blood.

SIGNIFICANCE OF TEST RESULTS

Elevated Values

Ovarian tumor
Adrenal tumor

Hyperthyroidism
Congenital adrenal hyperplasia
Testicular tumor
Idiopathic precocious puberty
Central nervous system lesion

Decreased Values
Testicular insufficiency

INTERFERING FACTORS

- Recent radioactive isotope scan

NURSING CARE

Nursing measures includes care of the venipuncture or capillary puncture site as described in Chapter 2, with the following additional measures.

Pretest

- The nurse schedules this test before or 7 days after any radioisotope scan because radioisotopes can interfere with the laboratory method of analysis.

Posttest

- The patient often presents with symptoms that he or she may find embarrassing or difficult to accept because they involve changes in the physical appearance and a disturbance in body image. For the female, manifestations may include male pattern baldness, acne, and hirsutism. For the male, infertility may exist. For the child with precocious puberty, both physical and sexual organs are developed beyond the age-related norms. The nurse can help the patient by using an open and calm approach in interactions and using listening skills if the patient verbalizes his or her feelings.

Thallium Testing

thal-ee-uhm tes-ting

Also called: Thallium Scan; Thallium Exercise Imaging; Resting Thallium Scan

SPECIMEN OR TYPE OF TEST: Radionuclide imaging

PURPOSE OF THE TEST

Thallium imaging is used to assess coronary blood flow to determine areas of infarction and ischemia. It is used to diagnose coronary artery disease (CAD) and assess revascularization after coronary artery bypass surgery.

BASICS THE NURSE NEEDS TO KNOW

Thallium is a radioactive analog of potassium, which is rapidly taken up by myocardial cells. After thallium-201 is given, almost 90% of it is extracted by the myocardium within seconds. For this to occur, two factors are essential: (1) adequate perfusion, and

(2) cellular extraction efficiency. Because cellular ischemia does not seem to affect thallium uptake in the myocardium, its lack of uptake is an indication of an infarction.

Instead of thallium, technetium Tc 99m (sestamibi), a different tracer agent, can be used. It has a shorter half-life than thallium. *Dual isotope studies* also can be performed using thallium and sestamibi.

Uptake of sestamibi is similar to that of thallium, but it does not redistribute within the myocardium as quickly. This allows for poststress imaging to be done for up to 1 to 2 hours after the injection.

NORMAL VALUES Normal myocardial perfusion; no "cold" spots

HOW THE TEST IS DONE

Thallium scanning is performed with an Anger gamma camera combined with a computer. Continuous counts of emitted photons are made during the cardiac cycle. The scan identifies "cold" spots, areas of decreased thallium uptake. Cold spots identify areas of ischemia and infarction. Thallium can be given under a state of no physical demand, which is known as a *resting thallium study,* or it can be part of a stress test, in which case it is called *exercise thallium imaging*. Exercise thallium imaging distinguishes ischemic sites from infarcted areas. Thallium scans are repeated, once during stress testing and then 3 to 4 hours after the thallium was given and the stress test was completed. With the second imaging, if a cold spot remains, it is assumed to be an infarcted area. If the cold spot disappears, it is recognized as an ischemic area.

SIGNIFICANCE OF TEST RESULTS

Abnormal Values

Cold spots indicate and distinguish areas of infarction and ischemia.

INTERFERING FACTORS

- See section on stress testing.

T

NURSING CARE

Nursing care is similar to that in stress testing, except as follows.

Pretest

- Ensure that the patient is not pregnant.
- Usually, long-acting nitrates are held for 8 to 12 hours before the test.
- The patient fasts for 4 to 6 hours before the test but may drink water.
- An infusion is started for intravenous access.
- The nurse informs the patient of the need to go to the nuclear medicine department twice.
- If a single photon emission computed tomography (SPECT) scan is planned, the nurse assesses the patient for claustrophobia.

Continued

NURSING CARE—*cont'd*

During the Test

- The thallium or adenosine is given intravenously about 1 minute before the completion of the stress test.
- After the completion of the stress test, the patient is placed supine on the table and multiple scintigraphic images are taken.
- If a SPECT scan is done, the patient lies supine with arms over the head.
- Between the two scans, the patient may drink clear, noncaffeinated fluids.

Posttest

- Assess the patient's response.
- Three to 4 hours later, the patient returns for repeat films.

Thoracentesis, Pleural Fluid Analysis, and Pleural Biopsy

thor-uh-sen-tee-sis, plur-uhl floo-id uh-nal-uh-sis, and plur-uhl bai-op-see

Also called: Pleural Tap

SPECIMEN OR TYPE OF TEST: Pleural fluid; possible pleural biopsy tissue

PURPOSE OF THE TEST

Thoracentesis is performed to remove fluid from the pleural space for diagnostic or therapeutic reasons. Examination of pleural fluid identifies or confirms diagnoses of cancer, infection, or severe fluid overload (congestive heart failure, liver failure, and systemic or pulmonary hypertension). The biopsy tissue is used to identify cancer or other pathologic change of the pleural tissue.

BASICS THE NURSE NEEDS TO KNOW

T

An accumulation of fluid in the pleural space is abnormal. Thoracentesis is an invasive procedure used to remove fluid from the pleural space. It may be performed for diagnostic or therapeutic reasons, or both. During thoracentesis, pleural fluid is removed. In addition, a percutaneous needle biopsy of the pleura may be performed.

Pleural Fluid Analysis

Pleural effusions (accumulation of fluid in the pleural space) may be a result of neoplastic or infectious processes or of leakage of fluid from the vascular system. If the effusion is due to neoplasm or infection, the fluid is usually called an *exudate*. If the fluid is due to leakage from the blood vessels, it is called a *transudate*. To distinguish between exudates and transudates, pleural fluid is evaluated for protein, specific gravity, glucose, and a blood cell count with differential. Pleural fluid is also obtained for cultures to identify tuberculosis, fungal, and various bacterial infections. Cytologic examination of the pleural fluid is performed to rule out malignancy.

Pleural Biopsy

If tissue samples are removed from the pleura during the thoracentesis, they will be examined microscopically to identify the cell types. Malignancy of the pleura can be detected.

NORMAL VALUES
Normal pleural fluid
No pathogens or malignant cells are present

HOW THE TEST IS DONE

Thoracentesis and Pleural Fluid Collection

After the patient is positioned in a seated, upright position, the lower posterior chest is exposed and prepared, and a local anesthetic is given. A needle is inserted into the pleural space, and the fluid is aspirated. The fluid is placed in a sterile container. The nurse affixes the label containing the patient's identification data, date, and the type of fluid. The container is sent to the laboratory immediately.

Pleural Biopsy

A pleural biopsy may be performed at this time. If a *pleural biopsy* is planned, a special biopsy needle with a hooked biopsy trocar is used. Usually, three tissue specimens are obtained from three pleural sites. Specimens are placed in a sterile container with fixative and labeled with the patient's identification data, date, and the source of the tissue specimen. The container is sent to the lab immediately.

SIGNIFICANCE OF TEST RESULTS

Bacterial, viral, or fungal infection
Malignancy
Collagen disease
Lymphoma
Systemic lupus erythematosus
Liver failure
Nephrotic syndrome
Myxedema
Pancreatitis

INTERFERING FACTORS

- Uncooperative patient

NURSING CARE

Pretest

- Explain the procedure and the purpose of the test to the patient.
- Ensure that a signed consent form has been obtained.
- Perform and document a baseline assessment. A blood pressure cuff is left in place to permit easy monitoring of the blood pressure during the procedure. Check the patient's recent laboratory values of the prothrombin time (PT), partial thromboplastin time (PTT), and platelet count to identify the potential for bleeding problems.

Continued

NURSING CARE—*cont'd*

Pretest—*cont'd*

- Check for allergy to local anesthetic.
- If prescribed, initiate supplemental O_2 and attach a pulse oximeter.
- Warn the patient not to cough or move during the procedure.
- Obtain a thoracentesis tray from the supply room.

During the Test

- The nurse continuously monitors the patient's response to the procedure.
- If it is in use, the nurse observes the pulse oximeter readings for changes in SaO_2.
- The patient is positioned in an upright position, seated on the side of the bed with the legs resting on a footstool. The patient's arms should be supported on a padded overbed table (Figure 81). If the patient is unable to sit up, he or she may lie on the unaffected side with the back flush with the edge of the bed. The head of the bed may be elevated 30 to 45 degrees.
- The nurse provides emotional support to the patient, because pressure pain may be experienced even though local anesthesia is given.
- After the physician inserts a thoracentesis needle with a stopcock attached, fluid is drawn off for analysis. A catheter may be inserted at this point if a large amount of fluid is to be drained.
- When the physician performs a biopsy, the nurse instructs the patient to exhale fully and perform the Valsalva maneuver. This prevents air from entering the pleural space when the tissue sample is taken.

Posttest

- The nurse checks vital signs every 15 minutes until they are stable and assesses for bilateral breath sounds.
- In the patient's record, the nurse documents the amount, color, and character of the fluid obtained and a notation of how the patient tolerated the procedure.
- If it is ordered, the nurse schedules a chest x-ray that would assess for potential pneumothorax.
- The nurse encourages the patient to lie on the uninvolved side for 1 hour to improve oxygenation. The nurse continues assessments by observation of the small dressing over the site for bleeding or drainage and palpation around the site for subcutaneous emphysema.

T

◇ Nursing Response to Complications

The major complication after thoracentesis is pneumothorax. Another complication the nurse needs to observe for is re-expansion pulmonary edema. It occurs when large amounts of pleural fluid are removed, causing an increase in negative intrapleural pressure. If the lungs do not re-expand to fill the space, edema can result. Bleeding is a rare complication. Because thoracentesis is an invasive procedure, infection is possible, but extremely rare, because thoracentesis is performed with sterile technique.

Pulmonary edema. The nurse will assess for pulmonary edema by checking bilateral breath sounds and observing for indications of hypoxia. The nurse will report crackles and hypoxia immediately. The nurse will anticipate the physician's orders for oxygen, diuresis, intubation, and mechanical ventilation.

NURSING CARE—*cont'd*

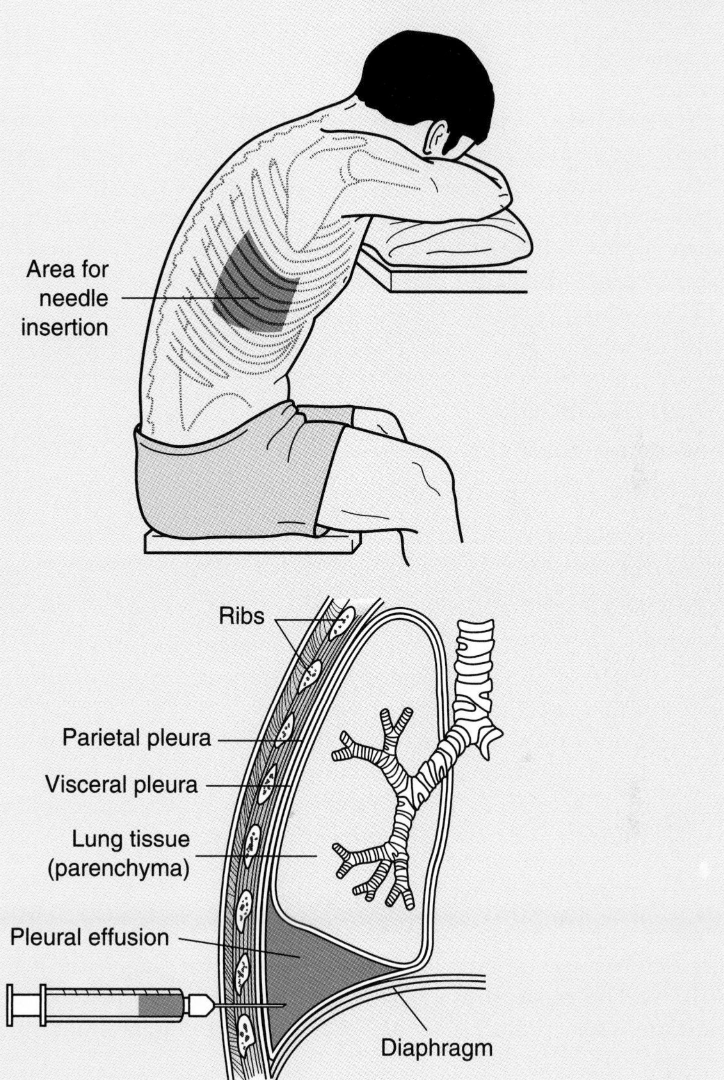

Figure 81. Thoracentesis. *A*, Thoracentesis position. Arms are raised and crossed. Head rests on folded arms. This position allows the chest wall to be pulled outward in an expanded position. If an overbed table is not available, the arms may be left down but positioned forward of the hips or crossed in front of the chest. *B*, The usual site for the insertion of a thoracentesis needle for a right-sided effusion. The actual site varies with each patient, depending on the location and volume of the effusion. The physician tries to keep the needle as far away from the diaphragm as possible, while at the same time inserting the needle close to the base of the effusion so that gravity can help with drainage.

Continued

NURSING CARE—*cont'd*

Bleeding. The nurse assesses for indications of bleeding: tachycardia, restlessness, hypotension, and bloody drainage. The nurse reports indications of bleeding immediately.

Pneumothorax. Anxiety, restlessness, dyspnea, tachypnea, pallor, and decreased breath sounds are indications of pneumothorax. If a tension pneumothorax has occurred, there will be a mediastinal shift to the unaffected side. Notify the physician immediately and anticipate an order for chest x-ray to evaluate the size of the pneumothorax. If a tension pneumothorax is present, the nurse needs to assess the patency of any chest tube that was inserted.

Thoracoscopy

thor-uh-kos-koh-pee

Also called: (VATS); Videoscopic or Video-Assisted Thoracic Surgery

SPECIMEN OR TYPE OF TEST: Endoscopy

PURPOSE OF THE TEST

Thoracoscopy is used to identify causes of pleural thickening and recurrent effusions, to remove pleural fluid for diagnostic or therapeutic reasons (cultures, cytology), and to biopsy pleural or peripheral lung tissue.

Therapeutic uses of thoracoscopy include insertion of anti-infective or fibrinolytic agents, reinflation of the lungs by inserting chest tubes, removal of adhesions, and treatment of pleurodesis. It may also be used to remove blebs and bullae, to make pericardial windows, and to perform sympathectomy.

BASICS THE NURSE NEEDS TO KNOW

T

A *thoracoscopy* is a surgical procedure that uses fiberoptic scopes inserted through small incisions in the chest wall. It may be performed for diagnostic or therapeutic reasons, or both. The procedure is used as an alternative to an open chest thoracotomy. Indications for a thoracoscopy and open thoracotomy are similar, but a thoracoscopy is less traumatic.

A thoracoscopy has an advantage over a thoracentesis in that direct visualization of the pleura and pulmonary tissue is possible.

NORMAL VALUES
No pleural fluid
No pathogens or malignant cells
Normal tissue

HOW THE TEST IS DONE

Thoracoscopy is an invasive procedure performed in the operating room under general anesthesia. Two or three 1- to 2-cm incisions are made between the ribs, and short, hollow pleural trocars are inserted. For visualization through one trocar, a telescope is inserted with a side portal attached to a video camera. Through the other trocars, endoscopic instruments can be inserted depending on the tests to be performed (suction tubes, forceps, aspiration needles). At the completion of the procedure, a chest tube is attached for suction.

SIGNIFICANCE OF TEST RESULTS

Bacterial, viral, or fungal infection
Malignancy

INTERFERING FACTORS

- Poor surgical risk

NURSING CARE

Follow hospital protocol for preoperative and postoperative care of a patient requiring open chest surgery. In addition, perform the following:

Pretest

- Administer prophylactic antibiotics, if ordered.

During the Test

- Position the patient in the lateral decubitus position with the unaffected lung down.

Posttest

- Monitor chest tube drainage. Large amounts of straw-colored drainage are expected initially in patients with recurrent effusions.

◆ **Nursing Response to Complications**

Following a thoracoscopy, the nurse assesses for possible pulmonary complications, which include atelectasis, pneumothorax, and pneumonia.

Atelectasis. Atelectasis may result from positioning the unaffected lung down during the procedure. Atelectasis refers to parts of the lung that are not ventilated. Assessments to identify atelectasis include diminished or absent breath sounds and dyspnea. The severity of the clinical manifestations is determined by the amount of lung not being aerated. If the atelectasis is severe, the nurse can anticipate that respiratory therapy will be ordered.

Pneumothorax. Anxiety, restlesssness, dyspnea, tachypnea, pallor, and decreased breath sounds are indications of pneumothorax. Notify the physician immediately and anticipate an order for chest x-ray to evaluate the size of the pneumothorax.

Pneumonia. The nurse assesses for manifestations of fever, sweating, chills, fatigue, dyspnea, pleuritic pain, and a productive cough. Auscultation of the chest reveals bronchial breath sounds and crackling sounds in alveolar tissue. The physician is notified of the abnormal findings and the nurse anticipates an order for oxygen, antibiotics, intravenous fluids, and chest x-ray.

Thyrocalcitonin

See Calcitonin on p. 162.

Thyroglobulin Autoantibodies

thai-roh-glob-yuh-lin aw-toh-an-ti-bod-eez

Also called: Antithyroid Antibodies

SPECIMEN OR TYPE OF TEST: Serum

PURPOSE OF THE TEST

Thyroglobulin antibodies are evaluated to detect autoimmune-based thyroid disease.

BASICS THE NURSE NEEDS TO KNOW

Some thyroid disorders may be autoimmune in origin. To evaluate this potential cause, antithyroid antibodies are measured. One of these antibodies is thyroglobulin autoantibody. The thyroglobulin autoantibodies act on the antigen *thyroglobulin*, the storage form of thyroid hormones. The presence of these antibodies helps confirm the diagnosis of autoimmune disease; however, their absence does not rule out the potential diagnosis.

NORMAL VALUES

Immunofluorescence method: Titer less than 1:100
Hemagglutination method: Negative

HOW THE TEST IS DONE

Venipuncture is performed to obtain 7 mL of blood in a red-topped tube.

SIGNIFICANCE OF TEST RESULTS

Elevated Values

Graves' disease
Hashimoto's thyroiditis
Hyperthyroidism
Hypothyroidism
Nontoxic nodular goiter
Pernicious anemia
Rheumatoid arthritis
Systemic lupus erythematosus
Thyroid cancer

INTERFERING FACTORS

- Oral contraceptives

T

NURSING CARE

The nursing actions are similar to those of other venipuncture techniques presented in Chapter 2.

Thyroid-Stimulating Autoantibody

See Long-Acting Thyroid Stimulator on p. 434.

Thyroid-Stimulating Immunoglobulins

See Long-Acting Thyroid Stimulator on p. 434.

Thyroid-Stimulating Hormone

thai-royd stim-yu-lay-ting hohr-mohn

Also called: (TSH); Thyrotropin

SPECIMEN OR TYPE OF TEST: Serum

PURPOSE OF THE TEST

Thyrotropin (thyroid-stimulating hormone [TSH]) levels are obtained to (1) diagnose hypothyroidism, (2) distinguish between primary and secondary hypothyroidism, and (3) monitor patient response to thyroid replacement therapy.

BASICS THE NURSE NEEDS TO KNOW

TSH is secreted by the anterior pituitary gland by a negative feedback mechanism (see Figure 82). Thyrotropin causes the thyroid gland to increase its production and secretion of thyroid hormones.

Because of the thyrotropin regulatory mechanism with the thyroid hormones, its level will be affected by primary thyroid abnormalities. If the patient has hyperthyroidism, thyrotropin will be suppressed. If the patient has primary hypothyroidism,

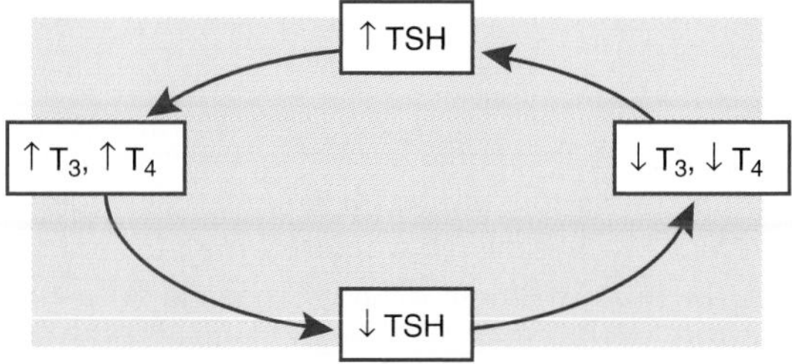

Figure 82. Thyroid hormone regulation. Thyroid hormone production and secretion are based on a negative feedback mechanism, with thyroid-stimulating hormone (TSH) secreted by the anterior pituitary gland. T3, triiodothyronine; T4, thyroxine.

T

thyrotropin secretion will become significantly elevated. This elevation may create a compensatory euthyroid state. Exogenous thyroid hormones will also suppress thyrotropin secretion. TSH varies very little with age.

NORMAL VALUES

Adult: 0.4–4.2 mL/U/L
Newborn: <7 mL/U/L

HOW THE TEST IS DONE

Venipuncture is performed to obtain 7 mL of blood in a red-topped tube. If the test is required on a newborn, a heelstick is performed and the blood is collected on filter paper.

SIGNIFICANCE OF TEST RESULTS

Elevated Values

Addison's disease
Goiter (some forms)
Hyperpituitarism
Pituitary adenoma
Primary hypothyroidism
Thyroid cancer

Decreased Values

Hyperthyroidism
Overdose of exogenous thyroid replacement
Secondary hypothyroidism
Tertiary hypothyroidism
Thyroiditis

INTERFERING FACTORS

- Radioisotope administration within 1 week
- Extreme stress
- Medications such as aspirin, corticosteroids, dopamine, heparin, lithium, potassium iodide, and thyroid replacement therapy
- If newborn is tested too soon after birth, false positive results can occur

NURSING CARE

- ***Health Promotion.*** The nurse encourages all women older than age 65 to have their TSH level checked every 3 to 5 years. If a woman complains of fatigue and has loss of hair or husky voice, the nurse would encourage medical follow-up with a TSH level. Screening with a capillary blood collection and special filter paper is done on all newborn babies to assess for congenital hypothyroidism. In the newborn, early detection of hypothyroidism allows for early medical treatment and prevention of the onset of mental retardation and physical deformities.

NURSING CARE—*cont'd*

Nursing actions related to venipuncture and capillary puncture are presented in Chapter 2, with the following additional measures.

Pretest

- The nurse assesses for and reports any clinical states that would increase the patient's endogenous glucocorticoid levels.
- Check with the physician regarding withholding medications that may interfere with test results.

Thyrotropin Receptor Antibodies

See Long-Acting Thyroid Stimulator on p. 434.

Thyrotropin-Releasing Hormone Test

thai-roh-troh-pin ree-lee-sing hohr-mohn test

Also called: TRH Test; TSH-Releasing Hormone

SPECIMEN OR TYPE OF TEST: Serum

PURPOSE OF THE TEST

Thyrotropin-releasing hormone (TRH) determinations are rarely performed today because the thyrotropin (TSH) test is usually adequate to support the diagnosis. TRH testing is performed when clinical manifestations of thyroid dysfunction are evident, but other tests are not clear.

BASICS THE NURSE NEEDS TO KNOW

TRH is produced and secreted by the hypothalamus. It acts as moderator of the thyroid hormone–thyrotropin negative feedback mechanism. In response to synthetic TRH being given intravenously, the anterior pituitary gland will normally increase its secretion of thyrotropin within 5 minutes. The thyrotropin levels peak in 20 to 30 minutes and will return to baseline within 2 to 4 hours.

NORMAL VALUES

After TRH is given, TSH increases.
Male: 14–24 µU/mL *or* SI: 14–24 mU/L
Female: 16–26 µU/mL *or* SI: 16–26 mU/L

HOW THE TEST IS DONE

TRH determinations may be performed in a number of ways, with the dose and route of the TRH varying. The most common method is the bolus intravenous administration of synthetic TRH after blood is drawn for a baseline thyrotropin level. After 30 minutes (and sometimes again after 60 minutes), when the thyrotropin response is normally peaking, a second specimen is drawn for a thyrotropin determination.

T

SIGNIFICANCE OF TEST RESULTS

Elevated Values

Normal response
Hypothyroidism

Decreased Values

Cushing syndrome
Depression
Hyperthyroidism
Multinodular goiter
Pituitary lesions
Renal failure

INTERFERING FACTORS

- Corticosteroids
- Levodopa
- Salicylates (high dose)

NURSING CARE

The nursing implementation for this test is similar to that for Thyroid-Stimulating Hormone (see p. 613), with the following additional measure.

Pretest

- Inform the patient of the need for multiple venipuncture procedures.

Thyroxine, Total

thai-rok-sin, toh-tuhl

Also called: T_4; Total T_4; Total Thyroxine

T

SPECIMEN OR TYPE OF TEST: Serum

PURPOSE OF THE TEST

Thyroxine levels are obtained to evaluate thyroid function, confirm the diagnosis of hyper- or hypothyroidism, and evaluate therapy for hyper- or hypothyroidism.

BASICS THE NURSE NEEDS TO KNOW

The thyroid gland produces and secretes the hormones *thyroxine* (T_4) and *triiodothyronine* (T_3). This gland takes up iodide from the extracellular fluid and uses it to produce thyroglobulin, the precursor of all thyroid hormones. The thyroglobulin is stored in the thyroid gland until thyroxine and triiodothyronine are processed before secretion from the gland. Secretion of triiodothyronine and thyroxine is primarily regulated by a negative feedback mechanism with thyrotropin. (Figure 82). Thyrotropin is secreted by the anterior pituitary gland.

Once secreted by the thyroid gland, triiodothyronine and thyroxine are bound primarily to thyroid-binding globulin and to a lesser degree to albumin and prealbumin.

The small amount of the hormones not bound to protein is called *free thyroxine* and *free triiodothyronine*. It is the free hormones that are biologically active. The bound hormones are released from the protein as the hormones are needed. In the peripheral circulation, thyroxine will lose one of its iodide molecules and become triiodothyronine, the more potent of the thyroid hormones.

Because the majority of the thyroid hormones are bound to protein, the evaluation of thyroid hormone levels should include the person's protein levels. If the patient has decreased proteins to carry the hormone, a greater amount of the hormone will be in the free state or active form. RIA measures both bound and unbound thyroxine.

NORMAL VALUES	Adult: 5–12 mcg/dL *or* SI: 64.4–154.4 nmol/L Children: 10–20 years: 4.2–11.8 mcg/dL *or* SI: 54.11–151.9 nmol/L 1–10 years: 6.4–15 mcg/dL *or* SI: 82.41–93.1 nmol/L 2–10 months: 7.8–16.5 mcg/dL *or* SI: 100.4–212.4 nmol/L Newborn: 6.4–23.2 mcg/dL *or* SI: 82.4–298.6 nmol/L
▼ Critical Values	<2.0 mcg/dL (SI: <26 nmol/L) and >20 mcg/dL (SI: >257 nmol/L)

HOW THE TEST IS DONE

Venipuncture is performed to obtain 5 mL of blood in a red-topped tube.

If a thyroxine determination is ordered on a newborn, umbilical cord blood may be used or a heelstick can be performed. With the heelstick method, special filter paper is used to blot the blood, and the filter paper is sent to the laboratory in a container that protects against light.

SIGNIFICANCE OF TEST RESULTS

Elevated Values

Hyperthyroidism
Acute or subacute thyroiditis

Decreased Values

Hypothyroidism
Chronic or subacute thyroiditis
Myxedema
Cretinism

INTERFERING FACTORS

- Liver disorders, which affect blood protein levels.
- Protein-wasting diseases such as chronic renal failure.
- Medications such as androgens, aspirin, chlorpropamide, chlorpromazine, estrogen, heparin, iodides, thyroid replacement medications, lithium, methadone, phenothiazines, phenytoin, reserpine, steroids, sulfonamides, sulfonylureas, and tolbutamide.

NURSING CARE

Nursing actions are similar to those used in other venipuncture or capillary puncture procedures (see Chapter 2) with the following additional measures.

During the Test

- If a heelstick is performed, the heel is first cleansed with antiseptic and the skin is pierced with a sterile lancet. Completely saturate the circles on the filter paper.
- Because pregnancy will normally cause an increase in thyroxine levels, indicate the pregnancy on the requisition slip, as applicable.

Posttest

- Send the filter paper to the laboratory in a container that protects against light.

Nursing Response to Critical Values

For very low thyroxine levels, assess the patient for myxedema coma. For very high thyroxine levels, assess the patient for thyroid storm. Assessments for both extremes of thyroxine levels include careful evaluation of the patient's mental status. Report change in mentation to the physician immediately.

Thyroxine-Binding Globulin

thai-rok-sin-bain-ding glob-yuh-lin

Also called: (TBG); T_4-Binding Globulin

SPECIMEN OR TYPE OF TEST: Serum

PURPOSE OF THE TEST

Thyroxine-binding globulin (TBG) is evaluated when clinical manifestations of thyroid dysfunction and thyroid hormone levels do not correlate.

BASICS THE NURSE NEEDS TO KNOW

TBG is the primary protein carrier of thyroxine and triiodothyronine. The thyroid hormones bound to TBG provide a storehouse of the hormones, which are released from the protein as needed. Because TBG carries approximately 70% of the total amount of thyroid hormones in the circulation, TBG levels significantly affect total hormone concentrations. TBG levels will affect the free forms of triiodothyronine and thyroxine.

T

NORMAL VALUES

Adult: 1.2–3.0 mg/dL *or* SI: 12–30 mg/L
Child: 2.9–5.0 mg/dL *or* SI: 29–50 mg/L
Infant: 1.6–4.2 mg/dL *or* SI: 16–42 mg/L

HOW THE TEST IS DONE

Venipuncture is performed to collect 7 mL of blood in a red-topped tube.

SIGNIFICANCE OF TEST RESULTS

Elevated Values

Congenital abnormality
Estrogen therapy

Hepatitis, acute
Hypothyroidism
Pregnancy

Decreased Values
Androgens
Cirrhosis of the liver
Congenital abnormality
Glucocorticoids
Hyperthyroidism
Recent surgery
Renal failure
Starvation

INTERFERING FACTORS

- Heparin
- Phenylbutazone
- Phenytoin
- Salicylates

NURSING CARE

Nursing actions related to venipuncture are presented in Chapter 2, with the following additional measures.

Pretest

- Obtain a medication history to determine if any drug is being taken that affects normal thyroid binding.

Tolbutamide Stimulation Test

tohl-byoo-tuh-maid stim-yu-lay-shun

SPECIMEN OR TYPE OF TEST: Serum

PURPOSE OF THE TEST

The tolbutamide stimulation test is performed to identify insulin-producing tumors of the pancreas.

BASICS THE NURSE NEEDS TO KNOW

Tolbutamide (Orinase) is an oral hypoglycemic agent. Its duration of action is short, being rapidly inactivated by the liver. For this reason, tolbutamide is used in stimulation tests to evaluate exaggerated and prolonged insulin secretion. This condition may occur with insulinoma, which is an insulin-secreting tumor of the pancreatic islets of Langerhans. It presents with spontaneous fasting hypoglycemia.

The goal in giving tolbutamide is to create a hypoglycemic state and see the insulin response to the induced hypoglycemia. Normally, insulin secretion decreases with hypoglycemia. If the insulin secretion stays at high levels and is prolonged, the test result is positive.

NORMAL VALUES

Serum insulin level: <195 μU/mL *or* SI: <1354 pmol/L

HOW THE TEST IS DONE

The tolbutamide stimulation test is performed by administering tolbutamide intravenously over a 2-minute period. Serum insulin levels are obtained every 5 minutes for 15 minutes. Each specimen is obtained by venipuncture and collected in either an anticoagulated or red-topped tube depending on the laboratory.

SIGNIFICANCE OF TEST RESULTS

If the insulin level is maintained or prolonged, the test confirms the diagnosis of insulinoma.

INTERFERING FACTORS

- Liver disorders
- Renal failure
- Medications such as chloramphenicol, dicumarol, MAO inhibitors, phenylbutazone, salicylates, and sulfonamides

NURSING CARE

See section on Insulin (p. 405). Nursing actions related to venipuncture are presented in Chapter 2, with the following additional measures.

Pretest

- Explain to the patient the need for several venipuncture procedures.

During the Test

- Observe the patient for a reaction to tolbutamide, which is most commonly a skin rash.

Posttest

- Observe the patient for prolonged hypoglycemia, especially in elderly individuals.

◆ Nursing Response to Complications

Prolonged hypoglycemia may occur with the administration of tolbutamide.

Hypoglycemia. The nurse needs to assess for hypoglycemia: Hunger, diaphoresis, palpitations, anxiety, tremulousness, vagueness and, if extreme, convulsions and coma. The physician should be notified immediately. If the patient is awake and able to swallow, oral glucose may be given.

Total Iron Binding Capacity

See Iron Studies on p. 411.

Total Triiodothronine

See Triiodothyronine on p. 626.

Toxoplasmosis Serology

tok-soh-plaz-mo-sis ser-ol-oh-jee

Also called: Toxoplasmosis Titer

SPECIMEN OR TYPE OF TEST: Blood, fetal blood

PURPOSE OF THE TEST

The antibody tests help in the diagnosis of toxoplasmosis, a parasitic infection.

BASICS THE NURSE NEEDS TO KNOW

Toxoplasma gondii is a protozoan parasite that infects household cats as well as domestic food animals (e.g., sheep, pigs). Oocysts in the feces of the infected animal are deposited in the environment. The infection is transmitted to people by the fecal-oral route. This includes ingestion of contaminated water or food, or having the oocysts on the hands after casual contact with contaminated soil or kitty litter. The individual also may become infected after eating undercooked meat of an infected animal. In pregnancy, maternal infection can be transmitted to the fetus via placental blood (Figure 83).

In acute toxoplasmosis, immunoglobulin (IgM) antibodies appear in 1 to 2 weeks, and the titer peaks at 6 to 8 weeks. Many individuals already have IgG antibodies from a previous asymptomatic infection, and the low or insignificant elevations persist for months to years. A rising IgG titer may be evidence of recovery from acute infection. The specific laboratory titers are dependent on the methodology used.

When the woman develops acute toxoplasmosis within the first 4 or 5 months of her pregnancy, congenital infection of the fetus can result in intrauterine death or cause fetal brain damage, central nervous system disturbance, or chorioretinitis. Testing may be performed on the fetus's blood, obtained by fetal blood sampling of the umbilical vein (see also Periumbilical Blood Sampling). An elevated IgM antibody in the cord blood is considered diagnostic for congenital toxoplasmosis.

NORMAL VALUES

IgM antibodies: Negative
IgG antibodies: Negative; <1:4

HOW THE TEST IS DONE

A red-topped tube is used to collect 10 mL of venous blood.

T

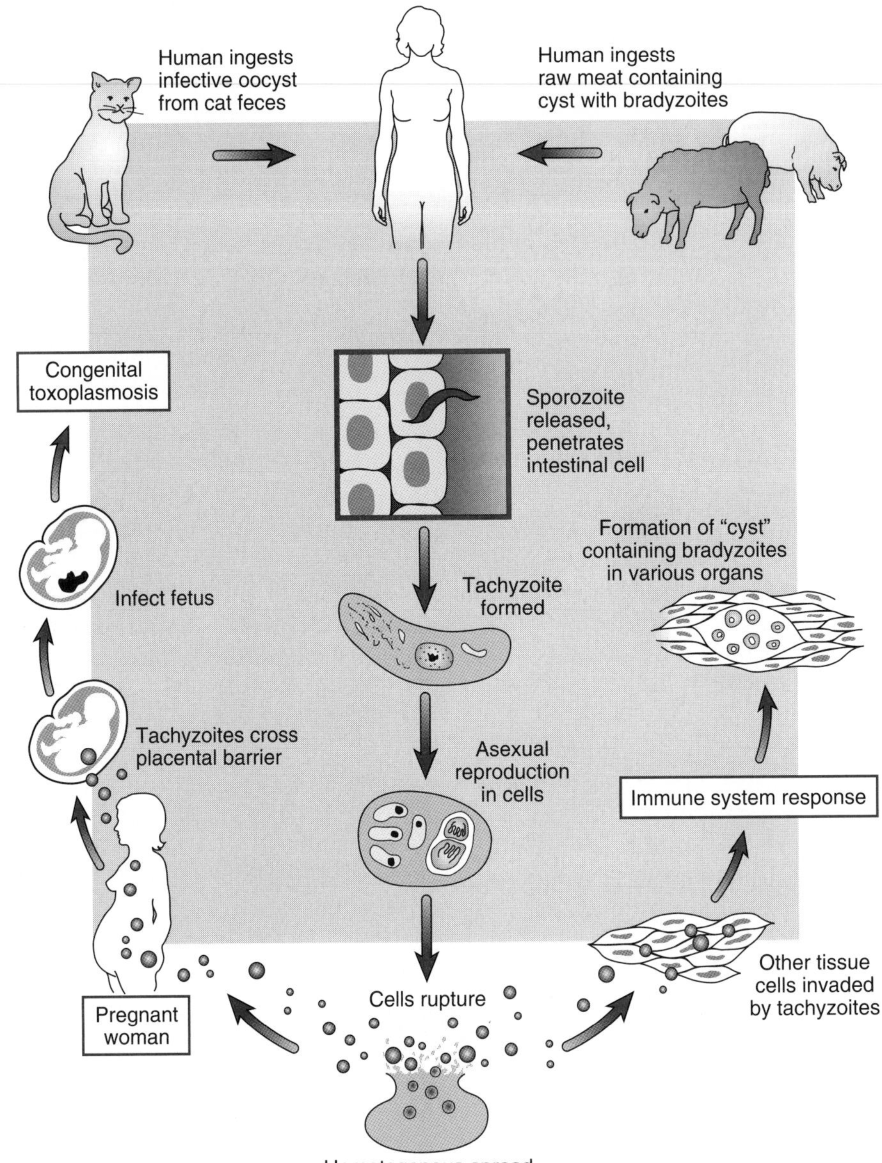

Figure 83. Life cycle of *Toxoplasma gondii*. The person ingests the infective stage of the parasite from infected feline fecal contamination on the hands or by eating raw or undercooked meat of an infected animal. In the person, the parasite passes through several maturation stages and infects cells and organs of the body. If the person is pregnant, the infection passes from the mother to the fetus. *(Reproduced with permission from Mahon, C., & Manuselis, G. [1995].* Textbook of diagnostic microbiology *[Fig. 24–35, p. 761]. W. B. Saunders.)*

T

SIGNIFICANCE OF TEST RESULTS

Positive Values

Toxoplasmosis infection

INTERFERING FACTORS

- None

NURSING CARE

Nursing measures include care of the venipuncture or capillary puncture site as described in Chapter 2, with the following additional measures.

Pretest

- Schedule the test to be performed at the onset of illness and 2 to 3 weeks later during the convalescent phase.

Posttest

- ***Health Promotion.*** The nurse can teach people the importance of cooking meat thoroughly, to eliminate this source of potential infection. The parasite can remain on the hands after touching contaminated soil or cleaning a kitty litter box used by an infected cat. Therefore, people should be reminded of the importance of hand-washing, particularly before preparing or eating food. Pregnant women should not clean the kitty litter box.

Transbronchial Biopsy

See Bronchoscopy on p. 158.

Transcatheter Bronchial Brushing

See Bronchoscopy on p. 158.

Transesophageal Echocardiography

tranz-ee-sof-uh-jee-uhl e-koh-kar-dee-o-gruh-fee

Also called: TEE

SPECIMEN OR TYPE OF TEST: Ultrasonography

PURPOSE OF THE TEST

Indications for transesophageal echocardiography include diagnosis of (1) a thoracic aortic pathologic condition, including suspected aneurysms, (2) mitral valve disease, (3) suspected endocarditis, (4) congenital heart disease, for example, atrial septal defect, (5) left atrial intracardiac thrombi, and (6) cardiac tumors. It also is used to assess cardiac function during minimally invasive cardiac surgery (MICS) and to assess prosthetic valves.

BASICS THE NURSE NEEDS TO KNOW

A transesophageal echocardiogram is an invasive procedure that uses ultrasound techniques to detect enlargement of cardiac chambers and variations in chamber size during the cardiac cycle. It also assesses valvular function, septal defects, and pericardial effusion. Although these functions can be accomplished with a transthoracic echocardiogram, transesophageal echocardiography permits a better view of the posterior atrium and aorta. Transesophageal echocardiography also is indicated when a transthoracic approach is inadequate, such as when the patient is obese or has chest wall structure abnormalities.

NORMAL VALUES

No anatomic or functional abnormalities

HOW THE TEST IS DONE

Transesophageal echocardiography is similar to transthoracic echocardiography except that the ultrasound probe is fitted into the end of a flexible gastroscopy tube and advanced down the esophagus behind the heart.

SIGNIFICANCE OF TEST RESULTS

Abnormal Values

Abnormal heart valves
Aneurysm
Cardiomyopathy
Congenital heart disorders
Congestive heart failure
Idiopathic hypertrophic subaortic stenosis
Mural thrombi
Myocardial infarction
Pericardial effusion
Restrictive pericarditis
Tumor of the heart

INTERFERING FACTORS

- Transesophageal echocardiography should not be performed if the patient has a history of irradiation of the mediastinum, esophageal dysphagia, or structural abnormalities

NURSING CARE

Pretest

- Ensure that a signed informed consent has been obtained.
- The nurse questions the patient about any disorder of the esophagus, stomach, throat, or vocal cords. The nurse also inquires if the patient has dentures, bridges, or plates.
- The nurse reports to the physician any history of arthritis of the neck, respiratory problems, or anticoagulation therapy.

NURSING CARE—*cont'd*

- Maintain the patient on a nothing-by-mouth status for 6 to 8 hours.
- The nurse describes the procedure to the patient, especially the need for a mouth-guard, positioning, and the need to swallow when asked.
- If the patient has prosthetic heart valves, the nurse administers prophylactic antibiotics, as prescribed.
- Report any indications of infection in the mouth or throat.
- The nurse administers antianxiety medication, as prescribed.

During the Test

- Administer medication to decrease secretions, as ordered.
- A topical anesthetic is sprayed into the throat.
- The nurse instructs the patient to gargle with viscous lidocaine and then to swallow it. Warn the patient that it will make the tongue and throat feel "swollen."
- A mouthguard is placed to prevent the patient from biting down on the endoscope.
- The patient is positioned on the left side in the chin-chest position. The head may be supported with a small pillow.
- The probe is lubricated with lidocaine jelly and the physician slowly inserts it as the patient swallows.
- The nurse monitors the patient for a vasovagal response from the medication given to dry up secretions. The patient also is assessed for gagging. The nurse observes the oximeter for oxygen saturation readings.

Posttest

- Assess the patient for return of the gag reflex before resuming oral intake.
- The nurse instructs the patient to avoid hot liquids or foods for 2 hours.
- If in an outpatient setting, the nurse ensures the patient is accompanied home by another person.
- Give lozenges for relief of throat discomfort.

Nursing Response to Complications

Transesophageal echocardiography has several complications that are related to the placement of the probe in the esophagus, including esophageal perforation, transient hypoxia, dysrhythmias, and a vasovagal response.

Esophageal perforation. An esophageal perforation will be evident during the procedure. Bleeding and pain will occur. The nurse will assist the physician as directed.

Transient hypoxia. Transient hypoxia may be noted with the insertion of the ultrasound probe. The nurse maintains the patient on a pulse oximeter and administers oxygen as ordered.

Dysrhythmias. During the procedure the patient is kept on a cardiac monitor. The nurse needs to monitor for dysrhythmias and response to possible lethal dysrhythmias. Dysrhythmias may also occur due to a vasovagal response. Notify the physician and anticipate treatment based on established protocols.

Transferrin and Transferrin Saturation

See Iron Studies on p. 411.

Transthoracic Needle Biopsy

See Biopsy of the Lung, Percutaneous, Needle on p. 138.

Triglycerides, Serum

See Lipid Profile on p. 431.

Triiodothyronine

trai-ai-oh-doh-thai-roh-neen

Also called: T_3; T_3 Total; Total T_3

SPECIMEN OR TYPE OF TEST: Serum

PURPOSE OF THE TEST

Triiodothyronine levels are obtained as part of the diagnostic process to determine hyper- or hypothyroidism and to diagnose triiodothyronine toxicosis.

BASICS THE NURSE NEEDS TO KNOW

The thyroid gland produces and secretes the hormones thyroxine and triiodothyronine. This gland takes up iodine from the extracellular fluid and uses the iodine to produce thyroglobulin, the precursor of all thyroid hormones. The thyroglobulin is stored in the thyroid gland until thyroxine and triiodothyronine are processed before secretion from the gland. Secretion of triiodothyronine and thyroxine is primarily regulated by a negative feedback mechanism with thyrotropin (Figure 82). Thyrotropin is secreted by the anterior pituitary gland.

Once secreted by the thyroid gland, triiodothyronine and thyroxine are bound primarily to thyroid-binding globulin and, to a lesser degree, to albumin and prealbumin. The small amount of the hormones not bound to protein is called *free thyroxine* and *free triiodothyronine*. It is the free hormones that are biologically active. The bound hormones are released from the protein as the hormones are needed. In the peripheral circulation, thyroxine will lose one of its iodine molecules and become triiodothyronine, the more potent of the thyroid hormones.

Because the majority of the thyroid hormones are bound to protein, the evaluation of thyroid hormone levels should include the person's protein levels. If the patient has decreased proteins to carry the hormone, a greater amount of the hormone will be in the free state or active form.

NORMAL VALUES

Adult: 40–204 ng/dL *or* SI: 0.6–3.1 nmol/L
Children:
10–20 years: 80–213 ng/dL *or* SI: 1.2–3.3 nmol/L
1–10 years: 105–269 ng/dL *or* SI: 1.6–4.1 nmol/L
1–12 months: 105–245 ng/dL *or* SI: 1.6–3.7 nmol/L
Newborn: 100–740 ng/dL *or* SI: 1.5–11.4 nmol/L

HOW THE TEST IS DONE

Venipuncture is performed to obtain 3 mL of blood in a red-topped tube.

SIGNIFICANCE OF TEST RESULTS

Elevated Values

Hyperthyroidism
Pregnancy
Toxic adenoma of the thyroid gland
Toxic nodular goiter

Decreased Values

Hypothyroidism
Liver disease
Recent surgery
Renal disease
Sick euthyroid syndrome

INTERFERING FACTORS

- Significant increase or decrease in thyroxine-binding globulins
- Medications such as estrogen, heparin, iodides, triiodothyronine replacement therapy, lithium, methadone, methimazole, methylthiouracil, phenylbutazone, phenytoin, progestins, propranolol, propylthiouracil, reserpine, salicylates, steroids, and sulfonamides

NURSING CARE

Nursing actions are similar to those for other venipuncture procedures, as presented in Chapter 2.

T

Troponin, Serum

See Cardiac Markers on p. 178.

Type and Crossmatch

taip and kros-mach

Also called: Blood Compatibility Testing; Crossmatch

SPECIMEN OR TYPE OF TEST: Blood

PURPOSE OF THE TEST

In preparation for transfusion, these tests are performed to determine the major blood groups, to screen for antibodies, and to determine the compatibility of the blood of the recipient and that of the potential donor.

BASICS THE NURSE NEEDS TO KNOW

Human blood is typed by group, based on the presence or absence of A, B, AB, O, and Rh antigens. Blood group A has A antigens on the erythrocytes and anti-B antibodies in the serum. Blood group B has B antigens on the erythrocytes and anti-A antibodies in the serum. Blood group AB (universal receiver) has a double set of antigens on the erythrocytes and no antibodies in the serum, whereas blood group O (universal donor) has no antigens on the erythrocytes and a double set of antibodies in the serum (Table 14). When Rh antigens also are present on the erythrocytes, the person is classified as Rh positive. With no Rh antigens on the erythrocytes, the person is classified as Rh negative.

In preparation for blood transfusion, the intended recipient's blood is tested for ABO/Rh_O(D) type and antibody screening. In the crossmatch part of the test, the donor's blood type is determined and the blood is screened to identify antibodies. In selecting a donor's blood that matches that of the recipient, a compatibility of antigens and antibodies must exist so that the transfusion is safe for the recipient. Incompatibility results in agglutination (clumping) and hemolysis of the erythrocytes. Incompatible blood must not be administered to the patient.

The process of typing and crossmatching the blood determines a probable compatibility between the blood of the donor and that of the recipient. Despite careful work, some incidence of transfusion reaction occurs. The process of typing and crossmatching cannot detect all possible antibodies, nor can it detect reactions to components other than erythrocytes. Most cases of severe transfusion reaction are a result of clerical error, including administration of the wrong unit of blood to the patient or identification of the wrong patient. Complications of a severe transfusion reaction include a shortened lifespan or hemolysis of the erythrocytes, anaphylaxis, or sudden death.

NORMAL VALUES Not applicable

TABLE 14 Erythrocyte Antigens and Antibodies: ABO System

Blood Group	Erythrocyte Antigens	Serum Antibodies
A	A	Anti-B
B	B	Anti-A
AB	AB	None
O	None	Anti-A, anti-B

HOW THE TEST IS DONE

Intended recipient's blood: Two red-topped tubes and one lavender-topped tube are used to collect 7 mL of venous blood in each tube.

SIGNIFICANCE OF TEST RESULTS

Positive Crossmatch

Incompatibility between the donor's blood and the recipient's blood

Negative Crossmatch

Probable compatibility between the donor's blood and the recipient's blood
The donor unit of blood is considered safe for transfusion to the recipient

INTERFERING FACTORS

- Hemolysis
- Inadequate identification procedure

NURSING CARE

Nursing measures include care of the venipuncture or capillary puncture site as described in Chapter 2, with the following additional measures.

Pretest

- Ask the intended recipient about a history of blood transfusion in the past 3 months because antibodies from a previous transfusion may be present. Additional laboratory testing is needed when the antibody screen is positive.

During the Test

- When blood is to be drawn, the intended recipient must be identified with absolute certainty by the person who draws the blood using the following steps: the intended recipient states his or her name, and the hospital wristband is compared with the verbal identification.
- A transfusion wristband is also applied to the recipient's wrist. This wristband contains the recipient's name and hospital identification number and the date and initials of the phlebotomist. The specimen tubes and the requisition form also are labeled with the same identification information.
- The requisition form is signed by the phlebotomist, indicating that all identification information has been verified on the two wristbands and by the intended recipient.

Posttest

- Once the type and crossmatch is completed, the donor blood units are available for the recipient. Donor blood that has been crossmatched is usually held for no more than 24 hours.
- Use the same careful identification procedure when the blood is to be administered. The consequences of an error in identification are profound. When error occurs, it can result in the death of the patient.

Ultrasound

ul-truh-sound

Also called: Sonogram

SPECIMEN OR TYPE OF TEST: Sound wave imaging

PURPOSE OF THE TEST

Ultrasound examines organs, blood vessels, and structures of the body to identify malposition, malformation, malfunction, or the presence of a foreign body. It also may be used as a visual guide for accurate placement of a needle in a biopsy or aspiration procedure. In pregnancy ultrasound, the test is used to determine the age of the fetus and gestation of the pregnancy, as well as to assess for possible congenital malformation (see Figure 12 on p. 61).

BASICS THE NURSE NEEDS TO KNOW

Ultrasound is a scanning procedure that transmits sound waves in a directed path through the skin and into body tissues. The sound waves quickly bounce back or "echo" when they encounter a solid structure or tissue of different density. The sound waves are converted to a visual image that can be analyzed for abnormality (Figure 84).

The ultrasound pulsations transmit through fluid and body tissue, but do not transmit through air, bone, or barium. When the sound wave signals pass through tissues of varying densities, one method of imaging produces images in varying shades of white, gray, and black that correspond to the tissue size, shape, structure, and density.

Doppler ultrasound is a different method of ultrasound. It detects the presence, direction, speed, and character of arterial or venous blood flow within the vascular lumen. The Doppler pulses echo off the moving erythrocytes in the blood in patterns that correlate with the flow of the blood. The echoes are converted to an audio signal or a linear graphic reading on a paper strip, similar to an electrocardiogram strip. The audio signal changes according to the character of the blood flow. The blood flow may be characterized as *normal; disturbed*, as at the bifurcation of a blood vessel; or *turbulent*, as encountered beyond the point of a partial obstruction. Severely obstructed circulation produces a weak signal or silence. This type of ultrasound is very helpful in assessing the circulation in a vascular graft after bypass or transplant surgery has been done (see also Ultrasound, Doppler, Vascular, p. 635).

Transducer

The transducer, in the form of a scan head or probe, is the instrument used to generate and transmit the ultrasound energy and then receive the echo sound waves that bounce back from the tissue within. The returning sound waves are converted to audio signals or visual images. When the transducer is used externally, the scan head is moved over the skin in defined patterns, according to the anatomic location of the target tissue and the viewing plane that is desired. Other transducers are specialized probes used within the body. These probes can be used in the esophagus, vagina, rectum, or lumen of a blood vessel. The internal application is useful because the sound waves are placed

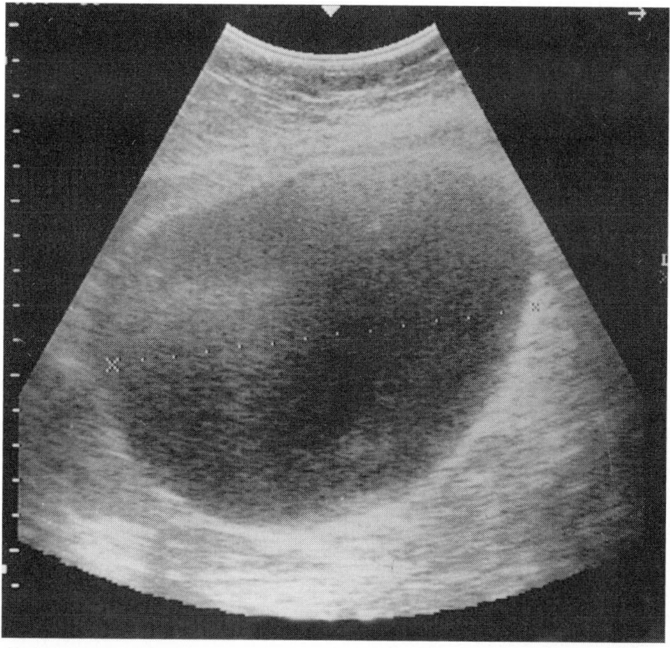

Figure 84. Abdominal ultrasound, liver. A hepatic cyst was the cause of the patient's pain in the right upper quadrant. The core of the cyst appears black because it is filled with fluid. *(Reproduced with permission from Schlager, D. [1997]. Ultrasound detection of foreign bodies and procedure guidance.* Emergency Medicine Clinics of North America, *15[4], 910.)*

near to the particular organ or tissue. The procedure reduces or eliminates the interference of other tissues and of the air of the lungs or bowel.

Many different ultrasound scans are used to examine organs, tissues, lymph nodes, and the vascular circulation. The more common scans are listed in Box 5.

Abdominal Ultrasound

Ultrasound is a major diagnostic tool for the examination of the liver, hepatobiliary tract, spleen, and pancreas. In the liver, it can detect a cyst, abscess, hematoma, primary neoplasm, and metastatic tumor. It is the best diagnostic tool to detect gallstones (Figure 85). It also may show thickening of the gall bladder walls associated with acute cholecystitis or dilation of the biliary tract associated with obstruction. An enlarged or edematous pancreas is measurable by ultrasound. Pancreatic abscess, pseudocyst, and pancreatic tumor are readily identified. Ultrasound identifies a congenital absence of the spleen or the existence of multiple spleens. It can also identify the presence and size of space-occupying lesions, such as cysts or tumors, and is accurate in the measurement of the size of the spleen.

BOX 5 Ultrasound Procedures

Popliteal artery scan
Inferior vena cava scan
Abdominal aorta scan
Carotid artery scan
Abdominal scan
Liver scan
Gall bladder, biliary tract scan
Pancreas scan
Renal scan
Spleen scan
Pelvic scans
- Female pelvic scan
- Obstetric scan
- Endovaginal scan
- Male pelvic scan

Thyroid scan
Scrotum scan
Breast scan
Transesophageal echocardiography
Echocardiography

Cardiac Ultrasound

Two cardiac ultrasound procedures are covered separately in detail in this text: Transesophageal Echocardiography (p. 623) and Echocardiogram (p. 281).

Renal Ultrasound

Renal ultrasound clearly defines the kidneys, including their size, shape, position, collecting systems, and surrounding tissues. Renal masses that are greater than 2 cm are readily detected, and renal cysts are a frequent finding. Ultrasound can identify the location and severity of obstruction. Renal ultrasound may be used as a guide for needle placement in renal biopsy, for drainage of a renal abscess, or for placement of a nephrostomy tube.

Pelvic Ultrasound

In the diagnosis of gynecologic problems in the female, one use of ultrasound is to identify an ovarian malignancy at an early stage. In the case of abnormal uterine bleeding, ultrasound will identify submucous leiomyomas and evaluate the thickness of the uterine wall. Pelvic ultrasound often precedes any invasive gynecologic diagnostic test, such as dilation and curettage. The procedure may also be used to monitor ovulation in the diagnosis and treatment of infertility and in follow-up after treatment for pelvic

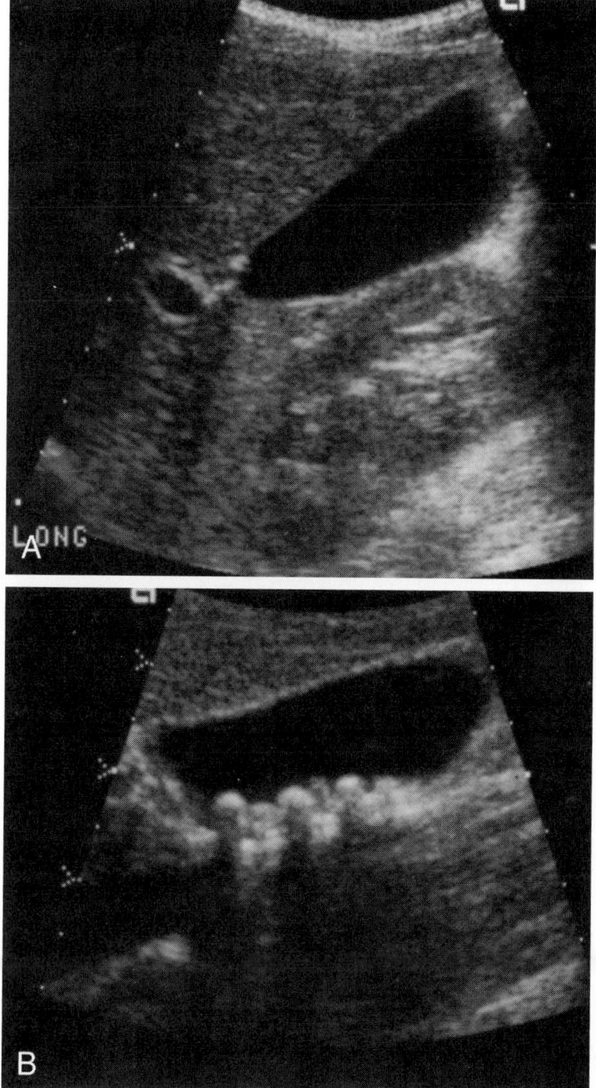

Figure 85. Abdominal ultrasound, gallbladder. *A*, Normal gallbladder. *B*, Gallbladder with gallstones. *(Reproduced with permission from Godderidge, C. [1995].* Pediatric imaging *[p. 193]. Philadelphia: W. B. Saunders.)*

inflammatory disease. For the female, the examination consists of imaging from both transabdominal and transvaginal approaches to obtain complete visualization.

Ultrasonography in the male is used to assess the texture, size, and condition of the prostate gland, prostatic urethra, seminal vesicles, and vas deferens. It is also used to guide the placement of the needle during biopsy of the prostate gland. Ultrasound is part of the diagnostic work-up to detect and stage prostate cancer.

Pregnancy Ultrasound

In conditions related to pregnancy, ultrasound identifies an early ectopic pregnancy, a multiple pregnancy, possible fetal abnormality, and assessment of fetal growth. It is also used to guide aspiration procedures such as amniocentesis, cordocentesis, and the aspiration of multiple oocytes for in vitro fertilization.

NORMAL VALUES

No anatomic or functional abnormalities exist. The organs are normal in size, shape, contour, and position. The internal structures of the organs and nearby tissues are within normal limits.

HOW THE TEST IS DONE

High-frequency sound waves from the transducer are directed into an area of the body in a specific pattern. The echoes of the ultrasound are converted to visual images, linear tracings, or audible sounds.

SIGNIFICANCE OF TEST RESULTS

Abnormal Values

Cyst
Tumor
Hypertrophy
Obstruction or stricture
Calculus
Aneurysm
Foreign body
Vascular occlusion
Venous thrombosis
Atherosclerotic plaque
Abscess
Congenital anomaly
Hematoma, bleeding
Pregnancy, fetal development

INTERFERING FACTORS

- Air
- Overlying bones
- Bowel gas
- Barium
- Obesity

NURSING CARE

Pretest

- Obtain a written consent, particularly for any ultrasound procedure that involves insertion of a transducer into a body cavity or blood vessel.
- The nurse schedules the ultrasound examination before or several days after any barium studies. Barium is an opaque substance that would block the transmission of ultrasound impulses. Residual barium causes an ultrasound problem for about 24 hours after a barium x-ray examination.
- ***Patient Teaching.*** The nurse or ultrasound technician instructs the patient about any dietary restrictions or modifications. Any abdominal ultrasound examination requires fasting from food for 12 hours. If the patient has a tendency toward bowel gas, a low-residue diet is implemented for 24 to 36 hours, followed by a 12-hour fast from all foods. Some abdominal ultrasound protocols require an enema before the examination because intestinal gas and feces must be removed from the colon. Gynecologic ultrasound procedures often require drinking 40 oz of water without voiding before the test. This fills the urinary bladder and moves it upward and away from the uterus.
- ***Patient Teaching.*** The nurse also instructs the patient that the examination is safe and painless. To alleviate anxiety, the nurse or examiner provides reassurance before and during the test.
- A small child or an agitated, anxious adult patient may be accompanied by a calming parent or other adult.

During the Test

- Assist the patient in removing all clothes, jewelry, and metallic objects. A hospital gown is worn. The patient is positioned on the examining table and is instructed to remain still during the examination. Neonates and infants are kept warm during the examination. Neonates are particularly prone to hypothermia, so a warming lamp may be used. The dark room, a pacifier, and gentle touch help keep the infant calm.
- The examiner applies the acoustic gel to the skin surface in the area to be examined. The gel serves as a conducting agent and eliminates the thin layer of air that would cause a barrier to the transmission of impulses. As the sound waves are transmitted, the image appears on a video screen or as an audible signal of vascular blood flow.

Posttest

- Remove the acoustic gel from the skin. This prevents soiling of the patient's clothes.

Ultrasound, Doppler, Vascular

ul-truh-sound, dop-ler, vas-kyuh-luhr

Also called: Doppler Flow Studies

SPECIMEN OR TYPE OF TEST: Ultrasound

PURPOSE OF THE TEST

In vascular studies, Doppler ultrasound detects stenosis or occlusion in an artery or vein, assists with the diagnosis of peripheral vascular or cerebrovascular disease, evaluates the results of arterial reconstruction or vascular bypass surgery, and assesses for possible trauma to an artery.

BASICS THE NURSE NEEDS TO KNOW

The Doppler ultrasound transducer transmits low-intensity sound waves that are directed at a specific blood vessel. The transmitted sound waves strike moving red blood cells and bounce back to the transducer-receiver. The received impulses are translated into an audible signal or a waveform recording on graph paper. Additionally, the systolic pressure in the upper and lower extremities can be measured.

Using the *audible signal*, changes in the pitch and volume of the blood flow can be heard. When the blood flow is normal, the sound is loud and of higher pitch. Conversely, when blood flow is constricted or partially obstructed, the sound is softer or fainter and the pitch is low. Total obstruction in a blood vessel produces no sound at all.

Waveform recordings are used to evaluate the circulation in lower extremities. The waveform recordings are Doppler signals that are transformed into a linear image. The waveforms are recorded on a graph-paper strip. In abnormal venous flow, as in partial or total venous occlusion, the augmentation signal of an upward spike is absent. Reflux flow, such as that caused by incompetent venous valves, is also evident on the waveform. The normal arterial waveform is characterized by three phases called the *systolic*, *diastolic*, and *wall rebound* phases (Figure 86). When the artery is stenosed, the waveform pattern diminishes in height. In severe obstruction, the diastolic phase and wall rebound phase are absent.

The *ankle-brachial index (ABI) and segmented pressures* are two measures that assess systolic pressures within the arteries of the extremity. Both tests use blood pressure cuffs and the Doppler probe to obtain exact systolic readings at different levels of the extremities. Stenosis or occlusion of the artery causes a drop in blood pressure distal to the site of the obstruction. The arterial pressure of the arteries of the ankle and upper arm should be approximately the same. An ABI of less than 0.9 indicates stenosis or occlusion of an artery. In segmented pressure readings, the purpose is to locate the site of the diminished circulation in the extremity. Normal pressure differences should not exceed 30 mm Hg between the right and left limbs or between the upper and lower segments of the extremity. A drop in pressure that exceeds the normal value locates stenosis or occlusion of an artery in a particular segment of the extremity.

Color-flow Doppler imaging demonstrates the change in blood flow in various colors. Blood flow that moves toward the transducer is imaged as a shade of red. Blood flow that moves away from the transducer is imaged as a shade of blue. When blood flow within the artery or vein is normal, the color is intense, and the lumen of the blood vessel should be filled with color. With obstruction of the blood flow, such as with deep vein thrombosis, the color fades from red to orange or yellow or from blue to aqua or white. This method may be used to assess cranial neck vessels and is also used to assess the abdominal aorta and the peripheral vascular system. The technique can detect an embolus, stenosis, a thrombus, an aneurysm, and venous insufficiency.

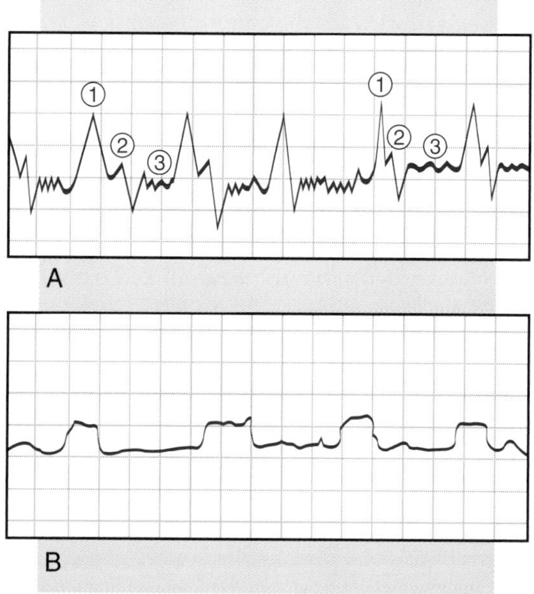

Figure 86. Normal versus abnormal Doppler arterial waveform patterns. *A*, Normal waveform with triphasic pattern of sharp upstroke and downstroke and good amplitude: *1*, systolic component; *2*, diastolic component; and *3*, elastic wall rebound. *B*, Abnormal waveform with monophasic pattern of low amplitude and flat waves. This pattern indicates severe arterial obstruction.

NORMAL VALUES

Arterial or venous examination: Normal frequency and volume of audio signal, normal waveform pattern, and normal color for blood flow velocity. There is no evidence of vascular stenosis or obstruction from a thrombus or embolus.

ABI: 0.9–1

Segmented pressures: <30 mm Hg difference in systolic pressure between the upper and lower segments of same extremity or between the right and left extremities

HOW THE TEST IS DONE

Venous and Arterial Doppler Tests

Acoustic gel and the Doppler probe are placed on the skin at the desired vascular sites. Audible signals are heard and interpreted. Three to five waveforms are recorded at each vascular site. The specific vascular sites and sides of the body (right or left) are identified to avoid confusion and error.

Venous sites of the lower extremities are the posterior tibial, greater saphenous, common femoral, superficial femoral, and popliteal veins. Venous sites of the upper extremities and neck are the brachial, axillary, subclavian, and jugular veins. Arterial pulse sites of the lower extremities are the common femoral, popliteal, dorsalis pedis, and posterior tibial pulses. Arterial pulse sites in the upper extremities and neck are the brachial, radial, ulnar, and carotid pulses.

Segmented Pressures

Blood pressure cuffs are applied to both upper thighs, above and below the knees, and above the ankles. Gel is applied to the skin. The pressure cuffs are inflated one at a time. On deflation of each, the Doppler probe identifies the systolic pressure by audio signal, and the numeric value is recorded. The ABI is calculated from the ankle and brachial pressures.

SIGNIFICANCE OF TEST RESULTS

Abnormal Values

Arterial stenosis or occlusion
Venous thrombosis
Incompetent venous valves
Atherosclerotic plaque

INTERFERING FACTORS

- Nicotine, alcohol, and caffeine
- Anxiety
- Uncooperative patient behavior

NURSING CARE

Pretest

- After the physician has informed the patient about the test, obtain a written consent from the patient.
- ***Patient Teaching.*** The nurse instructs the patient to avoid nicotine, alcohol, caffeine, and other stimulants and depressants that will cause vasoconstriction. To help control the patient's anxiety, the nurse reassures the patient that the test is painless.
- In most cases, vascular testing will be done in a radiology setting or a vascular laboratory. The room lighting should be reduced to promote relaxation. The patient will put on a hospital gown. For arterial tests, the patient is in the supine position. For venous tests of the lower extremities, the patient is placed in the supine position with two pillows under the legs to elevate them above the heart. The leg and hip are externally rotated, and the knee is flexed.

During the Test

- The nurse may perform ongoing audio Doppler assessments of pulses, particularly on the patient who has lower limb ischemia and pulses that are too faint to be palpated. The assessments may also be done to check the distal blood flow after a vascular graft or bypass graft is in place.

NURSING CARE—*cont'd*

- The procedure is to locate the pulse points on the upper or lower extremities and apply acoustic gel. At each pulse point, apply the transducer head to the skin and listen to the blowing sounds produced by the audio mode of the Doppler instrument.

Posttest

- Remove the acoustic gel from the skin. Record the findings in the patient's record.

Ultrasound, Pancreatic

ul-truh-sound, pan-kree-a-tik

Also called: Pancreatic Sonogram

SPECIMEN OR TYPE OF TEST: Ultrasound

PURPOSE OF THE TEST

An ultrasound of the pancreas is performed to support the diagnosis and progression of pancreatitis and to identify tumors, cysts, and pseudocysts. Ultrasound may be used as a guide for fine needle biopsy of the pancreas.

BASICS THE NURSE NEEDS TO KNOW

The pancreas is both an exocrine organ and an endocrine organ. The exocrine function consists of the production and excretion of digestive enzymes required for the absorption of ingested food. The endocrine function consists of the production and secretion of hormones necessary for cellular nutrition.

A pancreatic sonogram assesses the size, shape, and positioning of the organ. Inflammation of the pancreas, as well as calculi, cyst, pseudocyst, and tumor can be identified by ultrasound.

NORMAL VALUES Normal size and morphologic features

HOW THE TEST IS DONE

High-frequency sound waves from the transducer are directed into an area of the body in a specific pattern. The echoes of the ultrasound vary with the densities of the different tissues and organs. The echoes are converted to visual images.

SIGNIFICANCE OF TEST RESULTS

Abnormal Values

Abscess
Acute or chronic pancreatitis
Cancer
Cyst
Pseudocyst

INTERFERING FACTORS

- Barium or gas in the bowel
- Dehydration
- Noncompliance with fasting
- Obesity

NURSING CARE

- Review section on Ultrasound, p. 630, with the following additional measures.

Pretest

- Schedule any barium studies to be done after the sonogram. If a barium study was done prior to this test, the retained barium would interfere with the ultrasound imaging
- ***Patient Teaching.*** The nurse instructs the patient not to eat or drink for 12 hours before the test.
- ***Patient Teaching.*** Explain to the patient the need to distend the stomach to visualize the entire pancreas.

During the Test

- The nurse encourages the patient to drink the prescribed fluid (500 to 1000 mL of juice).
- Place the patient in the supine position. The patient is usually repositioned during the procedure to a sitting position.
- The examiner places acoustic gel on the skin to reduce interference from air and promote contact of the transducer head with the skin. As the transducer is moved along various planes of the abdomen, the images of the pancreas are visualized.

Posttest

- The acoustic gel is removed. The patient resumes a normal diet.

Upper Gastrointestinal Series and Small Bowel Series

U

u-per gas-troh-in-tes-tin-uhl seer-eez and smahl bow-el seer-eez

Also called: Upper GI Series; Small Bowel Follow-Through

SPECIMEN OR TYPE OF TEST: Radiography

PURPOSE OF THE TEST

The upper GI series detects disorders of structure or function of the esophagus, stomach, and duodenum. One week postoperatively, it is used to evaluate the results of gastric surgery. As an extension of the upper GI series, the small bowel series detects disorders of the jejunum and ileum.

BASICS THE NURSE NEEDS TO KNOW

The upper GI series involves a radiologic examination from the oral part of the pharynx to the duodenojejunal junction. When the small bowel requires examination, the small bowel series often follows the upper GI series directly, but it can be performed as a single procedure. The common sources of abnormality in the upper GI tract are stricture, inflammation, swelling, ulcers, tumors, motility disorders, or structural changes in the wall of the intestine.

The barium liquid is a radiopaque contrast medium that outlines the size, shape, and contour of the intestinal lumen. Air may be instilled to provide double contrast and better visualization of the lumen of the esophagus, stomach, and duodenum. Fluoroscopy and x-ray films are used at intermittent intervals to obtain the gastrointestinal images.

NORMAL VALUES No structural or functional abnormalities are found.

HOW THE TEST IS DONE

Upper Gastrointestinal Series

The patient drinks a barium solution to provide contrast views during swallowing and peristaltic action in the esophagus. As the barium coats the mucosal lining of the stomach, additional films are taken to outline the shape and contour of the organ (Figure 87).

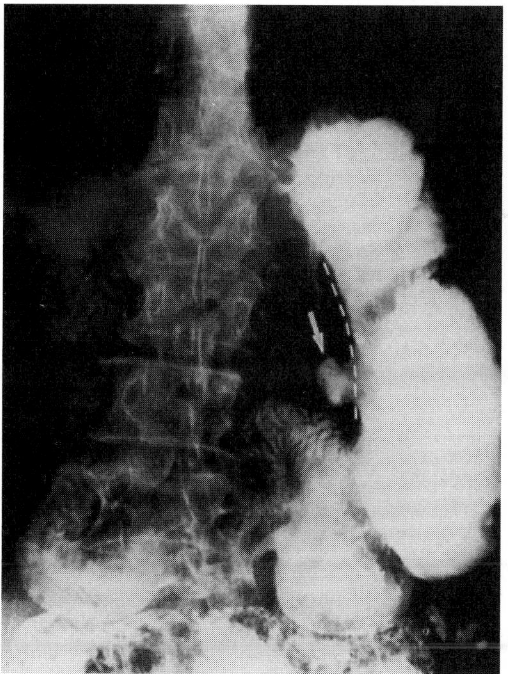

Figure 87. Upper gastrointestinal series view of a benign gastric ulcer. A large ulcer (*arrow*) is seen along the lesser curvature of the stomach. Notice that the ulcer projects out beyond the normal expected lesser curvature (*dotted line*). *(Reproduced with permission from Mettler, F. A. [1996].* Essentials of radiology *[p. 191]. Philadelphia: W. B. Saunders.)*

The patient's positional changes (vertical, supine, prone, and lateral) help coat the mucosa throughout the organ.

Small Bowel Series

When a small bowel series is included in this radiologic study, the transit time of the barium can be from 30 minutes to 6 hours before it reaches the colon. At the start of the small bowel series, additional barium is taken orally. The transit time can be shortened by having the patient drink 200 mL of iced water or eat a light meal after all the additional barium has left the stomach. Fluoroscopic views are taken three times in the first hour and every 30 minutes thereafter. Radiographic films are taken of any abnormality.

Enteroclysis Method

When the small bowel series is performed separately, enteroclysis may be used to instill the barium. A radiopaque catheter is passed through the nose or mouth and advanced past the pylorus and into the duodenum. Barium, followed by methylcellulose solution, is instilled by the catheter route directly into the small bowel. Views of the total small bowel can be completed in 20 to 30 minutes.

SIGNIFICANCE OF TEST RESULTS

Abnormal Values

Esophagus

Reflux esophagitis
Esophageal scarring or stricture
Barrett's esophagus
Infectious esophagitis

Stomach-Duodenum

Peptic ulcer (gastric, duodenal)
Cancer (stomach, duodenum)
Pyloric obstruction
Benign tumor
Gastric inflammatory disease
Perforation
Diverticula

Small Bowel

Malabsorption
Crohn's disease
Chronic appendicitis
Stricture
Hodgkin's disease
Cancer
Diffuse sclerosis
Surgical resection
Congenital abnormality
Intussusception
Perforation

INTERFERING FACTORS

- Failure to maintain nothing-by-mouth status
- Excess air in the small bowel

NURSING CARE

Pretest

- After the physician explains the test to the patient, a patient consent form must be signed. The nurse ensures that the signed form is entered into the patient's record.
- ***Patient Teaching.*** The nurse instructs the patient to fast from all food for 8 hours and all liquids for 4 hours before the test. In addition, most oral medications are withheld in the 8 hours before the test. Narcotics and anticholinergics are withheld for 24 hours before the test because they slow the motility of the intestinal tract.

During the Test

- The hospitalized patient may return to the nursing unit for an interval before the small bowel filming begins. The nurse obtains instructions from the radiology department about the nothing-by-mouth status or about a prescribed meal.

Posttest

- A laxative is given to the patient to help evacuate the barium promptly. Retained barium can cause constipation, obstruction, or fecal impaction.
- ***Patient Teaching.*** The nurse informs the patient that the feces will be gray or whitish for 24 to 72 hours until all barium has been evacuated. The patient is advised to rest for the remainder of the day because the test is tiring.

Urea Nitrogen, Blood

yuh-ree-uh nai-troh-gen, blud

Also called: (BUN); Blood Urea Nitrogen

SPECIMEN OR TYPE OF TEST: Serum

PURPOSE OF THE TEST

The blood urea nitrogen (BUN) level is used to evaluate renal function. With the serum creatinine level, it is used to monitor patients in renal failure or the patients receiving dialysis therapy.

BASICS THE NURSE NEEDS TO KNOW

BUN is the major nitrogenous end product of protein and amino acid catabolism. It is produced in the liver and distributed throughout intracellular and extracellular fluid. Urea nitrogen is excreted from the body primarily by the kidneys; lesser amounts are excreted in sweat or degraded by intestinal bacteria.

In the kidneys, almost all urea is filtered out of the blood by glomerular function. Some urea is resorbed with water in the renal tubules, but most is removed from the body in urine. The amount of urea excreted is dependent on the state of hydration and renal perfusion. If the patient is dehydrated, low tubular flow of urinary filtrate occurs, and more urea is absorbed. If overhydration and a high tubular flow rate exist, less urea is resorbed, resulting in a lower serum level.

Urea nitrogen level can rise from renal and nonrenal factors. Nonrenal factors include increased urea production associated with increased dietary protein intake and increased catabolism, such as occurs with corticosteroid therapy or muscle-wasting diseases. When excess urea is produced, the serum level rarely rises above 40 mg/dL (SI: >14.2 mmol/L). Some medications will cause a *slight* increase in the BUN level.

Renal causes of an elevated BUN level may result from prerenal, intrarenal, or postrenal problems. Prerenal disease includes poor renal blood flow, as in shock or renal artery stenosis with resulting decrease in glomerular filtration rate. Intrarenal disease includes damage to the renal parenchyma. Renal causes of azotemia result in a dramatic rise in the BUN level. Postrenal problems are related to obstruction in the kidney or in the urinary tract.

NORMAL VALUES	Older adult (>60 years): 8–23 mg/dL *or* SI: 2.9–8.2 mmol/L Child to adult (1–60 years): 5–20 mg/dL *or* SI: 1.8–7.1 mmol/L Infant (birth–1 year): 4–19 mg/dL *or* SI: 1.4–6.8 mmol/L
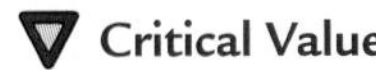 Critical Value	100 mg/dL or higher (SI: 35.7 mmol/L or higher)

HOW THE TEST IS DONE

A red-topped tube is used to obtain venous blood.

SIGNIFICANCE OF TEST RESULTS

Elevated Values

Acute or chronic renal failure
Shock
Renal artery stenosis
Hemorrhage
Postrenal syndrome
Stress
Congestive heart failure
Burns
Increased protein intake
Dehydration
Hyperalimentation
Ketoacidosis
Long-term steroid therapy
Diabetes mellitus

Decreased Values

Overhydration
Starvation
Intravenous therapy
Low-protein diet

Acromegaly
Severe liver damage

INTERFERING FACTORS

- None

NURSING CARE

Care of the patient is similar to that for other venipunctures, as described in Chapter 2.

▼ Nursing Response to Critical Values

Any BUN over 100 is extremely elevated and defines the condition of uremia. The patient will be stuporous or comatose. Usually, renal failure is identified at much lower levels. A patient with values at this level needs dialysis to remove the waste products of metabolism.

Uric Acid

yur-ik a-sid

Also called: Urate

SPECIMEN OR TYPE OF TEST: Serum

PURPOSE OF THE TEST

The elevated level of uric acid is used to confirm the diagnosis of gout and helps detect renal impairment that causes prerenal azotemia and renal failure.

BASICS THE NURSE NEEDS TO KNOW

Uric acid is the end product of protein metabolism and is excreted from the body by the kidneys and intestinal tract. The production of uric acid comes from a combination of dietary intake of protein and purine foods, purine biosynthesis, and catabolism of body tissues. The normal excretion of uric acid by the kidneys should eliminate two thirds of the uric acid from the blood daily. The remaining one third is in the bile and intestinal secretions. The level of uric acid in the blood is maintained by a balance between the amount that is produced and the amount that is excreted (Figure 88).

U

Elevated Values

Hyperuricemia is an elevated level of uric acid in the blood. It may occur from excessive production of uric acid but more frequently, it occurs because of impaired excretion. The conditions of abnormal overproduction include abnormal metabolism of purines and amino acids, excessive catabolism of body tissues, as in cancer before and after chemotherapy or radiation, some hemolytic disorders, and conditions that cause acidosis or lactic acidosis. Impaired excretion or urate retention is usually a result of renal disease that affects tubular secretion and reabsorption. It may also be caused by reduced renal blood flow and decreased renal filtration of the blood. Hyperurecemia exists when the serum urate level is >7.0 mg/dL (SI: >416 µmol/L).

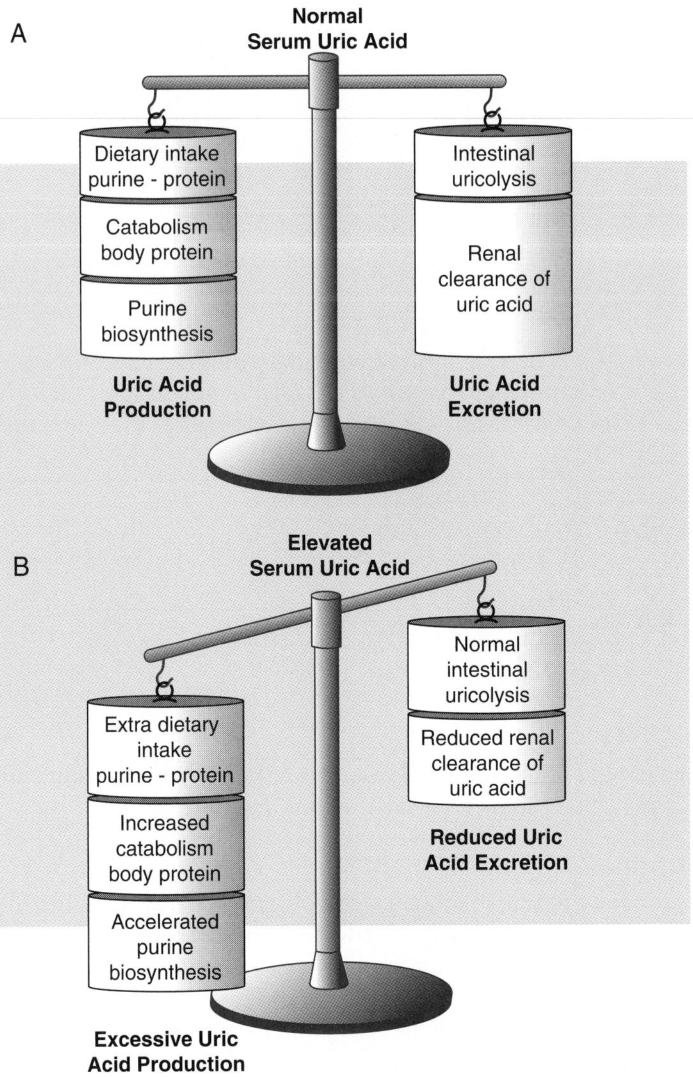

Figure 88. Uric acid production and excretion. *A*, Normal physiology. *B*, Pathophysiology of hyperuricemia.

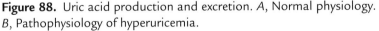

Gout produces an elevated level of uric acid in the blood. The condition may be asymptomatic or may cause acute gouty arthritis, often affecting the metatarsal joint of the big toe. The condition can cause acute attacks of pain, redness, and swelling, with quiet periods in between acute episodes. The urate crystals can form tophi, or nodular deposits of urate crystals in the joints, cartilage, bones, bursae, and subcutaneous tissue (Figure 89). The urate crystals also can accumulate in the renal pelvis and cause uric acid kidney stones to form. Some patients develop gout with lower elevations of serum uric acid and some have high levels of serum uric acid and do not acquire this inflammatory disease.

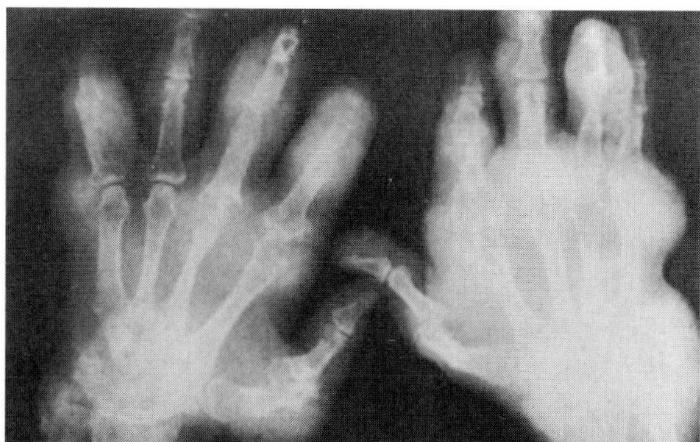

Figure 89. Radiographic visualization of bone changes in gout. Osteolytic changes have resulted from bone destruction owing to the disease process known as gout. Note the soft tissue swelling and bone destruction in the joints of both hands. *(Reproduced with permission from Thompson, M. A., Hattaway, M. P., Hall, J. D., & Dowd, S. B. [1994].* Principles of imaging science and protection *[Vol. 2, Slide 293]. Philadelphia: W. B. Saunders.)*

Decreased Values

Hypouricemia is an abnormally low level of uric acid in the blood. It usually results from defects in renal tubular absorption. The disorder can be congenital or acquired, but an increased urinary loss of urate and, therefore, a low level of uric acid in the blood occurs.

NORMAL VALUES	**Adult** Male: 3.4–7.0 mg/dL *or* SI: 202-416 μmol/L Female: 2.4–6.0 mg/dL *or* SI: 143-357 μmol/L
▼ Critical Value	>12 mg/dL *or* SI: >714 μmol/L

HOW THE TEST IS DONE

A red-topped tube is used to collect 10 mL of venous blood.

SIGNIFICANCE OF TEST RESULTS

Elevated Values

Gout
Diabetic ketoacidosis
Renal failure
Shock
Polycystic kidney disease
Leukemia
Tumor lysis syndrome
Lymphoma

Hemolytic anemia
Lead poisoning
Polycythemia vera
Pernicious anemia
Glycogen storage disease
Acute alcohol ingestion

Decreased Values
Fanconi syndrome
Wilson's disease
Hodgkin's disease
Multiple myeloma
Bronchogenic carcinoma

INTERFERING FACTORS

- Starvation
- High purine diet
- Stress
- Caffeine or vitamin C ingestion

NURSING CARE

Nursing measures include care of the venipuncture site, as described in Chapter 2.

Pretest

- On the requisition slip, list all medications taken by the patient. Many medications cause either a false-positive or a false-negative result.
- ***Patient Teaching.*** Instruct the patient to discontinue all food and fluids for 8 hours. Alcohol also should be discontinued before the test, because it will elevate the uric acid blood level.

Posttest

- ***Patient Teaching.*** When gout has been diagnosed, the nurse teaches the patient to drink adequate fluids daily. This will help flush urate crystals from the kidneys The patient is also instructed to reduce the intake of high purine foods, including organ meats, beef, and legumes, because high purine foods increase the level of uric acid. The intake of alcohol should be avoided because alcohol will increase the production of uric acid and alter the excretion of urate from the kidneys.

▼ Nursing Responsibility to Critical Values

If the serum level rises to 12 mg/dL (SI: 714 µmol/L) or higher, urate crystals can accumulate in the renal tubules and ureters, resulting in obstruction and renal failure. This crisis can occur after administration of cytotoxic drugs, after a malignancy is irradiated, as a result of acute alcohol ingestion, or with adult respiratory distress syndrome. The nurse must notify the physician of this critical elevation that is a marker of cell injury crisis. Specific interventions will depend on the cause of the problem.

U

Uric Acid, Urine

yur-ik a-sid, yur-in

Also called: Urine Urate

SPECIMEN OR TYPE OF TEST: Urine

PURPOSE OF THE TEST

The urinary uric acid test measures the urinary excretion of uric acid in patients with renal calculi or in those at risk for the development of a calculus. The test also is used to assess the effect of enzyme deficiency or metabolic abnormality that results in the overproduction of uric acid.

BASICS THE NURSE NEEDS TO KNOW

As an end product of protein metabolism, uric acid and urate crystals are excreted by the kidneys and bowel. *Hyperuricosuria*, a high level of uric acid in the urine, may be caused by excess secretion or excess production of uric acid.

When leukemia is treated with cytotoxic drugs or when malignant tumors are irradiated, tumor necrosis and a metabolic breakdown of nucleoprotein occur. This causes a massive amount of uric acid and urate crystal production that can result in elevation of the urine uric acid level. The urate crystals can block the renal tubules and ureters, resulting in renal failure.

NORMAL VALUES

Average diet (adult female): 250–750 mg/24 hr *or*
SI: 1.48–4.43 mmol/24 hr
Average diet (adult male): 250–800 mg/24 hr *or*
SI: 1.48–4.8 mmol/24 hr
Low purine diet (male): <420 mg/24 hr *or*
SI: <2.83 mmol/24 hr
Low purine diet (female): <400 mg/24 hr *or*
SI: <2.36 mmol/24 hr
High purine diet (adult): <1000 mg/24 hr *or*
SI: <5.9 mmol/24 hr

HOW THE TEST IS DONE

A 24-hour urine collection is used to measure the amount of daily uric acid that is excreted. The laboratory will provide a collection container with sodium hydroxide, which keeps the pH of the urine in an alkaline state. This prevents precipitation of urate crystals.

SIGNIFICANCE OF TEST RESULTS

Elevated Values

Uric acid nephrolithiasis
Viral hepatitis
Gout
Glycogen storage disease

Leukemia, chronic myeloid
Lesch-Nyhan syndrome
Acute leukemia of childhood
Radiation therapy
Lymphatic leukemia
Crohn's disease
Lymphosarcoma
Ulcerative colitis
Wilson's disease
Ileostomy
Cystinosis
Surgical jejunoileal bypass
Sickle cell anemia
Polycythemia vera
Tumor lysis syndrome

Decreased Values
Chronic glomerulonephritis
Collagen disease
Diabetic glomerulosclerosis
Lead toxicity
Folic acid deficiency
Renal failure
Xanthinuria

INTERFERING FACTORS

- Failure to collect all urine during the test period
- Failure to store the specimen properly
- High- or low-purine diet
- Many medications (including aspirin, antiinflammatory drugs, diuretics, vitamin C, and x-ray contrast medium)

NURSING CARE

Nursing actions related to the timed urine collection procedure are presented in Chapter 2, with the following additional measures.

Pretest

- Instruct the patient to collect all urine of the 24-hour test period and store it in a large container. Some laboratories require the specimen to be refrigerated or stored on ice during the test period. Other laboratories do not require refrigeration.

During the Test

- The nurse asks the patient to void at 8 AM. Discard the 8 AM specimen. All urine is collected for 24 hours thereafter, including the 8 AM specimen of the following morning.
- Ensure that the label and requisition slip contain the patient's name and the time and date of the start and finish of the test.

NURSING CARE—*cont'd*

Posttest

- List all medications taken by the patient on the requisition slip.
- Arrange for transport of the specimen to the laboratory on ice if required.

Urinalysis

yur-in-al-uh-sis

Also called: (UA)

SPECIMEN OR TYPE OF TEST: Urine

PURPOSE OF THE TEST

Urinalysis is performed to screen for urinary tract disorders, kidney disorders, urinary neoplasm, and other medical conditions that produce changes in the urine. This test also is used to monitor the effects of treatment of known renal or urinary conditions.

BASICS THE NURSE NEEDS TO KNOW

Urinalysis produces a large amount of information about possible diseases of the kidneys and lower urinary tract, as well as systemic diseases that alter the composition of the urine. Analysis of the urine consists of two parts: the chemical analysis and the microscopic analysis. The chemical analysis is usually performed by the dipstick method (Figure 90). Microscopic analysis may be done routinely, but also is done in response to a specific request or as a follow-up to abnormal results of the chemical analysis.

Color and Clarity

There are many possible causes of changes of color or clarity, some of which are presented in Table 15. In addition, some medications and chemicals are responsible for changes in urine color.

Specific Gravity

The specific gravity is a measurement of the ability of the kidneys to concentrate and excrete the urine. Concentrated urine has a higher specific gravity because the proportion of components to water in its composition is greater. Diluted urine has a lower specific gravity because it contains fewer components in proportion to the amount of water. When the specific gravity of urine remains *fixed* (unvarying over time) at 1.010, that value is an indication of severe renal damage. It indicates that the renal tubules cannot resorb water and effectively concentrate the urine (see also Specific Gravity, Urinary, p. 594).

pH

As part of the acid-base balance, the kidneys remove excess hydrogen ions from the blood and excrete them in the urine. In abnormal physiology, a urine pH greater than

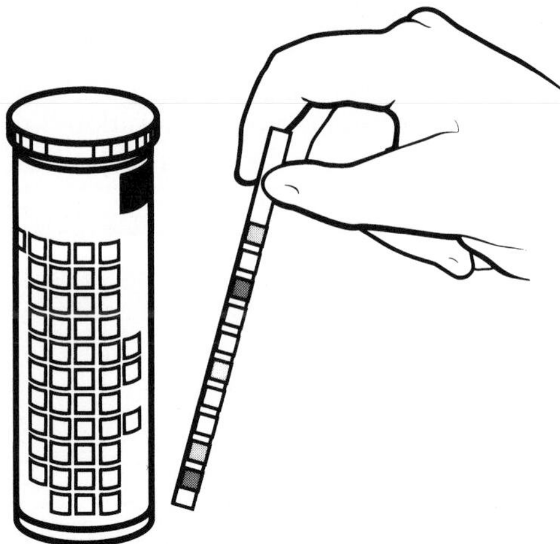

Figure 90. Urinalysis: dipstick method. A commercial reagent strip for urine chemistry testing and its container with color comparison chart. The reagent-impregnated test pads are fixed to an inert plastic strip. Once the strip has been wetted in a urine sample, a chemical reaction causes the reagent pad to change color. Results are obtained by comparing the color of the reagent pad to the appropriate analyte on the color chart. *(Reproduced with permission from Brunzel, N. A. [1994].* Fundamentals of urine and body fluid analysis *[p. 149]. Philadelphia: W. B. Saunders.)*

TABLE 15 Causes of Change in Urine Color and Clarity

Characteristic	Cause
Clarity	
Cloudy, smoky, hazy	Pyuria Bacteriuria Phosphates in the urine
Color	
Colorless	Overhydration Diuretic therapy Diabetes mellitus Diabetes insipidus
Dark red or pink	Acute intermittent porphyria Hematuria Ingestion of beets, berries, fava beans, red food coloring, rhubarb
Dark yellow or orange	Bile
Green	*Pseudomonas* bacteriuria Urinary bile pigments

6.5 indicates the presence of bicarbonate in the urine. Alkaline urine may occur because of systemic alkalosis (respiratory or metabolic) or because of a renal tubular disorder. If the renal tubules are damaged, metabolic acidosis and an inability to regulate acid-base balance will occur. A urinary pH less than 5.5 indicates the absence of bicarbonate ions in the urine. The cause of the problem may be systemic acidosis (respiratory or metabolic), with the excess hydrogen ions of the extracellular fluids spilling into the urine.

Protein

The presence of excess urinary albumin is an indicator of glomerular disease. The nephrotic syndrome produces a great loss of albumin in the urine. The renal loss also may be associated with systemic disease that causes glomerular damage.

Bilirubin

Bilirubinuria (bilirubin in the urine) is an abnormal finding that results from an increase in the serum conjugated (direct) bilirubin. The level of urine bilirubin rises in some conditions of hepatocellular jaundice and liver disease and in jaundice from conditions that result in biliary obstruction.

Glucose

Glycosuria (glucose in the urine) is usually an indicator of significant hyperglycemia and diabetes mellitus. When a fasting specimen is obtained, it is highly specific and accurate in the detection of glucose in the urine. The nonfasting random sample is much less specific.

Ketones

In starvation or abnormal carbohydrate metabolism, large quantities of ketone bodies appear in the urine before the serum levels of ketones are elevated. Urinalysis is useful in monitoring known diabetics, particularly when they are ill, hyperglycemic, or pregnant.

In children, ketonuria (ketones in the urine) can occur during febrile illness or as the result of severe diarrhea and vomiting.

Occult Blood

A positive result for occult blood in the urine occurs when intact erythrocytes, hemoglobin, or myoglobin are present. Hematuria is caused by diseases of the kidney or lower urinary tract or by a nonurinary problem of medical origin. When the occult blood test result is positive, a microscopic examination of the urine is performed to identify red blood cells (RBCs) and RBC casts. Additional laboratory or diagnostic tests are also indicated to diagnose and locate the cause of the bleeding.

Red Blood Cells

Normal urine may exhibit a few RBCs without any significant pathologic cause. The presence of a few cells is considered acceptable under high power field (HPF) microscopic visualization. Significant hematuria is indicated by one episode of gross hematuria or one episode of high-grade microhematuria, with an RBC count greater than 100 cells per HPF. Significant hematuria is an indicator for further diagnostic evaluation.

White Blood Cells

An elevated white blood cell (WBC) count in the urine indicates pyuria (pus in the urine). The microscopic urinalysis finding of 5 to 10 WBCs per HPF (5 to 10 WBCs/mm^3) is a significant elevation that indicates the presence of urinary tract infection.

Bacteria

Most urinary tract infections are characterized by a significant number of bacteria in the urine. The bacteria are visualized during high-power microscopic examination of the specimen. The finding of a bacteria count greater than 10^5 bacteria per milliliter is considered diagnostic of urinary tract infection. Bacteria also can be detected with the nitrite dipstick method. In the presence of most urinary bacteria, the dipstick turns pink (positive result) within 60 seconds. This method does not measure the severity of infection or identify the type of bacteria, but it is an effective method to screen for asymptomatic bacteriuria.

Leukocyte Esterase

The leukocyte esterase test is an indirect method used to detect bacteria in the urine. The dipstick method identifies lysed or intact WBCs. When these cells are present, the bacteria must also be present.

Casts

Casts are globulin protein structures that are precipitated in the renal tubules. They are found in the urine sediment, and the different types are identified during microscopic examination. The presence of a great number of casts is an indicator of renal parenchymal disease. Granular casts are associated with glomerulonephritis and renal pathologic conditions. Fatty casts are produced in the nephrotic syndrome. Cellular casts can have RBCs, WBCs, renal tubular cells, or a mix of these different cells. They are indicators of inflammation or infection of glomeruli, renal tubules, or renal interstitial tissue. Hyaline casts are the most common type of cast, but their presence may or may not be significant. Hyaline casts can appear after strenuous exercise, with fever, or in congestive heart failure. Persistent large numbers of hyaline casts are an indication of renal disease.

Crystals

Crystals are the end products of food metabolism and, when present, are found in urinary sediment. Crystals can be found in healthy urine, although most individuals have few or none present in urine. Crystals are seen commonly in patients with urolithiasis (kidney stones), toxic damage to the kidneys, or chronic renal failure. The presence of cellular elements or crystals, or both, causes the urine to become cloudy.

NORMAL VALUES

Color: Yellow, clear
Specific gravity: 1.003–1.029
pH: 4.5–7.8
Protein: Negative
Bilirubin: Negative

Glucose: Negative
Ketones: Negative
Occult blood: Negative
RBCs (male): 0–3 per HPF
RBCs (female): 0–5 per HPF
WBCs: 0–5 per HPF
Bacteria: Negative
Leukocyte esterase: Negative
Casts: 0–4 hyaline casts per low power field (LPF)
Crystals: Few

HOW THE TEST IS DONE

A clean container with a lid is used to collect 15 mL or more of urine. A random sample may be used, but the first-voided specimen of the morning is preferred. The urine is collected using the midstream clean-catch procedure.

SIGNIFICANCE OF TEST RESULTS

Elevated/Positive Values

Specific Gravity

Dehydration
Fever
Profuse sweating
Vomiting, diarrhea, or both
Glycosuria
Proteinuria
Congestive heart failure
Adrenal insufficiency
Altered secretion of antidiuretic hormone

pH

Metabolic alkalosis
Respiratory alkalosis
Bacteriuria (*Proteus* spp., *Pseudomonas*)
Vegetarian diet
Nasogastric suctioning
Prolonged vomiting
Fanconi syndrome
Milkman syndrome
Alkali therapy

Protein

Nephrotic syndrome
Renal disorders associated with hypertension, diabetes mellitus, systemic lupus erythematosus, or amyloidosis

Bilirubin

Hepatitis
Biliary obstruction

Glucose
Hyperglycemia
Diabetes mellitus
Ketones
Acidosis
Alcoholic ketoacidosis
Diabetic ketoacidosis
Fasting or starvation
Increased protein intake
Occult Blood
Glomerulonephritis
Urolithiasis
Urinary tract infection
Tumor, benign or malignant
Polycystic kidney
Renal infarct
Lupus nephritis
Benign prostatic hypertrophy
Blood dyscrasia, hemolysis of RBCs
Endocarditis
Leukemia
Poison (snake or spider bite)
Parasitic disease
Thermal or crush injury
Trauma
Severe exercise, jogging
Red Blood Cells
Benign tumor
Cancer
Urinary calculi
Glomerulonephritis
Lupus nephritis
Sclerosis
Urinary tract infection
Trauma from exercise
White Blood Cells
Urinary tract infection
Bacteria
Chronic urinary tract infection
Pyelonephritis
Cystitis, acute or chronic

Leukocyte Esterase
White blood cells in urine
Casts
Glomerulonephritis
Chronic renal disease
Nephrotic syndrome
Bacterial pyelonephritis
Renal failure
Crystals
Uric Acid Crystals
Gout
Rapid nucleic acid turnover
Urolithiasis
Calcium Oxalate Crystals
Chronic renal failure
Ethylene glycol ingestion
Urolithiasis
Triple Phosphate Crystals
Obstructive uropathy
Urinary tract infection
Urolithiasis

Decreased Values
Specific Gravity
Overhydration
Diuresis
Hypotension
Pyelonephritis
Glomerulonephritis
Renal tubular dysfunction
Severe renal damage
Diabetes insipidus
pH
Metabolic acidosis
Respiratory acidosis
Diabetes mellitus
Diarrhea
Starvation
Renal failure

INTERFERING FACTORS

- Insufficient quantity of urine
- Contamination of the specimen
- Warming of the specimen

NURSING CARE

Pretest

- ***Patient Teaching.*** The nurse instructs the patient to collect a sample of urine, preferably on arising in the morning. The specimen must not be contaminated by toilet paper, toilet water, feces, or secretions. Women should not collect urine during menstruation, to prevent contamination with bloody discharge. The patient also needs instruction on how to cleanse the urinary meatus and how to collect the urine. The information on the midstream clean-catch procedure is presented in Box 2, p. 36.

During the Test

- If the patient has an indwelling urinary catheter, the nurse collects the urine specimen from the port in the drainage tubing that is connected to the Foley catheter. The nurse cleanses the port with an alcohol swab and then uses a syringe with a 22- or 25-gauge needle to enter the port and aspirate the urine. If there is no visible urine in the tubing, a clamp may first be applied to the tubing just below the port. The urine is aspirated from the port after a few minutes. The specimen is placed in the specimen container and the clamp is then opened to reestablish drainage. Specimens are never removed from the collecting bag because the urine is not fresh. In addition, the collection tube is never separated (opened) from the Foley catheter to collect urine directly from the catheter. If the drainage system is opened, bacteria can enter and cause a urinary tract infection.

Posttest

- Label the container with the patient's name, the time, and the date of the voiding.
- Arrange for transport of the specimen to the laboratory as soon as possible, because the most accurate results are obtained from warm, fresh specimens. If there is delay, refrigeration of the specimen will preserve the elements in the urine, but crystals will precipitate. Allowing the specimen to stand at room temperature will cause decomposition of the bacteria and WBCs.
- The nurse may perform dipstick testing of the specimen. The procedure is presented in Box 6.

U

BOX 6 Accuracy in the Performance of Urinary Dipstick Testing

- Keep the container of test strips tightly closed when it is not in use. To prevent deterioration of the chemicals, protect the strips from exposure to light, heat, and moisture.
- Perform the test on a fresh sample of urine without delay.
- As the reagent strip is removed from the urine, tap the strip gently on the specimen container to remove excess urine.
- For each test, wait the required time before reading the results.
- Read the test results in a setting that has good lighting. Hold the strip in a horizontal position to prevent the mixing of chemicals from one pad to another.
- In comparing the test pad to the manufacturer's color chart, align the squares and tests accurately. Do not allow the moist strip to touch the chart and discolor the squares.

Urinary Glucose/Sugar

See Glucose, Urinary on p. 358.

Urobilinogen, Urinary

yur-oh-bai-lin-oh-jen, yur-i-nar-ee

Also called: Urinary Urobilinogen; 2-Hour Urine Urobilinogen

SPECIMEN OR TYPE OF TEST: Urine

PURPOSE OF THE TEST

This test is used to help detect hemolytic anemia and confirm the diagnosis of liver disease, including hepatitis and cirrhosis

BASICS THE NURSE NEEDS TO KNOW

Conjugated bilirubin exits from the liver as a component of bile. It flows through the biliary system and enters the intestine at the duodenum. In the small intestine, bilirubin is converted to urobilinogen by the bacterial flora of the intestine. About half the urobilinogen is excreted in fecal material and the remainder enters the portal vein circulation. Most of this circulatory portion of urobilinogen will return to the liver via the enterohepatic (portal vein) circulation and will be recycled into bile. The remainder of the circulatory portion is filtered out of the blood by the kidneys and is excreted in urine (Figure 91).

Urinary urobilinogen increases when there is excessive hemolysis of red blood cells that produces excess bilirubin formation by the liver and when there is liver disease that interferes with the enterohepatic circulation. Urinary urobilinogen decreases when there is obstruction in the flow of bile to the intestine and poor kidney function that impairs the filtration and removal of urobilinogen and bilirubin.

NORMAL VALUES

Male: 0.3–2.1 mg/2 hr *or* SI: 0.5–3.6 µmol/2 hr
Female: 0.1–1.1 mg/2 hr *or* SI: 0.2–1.9 µmol/2 hr

HOW THE TEST IS DONE

The 2-hour urine collection is scheduled for the afternoon, between 2 PM and 4 PM. This timing coordinates with the body's pattern for excretion of urine urobilinogen.

SIGNIFICANCE OF TEST RESULTS

Elevated Values

Moderate hepatocellular damage
Hepatitis
Hepatotoxicity from drugs or toxins
Hepatic anoxia
Portal vein cirrhosis
Hemolysis of erythrocytes
Intravascular hemolysis

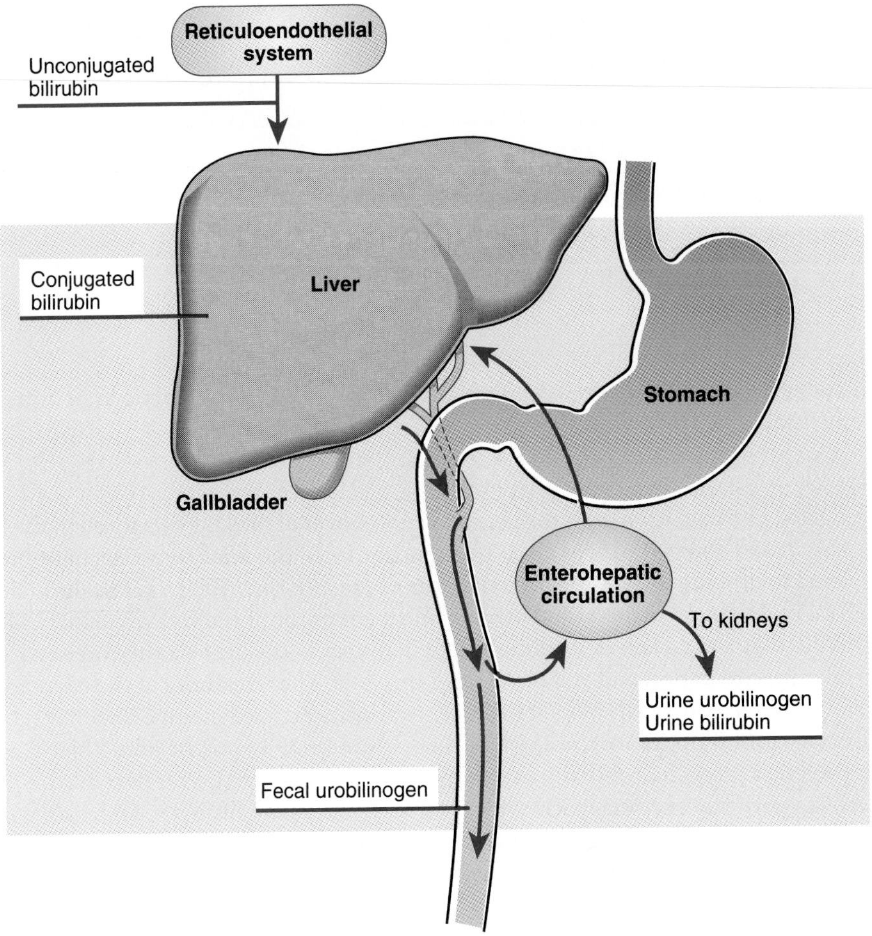

Figure 91. Pathways for bilirubin metabolism. Several organs and organ systems make different forms and amounts of bilirubin and urobilinogen.

Hemolytic anemia
Pernicious anemia

Decreased Values

Biliary tract obstruction
Massive hepatocellular damage
Renal insufficiency

INTERFERING FACTORS

- Failure to collect all of the urine in the collection period
- Exposure of the specimen to warmth or sunlight
- Recent or current use of antibiotics

NURSING CARE

Nursing actions are similar to those used in other timed urine collections (see Chapter 2), with the following additional measures.

Pretest

- ***Patient Teaching.*** The nurse explains the procedure to the patient to maximize the cooperation and accuracy in the collection of the specimen.

Schedule the test from 2 PM to 4 PM. The patient voids just before 2 PM, and this specimen is discarded because urine has been in the bladder for an unknown period.

Give the patient 500 mL of water to drink, all at once.

During the Test

- From 2 PM to 4 PM, the nurse collects all voided urine and places it in a dark-colored, sterile urine container. As an alternative, a clear container can be covered with aluminum foil to protect the urine from light. Keep the urine in the refrigerator. The reason for these measures is that urobilinogen is unstable and will convert to urobilin in the presence of sunlight, fluorescent light or warmth.

Posttest

- On completion of the collection, the nurse sends the specimen to the lab promptly. There should be no time delay before the lab prepares the specimen for analysis.

Uroflowmetry

yur-oh-floh-me-tree

Also called: Urodynamic Studies (UDS)

SPECIMEN OR TYPE OF TEST: Manometry

PURPOSE OF THE TEST

Uroflowmetry is used to help evaluate lower urinary tract dysfunction.

BASICS THE NURSE NEEDS TO KNOW

The broad category of urodynamic studies evaluates voiding and lower urinary tract function. Uroflowmetry is the initial test that is performed to assess bladder and sphincter function. This test is generally ordered for patients with incontinence or retention of urine.

Urinary incontinence is the involuntary leakage of urine through the urethral meatus. When incontinence is defined by its symptoms, the problem is called urge incontinence, stress incontinence, or total incontinence. When the incontinence is defined by its cause, the problem is one of bladder storage, bladder emptying, or urinary sphincter dysfunction. Urinary retention or obstruction may be classified as bladder or urethral dysfunction.

Determination of the urinary flow rate is a noninvasive procedure that provides measurable baseline data about the patient's ability to void. The data measure the volume of urine voided, the pattern of micturition, and the time and rate of voiding. The patient's data are compared with normal micturition patterns and numeric values of the flow rate. When the patient's values are higher than normal, the problem is one of incontinence. When the patient's values are lower than normal, the problem is one of impaired urinary flow.

In any person, the urinary flow rate varies with the volume of urine that is voided. The patient's results are compared with normal values based on the volume voided. The flow rate of any individual also varies from one voiding episode to another. The uroflowmetry test is repeated several times to obtain reliable data. Additionally, normal voiding rates vary between males and females and among different age groups across the life span. The interpretation of the patient's values is age- and gender-specific.

NORMAL VALUES

No anatomic or physiologic abnormalities are noted.

Urine Volume
66–80 years: >199 mL
46–65 years: >199 mL
14–45 years: >199 mL
8–13 years: >99 mL
4–7 years: >99 mL

Flow Rate
Male (66–80 years): 9 mL/sec
Female (66–80 years): 10 mL/sec
Male (46–65 years): 12 mL/sec
Female (46–65 years): 15 mL/sec
Male (14–45 years): 21 mL/sec
Female (14–45 years): 18 mL/sec
Male (8–13 years): 12 mL/sec
Female (8–13 years): 15 mL/sec
Male (4–7 years): 10 mL/sec
Female (4–7 years): 10 mL/sec

HOW THE TEST IS DONE

The patient urinates into a toilet that is equipped with a funnel and uroflowmeter. As voiding activates the uroflowmeter and its transducer, electronic data are received, transmitted, analyzed, and recorded. Specific variations in the procedure are based on differences in manufacturers' equipment and lab protocol. The total time for completion of the test is 10 to 15 minutes.

SIGNIFICANCE OF TEST RESULTS

Elevated Values

Conditions that cause reduced urethral resistance
Incontinence (stress, urge, or total)

Decreased Values
Urethral or bladder neck obstruction
Poor muscular contraction of the bladder

INTERFERING FACTORS

- Body movement during voiding
- Toilet tissue in the apparatus
- Straining during urination

NURSING CARE

Pretest

- ***Patient Teaching.*** The nurse instructs the patient to drink fluids and refrain from voiding for several hours before the test.

During the Test

- Ensure the patient's privacy for the test. The bathroom contains a toilet with the uroflowmeter installed in it.
- ***Patient Teaching.*** Instruct the patient to void into the urometer funnel without straining or body movement. The nurse also informs the patient not to dispose of the toilet tissue in the funnel or collection container.

Posttest

- No specific patient instruction or intervention is needed.

Vanillylmandelic Acid

See Catecholamines, Urinary on p. 185.

Varicella-Zoster Viral Antibody

var-ih-sel-uh–zos-tur vai-rul an-tib-od-ee

Also called: VZV Antibody

SPECIMEN OR TYPE OF TEST: Blood

PURPOSE OF THE TEST

The immunoglobulin (IgG) antibody test is used to confirm past infection or vaccination that provides immunity from future chickenpox infection. The IgM antibody test occasionally is used to identify current infection with the varicella-zoster virus.

BASICS THE NURSE NEEDS TO KNOW

The varicella-zoster virus is a herpesvirus that causes the primary infection of varicella (chickenpox) and years later, can cause the reactivated infection of shingles (herpes zoster infection). A negative result for varicella-zoster antibodies means that the person has no immunity from chickenpox and is susceptible to acquire this infection. If a person has positive IgG antibodies or a high IgG titer, it means there is immunity to future chickenpox infection, but there may not be immunity to shingles. A positive IgG antibody finding results from previous varicella infection or immunization with the varicella vaccine.

In the acute illness phase, the IgM antibody test becomes positive 1 to 3 days after the skin eruption occurs. In the convalescent phase, the IgG antibody becomes positive 9 to10 days after the skin eruption occurs. If the pregnant woman contracts this infection in the last 3 weeks of pregnancy, the fetus may develop chickenpox. Positive IgM antibodies in the amniotic fluid, cord blood, or in the neonate indicates the acute phase of chickenpox infection in the baby.

NORMAL VALUES

IgM: Negative
IgG: Negative; titer 1:4

HOW THE TEST IS DONE

A red-topped tube is used to obtain 10 mL of venous blood.

SIGNIFICANCE OF TEST RESULTS

Positive Values

Past or present varicella-zoster infection
Immunity to future varicella infection

INTERFERING FACTORS

- Infection with another type of herpesvirus

NURSING CARE

Nursing actions are similar to those used in venipuncture procedures (see Chapter 2), with the following additional measures.

Pretest

- Inform the adult patient that a positive IgG antibody titer indicates immunity from future chickenpox infection.

Posttest

- If the newborn baby has recent exposure to the varicella-zoster virus, the nurse maintains the infant in isolation in the newborn nursery. To determine the presence of perinatal infection, the physician may have the infant's blood tested for IgM antibodies. To reduce the severity of the infection in this newborn, the nurse prepares to administer varicella immunoglobulin to the baby, as prescribed by the physician.
- *Health Promotion.* To prevent chickenpox, vaccination with the live attenuated varicella vaccine is recommended for all children between the ages of 1 and 6 years and for patients who are immunocompromised. The vaccine is also recommended for people who attend or work in settings where infection rates are higher, including day care centers, schools, prisons, military settings, and colleges. The nonpregnant female also should be vaccinated to prevent severe illness during a future pregnancy and avoid potential risk to the fetus. The nurse can teach individuals and groups about the importance of early vaccination and encourage them to prevent this infection.

Vasopressin

va-zoh-pres-in

Also called: Antidiuretic Hormone (ADH), Arginine-Vasopressin (AVP)

SPECIMEN OR TYPE OF TEST: Plasma

PURPOSE OF THE TEST

A serum antidiuretic hormone (ADH) determination is obtained to diagnose diabetes insipidus and syndrome of inappropriate antidiuretic hormone.

BASICS THE NURSE NEEDS TO KNOW

Vasopressin (ADH) is produced by the hypothalamus and stored in the posterior pituitary gland. Its major function in the body is to act on the cells in the collecting ducts of the kidney, making them more permeable to water. The result is an increased reabsorption of water. This action is independent of electrolyte levels, and electrolytes are *not* reabsorbed with the water. The purpose of this action is to maintain normal plasma osmolality. ADH also has a vasopressor effect. It causes arteriole smooth muscles to constrict, thus elevating the blood pressure.

ADH is released from the posterior pituitary gland in response to several stimuli. The major stimulus is an increase in plasma osmolality. Whenever the osmoreceptors in the anterior hypothalamus sense even minor changes in plasma osmolality, neural stimulation of the pituitary gland will result in an increased secretion of ADH, which will result in an increased reabsorption of water at the renal collecting ducts. With the increase in water in the extracellular fluid, blood tonicity will decrease. Because the increase in water results in decreased blood osmolality, the osmoreceptors will cease the neural stimulation necessary for ADH secretion (Figure 92).

Another stimulant for ADH release is the extracellular fluid volume. A drop in blood volume is sensed by stretcher receptors primarily in the vena cava and right atrium. By way of the brainstem, these receptors tell the hypothalamus to stimulate the release of ADH from the posterior pituitary gland. The resultant increase in fluid volume from water retention results in a decrease in stretcher receptor stimulation. In addition, as arterial blood pressure drops, pressor receptors found in the aorta and coronary sinuses will stimulate the release of ADH to increase extracellular fluid volume and, thus, the patient's blood pressure.

ADH secretion may be increased by drugs (e.g., nicotine, opiates, barbiturates, chlorpropamide) and severe pain, stress, and hyperthermia. Decreased sensitivity of the kidneys to ADH occurs with the intake of lithium carbonate and demeclocycline.

NORMAL VALUES	
	If serum osmolality is >290 mOsm/kg: 2–12 pg/mL *or* SI: 1.85–11.1 pmol/L
	If serum osmolality is <290 mOsm/kg: <2 pg/mL *or* SI: <1.85 pmol/L

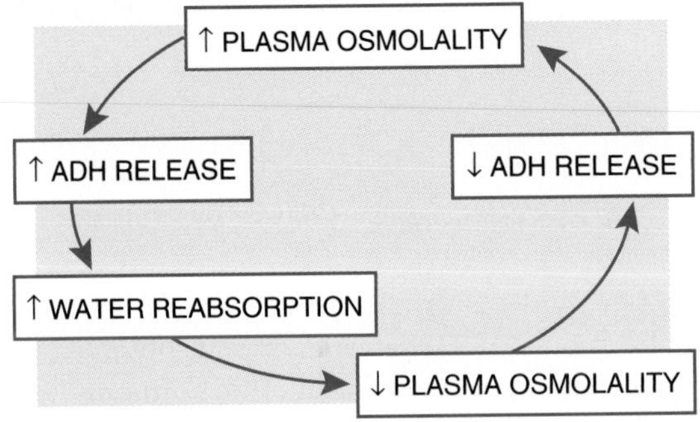

Figure 92. Vasopressin (ADH) regulation. ADH is secreted by the posterior pituitary gland primarily in response to an increase in plasma osmolality.

HOW THE TEST IS DONE

Venipuncture is performed; collect in a pre-chilled lavender-topped tube and send to the lab immediately.

SIGNIFICANCE OF TEST RESULTS

Elevated Values

Syndrome of inappropriate antidiuretic hormone

Decreased Values

Diabetes insipidus

INTERFERING FACTORS

- Noncompliance with diet, activity, and medication restrictions
- Pain
- Stress
- Mechanical ventilation
- Alcohol
- Medications such as anesthetics, carbamazepine, chlorothiazide, cyclophosphamide, estrogen, oxytocin, and vincristine

V

NURSING CARE

Nursing actions related to venipuncture are presented in Chapter 2, with the following additional measures.

Pretest

- *Patient Teaching.* The nurse instructs the patient not to eat or drink for 12 hours before the test.
- *Patient Teaching.* The nurse also instructs the patient to avoid substances that increase ADH secretion, such as nicotine, alcohol, caffeine, and diuretics. Instruct the patient to limit physical activity for 12 hours before the test. The patient should lie down and rest for 30 minutes before the blood is drawn.

NURSING CARE—*cont'd*

- Obtain a medication history to determine if any interfering drugs are being taken. In the pretest period, the nurse checks with the physician to determine if these drugs are to be withheld or continued.
- Assess the patient for pain and stress, which may interfere with results.

Posttest

- Send specimen to the lab immediately.
- Instruct the patient to resume normal activity and diet.
- The nurse administers prescribed medications that were withheld for the test.

Vectorcardiogram

vek-tuhr-kar-dee-oh-gram

Also called: VCG

SPECIMEN OR TYPE OF TEST: Electrophysiology

PURPOSE OF THE TEST

A vectorcardiogram is used to assess ischemia, conduction defects, and chamber enlargement (hypertrophy or dilation).

BASICS THE NURSE NEEDS TO KNOW

A vectorcardiogram is a graphic recording of electric forces of the heart. It is a noninvasive procedure that graphically records the direction and magnitude of the heart's electric forces by means of a continuous series of vector loops. Three planes of the heart are recorded (frontal, sagittal, and horizontal).

NORMAL VALUES Normal cardiac axis

SIGNIFICANCE OF TEST RESULTS

Abnormal Values

Myocardial ischemia
Conduction defects
Atrial and/or ventricular hypertrophy
Atrial and/or ventricular dilatation
Cardiomyopathy

INTERFERING FACTORS

- Patient who is unable to lie still

NURSING CARE

See section on electrocardiogram for nursing care (p. 289).

Venography

ve-nog-ruh-fee

Also called: Phlebography

SPECIMEN OR TYPE OF TEST: Radiography

PURPOSE OF THE TEST

Venography is used to investigate venous function, suspected obstruction, venous insufficiency, postphlebotic syndrome, and the source of pulmonary embolism. It also evaluates veins before and after bypass surgery, reconstructive surgery, or thrombolytic therapy to determine the effectiveness of treatment.

BASICS THE NURSE NEEDS TO KNOW

Venography is an invasive technique that provides radiographic visualization of the venous system, particularly in the lower extremities. Thrombosis (the formation of a blood clot) is the most common venous pathologic condition. Deep vein thrombosis and thromboembolism are caused by three general pathologic conditions: damage to the vein, venous stasis, and decreased fibrinolytic activity. As the thrombus enlarges, it occludes the lumen of the vein and ultimately destroys the venous valve or valves. In the early stage of formation, the thrombus is soft and friable. When located in the leg, a piece of the thrombus can break off, travel, and lodge as a pulmonary embolus in the arterial vasculature of the lungs.

Examination of the veins by venography is carried out by several methods. *Ascending venography* is used to identify the presence and location of deep vein thrombosis and to assess the patency of the deep venous system. *Descending venography* is used to assess valve competency. *Venography of the upper extremities* evaluates occlusion, lesions, or thrombosis in the subclavian or axillary veins. *Venacavography* evaluates the inferior vena cava for obstruction, malformation, traumatic injury, and placement of the inferior vena cava filter.

Venography is the best method to identify a deep vein thrombosis below the knee.

Other, noninvasive technologies such as ultrasound, plethysmography, and computed tomography also may be used to evaluate the venous vasculature, but when these procedures are inconclusive, venography is used to clarify the data.

NORMAL VALUES

No evidence of intraluminal filling defects, obstruction, incompetent venous valves, calcifications, or dilated collateral veins

HOW THE TEST IS DONE

Contrast medium is injected into the vein via a butterfly needle or an intravenous catheter. With use of a tilt table, fluoroscopy, and x-ray studies, the contrast medium illustrates the flow patterns of the venous circulation and identifies the site of occlusion in the vein.

In venography of the lower extremities, either ascending or descending venography may be used. Ascending venography uses a butterfly needle placed in a small vein on the dorsum of the foot (Figure 93). In descending venography, a catheter is placed in the common femoral vein via a percutaneous femoral approach.

SIGNIFICANCE OF TEST RESULTS

Abnormal Values

Deep vein thrombosis
Tumor
Vascular tumor
Venous compression syndrome
Venous insufficiency
Varicose veins
Congenital malformation
Traumatic injury to the vein

INTERFERING FACTORS

- Allergy to iodine or contrast medium
- Renal failure
- Congestive heart failure
- Severe pulmonary hypertension

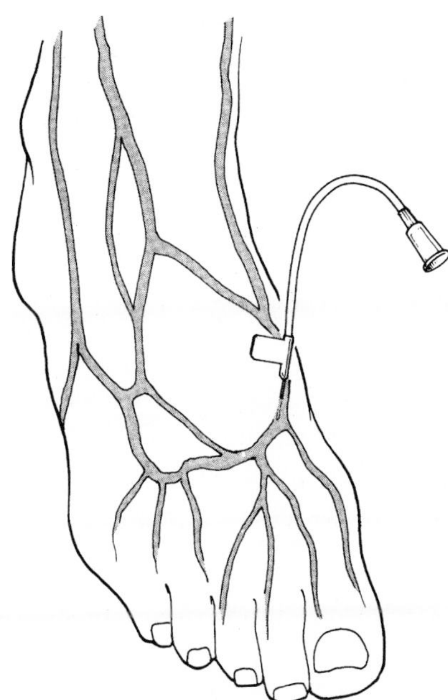

Figure 93. Technique of ascending venography. Diagrammatic representation of the ideal needle position to instill the contrast medium. *(Reproduced with permission from Kim, D., & Orron, D. E. [1992].* Peripheral vascular imaging and intervention. *St. Louis: Mosby–Year Book.)*

NURSING CARE

Pretest

- After the physician explains the procedure, obtain a written consent from the patient.
- Identify any allergy to iodine or shellfish or any allergic reaction to a previous x-ray study that used contrast medium.
- Ensure that the pretest blood urea nitrogen and creatinine determinations are performed and that the results are posted in the patient's chart. The kidneys must clear the contrast material from the blood, and these tests verify that renal function is adequate. Record the patient's baseline vital signs.
- ***Patient Teaching.*** Instruct the patient regarding the pretest preparation. Solid foods are omitted for 4 hours before the test, but water and clear liquids are permitted.

During the Test

- The patient is positioned according to the views required. Lower extremity views are done with the patient in supine position or tilted upward to a semi-erect position.
- Provide emotional support during the period of discomfort. The injection of contrast material is painful.
- On completion of the test, an intravenous solution of 200 to 300 mL of heparinized saline is administered. This flushes the contrast medium from the veins.

Posttest

- The nurse takes vital signs and records the results. The site where the contrast medium was injected should be assessed for swelling, pain, redness, ecchymosis, and hematoma.
- The nurse keeps the patient on bed rest for 2 hours. Food intake may be resumed. The nurse instructs the patient to drink extra fluids for 24 hours to help flush the remaining contrast medium from the veins and kidneys. Frequent urination is expected until the diuresis (increased excretion of urine) is complete.

◇ Nursing Response to Complications

The complications that can occur are related to the contrast medium that was used in the test. Although the incidence is not frequent, the nurse monitors the patient for potential problems and notifies the physician if they occur.

Cellulitis. During the test, if more than 5 to 10 mL of contrast material infiltrates the tissue, chemical cellulitis will result in the posttest period. The nurse assesses the tissue near the injection site for tenderness, pain, redness, and swelling.

Thrombophlebitis. The contrast medium can be irritating to the vein and cause phlebitis or thrombophlebitis. Along the path of the vein that received the injection of contrast, the nurse observes for redness, swelling, and pain. Like cellulitis, the manifestations often begin 2 to 12 hours posttest and usually subside in a few days.

Mild allergic reaction. Allergic reactions can range from mild to very severe (see p. 671). The mild reaction may begin during the test or shortly afterward. The patient develops a histamine response, including urticaria, itching, edema, and redness of the skin. When the reaction remains at this level of involvement, the nurse prepares to administer the antihistamine diphenhydramine hydrochloride (Benadryl), as prescribed. The nurse monitors the respirations of the patient because of the potential for a more severe allergic reaction.

NURSING CARE—*cont'd*

Severe allergic reaction. If the allergic reaction is severe, it can progress toward anaphylaxis in a very rapid manner. An anaphylactic response may occur during the test, very soon after injection of the contrast medium. The patient develops respiratory distress, wheezing, or stridor. Cyanosis develops as the airway becomes swollen, edematous, and increasingly obstructed. The patient develops tachycardia, hypotension, and chest pain. Cardiac arrest may occur. If the respiratory problems begin, the physician must be notified immediately. The nurse prepares to administer oxygen and prescribed medications that would help reverse the anaphylaxis and acute respiratory distress. These include epinephrine (Adrenaline) subcutaneously, and aminophylline intravenously. Benadryl may also be prescribed, intravenously.

Ventilation-Perfusion Scan

See Lung Scans on p. 443.

Vitamin D, Activated

vai-tuh-min dee, ak-ti-vay-ted

Also called: 1,25-Dihydroxycholecalciferol; Cholecalciferol

SPECIMEN OR TYPE OF TEST: Serum, plasma

PURPOSE OF THE TEST

Activated vitamin D levels are assessed to evaluate causes of hypocalcemia. They are usually obtained with parathyroid hormone levels.

BASICS THE NURSE NEEDS TO KNOW

Activated vitamin D is produced from vitamin D by the liver and kidneys. Vitamin D is derived from the action of ultraviolet light on a group of provitamins in the skin. Levels of vitamin D usually decrease in the winter months. Vitamin D is derived also from vitamin D-enriched foods. Vitamin D is first converted in the liver to 25-hydroxycholecalciferol and then to 1,25-dihydroxycholecalciferol in the kidney. Activated vitamin D elevates plasma calcium and phosphate levels by increasing intestinal absorption of calcium and phosphate and increasing the release of calcium from bone into blood.

NORMAL VALUES 25–45 pg/mL *or* SI 60–108 nmol/L

HOW THE TEST IS DONE

If a serum level test is ordered, 5 mL of blood is collected in a red-topped tube. If a plasma level is desired, 5 mL of blood is collected in a green-topped tube.

SIGNIFICANCE OF TEST RESULTS

Elevated Values

Hyperparathyroidism
Overdose of vitamin D
Sarcoidosis

Decreased Values

Anticonvulsants
Hepatic failure
Hypoparathyroidism
Isoniazid
Malabsorption syndrome
Osteomalacia
Pseudohypoparathyroidism
Renal failure

INTERFERING FACTORS

- Recent radioisotope administration
- Phosphorus deficiency
- Prolonged lack of exposure to sunlight

NURSING CARE

The nurse performs actions similar to those in other venipuncture procedures, as described in Chapter 2, with the following additional measures.

Pretest

- *Patient Teaching.* Instruct the patient not to eat or drink for 8 hours before the test.

Water Deprivation Test

waw-ter de-pri-vay-shun test

Also called: Dehydration Test; Concentration Test

SPECIMEN OR TYPE OF TEST: Urine

W

PURPOSE OF THE TEST

The water deprivation test is performed to diagnose diabetes insipidus (DI) and to assess the kidney's ability to concentrate urine based on extracellular fluid load.

BASICS THE NURSE NEEDS TO KNOW

Normally, as fluid intake is withheld, blood osmolality increases, urine output decreases, and urinary osmolality increases. The increase in serum osmolality causes an increase in antidiuretic hormone (ADH) secretion. In patients with DI, a normal response to increased plasma osmolality does not occur; instead, little or no increase in ADH occurs, resulting in little or no change in urinary output or osmolality.

DI may be caused by a defect in production, release, or utilization of ADH. If DI is a result of a problem in production (hypothalamic) or release (pituitary) of ADH, it is called *neurogenic* or *central* DI. If DI is caused by a failure of the kidney to respond to ADH, it is called *nephrogenic* DI. The water deprivation test supports the diagnosis of diabetes insipidus.

As part of the water deprivation test, a *vasopressin stimulation test* or *ADH stimulation test* may be performed to distinguish between neurogenic and nephrogenic DI. This distinction is important in determining appropriate treatment plans.

NORMAL VALUES	Specific gravity: 1.025–1.032 Osmolality: >800 mOsm/kg *or* SI: >800 mmol/kg

HOW THE TEST IS DONE

During the test, the patient is deprived of fluid intake, and periodic urine specimens are obtained for osmolality and specific gravity determinations. The urine is collected in separate clean containers and placed on ice or refrigerated. Strict urinary output measurements are maintained.

If a *vasopressin stimulation test* is included, hypertonic saline or nicotine is given to stimulate ADH release. If complete neurogenic DI is present, no change is noted in urinary output or osmolality. If partial neurogenic DI is present, only minor changes occur.

If desired, a *vasopressin test* may be performed. After vasopressin is given, no change will occur in urinary output or osmolality if nephrogenic DI is present. With central DI, the urine osmolality will increase and the urinary output will decrease.

SIGNIFICANCE OF TEST RESULTS

If no change in urine osmolality exists, the diagnosis of DI is supported.

INTERFERING FACTORS

- Noncompliance with fluid restrictions
- Inability to complete test because of hypovolemia
- Glucosuria
- Administration of radiopaque dyes within 7 days

NURSING CARE

W

Nursing actions related to timed urine collection and pediatric urine collection procedures are presented in Chapter 2, with the following additional measures.

Pretest

- The nurse assesses the patient's hemodynamic status. If a vasopressin test is planned, check for a history of coronary artery disease, because vasopressin may cause coronary artery spasm.
- Obtain baseline serum and urine specimens for osmolality determinations.
- Baseline weight is obtained before the evening meal on the day before testing.

Continued

NURSING CARE—*cont'd*

During the Test

- The nurse observes for early signs of hypovolemia (tachycardia, orthostatic hypotension).
- Observe the patient to ensure compliance with nothing-by-mouth status.
- Obtain a urine specimen every 2 hours. Label each specimen with the time and the amount obtained.
- The nurse weighs the patient every 2 to 4 hours. Maintain the patient on nothing-by-mouth status until 2% to 5% of the patient's weight is lost (this takes approximately 6 to 12 hours).
- After 2% to 5% of patient body weight is lost and urinary output continues with urinary osmolality plateauing, an ADH stimulation test may be performed by administering hypertonic saline (3% sodium chloride) or nicotine, as ordered.
- If a vasopressin test is to be performed, check the patient's blood pressure and document it; notify the physician if the patient is hypertensive. Aqueous vasopressin is given subcutaneously or intravenously. One hour after vasopressin administration, collect the urine specimen for amount and osmolality.

▼ Nursing Response to Critical Values

Hypovolemia may occur with the water deprivation test. Patients with DI will continue to put out urine, even though they have no intake. If a vasopressin test is performed, the administration of vasopressin may produce the complications of high blood pressure or coronary artery spasms, or both.

Hypovolemia. Tachycardia, restlessness, poor skin turgor, and hypotension are indications of hypovolemia. If these occur, the nurse notifies the physician and anticipates the test being discontinued and fluids being given.

Coronary artery spasms. With spasm of the coronary artery, perfusion will be affected. The patient may complain of chest pain. The physician is informed and the nurse anticipates that the order for vasopressin will be discontinued.

Water-Loading Test

waw-ter-loh-ding test

W

SPECIMEN OR TYPE OF TEST: Plasma, Urine

PURPOSE OF THE TEST

The water-loading test is performed to diagnose the syndrome of inappropriate secretion of the antidiuretic hormone (SIADH).

BASICS THE NURSE NEEDS TO KNOW

Review the discussion of Plasma Vasopressin (p. 665). Normally, with an increase in fluid intake, urinary output will increase to maintain a normal plasma osmolality. As the urine volume increases, its osmolality decreases. However, patients with syndrome of inappropriate antidiuretic hormone (SIADH) will not respond to increasing fluid intake.

NORMAL VALUES **Urinary output increases, and plasma and urine osmolality decrease.**

HOW THE TEST IS DONE

With the water-loading test, the patient orally ingests a water load of 20 to 25 mL/kg of body weight. Hourly serum and urine osmolality and urine outputs are recorded for 4 hours.

SIGNIFICANCE OF TEST RESULTS

Little or no change in urinary output or plasma and urine osmolality readings supports the diagnosis of SIADH.

INTERFERING FACTORS

- Patient is unable to drink the required volume of fluid.
- Medications such as demeclocycline, diuretics, and lithium carbonate.

NURSING CARE

Pretest

- The nurse assesses the patient for hyponatremia.
- Obtain the patient's cardiac history, the results of which may require that the test be canceled.
- Weigh the patient.

During the Test

- Instruct the patient to drink the required fluid.
- Obtain hourly output measurements and send blood and urine to the laboratory for osmolality determination. On the requisition slip, indicate the hour of the specimen, with zero hour being the time the patient ingested the fluid (see discussion of Osmolality, Plasma [p. 488] and Osmolality, Urine [p. 490] for the nursing procedures associated with the collection of these samples).
- The nurse observes the patient for water intoxication.

Posttest

- Weigh the patient.

Nursing Response to Critical Values

When patients with SIADH undergo the water-loading test, their output is not increased. The increased fluid load in the extracellular fluid can cause dilutional hyponatremia, also called *water intoxication*.

Dilutional hyponatremia. Indications of water intoxication are hyponatremia, lethargy, confusion, muscular twitching, stupor and, eventually, convulsions and death. The nurse will observe closely for changes in mental status and report these to the physician. The nurse should anticipate an order for a serum sodium level. If the sodium level is less than 120 mEq/L, the nurse would notify the physician immediately.

White Blood Cell Count

wait blud sel kount

Also called: (WBC); Leukocyte Count, White Count

SPECIMEN OR TYPE OF TEST: Blood

PURPOSE OF THE TEST

The white blood cell count indicates the possible presence and severity of infection or inflammatory response. This test may be part of the complete blood count, performed as a routine screening test or it may be performed separately to evaluate a specific problem. The leukocyte count is a general indicator of infection, tissue necrosis, inflammation, or bone marrow activity.

BASICS THE NURSE NEEDS TO KNOW

White blood cells, called leukocytes, maintain the general function of combating infection and inflammation. The five different types of white blood cells (neutrophils, eosinophils, basophils, lymphocytes, and monocytes), are included in the WBC count. Most of the white blood cells are manufactured by the bone marrow. Additional specific diagnostic information is obtained by the White Blood Cell Differential Count (p. 679), which identifies the numbers of each type of white blood cell.

Many of the white blood cells are phagocytic in their action. They are capable of rapid mobility to an area of infection or tissue damage, where they ingest many types of foreign cells, dead cells, or microorganisms. The used white blood cells will self-destruct and must be replaced. In the presence of infection or inflammation, the bone marrow activity increases greatly, and many leukocytes are produced to counteract the invasion by foreign cells or substances.

Variation in Normal Values

The leukocyte count can become falsely elevated with stress or exercise or after eating a heavy meal. The normal value is higher in children younger than age 5. The normal leukocyte count is lower in African Americans than in whites.

Elevated Values

W

Leukocytosis, an elevated number of white blood cells, occurs in response to infection and usually is directly proportionate to the degree of bacterial invasion. The elevated value may also be caused by necrosis of tissue or malignancy of the bone marrow. A white blood cell count of 11,000 to 17,000 cells ($11\text{–}17 \times 10^3/\mu L$ *or* SI: $11\text{–}17 \times 10^9/L$) is considered to be a mild to moderate leukocytosis.

Decreased Values

When the white blood cell count falls to less than normal limits, it is called *leukopenia*. Mild leukopenia is indicated by a white blood cell count of 3000 to 5000 cells ($3\text{–}5 \times 10^3/\mu L$ *or* SI: $3\text{–}5 \times 10^9/L$). Any marked decrease is usually in neutrophils, although all five forms of leukocytes may be decreased. Decreases in the leukocyte count are usually a result of bone marrow depression or overwhelming infection that has exhausted the supply of neutrophils and bone marrow reserves.

NORMAL VALUES	Adult: 4.5–11 × 10^3/μL *or* SI: 6–17.5 × 10^9/L Newborn: 18,000–22,000 cells/μL *or* SI: 18–22 × 10^9/L
Critical Values	<2500 cells/μL *or* SI: <2.5 × 10^9/L >30,000 cells/μL *or* SI: >30 × 10^9/L

HOW THE TEST IS DONE

A purple-topped tube with EDTA is used to collect 7 mL of venous blood. As an alternative, two purple-tipped capillary tubes can be used to collect blood from a heelstick, earlobe, or finger puncture. After the blood is collected, the tube is inverted gently five to ten times to mix the anticoagulant and prevent clotting.

SIGNIFICANCE OF TEST RESULTS

Elevated Values

Bacterial infection
Lymphoma
Leukemia
Chronic infection
Mumps
Cancer (liver, intestine)
Tissue necrosis (burns, gangrene, myocardial infarction)
Varicella
Rubeola
Leukemoid reaction

Decreased Values

Brucellosis
Typhoid fever
Viral infections (influenza, rubella, hepatitis)
Typhus
Dengue fever
Malaria
Gaucher's disease
Pernicious anemia
Aplastic anemia
Radiation
Antineoplastic drugs
Toxic ingestion of heavy metals or chemical poisons
Systemic lupus erythematosus
Felty syndrome

INTERFERING FACTORS

- Hemolysis
- Coagulation of the specimen
- Strenuous exercise
- Digestion of a heavy meal

NURSING CARE

Nursing actions are similar to those used in venipuncture or capillary puncture procedures (see Chapter 2), with the following additional measures.

Pretest

- The specimen should be obtained when the patient is calm and physically still.
- The nurse organizes the care of the neonate so that minimal disturbance occurs before drawing the blood. The crying infant should be comforted because with stress or distress, the patient's adrenaline causes a rise in the white blood cell count for 15 to 30 minutes.
- The nurse knows that infants and children usually have several white blood cell counts done on different days. The repetition of the tests helps provide an accurate count and limits the variations that occur from extraneous sources. The same vascular source (arterial, venous, or capillary) should be used each time.
- ***Patient Teaching.*** When the test is planned, the nurse instructs the patient to avoid strenuous exercise for 24 hours before the test. The exercise can cause a very high white blood cell count that is a false positive result. Instruct the patient to avoid a heavy meal before the test, because the digestion process causes a temporary rise in the white blood cell count.

Posttest

- The increase in the white blood cell count usually means that the patient has a bacterial infection and that the bone marrow has responded by manufacturing additional leukocytes. If the white blood cell count continues to rise, even after antibiotic therapy is administered, it is an indication that the infection is worsening or that there is a noninfectious cause of the elevation. Additional testing may be performed to determine the location of the infection.
- In noninfectious causes, bone marrow malfunction may be investigated, and leukemia is one cause of a dramatic rise in the white blood cell count.
- An elevated white blood cell count will recede and return to normal when the patient is recovering from infection. When infection is suspected or diagnosed, the nurse monitors the patient's temperature every 4 hours, administers extra fluids and fever measures, encourages the patient to rest, and administers the prescribed medications, such as antibiotics or antimicrobials.
- A decreased white blood cell count occurs because of the inability of the bone marrow to produce sufficient white blood cells. This can occur in response to severe infection, with leukemia, or depression of the bone marrow after radiation therapy, chemotherapy, or as a result of a toxic reaction to medication. Regardless of the medical cause, the patient has diminished ability to defend against infection. The nurse institutes precautionary measures to prevent the patient's exposure to germs. All visitors and

NURSING CARE—*cont'd*

employees who enter the patient's room must perform handwashing. Visitors should be limited and no one with an infection should enter the patient's room. If the count declines further, Reverse isolation procedures may be instituted.

Nursing Response to Critical Values

The physician should be notified immediately of either severe decline or severe elevation of the white blood count that is at or beyond the critical values. With severe leukopenia, the patient is at risk because there is little or no defense from infection. The cause may be severe infection or inflammation, but the cell count also may be abnormal because of a bone marrow disorder, such as leukemia or aplastic anemia.

Hyperleukocytosis is an extreme elevation of the white blood cell count and is a potential emergency. It is a value defined as >100,000 cells/µL *or* SI: >100 × 10^9/L. At this level, the patient may have a fatal hemorrhage in the lung or brain as the leukocytes clump or aggregate in the small blood vessels. Hyperleukocytosis is usually the result of leukemia in crisis stage.

White Blood Cell Differential Count

wait blud sel di-fer-en-shuhl kount

Also called: Differential Leukocyte Count; Peripheral Differential; White Blood Cell Morphology; WBC Differential

SPECIMEN OR TYPE OF TEST: Whole blood

PURPOSE OF THE TEST

The white blood cell differential assesses the ability of the body to respond to and eliminate infection. It also detects the severity of allergic reactions, parasitic infection, and other infection and identifies various stages of leukemia.

BASICS THE NURSE NEEDS TO KNOW

The white blood cell differential identifies the five different types of leukocytes. The test reports the percentages and cell counts of each type.

Neutrophils are the most active cells and respond to tissue damage or infection. The two types of neutrophils are segmented neutrophils and bands. They are phagocytes that provide an early, rapid removal of cellular debris and a large number of bacteria. Of all the leukocytes, the neutrophils are the largest group. An elevated value (neutrophilia) occurs in response to bacterial infection, inflammatory disease, or tissue necrosis. A decreased value (neutropenia) can be the result of a severe infection that used up all the reserved supply of neutrophils. It can also be caused by damage to the bone marrow that manufactures the neutrophils.

Eosinophils contain toxic substances that kill foreign cells in the blood. The eosinophils also participate in the inflammatory response by phagocytosis, and they digest the antigen-antibody complexes and clean up the late stages of inflammation. Elevated values occur when extra eosinophils are manufactured to respond to allergic disorders, inflammation of the skin, parasitic infection in the tissues, other infections, malignancy, and tissue necrosis. Decreased values occur with most infections that produce purulence.

Basophils are involved in modifying or calming systemic allergic reactions and anaphylaxis. The basophils release histamine, heparin, and serotonin into the circulation during an episode of inflammation. An elevated value occurs during the healing phase of inflammation and in chronic inflammation. It occurs in the presence of hypersensitivity reactions to foods, pollens, and injected protein substances. It also occurs after radiation therapy and in myeloproliferative disorders, including myeloid leukemia. A decreased value occurs during acute infection, hyperthyroidism, and stress.

Lymphocytes consist of the B cells and T cells that are responsible for the activities of the immune system. The B cells make antibodies and the T cells regulate the immune response. An elevated lymphocyte count occurs in response to bacterial, viral, and other types of infection. It also occurs in some hematologic disorders, including lymphocytic leukemia. A decreased value occurs with impaired lymphatic drainage, some advanced cancers, bone marrow failure, and immunologic deficiency that decrease the T lymphocytes.

Monocytes, in the blood, remove debris or foreign particles from the circulation. In the work of phagocytosis, monocytes perform the same work as neutrophils, but their numbers are greater, and they are capable of more work. They also participate in the immune response. An elevated value occurs in response to infection of all kinds. A decreased value occurs because of bone marrow failure and in some forms of leukemia.

NORMAL VALUES

Neutrophils

Segmented Neutrophils

Mean percent: 56% *or* SI: 0.56 (mean number fraction)
Cell count (range): 1800–7800 μL *or* SI: 1.8–7.8 × 10^9/L

Bands

Mean percent: <11% *or* SI: 0.11 (mean number fraction)
Cell count (range) <620/μL *or* S: <0.062 × 10^9/L

Eosinophils

Mean percent: 2.7% *or* SI: 0.027 (mean number fraction)
Cell count (range): 0–450/μL *or* SI: 0–0.45 × 10^9/L

Basophils

Mean percent: 0.3% *or* SI: 0.003 (mean number fraction)
Cell count (range): 0–200/μL *or* SI: 0–0.2 × 10^9/L

Lymphocytes

Mean percent: 34% *or* SI: 0.34 (mean number fraction)
Cell count (range): 1000–4800/μL *or* SI: 1–4.8 × 10^9/L

Monocytes

Mean percent: 4% *or* SI: 0.04 (mean number fraction)
Cell count (range): 0–800/μL *or* SI: 0–0.8 × 10^9/L

HOW THE TEST IS DONE

A purple-topped tube with EDTA is used to collect 7 mL of venous blood. As an alternative, two purple-tipped capillary tubes can be used to collect blood from a heelstick, earlobe, or finger puncture.

For the peripheral blood smear, two slides with coverslips are prepared immediately using drops of venous or capillary blood.

SIGNIFICANCE OF TEST RESULTS

Elevated Values

Neutrophils

Chronic myelogenous leukemia
Bacterial infection
Severe burns
Rheumatic fever
Ketoacidosis
Cancer
Down syndrome

Eosinophils

Skin diseases (pemphigus, eczema, exfoliative dermatitis)
Trichinosis, *Echinococcus* disease
Scarlet fever
Chronic myelogenous leukemia
Myeloproliferative diseases
Hodgkin's disease
Malignancy
Rheumatoid arthritis
Sarcoidosis
Allergic reaction to drugs
Allergies (hay fever, hives, and asthma)

Basophils

Hypersensitivity reactions
Ulcerative colitis
Chronic hemolytic anemia
Hodgkin's disease
Myxedema
Chronic myelogenous leukemia
Polycythemia vera

Lymphocytes

Infectious mononucleosis
Infectious hepatitis
Cytomegalovirus infection
Pertussis
Brucellosis
Tuberculosis
Syphilis
Lymphocytic leukemia

Monocytes
Acute infection (bacterial, viral, mycotic, rickettsial, protozoan)
Tuberculosis
Syphilis
Brucellosis
Sarcoidosis
Ulcerative colitis
Chronic myeloid leukemia
Myeloproliferative diseases
Multiple myeloma
Hodgkin's disease
Non-Hodgkin's lymphoma
Acute monocytic leukemia
Myelomonocytic leukemia
Lupus erythematosus
Polyarteritis nodosa
Rheumatoid arthritis

Decreased Values

Neutrophils
Infection
Drug reaction
Autoimmune neutropenia
Maternal antibody production
Aplastic anemia
Radiation or chemotherapy
Megaloblastic anemia
Hypersplenism
Cancer of the bone marrow
Eosinophils
Allergies
Pyogenic infection
Shock
Postsurgical response
Basophils
Hyperthyroidism
Pregnancy
Stress
Cushing syndrome
Lymphocytes
Thoracic duct drainage
Right-sided heart failure
Hodgkin's disease
Systemic lupus erythematosus

Aplastic anemia
Human immunodeficiency virus infection
Miliary tuberculosis
Renal failure
Terminal cancer
Monocytes
Hairy cell leukemia
Bone marrow failure
Aplastic anemia

INTERFERING FACTORS

- Temperature changes
- Exercise
- Pregnancy
- Pain
- Mental or physical stress
- Heightened emotion

NURSING CARE

Nursing actions are similar to those used in venipuncture or capillary puncture procedures (see Chapter 2), with the following additional measures.

Pretest

- Because the differential count rises falsely in conditions of mental and physical stress, prepare the patient as follows:
- Instruct the physically active patient to avoid strenuous activity for 24 hours before the test because it will cause a false positive result for neutrophils and lymphocytes.
- Calm the crying infant. Organize the care of the neonate so that he or she is calm at the time of the test.
- Relieve the pain or distress experienced by the older patient. To minimize the patient's apprehension, provide reassurance about the simplicity of the procedure.

Posttest

- Arrange for prompt transport of the blood to the laboratory. If the blood remains standing in the tube, deterioration of the leukocytes begins within 30 minutes.

X-Ray Studies

eks ray stu-deez

Also called: Plain Film

SPECIMEN OR TYPE OF TEST: Radiography

PURPOSE OF THE TEST

An x-ray provides a radiographic image of the organs or tissues, to detect abnormality such as tumor, perforation, abscess, infection, foreign body or fracture.

BASICS THE NURSE NEEDS TO KNOW

The source of x-ray emissions is a high-voltage electric current that passes through a special vacuum tube in the x-ray machine. Within the vacuum tube, the electric current is converted to x-ray waves. As the x-ray beams are emitted from the machine, they pass through the patient and onto a photographic plate called an x-ray film (Figure 94).

The varying densities and composition of the tissues permit different amounts of x-ray emissions to pass through and make photographic images on the film. Dense, thick tissue is more radiopaque, resulting in lighter shades of image. Bone contains calcium, a mineral that is radiopaque. In addition, some tissues are thicker or dense and appear whiter or radiopaque on x-ray. Other tissues are thinner and, therefore, more radiolucent or gray. The size, shape, and position of the organs or tissues are accurately visualized because of the differences in the densities and composition of the tissues.

Metal objects absorb or block x-ray emissions and will appear white on the film. Before the x-ray is taken, patients must remove all metal objects and jewelry so that the underlying tissue can be visualized. X-rays are also very useful to image a metallic foreign body that is swallowed or aspirated (Figure 95).

The radiopacity of metals is useful for protection against unwanted exposure to radiation. The x-ray emissions cannot pass through lead of particular thickness. The patient and staff members wear a lead protective shield or apron to protect reproduc-

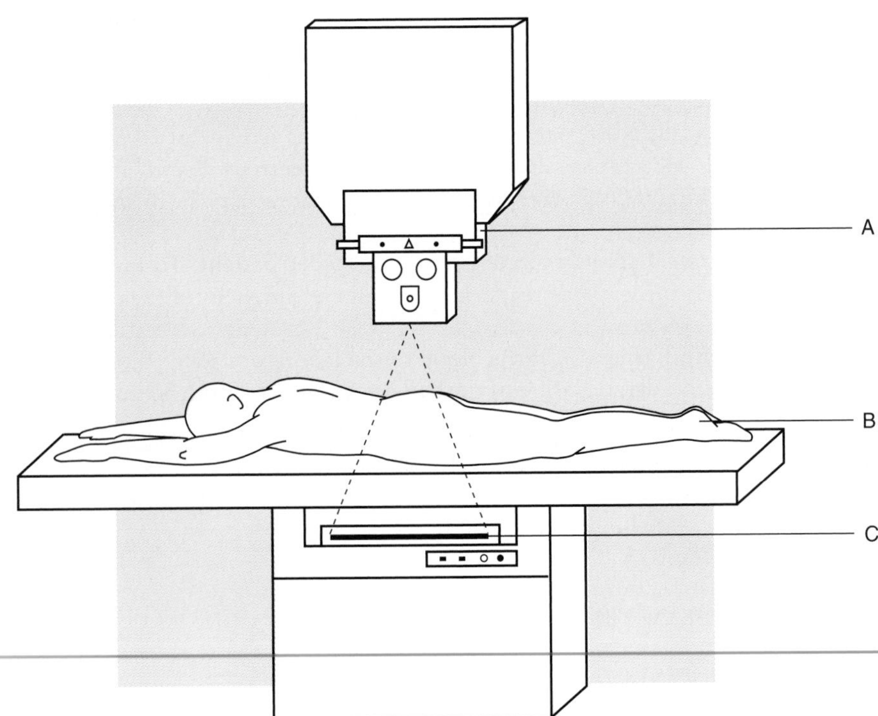

Figure 94. Simple radiograph. *A*, X-ray machine. *B*, Patient. *C*, X-ray film.

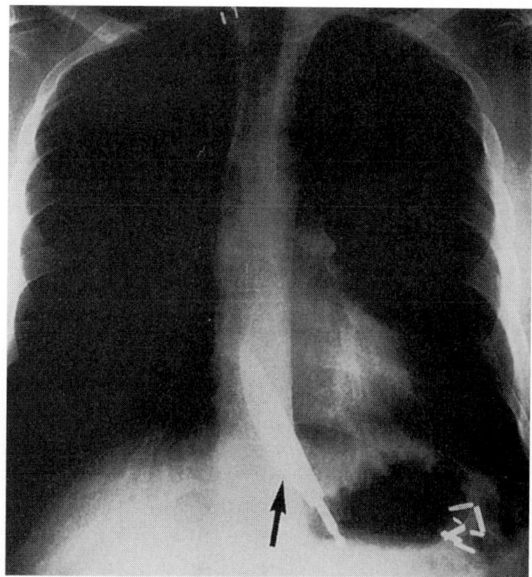

Figure 95. Steak knife lodged at the esophagogastric junction. This mentally ill patient claimed to have swallowed his steak knife at dinnertime. The chest x-ray shows the metallic blade *(arrow)* at the gastroesophageal junction. The wooden handle of the knife, which is down in the stomach, is not seen because wood typically is not visible on an x-ray. Metallic surgical clips are seen to the left of the stomach air bubble. These are from previous surgery to remove other swallowed objects. *(Reproduced with permission from Mettler, F. A. [1996].* Essentials of radiology *[p. 185]. Philadelphia: W. B. Saunders.)*

tive organs and other radiosensitive tissue. For example, nurses would wear a lead shield in the operating room when x-rays of the patient are taken. Lead is also used to line the walls of the x-ray rooms so that radiation energy cannot pass into the corridors or nearby offices. This protects workers and others from unwanted exposure.

Three-dimensional (3-D) views of the tissue are obtained by filming from the front to the back of the body as well as from the side. In radiology, these views are called *anteroposterior* and *lateral* (AP and lateral). Other positions, such as oblique views, may be requested to image a particular section of anatomy that is less visible from a traditional position. All AP x-ray films are viewed as if the patient were facing you. This means that the patient's left side is on your right side. To prevent confusion and possible error in the interpretation of the film, the technician places the letters R and L on the film to indicate the *patient's* right and left sides.

Chest X-Ray

This film is obtained routinely for hospitalized and preoperative patients to screen for tuberculosis and other serious pulmonary or cardiac diseases. It also provides a preoperative comparison film for the postoperative patient in whom a pulmonary or cardiac complication develops, and it is a basic radiologic procedure for the patient with a suspected pulmonary disorder (Figure 96). The chest x-ray also provides data about the heart, including its size and shape. In congenital and acquired cardiac disease, the enlargement of the heart and its atria or ventricles provides information about the improper function of the cardiac valves, pulmonary or aortic arterial hypertension, and venous pulmonary conditions that affect heart size.

Abdominal X-Ray

Various abnormal findings on the abdominal film are useful in obtaining a diagnosis. The patterns of air and gas appear light and bright on the abdominal film. In normal

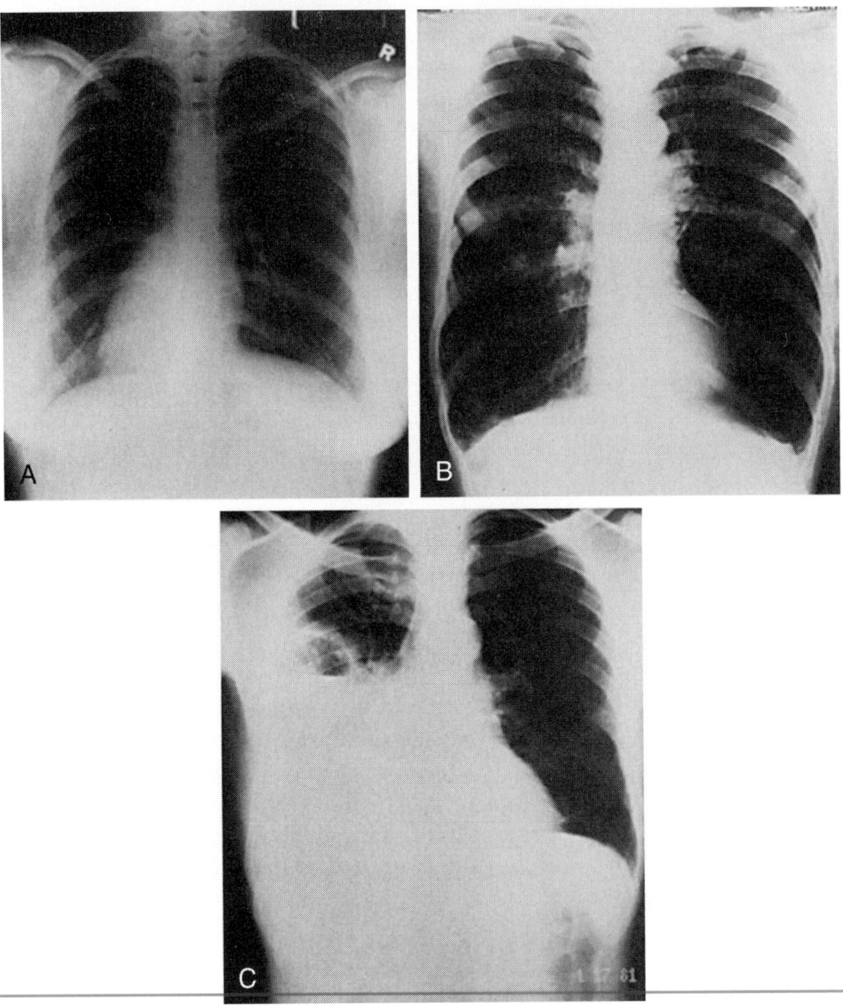

Figure 96. Chest roentgenogram. *A*, The normal chest x-ray film. *B*, Lung with emphysema. *C*, Lung with pneumonia. *(Reproduced with permission from Thompson, M. A., Hall, J. D., Hattaway, M. P., & Dowd, S. B. [1994].* Principles of imaging science and protection *[Vol. 2, Slides 207, 295, 296]. Philadelphia: W. B. Saunders.)*

findings, the air remains contained within the intestinal tract. With a perforation of either the stomach or the intestines, the gas escapes into the abdominal cavity. When the patient is seated or in an erect position, the air rises and gathers under the diaphragm, where it is visible on the abdominal x-ray film. In intestinal obstruction, air and fluid collect above the area of obstruction, distending the lumen of the intestine.

In the biliary tract, opaque stones or calculi produce a white, bright image on the abdominal film. The location of the stone is identified in the gallbladder or the cystic or common duct. Cholesterol stones are nonopaque, however, and cannot be seen on the abdominal film. This type of stone is visualized only on x-ray examination using contrast medium.

Kidney-Ureter-Bladder X-Ray

This x-ray film is also known as a flat plate of the abdomen. It images the structure, size, and position of the kidneys, ureters, and bladder, screening for abnormality in these organs and nearby tissues. Calcification of the renal calyces or renal pelvis is visible, as are any radiopaque calculi present in the upper urinary tract.

Bone and Joint X-Ray

X-ray studies are a vital tool in the assessment of bones and joints. In cases of trauma, the x-ray film is used to identify the presence, location, and type of fracture; the potential for injury to the surrounding soft tissue; and the healing activity after the fracture has been treated. Dislocation of a joint, a bone tumor, a bone infection, and a loss of bone mass are also visible. In arthritic disorders or metabolic diseases such as gout, x-ray studies are used to visualize the size and structure of the joints and soft tissues and the alignment of the bones that articulate at the joints (Figure 97).

Child Abuse

When child abuse is suspected as the cause of a skeletal injury, multiple x-ray studies of all parts of the skeleton are performed. In cases of child abuse, the incidence of bone fracture is high, and the sites of skeletal injury are often multiple, particularly in children younger than age 18 months. To differentiate between abuse and other causes of trauma, the radiologist compares the history of how and when the injuries occurred with the x-ray findings. Child abuse or suspected child abuse should be reported to authorities.

Skull-Vertebral X-Ray

The x-ray films of the skull can detect abnormality of shape, size, and contour, including skull fractures. Usually, computed tomography (CT) or magnetic resonance imaging (MRI) is used instead of skull radiographs, because these procedures are more accurate and detailed in the imaging of both skull and brain tissue. The vertebral x-ray films provide visualization of a fracture, dislocation, or deformity of the spine. X-ray also demonstrates degeneration or faulty alignment of the spinal vertebrae that causes a disorder in the intervertebral discs.

NORMAL VALUES The size, shape, appearance, thickness, and position of the organs and tissues are within normal limits for the patient's age. No anatomic abnormalities are noted.

Figure 97. Effects of calcium on bone density. *A*, Hand radiograph of a 28-year-old patient with good calcium deposits in bone. *B*, Hand radiograph of a 72-year-old patient whose bones appear transparent as the result of calcium loss. This radiographic appearance is also attributed to pathologic changes caused by rheumatoid arthritis. *(Reproduced with permission from Thompson, M. A., Hall, J. D., Hattaway, M. P., & Dowd, S. B. [1994].* Principles of imaging science and protection *[Vol. 2, Slide 290]. Philadelphia: W. B. Saunders.)*

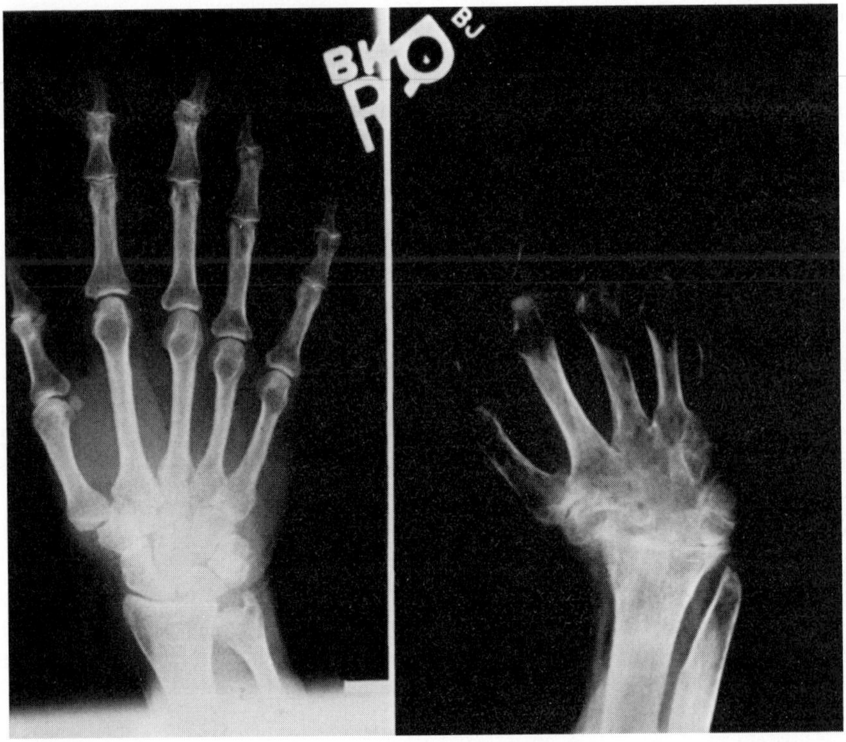

HOW THE TEST IS DONE

The patient is positioned between the x-ray machine and the photographic film. The machine emits the x-ray energy that passes through the patient's body and imprints the image on the film.

SIGNIFICANCE OF TEST RESULTS

Abnormal Values

CHEST AND HEART

Pneumothorax
Atelectasis
Pleural effusion

Pleurisy
Cystic fibrosis
Pulmonary fibrosis
Tumor or cyst
Atherosclerosis
Cor pulmonale
Cardiac hypertrophy
Pneumonia
Tuberculosis
Pulmonary abscess
Chronic obstructive pulmonary disease
Mediastinal nodes
Aortic aneurysm
Congestive heart failure
Adult respiratory distress syndrome
Fracture

Intestinal Tract

Perforation
Obstruction
Paralytic ileus
Volvulus
Intussusception
Subphrenic abscess
Foreign body
Biliary tract calculus

Urinary Tract

Renal abscess
Renal tuberculosis
Pyelonephritis
Glomerulonephritis
Polycystic renal disease
Hematoma
Congenital malformation
Tumor or cyst
Renal or ureteral calculus
Hydronephrosis
Amyloidosis

Bones and Joints

Fracture
Dislocation
Subluxation
Bone cyst or tumor
Congenital malformation
Vitamin D deficiency, rickets
Paget's disease

Osteoarthritis
Rheumatoid arthritis
Gout
Osteomyelitis
Osteoporosis
Osteomalacia

Skull

Congenital anomaly
Neoplasm, skull
Osteomyelitis
Fracture
Paget's disease
Acromegaly

Spinal Vertebrae

Ankylosing spondylitis
Scoliosis
Kyphosis
Tuberculosis
Fracture
Subluxation
Ruptured disc
Osteoarthritis
Osteoporosis
Paget's disease

INTERFERING FACTORS

- Excessive movement
- Failure to remove jewelry or other metal from the x-ray field
- Improper positioning
- For abdominal and kidney-ureter-bladder films: retained barium or contrast medium, feces, ascites, gas, obesity

NURSING CARE

Pretest

- For the patient who requires an abdominal or kidney-ureter-bladder film, schedule the x-ray study before any radiologic study that uses barium or contrast medium. The contrast medium is radiopaque, and the residual contrast interferes with the visualization of the underlying tissues.
- For most imaging procedures, instruct the patient to remove all clothes and put on a hospital gown. The exceptions are skull radiographs and x-ray films of the distal extremities.
- Instruct the patient to remove all jewelry and metal objects from the area that is to be imaged.

NURSING CARE—*cont'd*

- Provide reassurance to the patient. Young children often fear the equipment, strange room, isolation, and separation from their parents. Adults also may feel somewhat apprehensive.

During the Test

- Ensure the patient's safety at all times, particularly when there is a risk of the patient falling. The radiography table has no siderails. A Velcro waist restraint may be used, but sometimes the restraint interferes with the positioning and imaging needed.
- Position the patient for the specific views needed.
- Instruct the patient to remain motionless during the imaging. Sometimes the patient is instructed to inhale deeply and hold the breath until the image is taken.
- The patient must often wait in the imaging area as the decision is made concerning whether to take additional x-ray films. Provide a blanket or extra gown for the patient who is chilled in the cool room.

Posttest

- Assist the patient in dismounting from the radiography table and getting dressed, as needed.

APPENDIX A

Therapeutic Drug Monitoring

Therapeutic drug monitoring provides exact information about the quantity of medication that is in the blood. This testing is performed for several reasons. In the patient with a normal metabolism, the standard dose and schedule of a particular medication usually results in a therapeutic blood level of the medication within a specific period. In other patients, such as elderly individuals, neonates, and obese persons, the standard dose may produce a diminished or excessive clinical result because of abnormal metabolism or diminished renal or hepatic function. Therapeutic drug monitoring is used to adjust the dose and schedule of medications as needed.

For a variety of reasons, many patients do not take their medication in the same amount as was prescribed. Therapeutic drug monitoring provides data to alert the physician or nurse about the need to investigate the problem.

Some medications have a narrow range of values for a therapeutic effect. A small increase beyond that range can have a toxic result. Therapeutic drug monitoring is carried out to protect the patient from the harm of excess medication.

With some medications, the therapeutic value and the critical value are reported as peak and trough values. *Peak value* refers to the highest therapeutic level of medication in the blood. This usually occurs at a particular time interval after the medication has been taken. For some drugs, the peak value occurs a few hours after it is taken. Other drugs do not reach their peak value in the blood for days after continuing the medication regimen. The *trough value* identifies the level of medication in the blood, usually just before the next dose. Because of the variations of timing, the nurse should consult the laboratory as to when the blood specimen should be drawn for a peak or trough value, as needed.

In the case of overdose (accidental or deliberate), lab testing can identify the medication and the amount that is in the blood. The patient may be comatose, psychotic, or agitated from the effect of the overdose and may be unable to describe what was ingested. The test results provide data for corrective action.

The following table provides the range of blood values of selected medications to measure for therapeutic effect and for toxicity. For therapeutic drug monitoring, the tests are ordered at planned intervals to establish and maintain an effective medication level in the blood. To identify a critical value or a toxic level of the medication, the laboratory test also may be ordered when the patient demonstrates side effects to the medication or when an unexplained change in behavior, such as agitation, seizures or loss of consciousness can be caused by toxicity.

The classes of medications that are commonly monitored include: analgesics, antiarrhythmics, antiasthmatics, antibiotics, anticonvulsants, antidepressants, antipsychotics, and immunosuppressants.

Therapeutic Drug Monitoring

Drug	Collection Tube	Therapeutic Range	Critical Value (Toxic Value)
Acetaminophen (Tylenol)	Red	10–30 mcg/mL SI: 66–169 µmol/L	*4 hours after ingestion* >150 mcg/mL SI: >990 µmol/L *12 hours after ingestion* >50 mcg/mL SI: >330 µmol/L
Amikacin (Amikin)	Red	*Peak* 15–30 mcg/mL SI: 25–51 µmol/L *Trough* 5–10 mcg/mL SI: 8.5–17.1 µmol/L	*Peak* >35 mcg/mL SI: >74 µmol/L *Trough* >8 mcg/mL SI: >17 µmol/L
Amiodarone (Cordarone)	Red	1.0–2.5 mcg/mL SI: 1.6–3.9 µmol/L	>2.5 mcg/mL SI: >4 µmol/L
Amitriptyline (Elavil)	Red, green	80–200 ng/mL SI: 289–722 nmol/L	>300 ng/mL SI: >1080 nmol/L
Amobarbital (Amytal)	Lavender, green, red	5–15 mcg/mL SI: 22–66 µmol/L	>20 mcg/mL SI: >86 µmol/L
Amoxapine (Asendin)	Red, green	20–100 ng/mL SI: 64–319 nmol/L	>600 ng/mL SI: >1913 nmol/L
Bupropion (Wellbutrin, Zyban)	Red, lavender	50–100 ng/mL	>170 ng/mL
Carbamazepine (Tegretol)	Red	8–12 mcg/mL SI: 34–51 µmol/L	>12 mcg/mL SI: >51 µmol/L
Chloramphenicol (Chloromycetin)	Red	10–25 mcg/mL SI: 31–77 µmol/L *Trough* <5 mcg/mL SI: <15 µmol/L	>25 mcg/mL SI: >77 µmol/L

Therapeutic Drug Monitoring—*cont'd*

Drug	Collection Tube	Therapeutic Range	Critical Value (Toxic Value)
Chlordiazepoxide (Librax, Librium)	Red	0.7–1.0 mcg/mL SI: 2.3–3.3 μmol/L	>5 mcg/mL SI: >17 μmol/L
Chlorpromazine (Thorazine)	Red	50–300 ng/mL SI: 157–942 nmol/L	>750 ng/mL SI: >2355 nmol/L
Diazepam (Valium)	Red	0.2–1.0 mcg/mL SI: 0.7–3.5 μmol/L	>3 mcg/mL SI: >10.5 μmol/L
Digoxin (Lanoxin)	Red	0.8–2.0 ng/mL SI: 1.0–2.6 nmol/L	>2.5 ng/mL SI: >3.2 nmol/L
Disopyramide (Norpace)	Red, green, lavender	**Atrial arrhythmias** *Trough* 2.8–3.2 mcg/mL SI: 8.3–9.4 μmol/L **Ventricular arrhythmias** *Trough* 3.3–5.0 mcg/mL SI: 9.7–15 μmol/L	 *Trough* >7 mcg/mL SI: 20.6 μmol/L *Trough* 7 mcg/mL SI: >20.6 μmol/L
Ethchlorvynol (Placidyl)	Red, green	2–8 mcg/mL SI: 14–55 μmol/L	>20 mcg/mL SI: >138 μmol/L
Flucytosine (Ancobon)	Red	25–100 mcg/mL SI: 194–775 μmol/L	100–125 mcg/mL SI: 775–970 μmol/L
Fluoxetine (Prozac)	Red, green	100–800 ng/mL SI: 289–2314 nmol/L	>2000 ng/mL SI: >5784 nmol/L
Flurazepam (Dalmane)	Red	0.4 ng/mL SI: 0–9 nmol/L	200 ng/mL SI: 500 nmol/L
Gentamycin (Garamycin)	Red	*Peak* 4–10 mcg/mL SI: 8.3–40 mmol/L *Trough* 1–2 mcg/mL SI: 2–4 μmol/L	*Peak* >12 mcg/mL SI: >12 μmol/L *Trough* >2 mcg/mL SI: >4.1 μmol/L
Haloperidol (Haldol)	Red, green	5–20 ng/mL SI: 10–40 nmol/L	>42 ng/mL SI: >84 nmol/L
Imipramine (Tofranil)	Red, green	100–300 ng/mL SI: 350–1070 nmol/L	>500 ng/mL SI: >1780 nmol/L
Isoniazid (Laniazid)	Red, green	2–5 mcg/mL SI: 14.6–36.4 μmol/L	>20 mcg/mL SI: >145 μmol/L

Continued

Therapeutic Drug Monitoring—*cont'd*

Drug	Collection Tube	Therapeutic Range	Critical Value (Toxic Value)
Lidocaine (Xylocaine)	Red, green, lavender	1.5–5.0 mcg/mL SI: 6.4–21.4 mmol/L	>6 mcg/mL SI: >25.6 mmol/L
Lithium (Eskalith)	Red	0.6–1.2 mEq/L SI: 0.6–1.2 mmol/L	>1.5 mEq/L SI: >1.5 mmol/L
Maprotiline (Ludiomil)	Red	200–400 ng/mL SI: 721–1442 nmol/L	>1000 mcg/mL SI: 3605 nmol/L
Meprobamate (Equagesic)	Red	6–12 mcg/mL SI: 28–55 µmol/L	>60 mcg/mL SI: >275 µmol/L
Methotrexate (Mexate)	Red, green, lavender	Variable (dosage dependent)	*Low dose* >0.02 µmol/L, 48 hr post dose *High dose* >1.0 µmol/L, 48 hr post dose
Mexiletine (Mexitil)	Red	0.75–2 mcg/mL S: 4–11 µmol/L	>2 mcg/mL SI: >9 µmol/L
Nortriptyline (Aventyl)	Red	50–150 ng/mL SI: 190–570 nmol/L	>500 ng/mL SI: >1900 nmol/L
Phenobarbital (Luminal)	Red, green, lavender	20–40 mcg/mL SI: 86–172 µmol/L	>40 mcg/mL SI: >172 µmol/L
Phenytoin (Dilantin)	Red, lavender	10–20 mcg/mL SI: 40–79 µmol/L	25–50 mcg/mL SI: 100–200 µmol/L
Procainamide (Pronestyl)	Red	4–10 mcg/mL SI: 17–42 µmol/L	>12 mcg/mL SI: 59.5 µmol/L
Propoxyphene (Darvocet-N, Darvon)	Red	0.1–0.4 mcg/mL SI: 0.3–1.2 µmol/L	>0.5 mcg/mL SI: >1.5 µmol/L
Propranolol (Inderal)	Red	50–100 ng/mL SI: 190–390 nmol/L	>1000 ng/mL SI: >3860 nmol/L
Quinidine (Cardioquin)	Red	2–5 mcg/mL SI: 6.2–15.4 µmol/L	>8 mcg/mL SI: >24.7 µmol/L

Therapeutic Drug Monitoring—*cont'd*

Drug	Collection Tube	Therapeutic Range	Critical Value (Toxic Value)
Salicylate (acetylsalicylic acid, aspirin)	Red, lavender	**For analgesia** <10 mg/dL SI: <0.72 mmol/L	 *Mild* 30 mg/dL SI: 2.17 mmol/L *Severe* >80 mg/dL SI: >3.62 mmol/L
		For anti-inflammatory effect 15–20 mg/dL SI: 1.09–1.45 mmol/L	 *Mild* 30 mg/dL SI: 2.17 mmol/L *Severe* >80 mg/dL SI: >3.62 mmol/L
Theophylline (Aminophylline, Elixophyllin)	Red	10–20 mcg/mL SI: 56–111 μmol/L	>20 mcg/mL SI: >111 μmol/L
Thiocyanate (nitroprusside, Nipride)	Red, lavender	1–4 mcg/mL SI: 17–69 μmol/L	>35 mcg/mL SI: >609 μmol/L
Tocainide (Tonocard)	Red, green	6–15 mcg/mL 32–78 μmol/L	>15 mcg/mL >78 μmol/L
Valproic acid (Depacon)	Red, green	50–100 mcg/mL SI: 350–690 μmol/L	>200 mcg/mL SI: >1390 μmol/L
Vancomycin	Red	*Peak* 20–40 mcg/mL SI: 14–27 μmol/L *Trough* 5–10 mcg/mL SI: 3.4–6.8 μmol/L	*Peak* >80 mcg/mL SI: >54 μmol/L *Trough* Not applicable
Verapamil (Isoptin, Calan)	Red, green	50–250 ng/mL SI: 100–510 nmol/L	>250 ng/mL SI: >510 nmol/L
Warfarin (Coumadin)	Red, lavender	2–5 mcg/mL SI: 6.5–16.0 μmol/L	>10 mcg/mL SI: 32.4 μmol/L

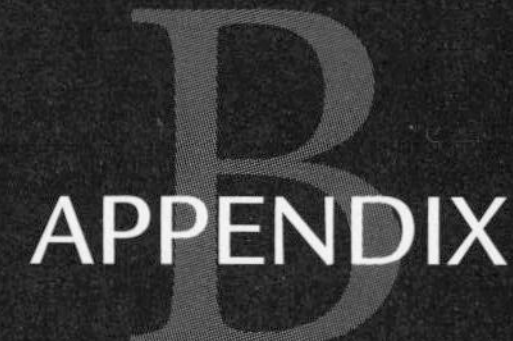

Toxic Substances

Screening for toxic substances is performed to identify the agent responsible for an acute, chronic, or possibly life-threatening illness. Some of these toxic substances are drugs of abuse and have been taken in an unknown quantity. The clinical effect of the substance varies among individuals who are occasional or habitual users. It can also vary with the preparation or mixture that was inhaled, injected, or eaten.

Some toxic substances are ingested by small children. The poisons commonly ingested include rat poison, antifreeze, and insecticide. Other toxic substances that can be identified by lab testing are toxic chemicals and metals that poison the individual from an environmental source, including inhalation of poisonous gases from a fire and exposure to hazardous industrial wastes. When the individual is acutely ill from any of these toxic substances, it is essential to identify the cause. Appropriate action can then be taken to reverse the effect and protect the organs from further damage. Some of the toxins pose a long-term threat because they cause mutation and eventual malignancy.

In the following table, the values for the normal range of a toxic substance vary from none to minute amounts. The values for toxicity levels are not always defined. The toxicity may vary among individuals, or its very presence may be considered toxic.

Toxic Substances

Substance	Specimen	Collection Tube	Normal Value	Critical Value (Toxic Level)
Alcohol (ETOH, ethanol)	Blood	Red, gray	Negative	>300 mg/dL SI: 65.1 mmol/L
Amphetamine	Urine (random)	Plastic cup	Negative	*Cutoff value* 1000 ng/mL SI: 7400 ng/mL
Arsenic	Blood (20 mL)	Trace metal-free container	<70 mcg/dL SI: <0.93 μmol/L	100–500 mcg/L SI: 1.33–6.65 μmol/L
	Urine (24 hr)	Plastic, acid-washed container	120 mcg/L SI: <1.59 μmol/L	>850 mcg/L SI: >11.3 μmol/L
	Hair, nails	Clean envelope	<1 ng/g SI: <0.13 nmol/g	>100 mcg/g 713.4 nmol/g
Cadmium	Urine (24 hr)	Plastic, acid-washed container	<1 mcg/L SI: 8.9 nmol/L	>10 mcg/L SI: >88.97 μmol/L
Cannabinoids (marijuana, hashish)	Urine (random)	Plastic cup	Negative	*Cutoff value* 50 ng/mL
Cocaine	Blood	Red, gray	Negative Negative	>1000 ng/mL >3300 nmol/L
	Urine (random)	Plastic cup	Negative	1–215 ng/mL
	Hair	Clean envelope	Negative	>1.2 ng/mL

Cyanide	Blood	Red, lavender	*Smoker* 0.041 mg/L SI: 1.57 mmol/L *Nonsmoker* 0.016 mg/L SI: 0.61 mmol/L	>1 mg/mL SI: 38.4 µmol/L
Ethylene glycol (antifreeze)	Blood	Red, green	Negative	>50 mg/L
Fluoride	Blood	Red (nonglass tube)	0.1–0.2 mg/dL SI: 0.5–10.5 mmol/L	Not well established
Lead	Blood	Lead-free tube with heparin	*Child* <10 mcg/dL SI: 0.5 µmol/L	>70 mcg/dL SI: >3.34 µmol/L
Mercury	Blood	Metal-free tube	<0.6–59 mcg/mL SI: <3–294 nmol/L	>50 mcg/mL SI: >250 nmol/L
	Urine	Plastic, acid-washed container	<20 mcg/L/24 hr SI: <100 nmol/L	>150 mcg/L SI: >748.5 nmol/L
Methadone	Urine	Plastic cup	Negative	*Cutoff value* 300 ng/mL
Opiates (codeine, morphine)	Urine	Plastic cup	Negative	*Cutoff value* 2000 ng/mL

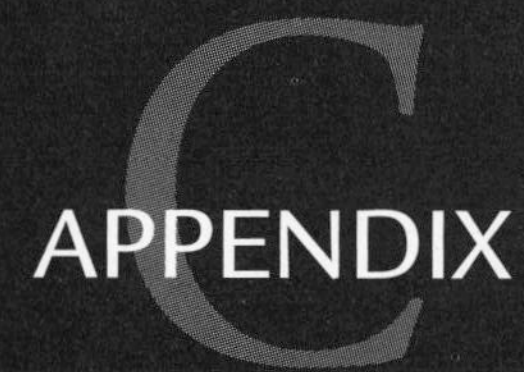

APPENDIX C

Abbreviations Associated with Laboratory Tests

Abbreviations	Complete Name
A-a	Alveolar-arterial
ABI	Ankle-brachial index
ACE	Angiotensin-converting enzyme
ACT	Activated clotting time
ACTH	Adrenocorticotrophic hormone
ADH	Antidiuretic hormone
AFAFP	Amniotic fluid alpha fetoprotein
AFP	Alpha fetoprotein
A/G	Albumin/globulin ratio
AGT	Antiglobulin test
ALB	Albumin
ALP	Alkaline phosphatase
ALT	Alanine aminotransferase
ANA	Antinuclear antibody
Anti-HAV	Hepatitis A antibody
Anti-HBc	Hepatitis B core antibody
Anti-Be	Hepatitis Be antibody
Anti-HCV	Hepatitis C virus antibody
APTT	Activated partial thromboplastin time
ART	Automated reagin test
AST	Aspartate aminotransferase
BAO	Basal acid output
BE	Barium enema

Continued

Abbreviations	Complete Name
BUN	Blood urea nitrogen
C&S	Culture and susceptibility
Ca, Ca^{2+}	Calcium
Ca_i	Calcium, ionized
CA 19-9	Carbohydrate antigen 19-9
CA 125	Cancer antigen 125
CAT	Computed axial tomography
CBC	Complete blood count
CCr	Creatinine clearance
CEA	Carcinoembryonic antigen
CH_{50}	Complement, total
CK	Creatine kinase
Cl^-	Chloride ion
CO_2	Carbon dioxide
CPK	Creatine phosphatase
CSF	Cerebrospinal fluid
CT	Calcitonin
CT	Computed tomography
cTnI	Cardiac troponin I
cTnT	Cardiac troponin T
CVS	Chorionic villus sampling
DAT	Direct antiglobulin test
DOPAC	Dihydroxyphenyl acetic acid
DSA	Digital subtraction angiography
DVI	Digital vascular imaging
E_2	Estradiol
E_3	Estriol
EA	Early antigen
EBNA	Epstein-Barr nuclear antigen
ECG	Electrocardiogram
ECHO	Echocardiogram
ECT	Emissions computed tomography
EEG	Electroencephalogram
EGD	Esophagogastroduodenoscopy
EIA	Enzyme immunoassay
EKG	Electrocardiogram
ELISA	Enzyme-linked immunoassay
EMG	Electromyography
EP	Erythropoietin
EPS	Electrophysiologic studies
ERC	Endoscopic retrograde cholangiography
ERCP	Endoscopic retrograde cholangiopancreatography
ER/PGR	Estrogen/progesterone assay

Abbreviations	Complete Name
ERV	Expiratory reserve volume
ESR	Erythrocyte sedimentation rate
EUG	Excretory urogram
EUS	Endoscopic ultrasound
FBP	Fibrin breakdown products
FBS	Fasting blood glucose
FDP	Fibrin degradation products
FEF	Forced expiratory flow
FEV	Forced expiratory volume
fFN	Fetal fibronectin
FNA	Fine needle aspiration
FNB	Fine needle biopsy
FOB	Fetal occult blood
FRC	Functional residual capacity
FSH	Follicle stimulating hormone
FSP	Fibrin-split products
FT_3	Free triiodothyronine
FT_4	Free thyroxine
FTA-ABS	Fluorescent treponemal antibody absorption test
FVC	Forced vital capacity
GB	Gall bladder
GEST	Graded exercise testing
GGT	Gamma-glutamyltransferase
GGPT	Gamma-glutamyltranspeptidase
GH	Growth hormone
GHb	Glycohemoglobin
GLU	Glucose
GPT	Glutamic pyruvic transaminase
G-6-PD	Glucose-6-phosphate dehydrogenase
GTP	Glutamyl transpeptidase
HAA	Hepatitis associated antigen
HAP	Haptoglobin
HAV, Ab	Hepatitis A virus antibody
HAVAB	Hepatitis A virus antibody
Hb	Hemoglobin
HBA_1	Glycosylated hemoglobin
HBcAb	Hepatitis B core antibody
HBeAb	Hepatitis Be antibody
HBeAg	Hepatitis Be antigen
HbF	Fetal hemoglobin
Hbg	Hemoglobin
HBsAb	Hepatitis B surface antibody
HBsAg	Hepatitis B surface antigen

Continued

Abbreviations	Complete Name
hCG	Human chorionic gonadotrophin
HCO_3	Bicarbonate
Hct	Hematocrit
HDL	High density lipoprotein
HLA	Human leukocyte antigen
HSV	Herpes simplex virus
IADSA	Intra-arterial subtraction angiography
I-ALP	Alkaline phosphatase isoenzymes
IAT	Indirect antiglobulin test
IC	Inspiratory capacity
IF	Intrinsic factor
IgG	Immunoglobulin G
IgM	Immunoglobulin M
INR	International normalized ratio
IRV	Inspiratory reserve volume
ITT	Insulin tolerance test
IUG	Intravenous urography
IVDSA	Intravenous digital subtraction angiography
IVFA	Intravenous fluorescent angiography
IVP	Intravenous pyelography
IVU	Intravenous urography
IVUS	Intravascular ultrasound
K^+	Potassium ion
17-KGS	17-Ketogenic steroid
17-KS	17-Ketosteroid
LAP	Leucine aminopeptidase
LATS	Long-acting thyroid stimulator
LDH	Lactate dehydrogenase
LDL	Low-density lipoprotein
LDM	Low-dose myelography
LH	Luteinizing hormone
LP	Lumbar puncture
L/S	Lecithin-sphingomyelin
Mb	Myoglobin
MBC	Maximum breathing capacity
MCH	Mean corpuscular hemoglobin
MCHC	Mean corpuscular hemoglobin concentration
MCV	Mean corpuscular volume
Mg, Mg^{2+}	Magnesium, magnesium ion
MHA-TP	Microhemagglutinin assay-*Treponema pallidum*
MMEF	Forced midexpiratory flow
MPV	Mean platelet volume
MRI	Magnetic resonance imaging

Abbreviations	Complete Name
MUGA	Multiple gated acquisition angiography
MV	Minute volume
MVV	Maximum voluntary ventilation
5′N	5′-Nucleotidase
Na^+	Sodium ion
NAP	Neutrophil alkaline phosphatase
NCS	Nerve conduction study
NH_3	Ammonia
NPO	Nothing by mouth
NST	Nonstress testing
O & P	Ova and parasites
O_2 sat	Oxygenation saturation
OF	Osmotic fragility
OGTT	Oral glucose tolerance test
P_4	Progesterone
PAP	Papanicolaou smear
PAP	Prostatic acid phosphatase
PCA	Parietal cell antibody
Pco_2	Partial pressure of carbon dioxide
P_{cr}	Plasma creatinine
PCR	Polymerase chain reaction
PCV	Packed cell volume
Pdi	Transdiaphragmatic pressure
PET	Positron emissions tomography scan
$PETco_2$	End tidal partial pressure of carbon dioxide
pH	Partial pressure of hydrogen
Phe	Phenylalanine
Pimax	Maximum intrathoracic pressure
PKU	Phenylketonuria
Po_2	Partial pressure of oxygen
Po_4^{3-}	Phosphate
PRA	Plasma renin activity
PSA	Phosphate specific antigen
PT	Prothrombin time
PTC	Percutaneous transhepatic cholangiography
PTH	Parathyroid hormone
PTT	Partial thromboplastin time
PUBS	Percutaneous umbilical cord sampling
Pvo_2	Partial pressure of oxygen in the venous system
RAIU	Radioactive iodine uptake
RBC	Red blood cell, erythrocyte
RDW	Red cell distribution width
RF	Rheumatoid factor

Continued

Abbreviations	Complete Name
RAI	Radioimmunoassay
RPR	Rapid plasma reagin
RT_3U	Resin triiodothyronine uptake
RV	Residual volume
SACE	Serum angiotensin-converting enzyme
SAECG	Signal-averaged electrocardiogram
SAo_2	Arterial oxygen saturation
SBGM	Self-blood glucose monitoring
SGOT	Serum glutamic-oxaloacetic transaminase
SGPT	Serum glutamate-pyruvate transaminase
SHBD	Serum hydroxybutyrate dehydrogenase
SI	Système International (International System of Units)
SMUG	Self-monitoring of urinary glucose
SPECT	Single positron emission computed tomography
STH	Growth hormone; somatotropin
Svo_2	Oxygen saturation in the venous system
T & C	Type and crossmatch
T-ALP	Total alkaline phosphatase
T_3	Triiodothyronine
T_4	Thyroxine
TBG	Thyroxine-binding globulin
tCO_2	Total carbon dioxide
TEE	Transesophageal echocardiography
TIBC	Total iron-binding capacity
TLC	Total lung capacity
TP	Total protein
TRH	Thyroid-releasing hormone
TSH	Thyroid-stimulating hormone
TUS	Transluminal ultrasound
TV	Tidal volume
UA	Urinalysis
VC	Vital capacity
VCA	Viral capsid antigen
VCG	Vectorcardiogram
Vds	Dead space volume
VDRL	Venereal Disease Research Laboratory
VMA	Vanillylmandelic acid
V/Q	Ventilation/perfusion
WBC	White blood cell

APPENDIX D

Common Laboratory and Diagnostic Tests for Frequently Occurring Medical Diagnoses

When caring for the patient, there are a number of laboratory tests and diagnostic procedures that the physician or nurse practitioner uses to make a diagnosis as to what has caused the illness and to determine the seriousness or extent of the disease. In Table 18, common medical conditions are listed, with the tests that are specific to that diagnosis. Generally, when particular tests can confirm and support the diagnosis, the list is somewhat shorter. In conditions where there are no specific tests, there is a longer list of tests that each provides partial information.

Essential parts of the diagnostic process begin with the patient's history and the physical examination. The physician or nurse practitioner uses this important, initial information as a guide to determine what is wrong. The diagnostic procedures and laboratory tests that are selected confirm or support the diagnosis by providing measurable, objective data. The physician or nurse practitioner uses all of the data, in totality, to arrive at a definitive diagnosis.

There are some tests that may provide similar information regarding the disease. For example, CT scan, MRI, ultrasound, and nuclear imaging all provide visualization of the particular organ. In cases of infection, culture, antigen/antibody tests, and PCR-DNA identification of the organism all identify or help identify the microbial cause of the infection. The physician or nurse practitioner selects some of the tests because they are the most useful or specific in the individual patient's circumstance. If the tests do not identify the cause, or they provide partial data only, additional tests or procedures will be ordered.

The nurse notes that there are some tests and procedures that are used to exclude or rule out other conditions that have presented similar symptoms. Additionally, some tests may be ordered which are supportive of the diagnosis or used to identify possible complications. In the following table, the tests listed are specific to the medical diagnosis and do not include tests to exclude other diagnoses or verify complications.

Clinical Guides to Diagnosis	
Common Medical Diagnoses	**Common Tests Used**
Acquired immune deficiency syndrome	Human immunodeficiency virus antibody screen/ELISA
	Western blot
	HIV antigen
	p24 antigen
	HIV-DNA amplification
	CD^4 (T) lymphocyte count
	Viral load
Addison disease	Adrenocorticotropic hormone, plasma
	Corticotropin stimulation test
	Cortisol, serum or plasma
	Electrolytes, serum
	Growth hormone, serum
	Osmolality, urine
	Sodium, urine
	Thyroid stimulating hormone, serum
	Thyroxine, serum
Aldosteronism	Adrenal vein catheterization for renin
	Aldosterone, serum or plasma
	Aldosterone, urine
	Computed tomography scan of the abdomen
	Electrolytes, serum
	Potassium, urine
	Renin, plasma
	Sodium, urine
Alzheimer's disease	Lumbar puncture
	Cerebrospinal fluid analysis
	Beta amyloid$_{(1\text{-}42)}$
	PET scan
Anemia	CBC
	Hemoglobin
	Hematocrit
	Red blood cell morphology, peripheral blood
	Red blood cell indices
	Reticulocyte count
	Biopsy, bone marrow
Anemia, iron deficiency	CBC
	Red blood cell morphology, peripheral blood
	Ferritin, serum
	Iron, serum
	Transferrin, serum
	Total iron binding capacity

Clinical Guides to Diagnosis—*cont'd*

Common Medical Diagnoses	Common Tests Used
Anemia, iron deficiency—*cont'd*	Biopsy, bone marrow
	Occult blood, feces
Anemia, sickle cell	Sickle cell test
	Hemoglobin electrophoresis
	CBC
	Red blood cell morphology, peripheral blood
	In pregnancy: Amniocentesis with amniotic fluid analysis for chromosome and genetic analysis
Aneurysm, aortic	X-ray, abdomen
	CT scan, abdomen
	Aortography
	MRI, abdomen
	Transesophageal ultrasound
Angina	Cardiac markers
	Cardiac catheterization
	Echocardiogram
	Electrocardiogram
	Holter monitoring
	Lipids, serum
	Stress testing, cardiac
	Thallium stress testing
Appendicitis	CBC
	White blood cell count
	White blood cell differential, peripheral blood
	CT scan, abdomen
	Ultrasound, abdomen
Arthritis, rheumatoid	CBC
	Erythrocyte sedimentation rate
	C-reactive protein
	Rheumatoid factor
	Arthrocentesis, with synovial fluid analysis
	X-ray, joint
Ascariasis	Ova and parasites, feces
	CBC
	Eosinophil count
Asthma	Allergen identification
	Arterial blood gases
	Eosinophil count
	Culture, sputum
	Pulmonary function studies
	X-ray, chest

Continued

Clinical Guides to Diagnosis—*cont'd*	
Common Medical Diagnoses	**Common Tests Used**
Bronchitis	Arterial blood gases Culture, bacterial, sputum Culture, viral, sputum X-ray, chest
Cancer, bone	X-ray, bone Bone scan, nuclear CT, bone MRI, bone, extremity Biopsy, bone
Cancer, bone marrow. *See* Leukemia.	
Cancer, breast	Mammography Biopsy, breast Estrogen and progesterone receptor assay Carcinogenic embryonic antigen, serum Cancer antigen 15-3 Bone scan
Cancer, cervix	Papanicolaou smear Cervicovaginal cytology Human papilloma virus-DNA probe Colposcopy Ultrasound, pelvic
Cancer, colorectal	Occult blood, feces Colonoscopy Sigmoidoscopy Barium enema Carcinogenic antigen 19-9 Carcinogenic antigen 125
Cancer, esophagus, stomach	Occult blood, feces Esophagogastroduodenoscopy (EGD) with biopsy for cytology Upper gastrointestinal series Carcinoembryonic antigen Carcinogenic antigen 19-9 CT scan, chest, abdomen
Cancer liver	Liver biopsy, with cytology studies Ultrasound, abdominal CT scan, abdominal MRI, abdominal Alkaline phosphatase Carcinoembryonic antigen

Clinical Guides to Diagnosis—*cont'd*

Common Medical Diagnoses	Common Tests Used
Cancer, lung	Bronchial brushings for cytology
	Bronchial washings for cytology
	Cytology, sputum
	CT scan, chest
	Fine needle biopsy, lung
	Open lung biopsy
	Transbronchial fine needle aspiration
	X-ray, chest
Cancer, pancreas	Percutaneous needle aspiration biopsy, pancreas, with cytology
	CA 19-9, serum
	CT scan, abdomen
	Carcinoembryonic antigen
	Ultrasound, pancreas
	ERCP with pancreatic cytology
	Bilirubin, serum, urine
	Alkaline phosphatase
Cancer, prostate	Alkaline phosphates, serum
	Biopsy, prostate
	Prostate specific antigen, serum
Cancer, renal	Fine needle aspiration biopsy, kidney
	MRI, abdomen
	Ultrasound, abdomen
Cancer, testicular	Ultrasound, testis
	Alpha fetoprotein, serum
	Beta human chorionic gonadotropin
	Chest x-ray
	CT, abdomen, pelvis
Cancer, thyroid	Calcitonin, serum or plasma
	Fine needle biopsy, thyroid
Cholecystitis/cholelithiasis	Ultrasound, gall bladder
	Liver-gall bladder radionuclide scan
	CT scan, abdomen
	MRI, cholangiography
	Oral cholecystography
	ERC
	PTC
Chronic obstructive lung (pulmonary) disease (COPD)	Arterial blood gas
	Electrocardiogram
	Complete blood count

Continued

Clinical Guides to Diagnosis—*cont'd*	
Common Medical Diagnoses	**Common Tests Used**
Chronic obstructive lung (pulmonary) disease (COPD)—*cont'd*	Culture, sputum Pulmonary function studies X-ray, chest
Cirrhosis, liver	Alanine aminotransferase Aspartate aminotransferase Protein, total, serum Albumin, serum Prothrombin time Sodium, serum Bilirubin, total, direct, indirect, serum Liver biopsy Liver-spleen scan Paracentesis, with peritoneal fluid analysis Ultrasound, liver CT, abdomen
Colitis, ulcerative	Occult blood, feces CBC Total serum protein Albumin, serum Sigmoidoscopy, with biopsy and cytology studies Barium enema Colonoscopy
Coronary artery disease (CAD)	Cardiac catheterization Cardiac markers Electrocardiogram Stress testing, cardiac
Coronary artery disease, risk for	Cholesterol total, serum or plasma C-reactive protein Homocysteine, plasma Lipids, serum
Crohn's disease	Barium enema Upper gastrointestinal series with small bowel series CBC Protein, total, serum Occult blood, feces
Cushing syndrome	Cortisol, free, urine Cortisol, serum or plasma Metyrapone test MRI, head Potassium, urine

Clinical Guides to Diagnosis—*cont'd*	
Common Medical Diagnoses	**Common Tests Used**
Cystic fibrosis	Chloride sweat test Cystic fibrosis DNA amplification Fat, fecal Chest x-ray Pulmonary function tests In pregnancy: Amniocentesis with amniotic fluid analysis and chromosomal analysis
Deep vein thrombosis. *See* Thrombophlebitis.	
Dehydration	Electrolyte panel, serum Sodium, serum, urine Urea nitrogen, serum Creatinine, serum Urinalysis Specific gravity, urine Osmolality, serum, urine CBC Hemoglobin Hematocrit
Diabetes insipidus	Albumin, serum Antidiuretic hormone, plasma Electrolytes, serum Fluid deprivation test MRI, pituitary and hypothalamus Osmolality, serum Osmolality, urine Specific gravity, urine
Diabetes mellitus	Anion gap Electrolytes, serum Glucose, fasting, whole blood Glycosylated hemoglobin assay Ketone bodies, blood Ketones, urine Osmolality, plasma
Disseminated intravascular coagulation (DIC)	Disseminated intravascular screen, serum D-dimer and fibrin split products Fibrinogen Partial thromboplastin time Prothrombin time CBC Platelet count Red blood cell morphology, peripheral blood

Continued

Clinical Guides to Diagnosis—*cont'd*

Common Medical Diagnoses	Common Tests Used
Fetal maturity	Fetal fibronectin, cervicovaginal secretions Amniocentesis with amniotic fluid analysis: Lecithin:sphingomyelin ratio Phosphatidylglycerol Pulmonary surfactant
Gastritis	*Helicobacter pylori* antibody, serum *Helicobacter pylori* antigen, serum EGD with biopsy for cytology
Gastroesophageal reflux disease (GERD)	Barium swallow Esophagoscopy, with esophageal biopsy and cytologic examination Esophageal manometry pH monitoring Bernstein acid perfusion test
Gonorrhea	Genital culture, *Neisseria gonorrhoeae* *Neisseria gonorrhoeae*-RNA detection, secretions Throat culture, *Neisseria gonorrhoeae* Rectal culture, *Neisseria gonorrhoeae*
Gout	Uric acid, serum, urine Urinalysis Arthrocentesis, with synovial fluid analysis
Heart failure (previously called congestive heart failure)	Albumin, serum Complete blood count Creatinine, serum or plasma Echocardiogram Electrolytes, serum Electrolytes, urine Thyroid stimulating hormone X-ray, chest
Hepatitis	Alanine aminotransferase Aspartate aminotransferase Bilirubin, total, direct, indirect, serum Hepatitis A antibody Hepatitis B, core antibody Hepatitis B DNA detection Hepatitis B surface antibody Hepatitis C virus serology Liver biopsy with cytology examination
Histoplasmosis infection	CBC Peripheral blood smear Fungal culture, blood, sputum, bronchial lavage, cerebrospinal fluid, urine

Clinical Guides to Diagnosis—*cont'd*

Common Medical Diagnoses	Common Tests Used
Histoplasmosis infection—*cont'd*	Cytology examination, oral ulcers or sores
	Bronchoscopy with transbronchial biopsy, fine needle aspiration and cytology studies
HIV infection. *See* Acquired Immune Deficiency Syndrome (AIDS).	
Hodgkin's disease	CBC
	Lymph node biopsy
	Liver biopsy
	Bone marrow biopsy
	CT scan, thorax, abdomen, pelvis
Hyperosmolar coma (HHNK)	Anion gap
	Arterial blood gases
	Electrolytes, serum
	Glucose, fasting, plasma
	Ketones, serum
	Ketones, urine
	Osmolality, serum
	Osmolality, urine
Hyperparathyroidism	Calcium, serum
	Calcium ionized, serum
	Calcium urine
	Parathyroid hormone, serum
	Phosphorus, serum
	Vitamin D, serum or plasma
Hypertension	Creatinine, serum or plasma
	Protein, urine
	Renal biopsy
	Renin, plasma
	Urea nitrogen, serum or plasma
	Sodium, serum or plasma
	Urinalysis
Hyperthyroidism	CT scan, thyroid
	MRI, thyroid
	Radionuclide scan (^{131}I, ^{123}I)
	Thyroid antibodies
	Thyroid stimulating hormone
	Thyroxine, free, serum
	Thyroxine, total, serum
	Triiodothyronine, serum

Continued

Clinical Guides to Diagnosis—*cont'd*	
Common Medical Diagnoses	**Common Tests Used**
Hypoparathyroidism	Calcium, ionized, serum
	Calcium, serum
	Calcium, urine
	Parathyroid hormone, serum
	Phosphorus, plasma
Hypopituitarism	Adrenocorticotropic hormone
	Cortisol, serum or plasma
	CT scan, head
	Follicle stimulating hormone
	Luteinizing hormone
	Metyrapone stimulation test
	MRI, head
	Thyroid stimulating hormone
Hypothyroidism	Cholesterol, serum or plasma
	Thyroid stimulating hormone
	Thyroid antibodies
	Thyroxine, free, serum
	Thyroxine, total, serum
	Triiodothyronine, serum
	Ultrasound of the thyroid
Kidney stones	Calcium, serum
	CT scan, kidneys
	Intravenous pyelogram
	Kidney stone analysis
	Phosphorus, serum
	pH, urine
	Retrograde pyelogram
	Ultrasound, renal
	Uric acid, serum
	Uric acid, urine
	Urinalysis
Leukemia	CBC
	White blood count
	White blood cell differential count, peripheral blood
	Platelet count
	Bone marrow aspiration and biopsy
	Chromosome analysis, bone marrow
Lyme disease	Lyme disease antibody
	Lyme disease-DNA detection
	Biopsy of lesion, with bacterial culture for *Borrelia burgdorferi*
	Arthrocentesis, with synovial fluid analysis and culture

Clinical Guides to Diagnosis—*cont'd*	
Common Medical Diagnoses	**Common Tests Used**
Lymphoma	CBC WBC differential, peripheral blood Biopsy, bone marrow Biopsy, lymph node(s) Lumbar puncture, with cerebral fluid analysis: chemistry analysis, protein electrophoresis, cytology
Melanoma	Biopsy, lesion or tumor, with microscopic pathology and chromosome analysis Biopsy, lymph node(s)
Meningitis	CT scan, brain Lumbar puncture, with cerebral fluid analysis Cerebrospinal fluid culture, fungal, bacterial Culture: blood, nasopharyngeal, sputum, urine, skin lesion
Multiple myeloma	CBC Erythrocyte sedimentation rate Urinalysis Protein electrophoresis, serum: immunoglobulins A, D, E, G, M Protein, total, serum Protein electrophoresis, urine Biopsy and aspiration, bone marrow X-rays, bones MRI, bones
Multiple sclerosis	MRI Lumbar puncture, with cerebrospinal fluid analysis Electroencephalogram
Myocardial infarction, acute	Cardiac markers Echocardiogram Electrocardiogram Thallium scan Erythrocyte sedimentation rate
Myocarditis	Culture, bacterial, blood Erythrocyte sedimentation rate Fine needle biopsy, myocardium White blood cell count
Nephrosis	Albumin, serum Antinuclear antibody Cholesterol, serum or plasma Complement components

Continued

Clinical Guides to Diagnosis—*cont'd*	
Common Medical Diagnoses	**Common Tests Used**
Nephrosis—*cont'd*	Creatinine clearance
	Glucose, plasma
	Glycosylated hemoglobin
	Osmolality, urine
	Protein electrophoresis, serum
	Protein, serum
	Protein, urine
	Urinalysis
Osteoporosis	Bone density scan (DXA, CT)
	Calcium, serum, urine
	Parathyroid hormone, serum
	X-ray, bone
Pancreatitis	Amylase, serum, urine
	Lipase, serum
	CBC
	White blood count
	Hematocrit
	Calcium, serum
	Glucose, plasma
	Urea nitrogen, serum
	Triglycerides, serum
	X-ray, abdomen
	CT, pancreas
Peptic ulcer	*Helicobacter pylori* antigen, serum
	Helicobacter pylori antibody, serum
	Occult blood, feces
	EGD, with biopsy
	Ulcer biopsy: urease test, culture, cytology, DNA identification
	Upper gastrointestinal series
Peripheral arterial occlusive disease	Duplex Doppler ultrasound
	Arterial plethysmography
	MR angiography, extremity
	Arteriography
Peritonitis, acute	Laparotomy, diagnostic
	Peritoneal aspiration and bacterial culture
	Peritoneal fluid analysis and cytology
	X-ray, abdomen
Pheochromocytoma	Catecholamines, plasma
	Catecholamines, urine
	Clonidine suppression test

Clinical Guides to Diagnosis—*cont'd*

Common Medical Diagnoses	Common Tests Used
Pheochromocytoma—*cont'd*	CT scan, chest and/or abdomen
	Cytology
	Glucagon stimulation test
	Metanephrines, urine or plasma
	MRI, chest and abdomen
	Vanillylmandelic acid, urine
	X-ray, chest and abdomen
Pneumonia	Complete blood count
	Culture, bacterial
	Abscess
	Biopsy
	Blood
	Sputum
	Culture, influenza viral
	Culture, viral
	Gram stain, sputum
	Sputum cytology
	X-ray, chest
Preeclampsia	CBC
	Urea nitrogen, serum
	Urinalysis
	Creatinine clearance, urine
	Albumin, serum, urine
	Protein, urine
	Electrolytes, serum
	Prothrombin time
	Partial thromboplastin time
	Alanine aminotransferase
	Aspartate aminotransferase
Prostatitis	Bacterial culture, urine and/or prostatic secretions
	Biopsy, prostate (transurethral)
	Culture, urine
	Prostate specific antigen
	Urinalysis
Renal failure (ESRD)	Albumin, serum
	Anion gap
	Biopsy, renal
	Calcium, serum
	Creatinine clearance
	Creatinine, serum or plasma
	Electrolytes, serum

Continued

Clinical Guides to Diagnosis—*cont'd*

Common Medical Diagnoses	Common Tests Used
Renal failure (ESRD)—*cont'd*	Erythropoietin, serum
	Osmolality, urine
	Protein, urine
	Sodium, urine
	Specific gravity, urine
	Ultrasound, kidney
	Urea nitrogen, serum or plasma
	Urea nitrogen-creatinine ratio
	Urinalysis
Rheumatic fever	CBC
	White blood count
	C-reactive protein, serum
	Culture, oropharyngeal (throat)
	Group A-beta hemolytic streptococcus screen, throat secretions
	Erythrocyte sedimentation rate
	Streptozyme, serum
	Electrocardiogram
	Antistreptolysin O antibody titer, serum
Sarcoidosis	CBC
	White blood count
	Calcium, serum
	Angiotensin converting enzyme, serum
	Alkaline phosphatase, serum
	Biopsy: liver, lymph node, or skin
	Fiberoptic bronchoscopy, with transbronchial fine needle biopsy or aspiration
	X-ray, chest
	Pulmonary function tests
Seizure	Electroencephalogram
	Glucose, plasma
	Sodium, serum
	Magnesium, serum
	Calcium, serum
	Osmolality, serum
	Toxicology, screen, urine
	MRI, brain
	Lumbar puncture, with cerebrospinal fluid culture: bacterial, viral
Severe acute respiratory syndrome (SARS)	SARS antibody titers, serum
	SARS PCR-RNA detection, blood, feces, sputum

Clinical Guides to Diagnosis—*cont'd*	
Common Medical Diagnoses	**Common Tests Used**
Severe acute respiratory syndrome (SARS)—*cont'd*	Nasopharyngeal swab, SARS PCR-viral RNA detection
	Oropharyngeal swab, SARS PCR-viral RNA detection
	Bronchoscopy, with bronchoalveolar lavage, tracheal aspirate: SARS PCR-viral RNA detection
	Thoracentesis, with plural fluid aspirate: SARS PCR-viral RNA detection
Syndrome of inappropriate secretion of antidiuretic hormone	Antidiuretic hormone, plasma
	Electrolytes, serum
	Osmolality, serum
	Osmolality, urine
	Sodium, urine
	Specific gravity, urine
	Urea nitrogen, serum or plasma
	Uric acid, serum
Syphilis	Darkfield examination, syphilis
	FTA-ABS, serum
	MHA-TP, serum
	VDRL, serum, cerebrospinal fluid
	Biopsy, skin lesion, lymph node
Systemic lupus erythematosus	CBC
	White blood cell count, blood
	White blood cell differential, peripheral blood
	Urinalysis
	Anti DNA
	Antinuclear antibody
	Complement, total, serum
	Complement C_3, serum
	Complement C_4, serum
	Antiphospholipid antibody, serum
	Smith (SM) and ribonucleoprotein (RNP) antibodies
	Creatinine, serum
	Creatinine clearance, urine
	Protein, urine
	Biopsy, kidney
Thalassemia	CBC
	Fetal hemoglobin, blood
	Hemoglobin electrophoresis

Continued

Clinical Guides to Diagnosis—*cont'd*

Common Medical Diagnoses	Common Tests Used
Thrombophlebitis	Duplex ultrasound, vein Venography Plethysmography, venous Hypercoagulation panel: Protein C, protein S, serum
Toxoplasmosis	*Toxoplasma gondii* antibodies (IgM, IgG), serum Biopsy, lymph node, with tissue culture PCR amplification-DNA, blood, amniotic fluid Bronchoscopy, with bronchoalveolar lavage, culture Lumbar puncture, with cerebrospinal fluid cytology
Tuberculosis, pulmonary	Acid-base stain, sputum Culture, sputum Bronchoscopy, fiberoptic Transbronchial biopsy/washing X-ray, chest
Urinary tract infection	Bacterial culture, urine Gram stain, urine Intravenous pyelogram (for recurrent infections) Urinalysis
Valvular heart disease	Cardiac catheterization Echocardiogram Transthoracic Transesophageal Electrocardiogram X-ray, chest
Wilson's disease	Ceruloplasmin, serum Cooper, serum, urine Liver biopsy Alanine aminotransferase Alkaline phosphatase Aspartate aminotransferase Bilirubin, total, serum

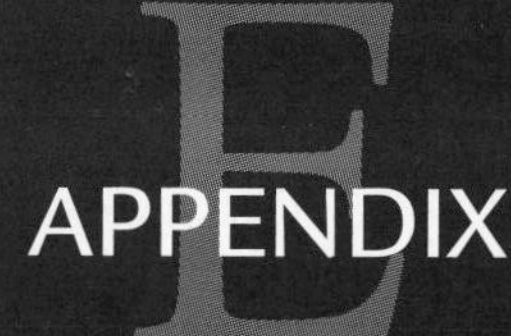

APPENDIX E

Tests by Body System with Test Purpose

Name of Test	Page	Primary Purposes
CARDIAC FUNCTION		
Biopsy, Endomyocardial	132	Determine rejection in a transplanted heart; diagnose cardiomyopathy; determine cause of restrictive heart disease
Cardiac Markers	178	Help diagnose acute myocardial infarction
Catheterization, Cardiac	187	Evaluate coronary artery disease, with unstable, progressive, or new-onset angina, or angina that is not responsive to medical therapy; diagnose atypical chest pain; diagnose complications from myocardial infarction, evaluate need for coronary artery surgery or angioplasty; diagnose aortic dissection; assess valvular function; determine the efficacy of a heart transplant
Echocardiogram	281	Evaluate abnormal heart sounds, heart size, chamber size; identify valvular function, tumor, pericardial effusion, and wall motion abnormality
Electrocardiogram	283	Diagnose myocardial infarction, injury, or ischemia; assist in identification of cardiac hypertrophy, axis deviation, and

Continued

Name of Test	Page	Primary Purposes
CARDIAC FUNCTION—*cont'd*		
Electrocardiogram—*cont'd*		electrolyte abnormalities; distinguish between left and right ventricular hypertrophy and between ventricular and supraventricular tachycardia
Electrocardiogram, Signal-Averaged	289	Detect conduction defects that may precede ventricular tachycardia
Electrophysiologic Studies, Cardiac	300	Identify cardiac dysrhythmia and conduction abnormality; guide appropriate medication therapy and evaluate the response to the medication
Ergonovine Provocation Test	309	Diagnose atypical angina when coronary artery spasm is suspected
Gated Blood Pool Studies	341	Assess ventricular function of the heart by evaluating wall motion and determining ejection fraction
Holter Monitoring	393	Detect cardiac dysrhythmia; help identify conduction defects; monitor cardiac response to therapy and daily activities
Homocysteine	395	Identify risk for heart attack or stroke
Lipid Profile	431	Identify the individual who is at risk for coronary heart disease; evaluate the effectiveness of "heart healthy" changes in lifestyle; health promotion screening test to identify coronary artery risk factors
Pericardiocentesis	512	Determine the cause and appropriate therapy for acute or subacute pericarditis, neoplastic pericardial disease, and pericardial effusion
Stress Testing, Cardiac	596	Assess the at-risk population; diagnose chest pain syndromes associated with ischemia; evaluate effectiveness of surgical or pharmacologic therapy; assess the patient's cardiac function before and after a cardiac rehabilitation program
Thallium Scan	604	Assess coronary artery blood flow; locate areas of infarction or ischemia; diagnose coronary artery disease; evaluate revascularization after coronary artery bypass surgery

Name of Test	Page	Primary Purposes
CARDIAC FUNCTION—*cont'd*		
Transesophageal Echocardiography	623	Diagnose thoracic aortic pathology, mitral valve disease, suspected endocarditis, congenital heart disease, intracardiac thrombus and cardiac tumor; assess cardiac function during minimally invasive cardiac surgery; assess prosthetic valves
Vectorcardiogram	667	Assess ischemia; conduction defect and cardiac hypertrophy or dilation
ENDOCRINE FUNCTION		
Adrenocorticotropic Hormone, Plasma	46	Diagnosis of Cushing's disease; differentiation of primary and secondary adrenal insufficiency
Adrenocorticotropic Hormone Stimulation	49	Diagnosis of primary or secondary adrenal insufficiency
Aldosterone, Serum	54	Used in workup for hypertension and diagnosis of aldosteronism
Aldosterone, Urinary	57	Help identify primary aldosteronism caused by adrenal adenoma
Biopsy, Thyroid	149	Identify and differentiate the cause of one or more thyroid nodules or lumps; diagnose benign lesion, follicular neoplasm, or malignant thyroid nodule
Calcitonin	162	Diagnose medullary carcinoma of the thyroid gland
Catecholamines, Plasma	183	Diagnose pheochromocytoma; identify extra-adrenal tumor
Catecholamines, Urinary	185	Diagnose pheochromocytoma; helps to identify the cause of hypertension
Cortisol, Total	239	Diagnose Cushing syndrome, Cushing's disease, and primary (Addison's disease) or secondary adrenal insufficiency
Dexamethasone Suppression Test	276	Assess the hypothalamic-pituitary-adrenal axis; identify Cushing's disease
Free Cortisol	331	Determine excessive production of glucocorticoids by the adrenal cortex
Free Thyroxine	332	Diagnose hyperthyroidism and hypothyroidism
Free Triiodothyronine	334	Diagnose hyperthyroidism and hypothyroidism

Continued

Name of Test	Page	Primary Purposes
ENDOCRINE FUNCTION—*cont'd*		
Glucagon	345	Assist with diagnosis of pancreatic tumor, chronic pancreatitis, and familial hyperglucagonemia
Glucose, Capillary	346	To assess and manage diabetes mellitus or other causes of hyperglycemia
Glucose, Fasting	350	Diagnose and manage diabetes mellitus; provide supportive data for many other disorders that influence glucose storage and use
Glucose, Postprandial	353	Support the diagnosis of diabetes mellitus; evaluate the management of diabetes mellitus
Glucose Tolerance Test	356	Confirm the diagnosis of diabetes mellitus
Glucose, Urinary	358	Determine insulin and dietary requirements when glucose monitoring is not possible
Glycosylated Hemoglobin Assay	360	Measure the patient's diabetic control over a period of weeks or months
Growth Hormone	362	Diagnose growth disorder and possible pituitary tumor
Growth Hormone Stimulation Test	364	Evaluate infants and children with retarded growth; support diagnosis of pituitary tumor
Growth Hormone Suppression Test	365	Assess an increase in growth hormone; confirm a diagnosis of giantism in the child or acromegaly in the adult
17-Hydroxycorticosteroids	401	Assess adrenal insufficiency
Insulin	405	Assess for insulin-producing tumors; confirm insulin-resistant states; help evaluate glucocorticoid insufficiency
Ketone Bodies, Blood	418	Determine the insulin requirements in patients with diabetes mellitus who have hyperglycemia
Ketones, Urinary	419	Evaluate the patient with diabetes mellitus and adjust insulin requirements; adjust insulin requirements in treatment of diabetes mellitus; diagnose carbohydrate deprivation; monitor patients on low carbohydrate diets
Long-Acting Thyroid Stimulator	434	Support the diagnosis of Graves' disease

Name of Test	Page	Primary Purposes
ENDOCRINE FUNCTION—*cont'd*		
Magnetic Resonance Imaging, Pituitary Gland	451	Identify hypothalamic-pituitary tumor, aneurysm, infarction, and vascular malformation
Metyrapone Stimulation Test	462	Diagnose secondary adrenal insufficiency; assess pituitary-adrenal reserves
Osmolality, Plasma	488	Determine a person's fluid status; identify antidiuretic hormone abnormalities
Osmolality, Urine	490	Assess the renal ability to concentrate or dilute the urine; identify antidiuretic hormone abnormalities
Parathyroid Hormone	500	Diagnose suspected parathyroid disorder; investigate cause of calcium and phosphate abnormalities
Radioactive Iodine Uptake Study	562	Assess thyroid function; confirm hyper- or hypothyroidism
Radioactive Thyroid Scanning	564	Help confirm diagnosis of hyper- or hypothyroidism, thyroid cyst, or thyroid cancer
Renin	573	Diagnose primary aldosteronism; help with hypertension workup
Resin Triiodothyronine Uptake	575	Diagnose hyper- and hypothyroidism
Thyroglobin Autoantibodies	612	Diagnose autoimmune-based thyroid disease
Thyroid Stimulating Hormone	613	Diagnose hypothyroidism; distinguish between primary and secondary hypothyroidism; monitor thyroid replacement therapy Health promotion screening test to detect hypothyroidism in infants and women older than age 65
Thyrotropin-Releasing Hormone Test	615	Evaluate thyroid dysfunction
Thyroxine, Total	616	Evaluate thyroid function; confirm diagnosis of hyper- or hypothyroidism; evaluate response to treatment of hyper- or hypothyroidism
Thyroxine-Binding Globulin	618	Help evaluate thyroid dysfunction
Tolbutamide Stimulation Test	619	Identify insulin-producing tumors of the pancreas
Triiodothyronine	626	Help diagnose hyper- or hypothyroidism; diagnose triiodothyronine toxicosis

Continued

Name of Test	Page	Primary Purposes
ENDOCRINE FUNCTION—*cont'd*		
Vasopressin	665	Diagnose diabetes insipidus and syndrome of inappropriate antidiuretic hormone
Vitamin D, Activated	671	Investigate the cause of hypocalcemia
Water Deprivation Test	672	Diagnose diabetes insipidus; investigate renal ability to concentrate the urine
Water-Loading Test	674	Diagnose syndrome of inappropriate secretion of antidiuretic hormone
GASTROINTESTINAL FUNCTION		
Barium Enema	114	Investigate and identify changes in the structure or function of the colon; health promotion screening test for cancer of the colon
Barium Swallow	118	Identify abnormalities of structure or function of the esophagus
Colonoscopy	214	Detect polyps and tumors of the colon; investigate the cause of chronic diarrhea, occult blood in the feces, or an abnormal result of a sigmoidoscopy or barium enema; health promotion screening tool to detect cancer of the colon
d-Xylose Absorption	279	Investigate the cause of steatorrhea; diagnose malabsorption; evaluate the ability of the duodenum and jejunum to digest carbohydrates
Esophageal Function Tests	314	*Esophageal manometry:* Investigate dysphagia; evaluate esophageal motor disorders; evaluate pre- and postoperative surgery that improves motility and prevents reflux *Esophageal pH:* Document esophageal reflux disease (GERD) *Acid perfusion test:* Investigate cause of heartburn pain
Esophagogastro-duodenoscopy	317	Identify and biopsy abnormal tissue; determine location of gastrointestinal bleeding; evaluate healing of gastric ulcers; investigate cause of dysphagia, dyspepsia, epigastric pain, or gastric outlet obstruction
Gastric Analysis	336	Assist in the diagnosis of Zollinger-Ellison syndrome and other conditions that produce hypersecretion of gastric acid

Name of Test	Page	Primary Purposes
GASTROINTESTINAL FUNCTION—*cont'd*		
Gastrin	338	Assist in the diagnosis of Zollinger-Ellison syndrome and pernicious anemia
Gastrointestinal Cytology Studies	339	Differentiate benign from malignant tissue of the esophagus, stomach, or colon
Lactose Tolerance Test	422	Identify lactose intolerance; investigate cause of malabsorption
Occult Blood, Feces	484	Detect small amounts of blood in the gastrointestinal tract; health promotion screening test for early detection of bowel cancer
Ova and Parasites, Feces	491	Identify specific parasites in the gastrointestinal system
Parietal Cell Antibody	502	Assist in diagnosis of pernicious anemia and atrophic gastritis
Sigmoidoscopy and Anoscopy	585	*Sigmoidoscopy:* Investigate the source of bleeding or infection of the lower colon; evaluate postoperative anastomosis of the lower colon; diagnose or monitor inflammatory bowel disease; health promotion screening test for cancer of the colon *Anoscopy:* Investigate anal symptoms, such as bleeding, pain, or prolapse
Upper Gastrointestinal Series and Small Bowel Series	640	*Upper GI series:* Detect disorders of structure or function of esophagus, stomach, and duodenum; evaluate postoperative repair of stomach *Small bowel series:* Detect disorders of the jejunum and ileum
HEMATOLOGIC FUNCTION		
Activated Clotting Time	44	Measure anticoagulation effect during administration of high doses of heparin
Antiglobulin Tests	95	*Direct antiglobulin:* Detect post-transfusion incompatibility of red blood cells of donor and recipient; help in diagnosis of erythroblastosis fetalis or hemolytic disease of the newborn; help confirm the diagnosis of hemolytic anemia *Indirect antiglobulin:* Antibody screen in type and crossmatch testing for blood transfusion; detect maternal-fetal incompatibility and predict risk to the fetus; help confirm diagnosis of hemolytic anemia

Continued

Name of Test	Page	Primary Purposes
HEMATOLOGIC FUNCTION—*cont'd*		
Biopsy, Bone Marrow	127	Evaluate hematopoiesis; diagnose malignancy of the bone marrow, evaluate progression of some hematologic anemias; evaluate bone marrow response to chemotherapy
Bleeding Time	151	Screen for platelet malfunction or vascular defect that interferes with clotting
Coagulation Inhibitors	209	Investigate antithrombin, protein C, and protein S as the cause of recurrent thrombus formation
Cobalamin	212	Identify vitamin B_{12} deficiency; investigate neurologic and hematologic symptoms that suggest cobalamin deficiency
Complement, Total	221	Evaluate or monitor systemic lupus erythematosus and response to treatment; detect autoimmune disease; diagnose complement deficiency
Complete Blood Count	222	Assess for anemia, infection, inflammation, polycythemia, hemolytic disease, hemolysis of ABO incompatibility, leukemia, dehydration; identify the cellular characteristics of the peripheral blood
D-dimer and Fibrin Degradation Products	274	Screening test for deep vein thrombosis; help to diagnose disseminated intravascular coagulation (DIC) and myocardial infarction; investigate hypercoagulable conditions that cause recurrent thrombus
Fibrinogen	325	Help diagnose bleeding disorders
Folic Acid, Serum	329	Detect folic acid deficiency; monitor folic acid replacement therapy; investigate megaloblastic anemia
Glucose-6-Phosphate Dehydrogenase (G-6-PD) Screen	355	Detect G-6-PD defect in erythrocytes; identify G-6-PD as cause of hemolytic anemia
Haptoglobin	367	Monitor conditions that cause hemolysis of erythrocytes
Hematocrit	371	Evaluate blood loss, anemia, hemolytic anemia, polycythemia, and dehydration
Hemoglobin	374	Measure the severity of anemia and polycythemia; monitor the response to treatment

Name of Test	Page	Primary Purposes
HEMATOLOGIC FUNCTION—*cont'd*		
Hemoglobin Electrophoresis	377	Detect genetic disorders of hemoglobin; identify the type of anemia caused by abnormal hemoglobin; differentiate between sickle cell anemia and sickle cell trait
Hemosiderin, Urinary	380	Identify hemolytic anemia associated with hemolysis of erythrocytes
Human Leukocyte Antigen	399	In organ transplantation, determine tissue compatibility between donor and recipient
International Normalized Ratio (INR)	407	Monitor the effect of oral anticoagulant therapy and adjust the medication according to the results; see Prothrombin Time, p. 555
Intrinsic Factor Antibodies	410	Differentiate between pernicious anemia and other causes of megaloblastic anemia; help determine the cause of cobalamin deficiency
Iron Studies	411	Measure serum iron, transferrin, total iron-binding capacity, transferrin saturation, and ferritin; estimate total iron storage; provide information about nutritional status; help distinguish between iron deficiency anemia and anemia of chronic disease; identify iron overload and hematochromatosis
Leukocyte Alkaline Phosphatase	428	Help differentiate chronic myelogenous leukemia from leukemoid reactions and other myeloproliferative disorders; help evaluate Hodgkin's disease and its response to therapy
Partial Thromboplastin Time (aPTT, PTT)	503	Identify bleeding or clotting disorder; monitor the effect of heparin anticoagulant therapy with adjustment of medication according to the test result
Platelet Aggregation	521	Evaluate platelet function; detect platelet bleeding disorder
Platelet Count	523	Assess bone marrow ability to produce platelets; help identify a decrease in platelets in blood; evaluate untoward effects of chemotherapy or radiation

Continued

Name of Test	Page	Primary Purposes
HEMATOLOGIC FUNCTION—*cont'd*		
Prothrombin Time	555	Evaluate extrinsic coagulation system; help screen for coagulation deficiency; investigate the effects of liver failure and disseminated intravascular coagulation (DIC); screen for vitamin K deficiency
Red Blood Cell Count	566	Evaluate anemia and polycythemia; monitor health problem that causes an altered number of erythrocytes
Red Blood Cell Morphology	568	Help identify cause of anemia; evaluate the function of the bone marrow
Reticulocyte Count	576	Evaluate erythropoiesis; distinguish among different types of anemia; assess severity of blood loss; evaluate bone marrow response to treatment of anemia
Sickle Cell Tests	583	Evaluate hemolytic anemia; help identify the cause of hereditary anemia; screening test to detect hemoglobin S, the sickling hemoglobin
Type and Crossmatch	627	Determine major blood groups; screen for antibodies; determine compatibility of donor blood with blood of proposed recipient of a transfusion
LIVER, BILIARY, AND PANCREATIC FUNCTION		
Alanine Aminotransferase		Detect hepatocellular injury; detect hepatitis
Alkaline Phosphatase	58	Nonspecific indicator of liver or bone disease, or hypoparathyroidism; tumor marker for malignancy of the liver or bone
Amylase, Serum	71	Help diagnose acute pancreatitis; investigate the cause of epigastric pain, with nausea and vomiting
Amylase, Urinary	73	Diagnose acute and relapsing pancreatitis
Aspartate Aminotransferase	111	Detect injury or inflammation of the liver
Bilirubin, Serum	121	*Total bilirubin:* Evaluate liver function; diagnose and monitor the progression of jaundice *Direct and indirect bilirubin:* Identify the underlying cause of elevated bilirubin levels
Carbohydrate Antigen 19-9	172	Tumor marker used to help stage cancer of the pancreas; monitor the course of pancreatic cancer and response to treatment; predict recurrence of pancreatic cancer

Name of Test	Page	Primary Purposes
LIVER, BILIARY, AND PANCREATIC FUNCTION—*cont'd*		
Ceruloplasmin	192	Evaluate chronic, active hepatitis, cirrhosis, and other liver disorders; helps diagnose Wilson's disease
Cholangiography, Percutaneous, Transhepatic	199	Diagnose the cause of obstructive jaundice; promote visualization of intrahepatic ducts and biliary ducts; evaluate location and changes in the biliary tree that cause obstruction
Cholecystography, Oral	202	Visualize the gall bladder and ducts to identify stones and other causes of obstruction; evaluate the gall bladder's ability to store and excrete bile
Endoscopic Retrograde Cholangiopan-creatography (ERCP) and Pancreatic Endoscopy, with Cytology	303	Investigate the cause of obstructive jaundice and persistent abdominal pain associated with pancreatic and biliary disorder; diagnose a bile stone in the common duct, chronic pancreatitis, and cancer
Fecal Fat	323	Identify steatorrhea; investigate the inability to digest fat, as in hepatobiliary, pancreatic, or intestinal disease
Gamma-glutamyl-transferase	335	Detect hepatobiliary disease
Hepatitis Tests (See Microbiologic tests for specific hepatitis tests)	381 to 391	Diagnose hepatitis; the type of virus, the stage of the disease, and the course of recovery
Lipase	430	Diagnose acute pancreatitis; identify pancreatic disease due to other diseases
5′-Nucleotidase	483	Help identify hepatobiliary diseases
Paracentesis and Peritoneal Fluid Analysis	497	Assist in the investigation of ascites; determine the effect of blunt abdominal trauma; help investigate the cause of an acute abdomen
Protein Electrophoresis, Serum	545	Detect hepatobiliary disease; detect monoclonal gammopathy; evaluate nutritional status
Protein Electrophoresis, Urinary	548	Identify different types of protein loss in urine; evaluate known or suspected multiple myeloma

Continued

Name of Test	Page	Primary Purposes
LIVER, BILIARY, AND PANCREATIC FUNCTION—*cont'd*		
Protein, Total, Serum	549	Help investigate the severity of diseases of the liver, bone marrow, and kidneys; investigate the cause of edema; evaluate nutritional status
Sweat Test	599	Diagnose cystic fibrosis
Ultrasound, Pancreatic	639	Help diagnose pancreatitis and pancreatic tumor, cyst, or pseudocyst; monitor progression of pancreatitis; guide needle placement in pancreatic biopsy
Urobilinogen, Urinary	659	Help confirm diagnosis of liver disease; detect hemolytic anemia
MUSCULOSKELETAL FUNCTION		
Anti-DNA	93	Confirm diagnosis of lupus erythematosus; monitor response to medication therapy for this disease
Antinuclear Antibody	97	Screen to detect systematic rheumatic diseases and lupus erythematosus; monitor response of lupus erythematosus to medication therapy
Arthrocentesis with Synovial Fluid Analysis	106	Help in diagnosis of rheumatic diseases, infection of joint, or other diseases that cause swelling of the joint with fluid
Arthroscopy	109	Detect damage or injury to tissues within the joint
Biopsy, Bone	124	Identify cell type of bone tissue; distinguish benign from malignant bone tissue
Bone Mineral Density	153	Measure the density of bones; diagnose osteopenia or osteoporosis; measure bone response to treatment with medication; health promotion screening test for osteoporosis
Bone Scan	155	Assess physiologic function of bone; assist in location and diagnosis of bone abnormality
C-Reactive Protein	241	Indicate inflammation or infection; monitor response to antibiotic or anti-inflammatory medication; possible marker of cardiovascular disease
Erythrocyte Sedimentation Rate	310	Identify or monitor disease activity in inflammatory or infectious conditions

Name of Test	Page	Primary Purposes
MUSCULOSKELETAL FUNCTION—*cont'd*		
Myoglobin, Urine	471	Identify myoglobinuria; investigate the cause of damaged muscle tissue
Rheumatoid Factor	578	Help with diagnosis and prognosis of rheumatoid factor
Uric Acid	645	Confirm diagnosis of gout; help investigate impairment of renal function
NEUROLOGICAL FUNCTION		
Angiography, Cerebral	75	Identify abnormalities of the arteries and blood flow to the neck and brain
Electroencephalography	290	Diagnose epilepsy and determine the type of epilepsy; help diagnose metabolic encephalography and brain injury
Electromyography and Nerve Conduction Studies	297	Investigate cause of muscle weakness or paralysis; distinguish nerve involvement from muscle disorder; identify muscle group or nerve involvement; evaluate severity of the problem
Lumbar Puncture and Cerebrospinal Fluid (CSF) Analysis	435	Detect and measure increased intracranial pressure; detect bleeding; detect blockage in the circulation of cerebrospinal fluid; diagnose or confirm inflammatory, autoimmune, or infectious disease of the brain
Myelography	468	Identify obstruction or abnormality that impinges on the spinal cord or its nerve roots
Single Photon Emission Computed Tomography (SPECT) Scan, Brain	588	Investigate, diagnose, or evaluate cerebrovascular diseases, dementia, epilepsy, and head trauma
PULMONARY FUNCTION		
Angiography, Pulmonary	81	Confirm diagnosis of pulmonary embolus; diagnose congenital or acquired abnormalities of the pulmonary vasculature
Angiotensin-Converting Enzyme	90	Evaluate possible cause of hypertension; diagnose sarcoidosis, assess its severity, and evaluate the response to treatment
Anion Gap	92	Determine the cause of metabolic acidosis

Continued

Name of Test	Page	Primary Purposes
PULMONARY FUNCTION—*cont'd*		
Arterial Blood gases	99	Provide information about acid-base balance, ventilatory ability, and oxygen status of the individual in many cardiovascular, pulmonary, and central nervous system disorders; use in management of patient on a mechanical ventilator and in the weaning process from the ventilator
Biopsy, Lung, Open	137	Diagnose pulmonary disorders, such as cancer or sarcoidosis of the lung; confirm diagnosis of fibrosis and degenerative or inflammatory disease of the lung
Biopsy, Lung, Percutaneous, Needle	138	Determine pathology of lung tissue, such as cancer, granuloma, infection, or sarcoidosis; stage the malignant tumor; diagnose cause of mediastinal mass
Bronchoscopy	159	Visualize tumor, obstruction, secretions, and foreign objects in the tracheobronchial tree; assess tumor for potential resection
Capnogram	170	Monitor alveolar ventilation; use in mechanical ventilation to evaluate ventilator changes and weaning parameters
Lactic Acid	420	Support diagnosis of cellular hypoxia; predict severity of illness and potential of survival
Lung Scans	443	Evaluate for decreased pulmonary function; V/Q scans diagnose pulmonary emboli
Mediastinoscopy	460	Determine metastasis of lung cancer into mediastinum; help stage the cancer and determine appropriate treatment; diagnose granulomatous, infectious, or other disease of the mediastinum
Mixed Venous Blood Gases	463	Assess the balance of oxygen supply and oxygen delivery
Pulmonary Function Studies	557	Evaluate respiratory status; evaluate treatment for or progression of obstructive or restrictive lung disease
Thoracentesis, Pleural Fluid Analysis, and Pleural Biopsy	606	Identify or confirm diagnosis of cancer, infection, or severe fluid overload, as in heart failure, liver failure, and systemic or pulmonary hypertension

Name of Test	Page	Primary Purposes
PULMONARY FUNCTION—*cont'd*		
Thoracoscopy	610	Identify causes of pleural thickening or recurrent effusion; diagnose cancer or infection
RENAL AND URINARY FUNCTION		
Albumin, Urinary	52	Assess renal function; differentiate renal disorders; determine effectiveness of therapy; screen for the renal complications associated with diabetes
Biopsy, Prostate	141	Determine cause of enlarged prostate gland; diagnosis of prostate cancer
Biopsy, Renal	143	Diagnose renal disorder, monitor progress of disease and evaluate response to treatment; assess for rejection of renal transplant
Calculus Analysis	166	Use in workup for nephrolithiasis; identify metabolic factors that cause kidney stones
Creatinine Clearance	243	Help assess renal function; assess creatinine excretion; monitor the progression of renal disease
Creatinine, Serum, Plasma	245	Evaluate renal function; estimate the effectiveness of glomerular filtration
Creatinine, Urine	247	Assess renal function
Cystoscopy	270	Diagnose and evaluate structural abnormality of the urinary bladder; identify tumors and source of bleeding
Electrolytes, 24-Hour Urine	293	Help monitor renal function, fluid and electrolyte balance, and acid-base balance; urinary calcium used to evaluate bone disease, parathyroid disorder, nephrolithiasis, and calcium metabolism
Erythropoietin	312	Investigate anemia in end-stage renal disease and cancer
Intravenous Pyelogram	408	Evaluate structure and function of the kidneys, ureters, and bladder; assess cause of nontraumatic hematuria; locate site of obstruction; investigate cause of renal colic

Continued

Name of Test	Page	Primary Purposes
RENAL AND URINARY FUNCTION—*cont'd*		
Prostate-Specific Antigen	541	A screening test to detect cancer of the prostate at an early stage; tumor marker for adenocarcinoma of the prostate; evaluate the postsurgical radical prostatectomy patient for recurrence or residual tumor; help identify the need for additional treatment
Prostatic Acid Phosphatase	543	Help with staging of metastatic adenocarcinoma of the prostate gland; after treatment of this malignancy, help evaluate for recurrence
Protein, Urine, 24-Hour	553	Help confirm renal disease
Specific Gravity, Urine	594	Measure the kidneys ability to concentrate or dilute the urine; assess renal function and hormone regulation of fluid balance
Urea Nitrogen, Blood	643	Evaluate renal function; help evaluate renal insufficiency or failure; help monitor patients receiving dialysis
Uric Acid, Urine	645	Support diagnosis of renal calculus; monitor patients who are at-risk to develop a renal calculus
Urinalysis	651	Screen for urinary tract disorder, kidney disorder, urinary neoplasm, and many other medical conditions that produce changes in the urine; monitor effect of treatment of known renal or urinary disease
Uroflowmetry	661	Evaluate urinary tract dysfunction of bladder incontinence or retention
REPRODUCTIVE FUNCTION		
Alpha-Fetoprotein	60	Help diagnose and evaluate treatment of primary cancer of the liver; help diagnose some testicular cancers and evaluate response to therapy; tumor marker for primary cancer of the liver and some testicular cancers *Pregnant patient:* Screening test helps detect neural tube defect of fetus; help detect Down syndrome in the fetus
Amniocentesis and Amniotic Fluid Analysis	65	Screening test for fetal abnormality; evaluate a problem pregnancy; assess fetal maturity or fetal distress

Name of Test	Page	Primary Purposes
REPRODUCTIVE FUNCTION—*cont'd*		
Biopsy, Breast	130	Differentiate benign from malignant tissue of the lesion or tumor of the breast
Cancer Antigen 125	168	Tumor marker for ovarian cancer; monitor the progression of ovarian cancer after surgical removal of the tumor; analyze body fluid for evidence of metastasis
Chorionic Gonadotropin, Human	204	*Blood and urine tests:* Detect pregnancy; help identify Down syndrome of the fetus *Blood test:* Help confirm the diagnosis of a germ cell or trophoblastic tumor; tumor marker to monitor the patient after surgical removal of tumor
Chorionic Villus Sampling and Genetic Abnormality Analysis	206	Diagnose genetic fetal abnormality
Colposcopy	219	Evaluation of an abnormal Papanicolaou smear; evaluate lesion of vagina or cervix; monitor for precancerous abnormality
Estriol, Unconjugated, Pregnancy	321	Evaluate fetal well-being and placental function in a high-risk pregnancy; help detect Down syndrome in the fetus
Fibronectin, Fetal	327	Determine the risk of a preterm delivery
Genetic Testing for Cystic Fibrosis	343	Screen for the genetic mutation of cystic fibrosis; identify carrier or disease status of cystic fibrosis; health promotion screening test for women early in their pregnancy
Hysterosalpingography	402	In infertility workup, assess patency of fallopian tubes; identify abnormal development of uterus; diagnose uterine fistula
Laparoscopy, Pelvic	424	Investigate cause of pelvic pain; detect endometriosis; detect ectopic pregnancy; identify pelvic mass; determine presence of cancer or metastasis
Mammography	456	Identify cyst or tumor; investigate any symptomatic changes in the breast tissue; health promotion screening test for early detection of breast cancer

Continued

Name of Test	Page	Primary Purposes
REPRODUCTIVE FUNCTION—*cont'd*		
Papanicolaou Smear	494	Detect inflammation, infection, premalignant changes, and malignancy of the cervix; health promotion screening test to detect cervical tissue changes at an early stage, before cancer develops or becomes advanced
Percutaneous Umbilical Cord Sampling	508	Assess for Rh isoimmunization; identify for chromosomal abnormality; detect fetal infection; measure acid-base abnormality; detect other fetal hematologic abnormalities
Progesterone	540	Assess ovulation; help investigate cause of first trimester bleeding, habitual abortion, and infertility
Testosterone, Total, Free	603	Diagnose precocious sexual development in a young boy; help diagnose deficient activity of testes or ovaries; help determine cause of male infertility or sexual dysfunction; help determine cause of female hirsutism or virilization
SENSORY FUNCTION		
Angiography, Fluorescein	79	Visualize the retinal circulation to help evaluate retinopathy
Biopsy, Skin	146	Differentiate a benign from a malignant growth
Patch Test, Skin	505	Identify cause of contact dermatitis; differentiate between contact dermatitis and eczematous disease
VASCULAR FUNCTION		
Angiography, Vascular	84	Identify abnormalities of arteries and arterial blood flow to specific tissues or organs
Plethysmography, Arterial	527	Help evaluate arterial blood flow in the extremities; detect peripheral arterial vascular disease
Plethysmography, Venous	530	Help detect deep vein thrombosis; screen patients who are at high risk for development of a venous thrombosis

Name of Test	Page	Primary Purposes
VASCULAR FUNCTION—*cont'd*		
Ultrasound, Doppler, Vascular	635	Detect vascular stenosis or occlusion; help diagnose peripheral vascular or cerebrovascular disease; evaluate postsurgical arterial reconstruction or vascular bypass; assess trauma to an artery
Venography	668	Investigate venous function, suspected obstruction, venous insufficiency, postphlebitic syndrome and the source of pulmonary embolism; evaluate veins before and after bypass surgery, reconstructive surgery, or after thrombolytic therapy
MICROBIOLOGY TESTS		
Chlamydia trachomatis Tests	194	Help detect infection with *C. trachomatis*
Culture, Blood	249	Confirm infection in the blood; identify the causative pathogen; identify susceptibility of the pathogen to various antibiotics
Culture, Genital	251	Confirm genital infection; identify the causative pathogen; identify susceptibility of the pathogen to various antibiotics
Culture, Nasopharyngeal	255	Identify the causative pathogen that caused upper respiratory tract infection; detect carriers of the organism; identify susceptibility of the pathogen to various antibiotics
Culture, Sputum	257	Diagnose respiratory infection; identify the pathogen responsible for the infection; identify susceptibility of the pathogen to various antibiotics
Culture, Stool	260	Identify the causative bacteria; identify susceptibility of the pathogen to various antibiotics
Culture, Throat	262	Identify bacteria of the oropharynx, pharynx, and tonsils; screen for asymptomatic carriers of infection; identify susceptibility of the pathogen to various antibiotics
Culture, Urine	265	Diagnose urinary tract infection; monitor the number of microorganisms; identify susceptibility of the pathogen to various antibiotics

Continued

Name of Test	Page	Primary Purposes
MICROBIOLOGY TESTS—*cont'd*		
Culture, Wound	268	Identify infection in the wound; identify the causative organism; identify susceptibility of the pathogen to various antibiotics
Darkfield Examination, Syphilis	272	Diagnosis of syphilis infection
Epstein Barr Virus Serology	307	Diagnosis of Epstein-Barr viral infection
Helicobacter pylori Tests	369	Establishes the presence of *H. pylori* infection that can cause gastric and peptic ulcers
Hepatitis A antibody	381	Identify hepatitis A virus as the cause of liver infection
Hepatitis B core antibody	382	Assess the stage of hepatitis B infection (acute, chronic, or a marker of past infection)
Hepatitis B_e Antibody	383	Help stage the course of illness; prognostic indicator for the future course of the infection
Hepatitis B_e Antigen	385	Diagnose the hepatitis B infection; provide prognosis for recovery
Hepatitis B Surface Antibody	386	Evaluate immunity or the need for vaccination against the hepatitis B virus; evaluate needlestick incidents involving health care personnel
Hepatitis B Surface Antigen	387	Diagnose the hepatitis B infection in acute or chronic stage; evaluate needlestick incidents involving health care personnel
Hepatitis B Virus DNA Assay	388	Help diagnose carrier state of hepatitis B infection; help establish the stage of the disease
Hepatitis C Antibody	389	Diagnose hepatitis C infection
Hepatitis C-RNA Assay	390	Diagnose hepatitis C infection; monitor the response to treatment
Histoplasmosis, Antigen and Antibody Tests	392	Help diagnose severe histoplasmosis infection; monitor response to therapy
Human Immunodeficiency (HIV) Tests	396	Diagnose HIV infection; monitor the progression of illness and the response to therapy
Infectious Mononucleosis Tests	404	Help diagnose infectious mononucleosis
Lyme Disease Tests	447	Help diagnose Lyme disease infection

Name of Test	Page	Primary Purposes
MICROBIOLOGY TESTS—*cont'd*		
Measles Antibody	459	*Blood test:* Diagnose a viral rash; document immunity to measles from immunization or past infection *Cerebrospinal fluid:* Diagnose the neurologic complications of measles infection
Mumps Antibody	466	*IgM test:* Acute infection with mumps (parotitis) *IgG test:* Immunity from past infection or after immunization
Rubella Antibody	580	*IgM test:* Diagnose acute infection with rubella *IgG:* Immunity from past infection or after immunization
Severe Acute Respiratory Syndrome (SARS) Tests	581	Identify SARS as the cause of the acute respiratory infection; distinguish SARS infection from other infectious organisms that cause respiratory infection or pneumonia
Syphilis Serology	601	Screen for or confirm the diagnosis of syphilis
Toxoplasmosis Serology	621	*IgM test:* Diagnose acute infection of toxoplasmosis *IgG test:* May indicate recovery from an acute infection
Varicella-Zoster Viral Antibody	663	*IgM test:* Diagnose acute infection with varicella-zoster virus *IgG test:* Immunity from past infection or after immunization
White Blood Cell Count	676	Identify presence and severity of infection or inflammation; assess bone marrow function; general screening test as part of complete blood count
White Blood Cell Differential Count	679	Assess the ability to respond to and eliminate infection; identify various stages of leukemia; measure the severity of allergic reactions and parasitic infections
MULTISYSTEM TESTS		
Calcium, Serum	164	Assist in the diagnosis of acid-base imbalance, coagulation disorder, pathologic bone disorder, endocrine disorder, cardiac arrhythmia, and muscle disorder

Continued

Name of Test	Page	Primary Purposes
MULTISYSTEM TESTS—*cont'd*		
Carbon Dioxide, Total	174	Help evaluate acid-base balance and the bicarbonate buffer system
Chloride, Serum	196	Help evaluate electrolyte levels, water balance, and acid-base balance; use in measure of anion gap
Computed Tomography	230	Visualize structure, size, and shape of soft tissue, bone, major blood vessels, and organs; distinguish between benign and malignant tissue; stage cancer tumors
Drugs of Abuse	277	Screen for the presence of drugs of abuse in suspected overdose or as a condition of pre-employment
Lead, Blood	426	Detect and measure the amount of lead in the blood; health promotion screening test for all children and for adults who are at risk for elevated lead levels
Magnesium, Serum	448	Evaluate electrolyte disorders and acid-base balance; monitor cardiac patients for hypomagnesemia; monitor the pregnant patient with toxemia during treatment with magnesium sulfate
Magnetic Resonance Imaging	451	Assess anatomic structures, organs, soft tissue, and visualize pathology that is present; distinguish between benign and malignant growth; stage cancer; evaluate response to treatment
Nuclear Scan	473	For a designated organ or tissue, assess physiologic function; assist in the localization of abnormality
Opiates, Urinary	487	Identify the presence of the opiate drugs of abuse
Phenylalanine, Blood	515	Detect the metabolic disease of phenylketonuria (PKU) and other causes of hyperphenylalanemia; monitor patients who have PKU and are treated with phenylalanine-restricted diet; a health promotion screening test for newborns to detect this metabolic disorder at an early stage
Phenylalanine, Urinary	517	Assist in the detection of hyperphenylalanemia, including phenylketonuria (PKU); monitor the effect of dietary treatment in patients who have PKU

Name of Test	Page	Primary Purposes
MULTISYSTEM TESTS—*cont'd*		
Phosphorus, Serum	518	Help diagnose kidney disorders and acid-base balance; detect disorders of calcium of bone or endocrine origin
Positron Emissions Tomography (PET Scan)	532	Images brain function and function of other targeted organs; detect areas of metabolic change at an early stage; guide treatment or management of disease; monitor tissue response to therapy; stage cancer
Potassium, Serum	535	Evaluate electrolyte balance, hypertension, renal disease and renal failure, and endocrine disease; monitor patients receiving treatment for ketoacidosis; monitor patients receiving hyperalimentation, hemodialysis, diuretic therapy, or intravenous therapy
Sodium, Serum	591	Monitor electrolyte levels, water balance, and acid-base balance; evaluate disorders of the central nervous system, musculoskeletal disorders, and diseases of the kidneys and adrenal glands
Ultrasound	630	Identify malposition, malformation, malfunction, and presence of a foreign body; visual guide for some biopsy or aspiration procedures *Pregnancy ultrasound:* Determine age of fetus and gestation of pregnancy; assess for fetal malformation
X-Ray Studies	683	Detect tumor, perforation, abscess, infection, foreign body, or fracture of bone

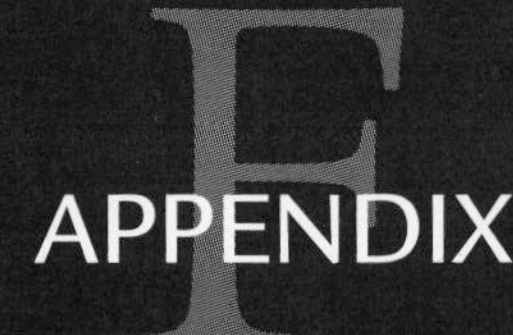

APPENDIX F

Brain Natriuretic Peptide Test

Brain Natriuretic Peptide Test

Also called: BNP, B-type Natriuretic Peptide

SPECIMEN OR TYPE OF TEST: Plasma

PURPOSE OF THE TEST

BNP levels may be used to differentiate between cardiac and pulmonary causes of dyspnea. The BNP test is rarely done because patient history, physical assessments, and other commonly performed tests are usually adequate for making the appropriate diagnosis. It has been proposed that BNP levels may be helpful in the prognosis and/or staging of heart failure.

BASICS THE NURSE NEEDS TO KNOW

BNP is a neurohumoral hormone produced primarily by the myocardial myocytes in the ventricles of the heart and to a lesser degree within the atria. BNP is secreted in response to ventricular stretching and increasing ventricular pressures. BNP causes a decrease in sodium retention, an increase in diuresis by improving glomerular filtration, and a decrease renin and aldosterone secretion. Exogenous use of this hormone is indicated in severe, uncompensated congestive failure.

NORMAL VALUES	<80 pg/mL *or* SI: <80 ng/L (values vary among laboratories)
Critical Values	Since values vary widely among laboratories, specific critical values will also vary. However, a value greater than 100 pg/mL *or* SI: 100 ng/L is highly suggestive of heart failure.

HOW THE TEST IS DONE

Depending on the laboratory, 1 to 5 mL of venous blood is collected in a purple- or red-topped tube. Specimen is placed on ice and sent immediately to the lab.

SIGNIFICANCE OF TEST RESULTS

Increased Values

Congestive heart failure
Acute myocardial infarction
Left ventricular hypertrophy
Hypervolemic states (e.g., renal failure)

INTERFERING FACTORS

- Kidney failure/dialysis
- Medications: cardiac glycoside, diuretics
- Not placing specimen on ice

NURSING CARE

Pretest

- ***Patient Teaching.*** Instruct patient to fast except for water for 8 to 12 hours before blood is drawn.

Check that the patient is not receiving nesiritide (Natrecor), which is an exogenous BNP.

Posttest

Check for results, which may be available within 30 minutes.

Nursing Response to Critical Values

Assess for indications of acute pulmonary edema and notify physician immediately of test result and clinical findings.

References

Chernecky, C.C. & Berger, B.J. (Eds) (2004). *Laboratory Tests and Diagnostic Procedures* (4th ed). St Louis: Elsevier.

Ford, C.M., Pruitt, R., Parker, V. & Reimels, E. (2004). CHF: Effects of cardiac rehabilitation and brain natriuretic peptide. *The Nurse Practitioner*, 99(3), 36-39.

Morton, P.G., Fontaine, D.K., Hudak, C.M. & Gallo, B.M. (2005). *Critical Care Nursing: A Holistic Approach* (8th ed). Philadelphia: Lippincott, Williams & Wilkins.

Sole, M.L., Klein, D.G. & Moseley, M.J. (2005). *Introduction to Critical Care Nursing* (4th ed). St Louis: Elsevier.

Bibliography

Abramson, N. (2000). Leukocytosis: Basics of clinical assessment. *American Family Physician, 62*(9), 2053–2061.

Adams-Hamonda, M. G., Caldwell, M. A., Scotts, N. A., & Drew, B. J. (2003). Factors to consider when analyzing 12-lead electrocardiograms for evidence of acute myocardial ischemia. *American Journal of Critical Care, 12*, 9–16.

Altender, R. R. (1998). The lived experience of women who undergo prenatal diagnostic testing due to elevated serum alpha-fetoprotein screening. *Maternal-Child Nursing, 23*(4), 180–186.

American Diabetes Association (2003). Standards of medical care for patients with diabetes mellitus. *Clinical Diabetes, 21*, 27–38.

American Diabetes Association (2002). Report of the expert committee on the diagnosis and classification of diabetes mellitus. *Diabetes Care, 25*(Suppl. 1), S5–S20.

Badenhop, D. T., Dunn, C. B., Eldridge, D., English, S. M., Hickey, A. P., Mayo, C. H, Gerardo, J. A., Pruitt, T. H., & Smith, R. (2001). Monitoring and management of cardiac rehabilitation patients with type 2 diabetes. *Clinical Exercise Physiology, 3*, 71–77, 113–115.

Balthazar, E. J. (2002). Staging of acute pancreatitis. *Radiologic Clinics of North America, 40*(6), 1199–1209.

Baum, J. (1998). Rheumatoid arthritis: How to make the most of laboratory tests in the workup. *Consultant, 38*(5), 1341–1344, 1347–1348.

Beattie, S. (2002). New biomarkers may predict CAD. *RN, 65*, 47–54.

Berg, A. O. (2003). Screening for prostate cancer: Recommendations and rationale. *American Journal of Nursing, 103*, 111.

Bergin, J. J. (2002). Anemia: A strategy for workup. *Consultant, 42*(7), 869–870, 872.

Blows, W. (2002). Diagnostic investigations part 3: Electroencephalography. *Nursing Times, 98*(38), 36–37.

Blows, W. (2002). Diagnostic investigations part 1: Lumbar puncture. *Nursing Times, 98*(36), 25–26.

Bock, J. L. (2002). Test strategies for the detection of myocardial damage. *Clinics in Laboratory Medicine, 22*, 357–375.

Bone, M., Diver, M., Selby, A., Sharples, A., Addison, M., & Clayton, P. (2002). Assessment of adrenal function in the initial phase of meningoccal disease. *Pediatrics, 110*, 563–569.

Braun, L. T. (2001). Lipid disorders in type 2 diabetes. *The Nursing Clinics of North America, 36*, 291–302.

Bruenwald, E., Fauci, A. S., Kasper, D. L., Hauser, S. L., Longo, D. L., & Jameson, J. L. (2001). *Harrison's principles of internal medicine* (15th ed.). New York: McGraw Hill.

Brunader, R. (2002). Radiologic bone assessment in the evaluation of osteoporosis. *American Family Physician*, 65(7), 1357–1364.

Burke, M. D. (2002). Selected endocrine test strategies. *Clinics in Laboratory Medicine, 22*, 421–434.

Burke, M. D. (2002). Liver function: Tests selection and interpretation of results. *Clinical Laboratory Medicine, 22*(2), 377–390.

Byrne, H. A., Tieszen, K. L., Hollis, S., Dornan, T. L., & New, J. P. (2000). Evaluation of an electrochemical sensor for measuring blood ketones. *Diabetes Care, 23*, 500–503.

Caroll, M. F. (2000). Proteinuria in adults: A diagnostic approach. *American Family Physician, 62*(6), 1333–1341.

Carroll, P. (2002). Using capnography effectively in critical care. *NTI News*, May 8, 1–3, 14–15.

Catheter-free esophageal pH monitoring is now feasible, (2002). *Family Practice News, 32*(13), 9.

Carr, M. W., & Grey, M. L. (2002). Magnetic resonance imaging: Overview, risks and safety measures. *American Journal of Nursing, 102*(12), 26–33.

Centeno, B. A. (1998). Fine needle aspiration biopsy of the pancreas. *Clinics in Laboratory Medicine, 18*(3), 401–428.

Clark, J. (2002). Positron emission tomography. *Images, 21*(4), 7–10.

Clark, S. J., Deming, D. D., Emery, J. R., Adams, L. M., Carlton, E. I. & Nelson, J. C. (2001). Reference ranges for thyroid function tests in premature infants beyond the first week of life. *Journal of Perinatology, 21*, 531–536.

Clearbrook, D. M., & Nuzzo, N. A. (2001). Effects of sustained moderate exercise on cholesterol, growth hormone and cortisol blood levels in three age groups of women. *Clinical Laboratory Science, 14*, 108–111.

Colorectal cancer screening: New recommendations. Primary care update, (2003). *Consultant, 43*(i3), 318–320.

Conlon, P. C. (2001). A practical approach to type 2 diabetes. *The Nursing Clinics of North America, 36*, 193–202.

Connolly, M. A. (2001). Chest x-rays: Completing the picture. *RN, 64*(6), 56–62.

Connolly, M. A. (1999). Postdural puncture headache. *American Journal of Nursing, 99*(11), 48–49.

Conquering claustrophobia during your MRI (2002). *Johns Hopkins Medical Letter, Health After 50, 14*(9), 3.

Conteh, A., & Henwood, S. (2000). Learning curve. Best practice in barium enemas, *Nursing Times, 96*(22), 34–35.

Cook, L. (1999). The value of lab values. *American Journal of Nursing, 99*(5), 66–69, 71, 73, 75.

Coombs, M. (2001). Making sense of arterial blood gases. *Nursing Times, 97*, 36–38.

Copp, K. (2001). Practical procedures for nurses, bone marrow aspiration and biopsy—3 . . . No.60.3 *Nursing Times, 97*(31), 45–46.

Corbett, J. V. (1998). Laboratory tests and diagnostic procedures in orthopedic nursing. *Nursing Clinics of North America, 33*(4), 685–700.

Coutts, A. (2002). Diagnostic investigation part 2, Computerized tomography. *Nursing Times, 98*(37), 41.

CT scans for kids: Guide to reducing radiation. (2002). *Health Facts, 27*(10), 3.

Culpin, D. G., & Chapman, A. H. (2002). Complications of radiographer-performed double contrast barium enema examinations. *Radiography*, 8(2), 91–95.

Cunningham, M. A. (2001). Glucose monitoring in type 2 diabetes. *The Nursing Clinics of North America, 36*, 361–374.

Curtas, S. (1999). Diagnosing gastrointestinal malignancies. *Seminars in Oncology Nursing, 15*(1), 10–16.

Custer, B. G. (2002). Management of acute myocardial infarction. *Physician Assistant, 26*, 21–44.

Czernin, J., & Phelps, M. E. (2002). Positron emission tomography screening: Current and future applications. *Annual Review of Medicine, 59*, 89–103.

Darovic, G. O. (1999). Understanding chest x-rays, part III. *Nursing 1999, 29*(3), 32cc6–7.

Darovic, G. O. (1998). Understanding chest x-rays, part II. *Nursing 1998, 28*(12), 32cc10–11.

Davidson, B. J., & Denger, L. F. (1997). Empowerment of men newly diagnosed with prostate cancer. *Cancer Nursing, 20*, 87–96.

Davis, J., Krasnewich, D., & Puck, J. M. (2000). Genetic testing and screening in pediatric populations. *Nursing Clinics of North America, 35*(3), 643–650.

Davis, M., & Houston, J. D. (2002). *Fundamentals of gastrointestinal radiology*, Philadelphia: W. B. Saunders.

Deane, K. A. (1998). Information needs, uncertainty, and anxiety in women who had a breast biopsy with benign outcome. *Cancer Nursing, 21*(2), 117–126.

De Koning, H.J. (2000). Assessment of nationwide cancer-screening programs. *Lancet, 355*, 80–81.

De Jong, M. J. (1998). Hyponatremia. *American Journal of Nursing, 98*(12), 36.

De Sanctis, J. T. (2001). Percutaneous interventions for lower extremity peripheral vascular disease. *American Family Physician, 64*(12), 1965–1973.

Dixon, L. R. (1997). The complete blood count: Physiologic basis and clinical usage. *The Journal of Perinatal and Neonatal Nursing, 11*(3) 1–18.

Djonret, L. L. (1998). Perspectives. An unexplained outcome of esophagogastroduodenoscopy. *Gastroenterology Nursing, 21*(3), 129–130.

Downes, K. A., & Yomtovovian, R. (2002). Advances in pretransfusion testing: Ensuring the safety of transfusion therapy. *Clinics in Laboratory Medicine, 22*(2), 475–491.

Doyle, B. (1997). Thrombocytopenia. *AACN Clinical Issues 8*(3), 469–480.

Dumler, J. S. (2003). Molecular methods for ehrlichiosis and Lyme disease. *Clinics in Laboratory Medicine, 23*, 867–884.

Durham, E. (2003). Growth hormone deficiency in children, *Advances for Nurse Practitioners, 11*, 41–42, 68.

Dybul, M., Bolan, R., Condoluci, D., Coy-Tyamu, R., Redfield, R., Hallahan, C. W., Folino, M., Sathasivam, K., Weisberger, M., Andrews, M., Hidalgo, B., Vasquez, J., & Fauci, A. S. (2002). Evaluation of CD4 + T cell counts in individuals with newly diagnosed human immunodeficiency virus infection by sex and race in urban settings. *Journal of Infectious Diseases, 185*(12), 1818–1821.

Ellett, M. L. C. (2000). Hepatitis C, E, F, G, and non A-G. *Gastroenterology Nursing, 23*(2), 67–72.

Enders, H. M. (2002). Evaluating iron status in hemodialysis patients. *Nephrology Nursing Journal, 29*(4), 366–371.

Expert Panel on Detection, Evaluation and Treatment of High Blood Cholesterol in Adults. (2001). Third annual report of the national cholesterol education program expert panel on detection, evaluation & treatment of high blood cholesterol in adults. *JAMA, 285*, 2486–2497.

Freda, M. C., Devore, N., Valentine-Adams, N., Bombard, A., & Merkatz, I. R. (1998). Informed consent for maternal serum alpha-fetoprotein in an inner city population: How informed is it? *Journal of Obstetrics, Gynecology, and Neonatal Nursing, 27*(1), 99–106.

Frolkis, J. P., Pothier, C. E., Blackstone, E. H., & Lauer, M.S. (2003). Frequent ventricular ectopy after exercise as a predictor of death. *New England Journal of Medicine, 348*, 781–790.

Gagnon, A. J. (2001). Indicators nurses employ in deciding to test for hyperbilirubinemia. *Journal of Obstetric, Gynecologic, and Neonatal Nursing, 30*(6), 626–633.

Gerard, M. J. (1998). Screening for prostate cancer in asymptomatic men: Clinical, legal, and ethical considerations. *Oncology Nursing Forum, 25*(9), 1561–1569.

Ginsberg, A. L. (2002). Liver enzyme abnormalities: What to do for the patient. *Consultant, 42*(3), 409–410, 413–414.

Goldstein, R. B. (2001). The role of sonography in the evaluation of pregnant women with high maternal serum alpha-fetoprotein. *Applied Radiology, 30*(3), 9–18.

Gollub, M. J. (2002). Virtual colonoscopy. *Lancet, 360*(9338), 964.

Goolsby, M. J. (2001). Urinary tract infection. *Journal of the American Academy of Nurse Practitioners, 13*, 395–398.

Gorlick, M. H. & Shaw, K. N. (1999). Screening tests for urinary tract infection in children: A meta-analysis. *Pediatrics, 104*, e54.

Gotzsche, P. C., & Olsen, O. (2000). Is screening for breast cancer with mammography justifiable? *Lancet, 355*, 129–134.

Goyen, M. (2002). MR angiography for assessment of peripheral vascular disease. *Radiologic Clinics of North America, 40*(4), 836–846.

Groen, K. A. (1999). Primary and metastatic liver cancer. *Seminar in Oncology Nursing, 15*(1), 48–57.

Guiliano, K. K. (2002). Blood analysis at the point of care: Issues and application in critically ill patients. *AACN Clinical Issues, 13*(2), 204–220.

Gunn, C. (2002). *Radiographic imaging* (3rd ed.). Edinburgh: Churchill Livingstone.

Gutman, P. D., & Henry, M. (1998). Fine needle aspiration cytology of the thyroid. *Clinics in Laboratory Medicine, 18*(3), 461–482.

Hasemeier, C. (1998). Critical care extra. Diagnostic tests. Cerebral angiography. Evaluating vessel patency. *American Journal of Nursing, 98*(9), 16ll–JJ.

Headley, J. M. (2003). Indirect calorimetry: A trend toward continuous metabolic assessment. *AACN Clinical Issues, 14*, 155–167.

Henry, J. B. (2001). *Clinical diagnosis and management by laboratory methods* (12th ed.). Philadelphia: W. B. Saunders.

Hilliard, N. J., & Waites, K. B. (2002). C-reactive protein and ESR: What can one test tell you that the other one can't? *Contemporary Pediatrics, 19*(6), 64–75.

Horrell, C. J., & Rothman, J. (2000). Establishing the etiology of thrombocytopenia. *The Nurse Practitioner, 25*(6), 68, 71–72, 74–75.

Huber, D. (2001). Does the "C" in hepatitis stand for complex? *Gastroenterology Nursing, 24*(3), 120–128.

Jeffrey, J., & Murphy, M. J., (2001). Ascitic fluid analysis: The role of biochemistry and haematology. *Hospital Medicine* (London), *62*(5), 282–286.

Jacobs, D. S., DeMott, W. R., & Oxley, D. K. (2001). *Laboratory test handbook* (5th ed.). Hudson, Ohio: Lexi-Comp.

Jenkins, T. L. (2002). Sickle cell anemia in the pediatric intensive care unit: Novel approaches for managing life threatening complications. *AACN Clinical Issues 13*(2), 154–168.

Kaplan, M. M. (2002). Alanine transferase levels: What's normal? *Annals of Internal Medicine, 137*(1), 49–51.

Kasper, C. E., Talbot, L. A., & Gaines, J. M. (2002). Skeletal muscle damage and recovery. *AACN Clinical Issues, 13*(2), 237–247.

Kenner C, & Dreyer, L. A. (2000). Prenatal and neonatal testing. A double-edged sword. *Nursing Clinics of North America, 35*(3), 627–642.

Keren, D. F. (2002). Antinuclear antibody testing. *Clinical Laboratory Medicine, 22*(2), 447–474.

Kerstein, M. D., & Reis, E. D. (2001). Lower extremity wounds 1: Vascular disease assessment. *Journal of Wound Care, 10*(10), 395–398.

Kessenich, C. R. (2001). Diagnostic imaging and biochemical markers of bone turnover. *Nursing Clinics of North America, 36*(3), 409–415.

Kumar, D. (1998). Diagnostic tests. Pet scanning. Applications for treating epilepsy. *American Journal of Nursing, 98*(7), 16 G–H.

Lane, S. K, & Gravel, J. J. (2002). Clinical utility of common serum rheumatologic tests. *American Family Physician, 65*(6), 1073–1080.

Lanes, R., & Jakubowicz, S. (2002). Is insulin-like growth factor-1 monitoring useful in assessing the response to growth hormone-deficiency children? *Journal of Pediatrics*, 141, 606–610.

Lasater, M., (2000). Impedence cardiography: A method of noninvasive cardiac output monitoring. *AACN News, 17*, 12–14.

Law, M. (2001). A study of adverse reactions to ophthalmic fluorescein angiography. *Ophthalmic Nursing: International Journal of Ophthalmic Nursing, 5*(2), 10–14.

Lawrence, B. L., & Tasota, F. J. (2003). Eye on diagnostics. Detecting neuromuscular problems with electromyography. *Nursing 2003, 33*(4), 82.

Lawson, H. W., Henson, R., Bobo, J. K., & Kaeser, M. K. (2002). Implementing recommendations for early detection of breast cancer among low-income women. *MMWR: Morbidity and Mortality Report 49* (RR-2), 35–55.

Leung, A. K. C., & Chan, K. N. (2001). Evaluating the child with purpura. *American Family Physician, 64*(3), 419–428, 363–365.

Levine, M. S., Rubesin, S. E., Laufer, I., & Herlinger, H. (2002). Barium studies. *Gastrointestinal Endoscopy, 55*(7), supp. S16–S24.

Lewis, C. D. (2001). Peripheral arterial disease of the lower extremity. *Journal of Cardiovascular Nursing, 15*(4), 45–63, 96–97.

Linekin, P. L. (2001). The challenge of diabetes as a secondary diagnosis. *Home Healthcare Nurse, 19*, 712–719.

Linekin, P. L. (2001). How the OASIS could include diabetes. *Home Healthcare Nurse, 19*, 659.

Litton, K., & Bauer, J. (2003). Defenses gone awry: Lupus. *R.N., 66*(3), 53–60.

Lizerbram, E., & Moffit, B. (2001). Neuroimaging in acute brain injury. *Topics in Emergency Medicine, 23*(2), 47–59.

London, D. G. (1997). Diagnostic tests. Antinuclear antibody testing. *American Journal of Nursing, 97*(12), 4–15.

Ly, J. N. (2002). MR imaging of the pancreas: A practical approach. *Radiologic Clinics of North America, 40*(6), 1289–1306.

Malchoff, C. D., Shoukre, K., Landu, J. I. & Buchert, J. M. (2002). A novel noninvasive blood glucose monitor. *Diabetes Care, 25*, 2268–2275.

McArthur, J. (2002). Review. Longer bedrest does not prevent more postpuncture headaches than immediate mobilization or short bedrest. *Evidenced-Based Nursing, 5*(3), 87.

McCormick, D. (2002). Colon cancer: Prevention, diagnosis, treatment. *Gastroenterology Nursing, 25*(5), 204–212.

Mitchell, R. (1999). Clinical snapshot. Sickle cell anemia. *American Journal of Nursing, 99*(5), 36–37.

Moreno, A. (2002). Assessment of platelet numbers and morphology in the peripheral blood smear. *Clinics in Laboratory Medicine, 22*(1), 193–213.

Moyad, M. A. (2002). Osteoporosis—part I: Risk factors and screening. *Urologic Nursing, 22*(4), 276–279.

Mushlin, A. I., Ruchlin, H. S., & Callahan, M. A., (2001). Cost effectiveness of diagnostic tests. *Lancet, 358*(9290), 1353–1356.

News briefs (2003). American Cancer Society updates guidelines on Pap tests. *Clinical Journal of Oncology Nurses, 7*(03), 269.

Nguyen, G. K., & Akin, M. R. (1998). Fine needle aspiration of the kidney, renal pelvis, and adrenal. *Clinics in Laboratory Medicine. 18*(3) 429–459.

Nuovo, J., Meinikow, J., & Howell, L.P. (2001). New tests for cervical cancer screening, *American Family Physician, 64*(5), 780–786, 723–725.

Ogedegbe, H. D. (2002). Your lab focus. Sickle cell disease: an overview. *Laboratory Medicine, 33*(7), 515–518, 539–543.

Onusko, E. (2003). Diagnosing secondary hypertension. *American Family Physician, 67*, 67–74.

Pachucki-Hyde, L. (2001). Assessment of risk factors for osteoporosis and fracture. *Nursing Clinics of North America, 36*(3), 401–406.

Palmer, J. B. (2000). Evaluation and treatment of swallowing impairment. *American Family Physician, 61*(8), 2453–2463.

Pearlstein, I. (1998). Diagnostic tests. The PSA test. *American Journal of Nursing, 98*(4), 14–15.

Peerschke, E. I. B. (2002). The laboratory evaluation of platelet dysfunction. *Clinics in Laboratory Medicine. 22*(2), 405–420.

PET scanning (patient page) (2002). *Radiologic Technology, 73*(6), 608.

Pitman, M. B. (1998). Fine needle aspiration biopsy of the liver: Principle diagnostic challenges. *Clinics in Laboratory Medicine, 18*(3), 483–506.

Planes, C., Leroy, M., Foray, E., & Raffestin, B. (2001). Arterial blood gases during exercise: Validity of transcutaneous measurements. *Archives of Physical Medicine and Rehabilitation, 82*, 1689–1691.

Pontieri-Lewis, V. (2002). Colorectal cancer: Prevention and screening. *Med-Surg, 9*(1), 9–17.

Porter, B. (2002). Role of the advanced practice nurse in anticoagulation. *AACN Clinical Issues, 13*(3), 221–233.

Portis, A. J., & Sundaran, C. P. (2001). Diagnosis and initial management of kidney stones. *American Family Physician, 63*, 1329–1338, 1387–1389.

Powell, L. L. (2003). Commentary on screening for prostate cancer: Recommendations and rationale. *American Journal of Nursing, 103*, 107–110.

Quinn, L. (2001). Type 2 diabetes: epidemiology, pathophysiology and diagnosis. *The Nursing Clinics of North America, 36*, 175–192.

Ratanalert, S. (2003). Preoperative education improves quality of patient care for endoscopic retrograde cholangiopancreatography, *Gastroenterology Nursing, 26*(1), 21–25.

Reiss, R. T. (2000). Hemostatic defects in massive transfusion: Rapid diagnosis and management. *American Journal of Critical Care, 9*(3), 158–167.

Ridker, P. M., Rifai. N., Rose, L., Buring, J. E., & Cook, N. R. (2002). Comparison of C-reactive protein and low density lipoprotein cholesterol levels in the prediction of first cardiovascular events. *New England Journal of Medicine, 347*(20), 1557–1565.

Rodak, B. F. (2002). *Hematology principles and applications* (2nd ed.). Philadelphia: W.B. Saunders.

Rolka, D. B., Narayan, K. M., Thompson, T. J., Goldman, D., Lindermayer, J., Alich, K., Bacal, D., Benjamin, E. M., Lamb, B., Stuart, D.O., & Engelgau, M. M. (2001). Performance of recommended screening tests undiagnosed diabetes and dysglycemia. *Diabetes, 24*, 1899–1904.

Rutecki, G. W., & Whittier, F. C. (1998). Decision points in hypocalcemia: Is emergent therapy required? Complications may include tetany, seizures, and arrhythmias. *Journal of Critical Illness, 13*(2), 84–86, 89–90.

Sacks, D. B., Bruns, D. E., Goldstein, D. D., Maclaren, N. K., McDonald, J. M., & Parrott, M. (2002). Guidelines and recommendations for laboratory analysis in the diagnosis and management of diabetes mellitus. *Diabetes, 25*, 750–787.

Sadowitz, P. D., Amanullah, S., & Souid, A. (2002). Hematologic emergencies in the pediatric emergency room. *Emergency Medicine Clinics of North America, 20*(1), 177–198.

Sargent, C., & Murphy, D. (2003). What you need to know about colorectal cancer. *Nursing 2003, 33*(2), 36–42.

Schell, H. M. (1999). The immunocompromised host and risk for cardiovascular infection. *The Journal of Cardiovascular Nursing, 13*(2), 31–48.

Schnitker, J. B., & Light, D. W. (2001). Nonneurologic indicators for MRI: Technological advances have broadened applications. Symposium: Second of four articles on radiology. *Postgraduate Medicine, 109*(6), 81–84, 87–89.

Sedrine, W. B. (2002). Risk indices and osteoporosis screening: Scope and limits. *Mayo Clinic Proceedings, 77*(7), 629–637.

Shafer, M. B., Tebb, K. P., Pantell, R. H., Wibbelsman, C. J., Neuhaus, J. M., Tipton, A. C., Kunin, S. B., Ko, T. H., Schweppe, D. M., & Bergman, D. A. (2002). The effect on clinical practice improvement intervention on chlamydial screening among adolescent girls. *Journal of the American Medical Association, 288*(22), 2846–2852.

Shanewise, J. S., Savage, R., Aronson, P., & Thys, D. M. (2003). Transesophageal echocardiography. In: *A practical approach to cardiac anesthesia*. (3rd ed.). Philadelphia: Lippincott Williams & Wilkins.

Shinopulos, N. (2000). Bedside urodynamic studies: Simple testing for urinary continence. *The Nurse Practitioner, 25*(6), 19–20, 22, 25–26, 28, 33–34, 37.

Shoop, N. M. (2001). Flexible endoscopes: Structure and function: The mechanical system. *Gastroenterology Nursing, 24*(6), 294–297.

Shoulders-Odom, B. (2000). Using an algorithm to interpret arterial blood gases. *DCCN: Dimensions of Critical Care Nursing, 19*, 36–41.

Shpritz, D. W. (1999). Neurodiagnostic studies. *Nursing Clinics of North America, 34*(3), 593–600.

Sivan, E., Weisz, B., Homko, C. J., Reece, E. A., & Schiff, E. (2001). One or two hours postprandial glucose measurements: are they the same? *American Journal of Obstetrics and Gynecology, 185*, 604–607.

Sjögren, M., Andreasen, N., & Biennow, K. (2003). Advances in the detection of Alzheimer's disease—use of cerebrospinal fluid biomarkers. *Clinica Chimica Acta, 322*(1–2), 1–10.

Slawson, D. (2000). How accurate is the GlucoWatch automatic glucose compared with serial blood glucose measurements? *Evidence-Based Practice, 3*, 6.

Sokolowsky, M. C. (2001). Hematuria. *Emergency Medicine Clinics of North America, 19*(3), 621–632.

Sparks, A. R., Johnson, P. L., & Meyer, M. C. (2002). Imaging of aortic aneurysms. *American Family Physicians, 65*(8), 1565–1570, 1509–1512.

Stern, M. P., Williams, K., & Haffner, S. M. (2002). Identification of persons at high risk for type 2 diabetes mellitus: Do we need the oral glucose tolerance test? *Annals of Internal Medicine, 136*, 575–581.

Stock, W., & Hoffman, R. (2000). White blood cells 1: Nonmalignant disorders. *Lancet, 355*(9212), 1351–1358.

Stoler, M. H. (2003). Testing for human papillomavirus: Data-driven implications for cervical neoplasia management. *Clinics in Laboratory Medicine, 23*(3), 569–583.

Sunderland, T., Luker, G., Mirza, H., Putnam, K. T., Friedman, D. L., Kimmel, D. L., Bergeson, J., Manetti, G. J., Zimmerman, M., Tang, B., Bartko, J. J., & Cohen, R. M. (2003). Decreased beta-amyloid 1-42 and increased tau levels in cerebrospinal fluid of patients with Alzheimer's disease. *Journal of the American Medical Association, 289*(16), 2094–2103.

Swagerty, D. L., Walling, D. D., & Klein, R. M. (2002). Lactose intolerance. *American Family Physician, 65*(9), 1845–1851.

Swaroop, V. S. (2002). Colonoscopy as a screening test for colorectal cancer in average risk individuals. *Mayo Clinic Proceedings, 77*(9), 951–956.

Szaflarski, N. L., & Hanson, W. H. (1997). Metabolic acidosis. *AACN Clinical Issues 8*(3), 481–496.

Szarka, L. A., DeVault, K. R., & Murrray, J. A. (2001). Diagnosing gastrointestinal reflux disease. *Mayo Clinics Proceedings, 76*(1), 97–101.

Tambyah, P. A., & Maki, D. G. (2000). The relationship of pyuria and infection in patients with indwelling urinary catheters: A prospective study of 761 patients. *Archives of Internal Medicine, 160*(5), 673–677, 718–719.

Tasota, F. J. (2000). Eye on diagnostics: Reading liver function values. *Nursing 2000, 30*(6), 73–75.

Tasota, F. J., & Tate, J. (2000). Assessing renal function. *Nursing, 30*, 20.

Tate, J. (2000). Eye on diagnostics. Looking at lumbar puncture in adults. *Nursing 2000, 30*(11), 91.

The New York City Department of Health and Mental Hygiene (2003). Severe acute respiratory syndrome: Preparing for the possibility of an outbreak. *City Health Information, 22*(8), 1–8.

Thorpe, A., & Neal, D. (2003). Benign prostatic hyperplasia. *Lancet, 361*, 1359–1367.

Tkacs, N. C. (2002). Hypoglycemia unawareness: Your patients with diabetes won't always know when their blood sugar is low. *American Journal of Nursing, 102*, 34–41.

Trewitt, K. G. (2001). Bone marrow aspiration and biopsy: Collection and interpretation. *Oncology Nursing Forum, 28*(9), 1409–1417.

Twombly, R. (2002). The new Pap test terminology, management guidelines published. *Journal of the National Cancer Institute, 94*(12), 878–880.

Urden, L. D., Stacy, K. M. & Lough, M. E. (2002). *Thelan's Critical Care Nursing* (4th ed.). St.Louis: Mosby.

U.S. Department of Health and Human Services (2000). *Healthy People 2010, Vol. I & Vol II.* Washington D.C.

U.S. Preventive Service Task Force (2003). Screening for osteoporosis in postmenopausal women: Recommendations and rationale. *American Journal of Nursing, 103*(1), 73, 75, 77.

U.S. Preventive Service Task Force (2002). Screening for chlamydial infection: Recommendations and rationale. *American Journal of Nursing, 102*(10), 87–89, 91–92.

U.S. Preventive Service Task Force (2002). Screening for colorectal cancer: Recommendations and rationale. *American Journal of Nursing, 102*(9), 107–108, 111, 113–114.

Virender, K., Sharma, V. K., & Howden, C. W. (2001). Colorectal cancer screening: What tests, how often? *Consultant, 41*(2), 173–176, 179.

Vissers, R. J., Abu-Laban, R. B., & McHugh, D. F. (1999). Amylase and lipase in the emergency department evaluation of acute pancreatitis. *Journal of Emergency Medicine, 17*(6), 1027–1037.

Vowden, D. (1998). The investigation and assessment of venous disease. *Journal of Wound Care, 7*(3), 143–147.

Ward, P. C. J. (2002). The modern approach to the investigation of vitamin B_{12} deficiency. *Clinics of Laboratory Medicine, 22*(2), 435–445.

Watts, S. A., Anselmo, J. M. & Smith, M. A. (2003). Combating hypoglycemia in the hospital and at home. *Nursing, 33*, 32hn1–2, 32hn4–5.

Webster, A., Brady, W., & Morris, F. (2002). Recognizing signs of danger: ECG changes resulting from an abnormal serum potassium. *Emergency Medicine Journal, 19*(1), 74–77.

Weissleder, R., Wittenberg, J., & Harisinghani, M. G. (2003). *Primer of diagnostic imaging* (3rd ed.). St. Louis: C.V. Mosby.

Wethers, D. L. (2000). Sickle cell disease in childhood: Part I. Laboratory diagnosis, pathophysiology and health maintenance. *American Family Physician, 62*(5), 1013–1021.

Wilbourn, A. J. (2002). Nerve conduction studies: Types, components, abnormalities, and value in location. *Neurologic Clinics, 20*(2), 305–338.

Wood, B. J., Razavi, P. (2002). Virtual endoscopy: A promising new technology. *American Family Physician, 66*(1), 107–112.

Worster, A., Preyra, I., Weaver, B., & Haines, T. (2002). The accuracy of noncontrast helical computed tomography versus intravenous pyelography in the diagnosis of suspected acute urolithiasis. *Annals of Emergency Medicine, 40*(3), 280–286.

Yaakob, W., & Gordon, L. (2003). Know your nukes: Which test(s) to order—and why. *Consultant, 43*(1), 82–83.

Yang, X., Hsu-Hage, B., Zhang, H., Zhang, C., Zhang, Y., & Zhang, C. (2002). Women with impaired glucose tolerance during pregnancy have significantly poor pregnancy outcomes. *Diabetes Care, 25*, 1619–1624.

Yoshida, E. M. (2003). Abnormal liver function tests: What to do for the patient. *Consultant, 43*(4), 505–512.

Zuber, T. J. (2001). Flexible sigmoidoscopy. *American Family Physician, 63*(7), 1375–1381.

Index

NOTE: Page numbers followed by b indicate boxes; f, figures; t, tables.

B

C

D

G

M

Q

R

S

U

W

X

Z